BSAVA Manual of Canine and Feline Endoscopy and Endosurgery
second edition

T0203140

Editors:

Philip Lhermette
BSc(Hons) CBiol FRSB BVetMed FRCVS
Elands Veterinary Clinic,
St John's Church, London Road,
Dunton Green, Sevenoaks TN13 2TE, UK

David Sobel
DVM MRCVS
Metropolitan Veterinary Consultants,
20 Dresden Road, Hanover, NH 03755, USA

Elise Robertson
BS BVetMed MANZCVSc(Feline) DipABVP(Feline) FHEA FRSB FRCVS
Feline & Endoscopy Vet Referrals,
Brighton, East Sussex BN1 6GE, UK

Published by:

British Small Animal Veterinary Association
Woodrow House, 1 Telford Way, Waterwells Business Park,
Quedgeley, Gloucester GL2 2AB

A Company Limited by Guarantee in England
Registered Company No. 2837793
Registered as a Charity

Titles in the BSAVA Manuals series

For further information on these and all BSAVA publications, please visit our website: **www.bsava.com**

Contents

Video extras

New to this edition are a series of videos that accompany the chapters. These videos are available from the BSAVA Library.

- **How to identify the videos in the text:** in the selected chapters, each video is identifiable by a still image with a 'play' symbol.
- **How to access the videos:** the videos can be accessed via a QR code, which can be found in the box at the end of each chapter with the list of available videos.
  You will need a QR code reader on your smart phone or tablet – a number of QR code reader apps are available. The videos can also be accessed by typing the web address provided at the end of the chapter into a web browser.

Flexible endoscopy: basic technique

Video 3.1
Escape of air bubbles during a leakage test of an endoscope.

Video 3.2
Single- and two-handed manipulation of steering wheels.

Video 3.3
Steering by tip deflection and torquing.

Flexible endoscopy: oesophagoscopy

Video 4.1
The endoscope in a j-flexed position looking at the lower oesophageal sphincter (abnormally dilated) in a patient presenting with chronic vomiting. A case of sliding hiatal hernia.

Flexible endoscopy: upper gastrointestinal tract

Video 5.1
Upper GI endoscopy.

Video 5.2
Video sequence recorded from an Alicam® video-endoscopy capsule, showing a bleeding gastric polyp.

Video 5.3
Upper GI endoscopy of a dog with a gastric carcinoma.

Video 5.4
Placement of a percutaneous endoscopic gastrostomy (PEG) tube in a cat.
- Severe oesophagitis.
- Identifying the PEG tube site.
- Insertion of a needle into the stomach.
- Passage of a wire loop into the stomach.
- Grabbing and pulling the wire loop out of the mouth.
- Positioning of the PEG tube mushroom.

Flexible endoscopy: respiratory tract

Video 7.1
Epiglottic retroversion – intermittent spontaneous retroflexion of the epiglottis during inspiration causing obstruction of the rima glottides.

Video 7.2
Bilateral laryngeal paralysis in a cat.

Video 7.3
Laryngeal carcinoma in a cat.

Video 7.4
Grade III collapsing trachea in a Chihuahua.

Video 7.5
Endoscopic removal of a grass stalk foreign body from the airway of a dog

Rigid endoscopy: otoendoscopy

Video 10.1
Foreign bodies: removal of plant awns using grasping forceps passed through the working channel of the video-otoscope.

Video 10.2
Removal of an inflammatory polyp from the ear canal of a cat.

Video 10.3
Flushing technique: flushing and suctioning cycles in the external ear canal of a dog with otitis externa.

Video 10.4
Flushing technique: appearance of the intact tympanic membrane after the flushing procedure.

Video 10.5
Myringotomy procedure: the incision into the caudoventral quadrant of the pars tensa is made with a 3.5 Fr tomcat catheter.

Rigid endoscopy: urethrocystoscopy and vaginoscopy

Video 11.1
Normal urethrocystoscopy of the neutered bitch.

Video 11.2
Normal urethrocystoscopy of the neutered male dog.

Rigid endoscopy: laparoscopy

Video 12.1
Passing instruments around the caudal edge of the falciform fat.

Rigid endoscopy: thoracoscopy

Video 13.1
Resection of a cranial mediastinal mass and removal from the thorax in a specimen retrieval bag.

Video 13.2
Demonstration of the correct bronchoscopically guided placement of an endobronchial blocker.

Video 13.3
Optical entry using a trocarless cannula (ENDOTIP, Karl Storz Endoscopy).

Video 13.4
Resection using an endoscopic stapler of a consolidated lung lobe in a dog secondary to pneumonia associated with chronic grass awn migration.

Video 13.5
Thoracic duct ligation with haemoclips.

Evolving trends and future developments

Video 17.1
Transvaginal approach to the abdomen using a flexible endoscope.

Video 17.2
Transvaginal ovariectomy in a dog.

Video 17.3
Transvaginal ovariectomy in a dog using an optical trocar.

Video 17.4
Transvaginal ovariohysterectomy in a dog.

Video 17.5
Transvaginal ovariectomy in a cat using a diode laser.

Video 17.6
Dog 1 year after transgastric laparoscopy with closure of the laparocentesis site using endoscopic clips.

Video 17.7
Closure of the transgastric laparocentesis site using an over-the-top technique.

Video 17.8
Transgastric ovariectomy in a dog.

Video 17.9
Transgastric cholecystectomy in a dog.

Video 17.10
Transgastric gastropexy in a dog (case 1).

Video 17.11
Transgastric gastropexy in a dog (case 2).

Video 17.12
Transanal laparoscopy in a dog.

Video 17.13
Peroral thoracoscopy in a cat.

Video 17.14
Transvaginal ovariohysterectomy in a dog using a hybrid NOTES procedure.

Video 17.15
Transgastric approach to the abdominal cavity in a dog using a hybrid NOTES procedure.

Contributors

Maurici Batalla
DVM
Endoscopia Veterinaria Móvil, Barcelona, Spain

Fausto Brandão
DVM MSc Cert Spec VEaMIS
Karl Storz SE & Co. KG, Lisbon, Portugal

Julie K. Byron
DVM MS DipACVIM
Department of Veterinary Clinical Sciences,
Ohio State University, 601 Vernon Tharp Street,
Columbus, OH 43210, USA

Christopher J. Chamness
DVM
Karl Storz SE & Co. KG,
5266 Hollister Avenue, Santa Barbara, CA 93111, USA

Alexander Chernov
DM DVM PhD
Endovet™ Veterinary Centre,
VetEndoSchool VESK™ and Karl Storz SE & Co. KG,
Kurgan, 640007, Russia

Michela De Lucia
DMV DipECVD
San Marco Veterinary Clinic and Laboratory,
Via Dell'Industria 3, Veggiano 35030, Italy

Gary C. W. England
BVetMed PhD DVetMed DVR DVRep DipECAR DipACT PFHEA FRCVS
School of Veterinary Medicine and Science,
University of Nottingham, Sutton Bonington Campus,
Sutton Bonington, Leicestershire LE12 5RD, UK

Edward J. Hall
MA VetMB PhD DipECVIM-CA FRCVS
Langford Vets, Bristol Veterinary School,
Langford House, Langford, Bristol BS40 5DU, UK

John F. Innes
BVSc CertVR PhD DSAS(Orth) FRCVS
ChesterGates Veterinary Specialists,
Units E & F, Telford Court, Gates Lane, Chester CH1 6LT, UK

Susan Kimmel
DVM DipACVIM
Veterinary Referral & Emergency Center of Westbury,
609-5 Cantiague Rock Road, Westbury,
New York 11590, USA

Diane M. Levitan
VMD DipACVIM
Peace Love Pets Veterinary Care,
6229 Jericho Turnpike, Commack, NY 11725, USA

Philip Lhermette
BSc(Hons) CBiol FRSB BVetMed FRCVS
Elands Veterinary Clinic,
St John's Church, London Road,
Dunton Green, Sevenoaks TN13 2TE, UK

Jody Lulich
DVM PHD DipACVIM
Minnesota Urolith Center, Department of Veterinary
Clinical Sciences, College of Veterinary Medicine,
University of Minnesota, St Paul, MN 55108, USA

Philipp D. Mayhew
BVMS DipACVS MRCVS
Department of Surgical and Radiological Sciences,
School of Veterinary Medicine, University of California-
Davis, 1 Shields Avenue, Davis, CA 95616, USA

Gerard McLauchlan
BVMS DipECVIM-CA FHEA MRCVS
Fitzpatrick Referrals Oncology and Soft Tissue Ltd.,
70 Priestley Road, Surrey Research Park,
Guildford, Surrey GU2 7AJ, UK

Eric Monnet
DVM PhD FAHA DipACVS DipECVS
College of Veterinary Medicine & Biomedical Sciences,
Colorado State University, 300 West Drake Road,
Fort Collins, CO 80521, USA

Laura Ordeix
Lda Vet MSc PhD DipECVD
Dermatology Service, Hospital Clínic Veterinari and Dept.
Medicina i Cirurgia Animals, Facultat de Veterinària,
Universitat Autònoma de Barcelona, 08193 Bellaterra
(Cerdanyola del Vallès), Barcelona, Spain

Rob Pettitt
BVSc PGCertLTHE DSAS(Orth) SFHEA FRCVS
Small Animal Teaching Hospital, Institute of Veterinary
Science, University of Liverpool, Leahurst Campus,
Chester High Road, Neston CH64 7TE, UK

Elise Robertson
BS BVetMed MANZCVSc(Feline) DipABVP(Feline) FHEA FRSB FRCVS
Feline & Endoscopy Vet Referrals,
Brighton, East Sussex BN1 6GE, UK

Fabia Scarampella
MSc DipECVD
Medico Veterinario,
Via Sismondi Giancarlo 62, 20133 Milano, Italy

Jimmy W. Simpson
BVM&S SDA MPhil FHEA MRCVS
Royal (Dick) School of Veterinary Studies, University of
Edinburgh, Roslin, Midlothian EH25 9RG, UK

David Sobel
DVM MRCVS
Metropolitan Veterinary Consultants, 20 Dresden Road,
Hanover, NH 03755, USA

David Twedt
DVM DipACVIM
College of Veterinary Medicine & Biomedical Sciences,
Colorado State University, 300 West Drake Road, Fort
Collins, CO 80521, USA

Foreword

Welcome to the second edition of the *BSAVA Manual of Canine and Feline Endoscopy and Endosurgery*. I hope that you are as excited to turn the pages as I was when I received the news that the new Manual was on its way. This book represents the pinnacle of endoscopic surgery. Thank you for taking the time to read the foreword.

We all know that one of the foundational pillars of the British Small Animal Veterinary Association (BSAVA) is their excellence in printed Manuals. It is not only the contribution of experts in the field but also the continuous improvement of the contents that keep on impressing me. I use BSAVA Manuals all the time because they are easy to work with, are extremely practical, and have excellent images and drawings to help readers along their educational journeys. The authors of this second edition are key opinion leaders in the field of flexible and rigid endoscopy, one of the few 'surgical' (by definition, the treatment of injuries or disorders of the body by incision or manipulation, especially with instruments) practises that both internal medicine and surgical-focused veterinarians alike seem to enjoy.

This time around, you should be even more excited, as this particular Manual has been updated and extended throughout with many more procedures in the laparoscopy section, including detailed step-by-step guidance on basic procedures and laparoscopic spays, as well as more information on feline endoscopy. New chapters on oesophagoscopy, interventional endoscopy and future developments have been added. The chapter on basic principles of endosurgery has also been extended.

The best news, however, is that many of the chapters have accompanying videos to show the techniques described; readers can download them from the BSAVA Library. In all, there are 41 videos featured in the Manual that will help the reader understand how a particular procedure should be performed.

Medical endoscopic procedures only got their start in the 1960–70s (Litynski, 1999). In the 1990s, I was personally involved in the 'laparoscopic revolution', which marked the end of many traditional open surgeries. It is extremely satisfying that so many veterinary surgeons nowadays consider this new perspective of endoscopic intervention as the mainstay of their practice.

Jolle Kirpensteijn
DVM PhD DipACVS DipECVS

Reference
Litynski GS (1999 Endoscopic surgery: the history, the pioneers. *World Journal of Surgery* **23(8)**, 245–753

Preface

"The second millennium has brought with it a new era of modern surgery. The creation of video surgery is as revolutionary to this century as the development of anesthesia and sterile technique was to the last one."

Marelyn Medina, MD
Rio Grande Regional Hospital (McAllen, TX)
Society of Laparoscopic Endosurgeons Public Relations Committee

The above quote puts into perspective the huge regard in which human surgeons hold minimally invasive techniques. Since the early beginnings in the late 1980s, there has been a massive paradigm shift in surgical care with the conversion of open surgical techniques to minimally invasive alternatives, to the great benefit of patients, surgeons and hospitals alike. The veterinary profession was initially slow to recognize the advantages and convert to these techniques, partly due to the cost of equipment and retraining. As equipment costs have reduced the number of veterinary clinics offering minimally invasive procedures has increased dramatically and many routine procedures are now done endoscopically.

Since the first edition of this Manual was published in 2008, many of the techniques have been modified and improved. As with the previous edition, this Manual is written as a hands-on guide for general practitioners, especially those starting out in this interesting field. Routine procedures are described in detail as these provide the foundation for practical experience and enable transferrable skills to be applied to more advanced procedures at the appropriate time. New techniques have been added for those more experienced in basic techniques who are keen to expand their repertoire. Many, if not most, of the open surgical procedures carried out in general practice can be performed endoscopically or be endoscopically-assisted, but all these techniques require practice and so we have once again tried to make this Manual as practical as possible, drawing on our own experience. Hints and tips that we find useful, both in terms of surgical technique and on the purchase of instrumentation without breaking the bank – and without compromising quality – are given in order to maintain high surgical standards.

The Manual is not meant as a substitute for qualified practical tuition, and we would urge the reader to take practical 'wet lab' courses with qualified instructors before embarking on these techniques for the first time. Endoscopy is a very practical skill and requires adequate training both in the use of the instrumentation and in working within a two-dimensional video environment. Having said that, most of what is contained in this Manual is relevant to general practice and any competent surgeon with good hand—eye coordination can, with practice, carry out most of these procedures.

As Hippocrates famously said 'first do no harm'. Unfortunately, as surgeons, we inevitably do harm with every incision we make, albeit with the intention of improving the welfare of our patients in the longer term. Surely if we can achieve the same or a better result and create much less trauma in the process, we should aspire to do so. Reduction in perioperative pain is a major benefit for all patients. At a time when the profession is becoming more and more aware of the need for postoperative pain relief, should we not give some thought to causing less pain and trauma in the first place? The advantages of minimally invasive techniques are well documented in humans and animals, and our clients actively seek out veterinary surgeons who can carry out these procedures as they are well aware of these benefits.

We rashly thought that updating this Manual would be easier than starting the first one afresh. How wrong we were. It has been a mammoth effort and we are extremely grateful to the authors who have given up their time so generously to contribute to this Manual. They are, without doubt, leaders and pioneers in their field and bring not only a depth of knowledge and experience but also an unbridled enthusiasm for their work that will hopefully inspire others to continue to develop techniques in the future.

Philip Lhermette
David Sobel
Elise Robertson
August 2020

Chapter 1

An introduction to endoscopy and endosurgery

Philip Lhermette, David Sobel and Elise Robertson

Introduction

The term 'endoscopy' is derived from two words: the Greek *endo*, meaning inside, and *scopein*, meaning to look at or view. Over the past decades there have been major advances in the ability to 'look inside' patients and to perform quite complex operations through tiny incisions. This has given rise to the term 'keyhole surgery'.

But endoscopy is not new. Mankind has seemingly always possessed an innate curiosity to look inside body cavities. The first reports of endoscopy come from Hippocrates (460–377 BC), who described the use of a rectal speculum. Roman, Greek and Arab physicians all made use of various primitive specula for peering into body cavities; indeed, three- and four-pronged vaginal specula (not dissimilar to modern instruments) were unearthed at the ruins of Pompeii, dating from AD 79. However, these devices used only natural light and no lenses or optics of any kind. No real advances on these initial attempts were made until the 19th century.

Endoscopists have had a difficult time throughout history convincing the critics. The modern era of endoscopy really started in the early 19th century with the introduction of the *Lichtleiter* (Figures 1.1 and 1.2), or light conductor, by Philipp Bozzini (Figure 1.3) of Frankfurt, Germany, in 1805. The breakthrough was the addition of a light source to improve visualization. The Lichtleiter utilized a beeswax candle as a light source, and reflected the light down a hollow tube using a mirror. The operator peered through a hole in the centre of the mirror. This device was used for looking at the rectum, vagina and urethra via a selection of different specula. However, visibility was still poor and the procedure was uncomfortable or even painful for the patient (with the additional risk of burns), so the device did not gain popularity at the time. Added to this, when Bozzini demonstrated his device to the Academy of Medicine of Vienna in 1806, he was ostracized for his 'undue curiosity', and his invention described as 'but a magic lantern'. He died a few years later, in 1809, but his work inspired some to continue in this field.

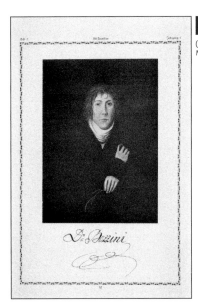

1.2 Attachable light-carrying tubes.
(Courtesy of Magister E Krebs)

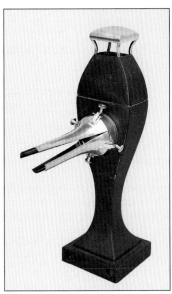

1.1 Restored light conductor with attached four-part light-carrying tube.
(Courtesy of Magister E Krebs)

1.3 Philipp Bozzini (1773–1809).
(Courtesy of the Collections of the Medical University of Vienna)

Half a century later, in 1853, the French surgeon Antonin Desormeaux (Figure 1.4), another urologist, designed the first functional cystoscope. This device used a gazogene lamp, burning a mixture of turpentine and alcohol, and was based on the Lichtleiter. This had all the drawbacks of Bozzini's apparatus, but prompted Desormeaux to write his monograph 'De l'endoscopie' in 1865, which greatly increased interest in endoscopy and resulted in the early commercial production of endoscopes in the USA.

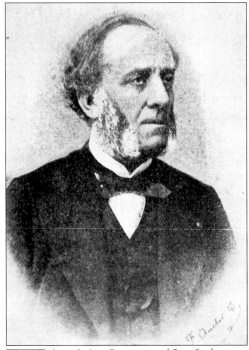

1.4 Antonin Jean Desormeaux (1815–1894).
(Courtesy of the Austrian Urological Society)

Up until then most attention had focused on cystoscopy and the urogenital tract. In 1868, a Desormeaux endoscope was used by Adolf Kussmaul in the first attempts to explore the oesophagus and the stomach. Since this device was essentially a hollow rigid tube, it was somewhat difficult to introduce into the stomach, especially in a conscious subject, so it was probably no coincidence that the 'patient' used for Kussmaul's demonstrations was a professional sword swallower. Although visualization was limited using this apparatus, the principle of gastroduodenoscopy was born.

When Thomas Edison invented the light bulb in 1879, it was immediately seen to be the answer to many of the problems of poor illumination in the early endoscopes. In the same year, Maximilian Nitze (Figure 1.5) and Josef Leiter (Figure 1.6) produced a rigid cystoscope with a built-in light source made from electrically heated platinum wire. The endoscope itself incorporated a working channel and a multi-lens system, and the whole apparatus was water-cooled, much to the relief of their patients. They followed this up with a crude gastroscope based on the same pattern.

In 1887, Nitze and Leiter improved the design by moving the light bulb to the distal end of the device, improving illumination further. The rigid nature of these devices limited the range of view and required great care and skill on the part of the endoscopist to prevent iatrogenic damage.

The limitations caused by blind spots were partly overcome by the introduction of a gastroscope with a flexible lower tip. This was developed in 1898 by Georg Kelling in

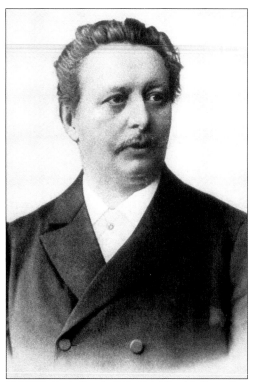

1.5 Maximilian Carl Friedrich Nitze (1848–1906).
(Courtesy of the Collections of the Medical University of Vienna)

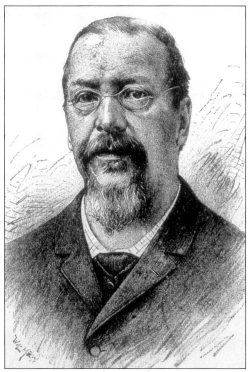

1.6 Josef Leiter (1830–1892).
(Courtesy of the Collections of the Medical University of Vienna)

Dresden, Germany, and was controlled by a system of wire pulleys operated from the proximal end. However, this instrument did not prove popular and was superseded by a modification of an earlier rigid instrument, a triple-tube gastroscope, originally invented by Theodore Rosenheim in Berlin in 1896. This consisted of an inner tube containing a number of short-focus lenses, a middle tube containing the lighting system, derived from a water-cooled platinum wire loop, and an outer sheath with a scale of measurement. This apparatus was modified by

Elsner in 1911 to include a rubber tip for introduction, and became the standard gastroscope for the next 20 years.

The first attempt at an endoscopic examination of the abdominal cavity was carried out by Dmitri Oskarovich Ott of Petrograd (now Saint Petersburg), Russia, in 1901. He used a head mirror and speculum to peer through an incision made in the posterior vaginal wall. In the same year, Georg Kelling performed the first true laparoscopy on a dog. He used a Nitze cystoscope and insufflated the animal's abdomen by injecting air through a sterile cotton filter. He published this work in 1902, terming his procedure 'coelioscopy'.

Working separately, Hans Christian Jacobaeus from Stockholm, Sweden, published his initial series of endoscopic examinations of patients with ascites and coined the term 'laparoscopy'. He went on to apply this technique to the thorax, and performed thoracoscopic lysis of pleural adhesions and chest drainage under local analgesia in a tuberculosis sanatorium. By 1912, Kelling and Jacobaeus had reported 160 examinations and described liver pathology, neoplasia and tuberculosis. In 1912, Victor Darwin Lespinasse, working in Chicago, USA, performed the first endoscopic neurosurgical procedure: intracranial intraventricular endoscopy and coagulation of the choroid plexus for the treatment of hydrocephalus in two children. Walter Dandy went on to improve the technique in 1932, with results similar to those of craniotomy. In 1911, the first laparoscopic procedure was carried out in the USA by Bertram Bernheim; the diagnostic use of laparoscopy expanded rapidly among internists and gynaecologists, but general surgeons lost interest as the therapeutic value appeared limited.

Over the following 20 years, many modifications to instrumentation and technique were made to facilitate exploration of the abdominal cavity. Sharp-tipped pyramidal trocars were introduced in 1920, and insufflation by syringe was supplanted by a manual insufflator operated by a foot pump, introduced in 1921 by Otto Goetze. A move to carbon dioxide as the insufflation gas was made popular in 1924 by Richard Zollikofer in Switzerland, as it was less flammable and more rapidly absorbed, and therefore less likely to result in embolism. Other major advances were the introduction of a rubber gasket by Stone in the USA, which dramatically reduced gas leakage through the trocar, and the introduction of a new needle for induction of pneumoperitoneum by Janos Veress from Hungary in 1938. The Veress needle was originally designed for the induction of pneumothorax before thoracoscopic treatment of tuberculosis, but it was quickly adopted by laparoscopic surgeons. It comprised a sharp needle containing a spring-loaded blunt trocar to minimize trauma to intraabdominal organs, and is still widely used today.

Up until the 1920s endoscopes had been almost entirely rigid instruments, often with an arrangement of angles and mirrors to negotiate around corners. In 1920, Rudolf Schindler, a physician from Munich, modified an old Elsner gastroscope by adding a channel for air insufflation, which greatly improved the image and reduced smearing of the lens with gastric contents and mucus. The rubber tip was inserted using a rigid inner tube that was then withdrawn and replaced with the lens and lighting system. In 1932, Schindler, in collaboration with George Wolf of Berlin, replaced the lower third of the gastroscope with a flexible bronze spiral covered in rubber. A system of short-focus lenses in the inner tube could be bent in any direction to an angle of 34 degrees without visual distortion, thus heralding an era of semi-flexible endoscopy, which remained dominant until 1957.

Schindler was an inspirational teacher and groundbreaking researcher, introducing photography and microphotography to his work and publishing widely. He became a world authority on endoscopy and inspired a medical student, Heinrich Lamm, to suggest that a bundle of flexible glass rods might conduct light and images better than the system of lenses traditionally used. John Logie Baird, renowned as the inventor of the television, coincidentally patented the idea of using curved glass rods to carry light around a curve at about the same time, but failed to develop his idea. Lamm spent 2 years developing his prototype, and in 1930 was able to photograph writing on a piece of paper placed in the stomach. In 1934, Schindler, a Jew, was arrested by the Gestapo and sent to Dachau concentration camp, where he remained for 6 months until the combined efforts of colleagues in the USA and Germany managed to get him released. He travelled to Chicago where, as a visiting professor, he established Chicago as the new world centre of endoscopy and was responsible for a renewed and serious interest in the manufacture of endoscopes in the USA.

By the 1950s antibiotic therapy had largely replaced the use of thoracoscopy in the treatment of tuberculosis, and over the next 20 years thoracoscopy developed as a mainly diagnostic procedure. It was still used in the management of pleural effusion and also for the management and biopsy of primary and metastatic tumours. It was not until 1954 that flexible endoscopes, as we know them today, were first conceived. Harold H. Hopkins, who invented the zoom lens in 1946, was a mathematician and professor of applied physics at Imperial College of Science in London. In 1929 Hopkins had thought of the idea of using flexible plastic rods, coated with a lowrefractive-index material and an outer layer of black paint, to transmit undistorted images from one end of the bundle to the other. Recent advances in chip technology and the introduction of complementary metal oxide semiconductor (chips have allowed increased miniaturization and the incorporation of video chips into endoscopes as small as 1.5 mm in diameter.

Instrument maker Karl Storz had suggested to Hopkins the idea of using optical fibres to transmit light, coupled with a rod-lens system within an optical shaft to transmit images. These improvements produced a much clearer, brighter image than had been possible before, with a more natural rendition of colours. An additional advantage was that the light source was removed from the tip of the instrument, decreasing the risk of burning the patient. Storz patented this idea in 1965, and this principle is still used today in most rigid endoscopes, giving a wider field of view and better light transmission with a smaller diameter of insertion tube than when using traditional thin lenses.

Hopkins was also interested in transmitting images via optical fibres, and together with his postgraduate fellow Narinder Singh Kapany, a physicist studying advanced optics, he researched ways of coating optical fibres and arranging them in a coherent bundle so that the spatial arrangement of fibres remained unchanged along the length of the bundle. In this way an image could be transmitted even if the bundle were bent through 360 degrees. In 1954, Hopkins and Kapany published a report of successful transmission of images through fibreoptic bundles in the journal *Nature*, entitled 'A flexible fibrescope, using static scanning'. A cardiology registrar at the Hammersmith Hospital in London, Timothy Counihan, read this paper and mentioned it to a colleague, Keith Henley.

Henley was a gastroenterologist, and Counihan, rightly as it turned out, suggested that fibreoptics might have a practical application in gastroenterology. A short while later, Henley was in the USA and discussed the idea over lunch with a fellow gastroenterologist, Basil Hirschowitz, a South African who had trained at the Central Middlesex Hospital in London. Hirschowitz was conducting research into a miniature camera that could be used to take diagnostic images of the gastric lumen, and he immediately saw the potential of this idea and contacted Kapany in London. The discussion convinced Hirschowitz that these techniques could be applied to endoscopy, and on his return to the USA he collaborated with two physicists from Michigan, C. Wilbur Peters and Lawrence E. Curtiss, to produce the first working flexible fibreoptic endoscope in 1957. This was manufactured commercially in 1960, and in 1962 a controllable directional tip was introduced following a suggestion by Liverpool gastroscopist Robert Kemp. Over the following 10 years or so further modifications were introduced, with the addition of water and air insufflation channels and provision for suction and passage of instruments.

Another leap forward came with the development in 1969 of the charge-coupled device (CCD) by Bell Laboratories in the USA. This device is common today in digital still and video cameras, and revolutionized endoscopy. CCDs are small, lightweight and very sensitive to light, and are ideal for capturing endoscopic images. By 1983 the first flexible video-endoscopes were being introduced with a CCD chip at the distal end. These had a much improved image quality as they did not produce a pixelated image, which results from fibreoptic transmission.

Even at this late stage, endoscopy was largely used by internists in a predominantly diagnostic role. Minor procedures, such as intestinal polyp removal, biopsies and bladder stone retrieval, were being performed, but general surgeons were still rather uninterested. The stimulus for advances in laparoscopy and endosurgery came from the German gynaecologist Kurt Semm (Figure 1.7), who is widely acknowledged as the father of modern laparoscopy. Semm developed an automatic carbon dioxide insufflator to monitor intra-abdominal pressure during laparoscopy, as well as tissue morcellators, suction/irrigation systems and various techniques for laparoscopic haemostasis. Above all, he was an enthusiastic teacher and innovator and, with the assistance of Karl Storz, developed the pelvi-trainer, a laparoscopic model that enabled surgeons to practise the vital hand–eye coordination and suturing techniques necessary for successful interventional laparoscopy.

However, laparoscopy was still widely viewed with considerable scepticism; indeed, it was variously thought of as unethical, reckless and even downright dangerous. On one occasion, Semm was in the middle of a slide presentation on ovarian cyst enucleation by laparoscopy when suddenly the projector was unplugged, with the explanation that such unethical surgery should not be presented. When he was appointed to the chair of the Department of Obstetrics and Gynaecology at the University of Kiel, Germany, in 1970, Semm introduced laparoscopic surgery into his department and, at the request of co-workers, had to undergo a brain scan because colleagues suspected that only a person with brain damage would perform laparoscopic surgery.

Upon requesting that surgeons at the University of Kiel in the years 1975–1980 perform laparoscopic cholecystectomy, Semm was greeted with laughter. Despite all this, he persisted with his vision. In 1980, Semm performed the

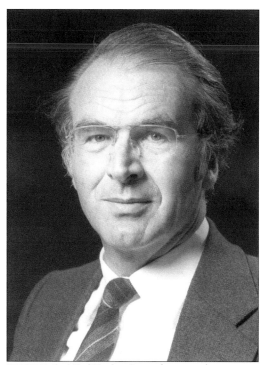

1.7 Kurt Karl Stephan Semm (1927–2003).
(Courtesy of L Metter, University of Kiel)

first laparoscopic appendectomy, making the first move from diagnostic to therapeutic laparoscopy. When he later told a surgical meeting what he had done, the President of the German Surgical Society called for his suspension. But the seed had been set.

Erich Muhe of Germany carried out the first laparoscopic cholecystectomy in 1985, amid severe criticism from the German Surgical Society. These procedures were difficult and awkward to perform because the surgeon had to hold the endoscope in one hand and peer through the oculus. Then came the development of the CCD television camera. For the first time, cameras were small enough to clip on to the eyepiece of an endoscope and transmit a magnified image to a monitor. Not only did this greatly increase the diagnostic and surgical capabilities of the endoscopist, it also allowed other members of the surgical team to view the procedure. Surgical assistants could operate the camera and endoscope, freeing the surgeon's hands to enable more delicate procedures to be carried out using two hands, and the maintenance of a sterile field was greatly enhanced. The first video-assisted cholecystectomy was carried out by Philippe Mouret of Lyon, France in 1987, and was rapidly followed by others. Despite the early scepticism, the advent of video-assisted endoscopy heralded a major paradigm shift in the view of general surgeons worldwide, and by 1991 there was an explosion of new techniques unparalleled in surgical history. In 1993 the National Institutes of Health in the USA held a consensus conference, which declared laparoscopic cholecystectomy the treatment of choice for uncomplicated cholelithiasis. Laparoscopic techniques were applied to almost every aspect of abdominal and thoracic surgery, as well as the arthroscopic exploration of joints. After being subjected to years of ridicule, Kurt Semm's vision had finally been vindicated.

Surgeons quickly appreciated the benefits of fewer abdominal adhesions, faster return of intestinal function after surgery, and fewer wound complications and postoperative infections. Patients were up and about more quickly, freeing hospital beds, and there was much less postoperative pain and scarring. This led to an added impetus from patients themselves, demanding minimally invasive procedures, and hospital authorities were quick to appreciate the benefits too. Laparoscopic hernia repairs and antireflux surgery were quickly followed by techniques for the removal of solid organs, such as the spleen, adrenal glands, liver lobes and kidneys. This not only benefited patients with organic disease but also increased the donor pool for transplantation, since donor organ removal became less traumatic. Initial laparoscopic procedures to resect colon cancer met with scepticism and worries that such techniques might increase recurrence through seeding at the operative site. However, these fears have not been realized, and indeed rates of recurrence have been similar or less with laparoscopic techniques compared with open techniques, whereas return of intestinal function and lack of adhesions have been greatly enhanced.

Veterinary surgeons (veterinarians) have also pioneered minimally invasive techniques since the early 1970s, but uptake has been slow, due in part to the considerable cost of instrumentation and the same scepticism that so inhibited the early pioneers in the human field. Flexible endoscopy was the first technique to gain acceptance in the veterinary field, given the obvious benefit that these instruments provide in the exploration of the tubular structures of the body, in particular the respiratory and gastrointestinal (GI) tracts. The first reports of bronchoscopy in small animals came from O'Brien in 1970 and were followed by descriptions of flexible endoscopy of the GI tract by Johnson *et al.* in 1976. Biopsy samples could be taken and foreign bodies removed without resorting to open surgery, and these procedures rapidly gained acceptance. Rigid endoscopy has taken longer to become established, despite the first reports from Dalton and Hill (1972) and Lettow (1972), working separately, on the use of laparoscopy for evaluation of the liver and pancreas.

Many veterinary surgeons were taught at college that 'wounds heal side to side, not end to end; make a big hole', the aim of which was to give the surgeon optimum exposure and visualization of the surgical field with minimal tension on the tissues. Video-assisted endoscopy has completely superseded this opinion by giving the surgeon a considerably enhanced, magnified and well illuminated view of almost the entire abdominal or thoracic cavity through a tiny 5 mm incision. Tension on tissues is minimal or absent because organs are operated on *in situ*, without the need to exteriorize them through an abdominal incision in order to visualize them adequately. It has enabled veterinary surgeons to directly visualize structures such as the urethra and nasal passages, which were previously impossible to access adequately without recourse to major open surgery, and to carry out endosurgical procedures without the need for any surgical incisions at all. The benefits to the patient are obvious and, much as has been the case in human surgery, the impetus for veterinary minimally invasive procedures may well become client driven, at least in part. As the necessary equipment has become cheaper, it has become economically viable to convert to minimally invasive procedures, and many manufactures of surgical equipment for the human field have formed veterinary divisions. Manufacturers are also producing equipment exclusively for the veterinary market with modifications that suit veterinary patients and techniques, as well as veterinary practices' budgets. A full range of equipment suitable for performing laparoscopy, thoracoscopy, rhinoscopy, urethrocystoscopy, otoscopy and arthroscopy is now available for less than the cost of a mid-range ultrasound machine.

Incorporating endoscopy into veterinary practice

The decision to incorporate minimally invasive surgery and diagnostics into a companion animal practice is a complicated one, which must take into account practice demographics, economics, staffing, physical plant considerations, practitioner interests and relative proximity to similar practices.

Make no mistake – endoscopic equipment is not cheap. It is expensive to purchase, delicate and prone to breakages, and so there are additional costs of maintenance and replacements to consider. For the purchase of instrumentation, both the used secondary equipment market and the new equipment market are viable sources. However, since the cost of instrumentation has reduced dramatically over the past 20 years or so, purchasing new equipment is recommended, especially in the first instance, as everything will be compatible, spare parts will be available and everything will be covered by a warranty for at least a year. Perhaps as importantly, most suppliers of new equipment will provide free training for the practice's veterinary surgeons and nurses on the care, sterilization and storage of the new equipment, which will minimize damage and reduce replacement costs.

In the USA, where human healthcare is largely in the competitive marketplace, the market for used medical equipment is thriving. At top US hospitals, when new and improved instrumentation becomes available, there is often a race to procure the latest technology. The resultant excess, high-quality equipment ends up on the secondary market, where it is either exported overseas or sold on to the veterinary market. In the UK, current National Health Service (NHS) regulations make it difficult for individual NHS hospitals to dispose of excess or redundant equipment to the veterinary community. The government does maintain a resource database of available used medical equipment, but it is limited, and navigating the NHS bureaucracy to obtain medical equipment can be frustrating. That being said, having a good working relationship with personnel in the operating theatres and storerooms of the local NHS hospital can be helpful. Surplus equipment from the NHS and the private sector is often sold off at medical auctions, and this can be a useful source for veterinary surgeons. However, here 'buyer beware' applies, since the equipment is sold with no warranty and it can be difficult to assess its functionality in the auction environment. Spare parts may no longer be available and it may be difficult or impossible to get items serviced.

The used medical equipment market, while variable in inventory and quality, can be an excellent place for the veterinary practitioner to obtain endoscopic equipment. However, there are some important considerations when navigating these resellers. It should be borne in mind that none of the human equipment sold on the secondary market was designed for small animal use and has often been 'retired' for a reason. The veterinary surgeon must have a solid understanding of what procedures they will be performing, and on which patients. For instance, buying a very inexpensive 12 mm sigmoidoscope will be of limited value for the feline practitioner looking to perform small intestinal endoscopy. Taking careful stock of what equipment is needed for the most common procedures intended to be performed is critical before going shopping.

The history of the equipment is difficult to obtain from the secondary market. How, where and for what procedures the equipment was used, and whether there is any relevant repair history, all affect the potential resale value of the equipment. Resellers often obtain equipment in bulk lots and have little information to pass on to their customers. As such, warranty information is often unavailable or warranties may be limited in duration or scope. Purchasing a 10-year-old video camera system without a warranty can be a risky proposition, especially if spare parts have been withdrawn from the market. It is wise to enquire from the secondary reseller as to whether they provide on- or off-site service, the service costs, and the availability of spare parts and repairs. A service contract may be available to purchase; the cost of the contract must be evaluated in light of the age and value of the equipment relative to its replacement cost. Resellers should always be asked to provide a warranty of at least 3 months to allow time to assess the equipment fully.

With the used equipment market thriving in the USA, more and more high-quality endoscopic equipment is making its way across the Atlantic, especially through websites such as eBay. This has made it much easier for practitioners to purchase equipment and has reduced the costs in the secondary market. However, it is prudent for the European veterinary surgeon to carefully evaluate the electrical and video compatibility of North American equipment with what is available in their countries. The electrical supply in the USA is based on a standard 110 V power source with country-specific mains power supply cords. Often, a power converter or phase transformer is needed to make the equipment usable in other countries. In addition, the video standard used in the USA is National Television Standards Committee (NTSC). It can be difficult to use NTSC video cameras with monitors and video-recording devices using the standard European PAL video format. Most equipment nowadays is compatible with both standards but sometimes converters are needed, decreasing image quality, complicating the set-up and increasing costs.

In response to the burgeoning need for endoscopic instrumentation in the veterinary market, new equipment, much of it specifically engineered for companion animal practices, has become more readily available. In the UK and worldwide, there are now many companies that specifically work with the veterinary community. New equipment almost invariably costs more. However, knowledgeable representatives from these companies can provide advice on the best equipment for the particular species and procedure. Often, these companies provide excellent warranties and service plans guaranteeing a high degree of 'up-time'. In addition, continuing professional development (CPD) and installation training to facilitate the integration of endoscopy into the practice are often available from these companies.

Financing the purchase of endoscopic equipment is beyond the scope of this Manual. Suffice to say that creative financing options, such as leases with low-cost buyouts, and many other options are available. The options should be discussed with the practice's tax advisers and other business professionals to make sure that the best financial option for the individual practice is chosen. As competition in the market increases, the cost of new equipment falls, and a basic set of rigid endoscopy equipment, including a camera and monitor, is now affordable by almost all practices. However, the cost of the equipment is only an abstract number without adequate planning and prediction of the number of procedures to be performed and the revenue expected to be generated. Many practices will incorporate routine procedures such as laparoscopic bitch spays into their repertoire at a cost premium over a traditional open spay. Since these procedures are carried out on a predictable weekly basis it may only take four or so procedures a month to recoup the cost of the equipment lease, at the same time broadening the scope of procedures the practice can offer to include other laparoscopic procedures, rhinoscopy, urethrocystoscopy and video-otoscopy.

Once a general figure for the start-up costs has been determined, it is possible to calculate the fees needed to be generated to justify the equipment purchase. Most practices will charge a higher fee for an endoscopic procedure than for the traditional open equivalent, to cover the additional equipment and training costs as well as the costs of cleaning, sterilization and replacements. It is a good idea to keep a log of the instances in which the surgeon would consider performing an endoscopic procedure. For example, when presented with a sneezing dog, a note should be made that this patient may be a potential rhinoscopy case. Similarly, when presented with a giant-breed bitch for ovariohysterectomy, a note should be made of the laparoscopic ovariectomy/ovariohysterectomy and gastropexy that might be performed. This information can then be extrapolated to come up with a prediction of how many of each type of procedure might be performed over the course of the fiscal year. These basic calculations can give a very rough approximation of the client costs for each procedure, although it is important to be sure to account for an appropriate profit margin. Questions to consider are: does this number correlate well with the fees currently generated by similar traditionally performed procedures in the surgery? Does it allow endoscopy to be a cost-competitive alternative to traditional approaches?

Consideration of the demographics of the human and animal clientele is also important. The clientele's level of income and education, proximity to large urban centres and proximity to advanced human healthcare centres are all somewhat predictive of their likelihood of availing themselves of advanced veterinary care. Careful observation of the type of pets seen in the practice is also important. Is the practice an urban small dog/cat/'pocket pet' practice? Or is it a 'green belt' suburban large dog practice? Is the predominant pet the farm dog or stable-yard cat? These observations play a role in determining the type of procedures to be performed, the equipment needed and the numbers of cases likely to be seen. It is important, however, to avoid jumping to conclusions and being overly pessimistic when assessing clients' willingness to pay for minimally invasive procedures. It is the authors' experience that clients are very often happy to pay a premium for procedures that reduce the pain and morbidity of surgery, even for routine procedures that are often more price sensitive, such as bitch spays.

Another important factor to consider is the physical plant. While most practices do not have a dedicated endoscopy suite, it is highly advantageous if one can be accommodated. Having a dedicated room to perform endoscopy is of huge benefit. Indeed, having a dedicated room for non-sterile endoscopy and a separate theatre for surgical endoscopy would be the best option of all. In reality, it is helpful to have a theatre of adequate size to allow movement of the equipment into and out of the room, and space in a non-sterile area of the building to perform non-sterile endoscopic procedures. A wet sink table is very beneficial when performing rhinoscopy, cystoscopy and colonoscopy. The ergonomics of the workspace need to be examined to allow adequate access of the anaesthetist to the patient, adequate visualization of the video monitor and adequate room to perform the procedures appropriately and comfortably. These factors are covered in the appropriate procedure chapters.

The practitioner's commitment to learning and performing endoscopy is another factor worth considering. Virtually all of the techniques described in this Manual can be performed by most practitioners with expertise. Aside from the financial commitment, the veterinary surgeon needs to evaluate their interest in spending the requisite time to learn and perfect the skills needed to become a competent endoscopist. Certainly in the initial phases of learning, procedures will take more time, and frustration levels can be high. But with practice and persistence, endoscopy will become easier and more time-efficient. Does the practice allow for enough time to learn these new techniques? Is the volume of consultations and surgical procedures so great that it makes introducing new procedures difficult? These questions must be answered by each practice individually, assessing the particulars of the desires of the veterinary staff and the time constraints placed on each veterinary surgeon.

Marketing the minimally invasive surgery programme to the clientele and local veterinary community should be an integrated component of any scheme to establish a successful endoscopy practice. The support staff of receptionists and veterinary nurses are often the first line in introducing these procedures to clients. Staff should be well trained in identifying the patients for which a particular endoscopic procedure might be appropriate when clients contact the practice with an enquiry or to make an appointment. The practice should be identified to the client as offering the most advanced diagnostics or treatments for the given problem. Staff should be equipped with the ability to answer clients' questions regarding the superiority of endoscopic intervention compared with traditional approaches, including the benefits to their pet of faster recovery and less pain. When the consultation with the veterinary surgeon is scheduled, additional time should be allotted to allow adequate discussion of the appropriateness of endoscopic interventions. Surgeons should be cautioned against overplaying the 'gee-whiz' factor of endoscopic surgery, but rather should focus on the very real physiological benefits of minimally invasive approaches.

Observations of the authors made over the past 10–20 years, from practising in the UK, the USA, Europe and Asia, have given the firm impression that when it comes to medical technology, the general public is quite savvy. Virtually every week clients come in for a consultation and enquire whether the particular procedure can be performed in a 'keyhole' (or, in the USA, a 'Band-Aid') fashion. Even on those occasions when a minimally invasive procedure might not be appropriate, it is interesting to note how aware clients are of the advances in surgical procedures. Often they will have had a 'keyhole' procedure themselves, or will know someone who has, and appreciate the advantages. With the advent of the internet, clients have become much more aware of the availability of these procedures for their pets. When clients are presented with surgical options that might result in less pain and trauma for their pets, and improve recovery, they are often very keen to explore those possibilities.

This is particularly true in feline practice, where many owners have traditionally declined invasive diagnostic procedures (e.g. exploratory laparotomy) for the sole purpose of biopsy sample collection. Offering the option of outpatient diagnostic laparoscopy to these clients addresses the expectation of an alternative, minimally invasive procedure. In addition, rapid technological improvements (e.g. digitization and the miniaturization of equipment) have enhanced the clinician's visualization, access and sampling capabilities and thus elevated medical investigations beyond using inappropriately sized equipment, repeated diagnostic tests and resorting to blind polypharmacy.

Client education brochures and pamphlets are very helpful in disseminating information to pet owners. Full-colour glossy productions, highlighting the unique offerings of the practice and the advanced level of care the patients receive, will be read carefully by owners and often distributed to their friends and colleagues. Similar information should also be provided on the practice's website and social media to reach clients who prefer to receive information in a digital format. The provision of material online has the added benefit of providing pet owners who like to research the potential treatment options before consultation with a readily accessible and reliable source of information. In addition, social media platforms are increasingly being used as a way for practices to advertising their services to both clients and potentially referring veterinary surgeons.

Practices can have 'open house' days at the surgery to allow the public to come in and see for themselves the impressive level of care that advanced endoscopic techniques make possible. Video presentations and tours of the endoscopic theatre are all very impressive to the general public. A laparoscopic dry lab trainer can be set up to allow clients to try their hand at simple laparoscopic manipulations and get involved in an entertaining and educational way.

Many practitioners are keen to use endoscopy and endosurgery to augment or establish a referral component to their practice. For the existing referral practitioner or specialist, the introduction and marketing of endoscopy is of critical importance. The referring veterinary clientele are expecting their referral and specialist sources to have access to the most current state-of-the-art techniques. They will be looking to the referral practitioner to provide access to these modalities for their patients. For the first-opinion practitioner, endoscopy offers an opportunity to break into the referral market. The first question for the practitioner in this situation to ask themselves is 'Do I have the requisite degree of expertise to offer referral services?' Since there is currently no recognized specialism in minimally invasive surgery, the surgeon must guard against referring to themselves as a 'specialist' unless they are suitably qualified in a related field, and must be careful not to take on cases that are beyond their expertise. Initially, it may be the case that a limited range of procedures is offered. Additional procedures can be added as the practitioner gains experience with different and more advanced techniques. It is important for first-opinion practices to have firm and well publicized policies regarding their referral practices. Often, competing local practices will be reluctant to send referrals to competitors that also provide first-opinion services, for fear of losing the client to the competitor. Each practice must make this decision for themselves, but careful consideration must be given to developing a policy that will encourage referrals for endoscopy and alleviate fears of losing clients.

Some practices will put on small informal CPD programmes to introduce their services to veterinary surgeons in the local area. Often, equipment or pharmaceutical manufacturers can be encouraged to help sponsor such CPD. This low-key, informal way of educating practitioners and marketing new referral services is a fun and easy way of answering questions and encouraging local participation in the new services provided by the practice.

Patient assessment and stabilization

The initial assessment of each patient presented for an endoscopic or endosurgical procedure is based on the clinical history, full clinical examination and relevant diagnostic tests (e.g. haematology/biochemistry/electrolytes/ TT4 (total thyroxine), radiographic and ultrasonographic imaging) to establish a baseline. It may be the case that after proceeding with these 'gold standard' tests, a diagnostic roadblock is reached that may be resolved by endoscopy, obviating the need for repeating tests, repeating blind treatments or referral. The general haemodynamic stability of the patient should be established, as well as its stability for the specific procedure being considered. Careful history-taking should be undertaken:

- The client should be asked about the animal's diet and housing
- Eating and drinking patterns should be evaluated, and examined in the consultation room if possible
- Urinary and defecatory patterns should be evaluated
- The duration of the clinical problem and the owner's perception of the progression of clinical signs should be ascertained
- Enquiries regarding animal housemates and/or littermates should be made.

For any endoscopic procedure, consideration must be given to the relative safety of general anaesthesia. The first consideration is haemodynamic stability. Careful auscultation of the heart and lungs is of paramount importance. Many endoscopic procedures have the potential to decrease ventilatory efficiency, so it is critical that the patient has an acceptable cardiovascular status. Ideally, the resting peripheral capillary oxygen saturation (S_pO_2) should be evaluated by pulse oximetry. In addition to the standard serum biochemistry analysis and complete blood count, blood gases (arterial if possible) should be evaluated. Thoracic radiographs should be obtained if clinically indicated and, if there is any clinical or historical indication of cardiac disease, an echocardiogram performed. The patient's hydration status should be evaluated via both clinical pathological analysis (packed cell volume, total solids and urine specific gravity) and clinical assessment.

A thorough general physical examination is indicated. The tendency to focus exclusively on body parts or organ systems related to the presenting problem should be avoided. However, special attention obviously needs to be given to the systems directly related to the presentation, as well as to the cardiovascular status, as noted above. A review of the previously performed clinical pathology needs to be undertaken and, if indicated, the diagnostic work-up should be completed before endoscopy. The underlying principle for any surgical or anaesthetic intervention is to perform the least invasive intervention needed to diagnose and manage the presenting problem effectively.

The patient should be stabilized in preparation for the subsequent intervention. Supportive management of the animal's hydration status via intravenous fluid therapy should be dictated by the findings of clinical assessment and clinical pathology. The patient's cardiovascular status needs to be monitored and maintained. Monitoring and correction of blood gas abnormalities, thoracocentesis, pericardiocentesis and abdominocentesis (as well as appropriate analysis of all fluid samples so obtained) should be performed if clinically indicated and needed to improve haemodynamic stability. Therapy for secondary or concomitant disease states should be undertaken, for example, managing infectious diseases, vomiting and diarrhoea, and endocrinological anomalies. Nutritional support in the form of total or partial parenteral nutrition or tube feeding should be considered where indicated.

In spite of the increasing use of endoscopy in veterinary practice, traditional diagnostic modalities have not been abandoned. Indeed, the ability to perform minimally invasive procedures has increased the use of other imaging and diagnostic modalities as well. Traditional and digital radiography are almost always the first imaging techniques used for evaluating both the pleural and the peritoneal space. Positive and negative contrast studies are still performed, albeit with less frequency than before the advent of endoscopy. Ultrasonography and echocardiography are excellent techniques for examining the internal structure and size of the viscera, and are commonly used before endoscopy.

Ultrasonography is very helpful in determining the size and structure of organs such as the liver, spleen, pancreas, intestine, adrenal glands, kidneys and bladder. The presence and location of free peritoneal fluid can easily be assessed. Echocardiography is ideal for evaluating the morphology and structure of the heart, determining both cardiovascular stability and disease states of the heart and surrounding structures. Thoracic ultrasonography is helpful in examining the pleural space, although it is less consistently valuable in assessing pathology of the pulmonary parenchyma.

When available, computed tomography (CT) and magnetic resonance imaging (MRI) are also very valuable. MRI is excellent for examining pathology of the nasal passages and sinuses, and CT is very helpful in evaluating the abdomen and central nervous system, particularly when considering extension of fungal disease via the cribriform plate or extension of otic disease. These modalities have limitations of accessibility and cost, meaning that they are less frequently used. However, this situation is rapidly changing with an increase in the number of static and mobile units in veterinary use in both private practice and teaching hospitals. It is important to remember that the more sensitive the test, the more likely it is to call attention to incidental lesions that may be of little clinical relevance.

The endoscopist must give constant consideration to the potential for the need for traditional open surgical approaches. In the author's [DS] experience, despite a keen interest in performing as much surgical and diagnostic work as possible using endoscopic techniques, there are limitations to what can be accomplished endoscopically. If during the diagnostic work-up it becomes apparent that a more invasive surgical intervention will yield more complete and timely information or therapeutic results, the veterinary surgeon must remain open to the possibility that endoscopy may not be the most reasonable approach. The best interests of the patient must always be the guiding principle.

Flexible *versus* rigid endoscopy

The flexible endoscope is essential for examining tubular structures that have a tortuous course, such as the GI tract or lower airways. Long flexible endoscopes allow structures deep within the lungs and digestive tract to be visualized, and biopsy samples to be taken, without the need for invasive surgery. This has obvious benefits for the patient. Their limitations, apart from expense and the problems of cleaning and maintenance, are due to light transmission and instrumentation.

Flexible endoscopes are complex instruments with channels for suction/irrigation and the passage of instruments, as well as light guide fibres and optical image fibres, and guidewires for the angulation of the tip. This complexity accounts for the initial expense of the instrument and the high maintenance costs, and also gives rise to numerous nooks and crannies where bacterial contamination can reside, making adequate cleaning difficult but essential. The majority of flexible endoscopes on the veterinary market are digital video-endoscopes. In older fibreoptic flexible endoscopes, the image is transmitted down a bundle of coherent optical glass fibres to the eyepiece. Light is transmitted from the light source to the tip of the insertion tube by an incoherent glass fibre bundle. This results in poorer light transmission than a rigid endoscope and a pixelated view of the operative site, since the final image is a composite of a large number of smaller images transmitted down each individual fibre. In addition, the glass fibres are very fragile and easily damaged; broken fibres lead to black spots within the image. Damage to the light fibre bundle can reduce light transmission and illumination, which further degrades the final image.

These problems have been largely overcome by video-endoscopes, which have a digital camera chip at the distal end, but at a significant cost penalty since essentially a separate camera is purchased with each endoscope. As the cost of equipment comes down this will be less of a problem, but at the moment the price premium is not inconsiderable. Damage to the light fibre bundle can still occur in video-endoscopes, so careful handling is required.

Instrumentation for a flexible endoscope has to pass down the instrument channel, which limits its size and requires it to be long and flexible. In particular, biopsy samples obtained endoscopically are necessarily small, and it is sometimes difficult to biopsy to an adequate depth to ensure that representative pathological tissue is obtained. This is particularly true where the mucosa overlying an area of pathology is inflamed and thickened.

Rigid endoscopes are simpler in construction, with no moving parts. Light transmission and image quality are much better than with a fibreoptic flexible endoscope, and cleaning, sterilization and maintenance are relatively simple. Their initial cost is also considerably less. Instrumentation for rigid endoscopy can be larger and more robust, since it does not always need to be passed through an instrument channel; it can be passed alongside the endoscope or through a separate operative port. This allows larger instrumentation, which not only enables the use of a variety of instruments akin to the familiar day-to-day surgical instruments, but also allows larger tissue samples to be taken, which can result in a higher diagnostic yield. Rigid endoscopy also enables instruments to be inserted in several ports, spaced apart and triangulated to the operative area. This can allow easier surgical manipulation than a strictly linear flexible endoscope would permit, so that many of the surgical operations that are currently performed through open surgery become possible endoscopically with appropriate instrumentation.

The advantages of this to the patient are obvious; smaller wounds mean less trauma and reduced postoperative pain, faster healing and fewer sutures to take out. Tissue handling is often more delicate and, with no manual handling of organs and tissues, release of inflammatory mediators is reduced, resulting in fewer adhesions. Much of the operative time in open surgery is taken up with closing the wound made in the first place. Surgical operating time is often shorter for endoscopic procedures, so the price differential with conventional open surgery need not be great despite the increased cost of instrumentation.

In some areas there may be overlap between the use of rigid and flexible endoscopes. Although flexible endoscopes are used widely in the respiratory and GI tracts, rigid endoscopes may be useful in some situations. Rigid endoscopes are used in tracheoscopy, where a view down as far as the carina is possible in most patients. Rigid instrumentation is more robust than the smaller forceps that must be passed through the instrument channel of a flexible endoscope and therefore may be better suited for removing some foreign bodies from the trachea or oesophagus. Rigid biopsy forceps are also larger in size for the same reason, and their use may result in a more diagnostic sample in sites such as the colon. Although access to the descending colon is limited when using a rigid endoscope, most colon pathology is fairly diffuse, and representative samples can usually be obtained from this site. Conversely, although rigid endoscopes are more commonly used in the nose and bladder, small flexible endoscopes can be used to access the sinuses and the male urethra.

Recent advances in endoscopic surgery

Flexible endoscopy of the GI tract is limited to some extent by the length of the insertion tube. Wireless endoscopic CCD camera systems have been developed, which can be swallowed in a capsule and collected after it has passed in the faeces. Images of the whole digestive tract can thus be obtained, and these devices are now available commercially for small animal veterinary patients (ALICAM®, Infiniti Medical Ltd). Propulsion devices attached to the capsule are being developed to allow its movement to be controlled by the surgeon. Eventually, with the incorporation of biopsy, cautery or laser instrumentation, minor procedures may be carried out without the need for any traditional insertion tube.

Rigid endoscopes with a variable angle of view of 0–30 degrees are now available, and flexible endoscopes have also been developed with zoom-enabled magnification of up to X100, allowing extremely detailed mucosal analysis for the diagnosis and management of mucosal disorders such as coeliac disease. The incorporation of ultrasound devices into the tip of the flexible endoscope enables detailed examination of structures such as the pancreas and hepatic portal system.

There is currently a great deal of research being carried out on endoluminal or natural orifice surgery. Natural orifice transluminal endoscopic surgery (NOTES) involves passing a dual operating port flexible endoscope via the mouth, vagina or colon and through the gastric/vaginal/colonic wall into the peritoneal cavity to carry out laparoscopic surgery, without making any external incision. An appendectomy has been carried out on a human patient in India with the appendix removed via the mouth and the gastric mucosa repaired from within. In 2007, at the University Hospital of Strasbourg, France, the first transvaginal cholecystectomy was performed. In 2009, a series of 10 NOTES ovariectomies in the bitch was described by Lynetta Freeman at Purdue University, USA. Various other procedures, from splenectomy to hernia repair, have been described in the pig model. With the development of improved optics, endosurgical sewing machines and electrocautery devices, NOTES is likely to become commonplace in future years. (For further information, the reader is referred to Chapter 17.)

Advances in surgical glues may render suturing or stapling redundant and greatly facilitate endosurgical procedures; the advent of electrosurgical instruments, such as Ethicon's HARMONIC® scalpel and ENSEAL™ and Valleylab's LigaSure™, has already improved haemostasis and reduced the length of surgical procedures.

The use of robotics has revolutionized many aspects of laparoscopic and thoracoscopic surgery. In 2001, Jacques Marescaux used the Zeus robot to perform a cholecystectomy on a patient in Strasbourg, with the surgical team located in New York. The year 2006 saw the first surgery performed entirely by a robot with no human assistance: the 50-minute operation for atrial fibrillation was carried out on a 34-year-old patient in Milan, Italy. The da Vinci robotic system is used in human heart and prostatic surgery, and is being applied to many other laparoscopic procedures. There are many advantages of robotic devices:

- The binocular endoscope provides high-definition, full-colour, magnified, three-dimensional images of the surgical site to the surgeon, who sits at a remote console
- The surgeon's hands are attached to manipulation controls, which have seven degrees of freedom of movement reflected in the articulated instrumentation to mimic the natural flexibility of the human hand and wrist
- As the surgeon moves their hands, the operative arm of the robot mimics the movement, and the addition of tremor filters (similar to those employed as 'anti-shake' filters in modern digital camcorders) eliminates excessive movement, which can be a problem at high magnification. This allows extremely precise manipulation of tiny instruments for intricate vascular surgery and neurosurgery.

The ability to record procedures into the computer's memory, coupled with the integration of MRI and CT scans of the patient, enables simulations – complete with tactile feedback – to be carried out for training purposes, much as an airline pilot practises in a flight simulator. A surgeon is able to carry out 'dummy runs' before performing a complex procedure on a live patient, and the superimposition of coloured MRI scans on live video-endoscopic images allows the surgeon to visualize enhanced borders of abnormal tissue to facilitate dissection.

The applications of minimally invasive surgery are being continually expanded as technology advances. The modern era of laparoscopy and minimally invasive surgery, championed by Kurt Semm and others, has revolutionized human surgery, and is set to do the same in the veterinary world. In the words of Dr Paul A. Wetter, chairman of the Society of Laparoendoscopic Surgeons: *'Someday in the future, people will look back at a regular surgical incision as something archaic and barbaric. We have Kurt Semm to thank for that'*.

References and further reading

Dalton JR and Hill FW (1972) A procedure for the examination of the liver and pancreas in dogs. *Journal of Small Animal Practice* **13**, 527–530

Doglietto F, Prevedello DM, Jane JA Jr *et al.* (2005) A brief history of endoscopic transsphenoidal surgery: from Philipp Bozzini to the First World Congress of Endoscopic Skull Base Surgery. *Neurosurgery Focus* **19**, E3

Freeman LJ, Rahmani EY, Sherman S *et al.* (2009) Oophorectomy by natural orifice transluminal endoscopic surgery: feasibility study in dogs. *Gastrointestinal Endoscopy* **69**, 1321–1332

Harrell AG and Heniford BT (2005) Minimally invasive abdominal surgery: *lux et veritas* past, present and future. *American Journal of Surgery* **190**, 239–243

Johnson GF, Jones BD and Twedt DC (1976) Esophagogastric endoscopy in small animal medicine. *Gastrointestinal Endoscopy* **22**, 226

Kalbasi H (2001) History and development of laparoscopic surgery. *Official Journal of the Association of Iranian Endoscopic Surgeons* **1**, 45–48

Kaushik D and Rothberg M (2000) Thoracoscopic surgery: historical perspectives. *Neurosurgery Focus* **9**, E10

Lettow E (1972) Laparoscopic examination in liver diseases in dogs. *Veterinary Medicine Review* **2**, 159–167

NIH Consensus Conference (1993) Gallstones and laparoscopic cholecystectomy. *Journal of the American Medical Association* **269**, 1018–1024

O'Brien JA (1970) Bronchoscopy in the dog and cat. *Journal of the American Veterinary Medical Association* **156**, 213–217

Sircus W (2003) Milestones in the evolution of endoscopy: a short history. *Journal of the Royal College of Physicians of Edinburgh* **33**, 124–134

Tuffs A (2003) Kurt Semm: a pioneer in minimally invasive surgery. *British Medical Journal* **327**, 397

Chapter 2

Instrumentation

Christopher J. Chamness

Introduction

Just a decade ago, the term 'endoscopy' would make most veterinary surgeons (veterinarians) think of a flexible endoscope being used to examine the upper or lower gastrointestinal (GI) tract. Nowadays, the general term endoscopy carries much more meaning for many veterinary surgeons, who are becoming increasingly aware of the vast array of applications that make use of both flexible and rigid endoscopes. To name a few, GI endoscopy, bronchoscopy, cystoscopy, vaginoscopy, rhinoscopy, arthroscopy, otoscopy, laparoscopy and thoracoscopy are all endoscopic procedures performed in both human and veterinary surgery with the use of flexible or rigid endoscopes, depending upon the anatomy, the available equipment and the preference of the surgeon.

Flexible endoscopes are more useful in anatomical regions where access requires an optical instrument that is able to turn corners, such as the gastrointestinal, respiratory and urinary tracts. Under certain conditions these procedures may also be performed using rigid endoscopes, but visual access may be limited. For example, a rigid endoscope can be used for gastroscopy but not duodenoscopy; a rigid endoscope may also be used for colonoscopy, but only to examine the distal portion of the colon. Rigid endoscopes are preferred for cystoscopy in female animals, but a flexible endoscope is needed for transurethral cystoscopy in male dogs. Either flexible or rigid endoscopes may be used for tracheobronchoscopy; however, a small-diameter flexible endoscope enables the operator to reach deeper into the bronchial tree.

Flexible endoscopes

Most flexible endoscopes designed for GI use consist of three sections (Figure 2.1):

- The **insertion tube** is the part of the endoscope that enters the patient

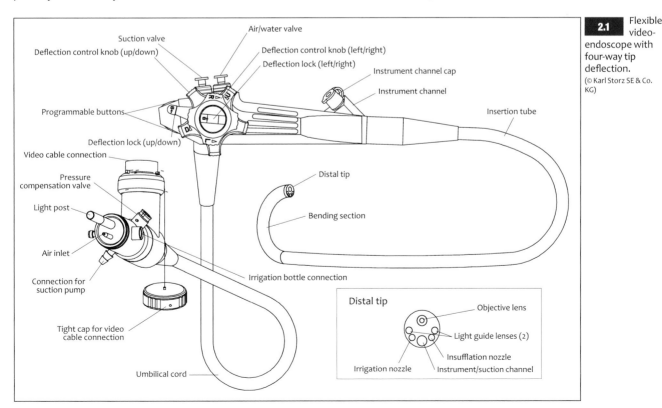

2.1 Flexible video-endoscope with four-way tip deflection. (© Karl Storz SE & Co. KG)

Suction valve
Air/water valve
Deflection control knob (up/down)
Deflection control knob (left/right)
Deflection lock (left/right)
Instrument channel cap
Instrument channel
Programmable buttons
Insertion tube
Deflection lock (up/down)
Video cable connection
Pressure compensation valve
Distal tip
Light post
Bending section
Air inlet
Connection for suction pump
Irrigation bottle connection
Tight cap for video cable connection
Umbilical cord

Distal tip
Objective lens
Light guide lenses (2)
Insufflation nozzle
Irrigation nozzle
Instrument/suction channel

- The **handpiece** contains the manual controls and working channel port (if present)
- The **umbilical cord** plugs into the light source.

Some flexible endoscopes, especially those designed for the respiratory and urinary tracts, have no umbilical cord; examples of these are shown in Figure 2.2. The fibrescope shown in Figure 2.2a requires a simple light-transmitting cable, like those used for rigid endoscopes, which attaches to the light post of the endoscope. The video-endoscope shown in Figure 2.2b contains a light-emitting diode (LED) light source integrated into the handle of the endoscope, so that no external light source is needed. The cable attached to the handpiece of the endoscope in Figure 2.2b is not for light transmission but for transmitting the electronic image information to the camera control unit.

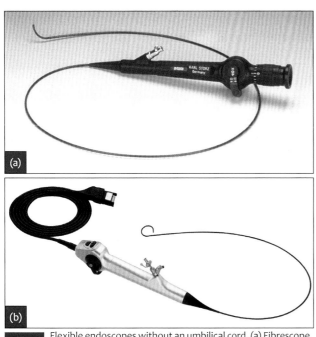

2.2 Flexible endoscopes without an umbilical cord. (a) Fibrescope (2.7 mm diameter, 100 cm long) with two-way tip deflection. (b) Video-endoscope with two-way tip deflection and a LED light source integrated into the handpiece.
(© Karl Storz SE & Co. KG)

Structure

The flexible endoscope most commonly used by veterinary surgeons is the gastroscope, sometimes also referred to as a multi-purpose flexible endoscope, since it has applications in various anatomical locations in both small and large animals. It can be used in the GI, respiratory and urinary tracts, depending upon patient size. Gastroscopes have four-way tip deflection (i.e. up/down and left/right), as shown in Figure 2.3. This deflection capability is very important for the successful manoeuvring of a gastroscope through the intestines, and particularly for the fine manoeuvres required to traverse the pylorus.

Deflection control

The deflection control knobs are located on the handpiece (Figure 2.4). When rotated, they cause the shortening or lengthening of cables within the insertion tube, which deflects the distally located bending portion of the insertion tube. The larger inner control knob controls up/down deflection and is operated using the left thumb. The smaller outer control knob controls left/right deflection and

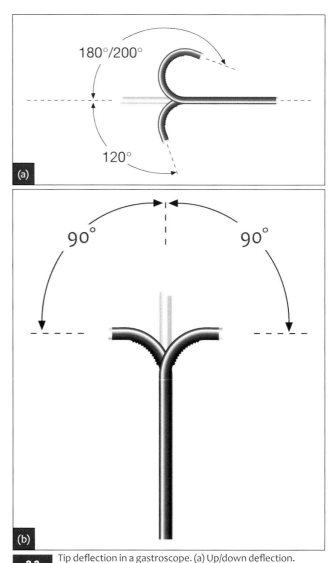

2.3 Tip deflection in a gastroscope. (a) Up/down deflection. (b) Right/left deflection.
(© Karl Storz SE & Co. KG)

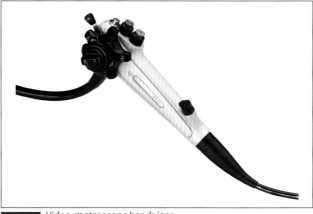

2.4 Video-gastroscope handpiece.
(© Karl Storz SE & Co. KG)

may be operated using either the right hand or the thumb of the left hand. Each deflection control knob also has a locking lever, which may be used to fix the deflection of the tip in any given position. The maximal deflection of a typical gastroscope is in the upward direction, and should be at least 180 degrees. Deflection capabilities in the other three directions (down, left and right) should be at least 90 degrees.

Insufflation, irrigation and suction

Other mechanical functions of a flexible endoscope include insufflation, irrigation and suction. Each of these mechanical functions is activated by touching or depressing one of the valves on the handpiece of the endoscope. Insufflation with either room air or carbon dioxide (CO_2) (see below) is required to expand the viscus and create a space between the distal lens of the endoscope and the mucosa to obtain a clear image. Irrigation is needed to clean the distal lens of the endoscope when mucus, debris or fogging obscures the view. Suction is applied to reduce insufflation as needed and also, in some cases, to remove fluid that may otherwise interfere with visibility. When suctioning fluid, care should be taken to suction from the surface of the liquid 'pool' and avoid suctioning from deep in the pool, which may contain grit or debris that could clog the channel.

Instrument channel

Many types of flexible endoscopes also contain an instrument channel, the proximal opening of which is usually located at the distal end of the handpiece. A variety of instruments, including biopsy forceps, foreign body graspers and cytology brushes, can be placed through this channel until they exit the tip of the endoscope. Care should be taken when passing instruments through the deflected tip of an endoscope (instruments should not be inserted while the endoscope tip is retroflexed), as forceful passage of any instrument could damage the inner lining of the instrument channel. It should be noted that the instrument channel also serves as the suction channel for the endoscope. This means that suction will be significantly reduced or abolished when an instrument is in the channel. This also means that suction will not be effective if the cap of the instrument channel is open.

Insertion tube and umbilical cord

Both the insertion tube and the umbilical cord of a flexible endoscope contain glass light fibre bundles. This is the case for both fibrescopes and video-endoscopes (see below). The light fibre bundle transmits light from the light source to the tip of the endoscope to illuminate the area being examined. The glass fibres are fragile and so the entire shaft of any endoscope should be handled with care, avoiding knocking, crushing or tight coiling. The distal tip of the endoscope should also be carefully protected, as it contains glass lenses and tiny nozzles for the exit of air and water.

The umbilical cord of a gastroscope contains the connector to the light source as well as fittings for insufflation, irrigation and suction. The insufflation and irrigation are both driven by an air pump, which is either integrated into the light source or is a self-contained unit that is connected via a length of tubing. Gastroscopes come with a small plastic bottle that provides the water for irrigation; the water used should always be demineralized or distilled to prevent the channel from becoming clogged with mineral deposits from hard water. A fluid line on the bottle cap connects directly to the water connector on the umbilical cord. A standard hospital suction unit is connected to the suction connector.

On video-endoscopes, a video cable connector is located at the distal end of the umbilical cord for connection to a video processor, which transmits the image to a monitor for viewing.

A pressure compensation valve is also typically found at the distal end of the umbilical cord. This valve is used for leakage testing as well as pressure compensation under high-pressure conditions, such as ethylene oxide gas sterilization. By attaching the pressure compensation cap or a leakage tester to this valve, the inside of the endoscope is opened to the external air. It is therefore critical that neither of these items is attached to the valve when the endoscope is immersed in fluids for cleaning.

Leakage testing

Endoscopes must be watertight in order to prevent damage by fluids leaking into the inner workings, which could corrode deflection cables and/or infiltrate glass fibre bundles, causing staining, brittleness and breakage. It is therefore highly recommended that a leakage test be performed before and after every endoscopic procedure. The leakage tester (Figure 2.5) is attached to the pressure compensation valve and the bulb on the tester is squeezed until the endoscope is pressurized to the appropriate level. The pressure should remain stable if no leaks are present. The cost of repairing a leak identified early is usually much less than for a leak that has been allowed to go undetected for a period of time.

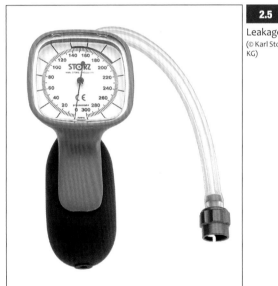

2.5

Leakage tester.
(© Karl Storz SE & Co. KG)

Other considerations

Gastroscopes can also be used for bronchoscopy in patients large enough to accept the diameter of the insertion tube in the respiratory tract (i.e. medium- and large-breed dogs). Sterility of the endoscope is a greater concern in bronchoscopy than it is for GI endoscopy. Any flexible endoscope used for respiratory endoscopy should be sterilized before use. Depending on the manufacturer's recommendations, this may be achieved either with ethylene oxide gas sterilization or by soaking in an approved cold sterilant solution (see below).

Most gastroscopes are in the range of 7.9–10 mm in diameter, and so there is a need for smaller diameter flexible endoscopes to examine the respiratory and urinary tracts of dogs and cats. Smaller diameter (≤5.9 mm) flexible endoscopes (see Figures 2.2 and 2.6) typically deflect in only one plane (i.e. up/down or up only). They also lack the dedicated insufflation and irrigation channels of a gastroscope. However, a small instrument channel is

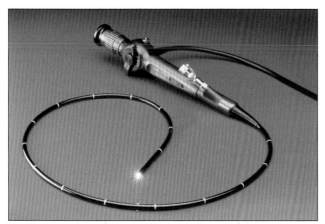

2.6 Fibrescope (5.2 mm in diameter, 85 cm long) with two-way tip deflection.
(© Karl Storz SE & Co. KG)

typically included, which can be used for the passage of instruments, suction, and even irrigation or insufflation when needed.

Video-endoscopes *versus* fibrescopes

Flexible endoscopes can be divided into two categories: fibrescopes and video-endoscopes. Both types of endoscope utilize a glass fibre bundle to transmit light from the light source to the tip of the insertion tube to illuminate the area being examined. However, they use different methods for transmitting the image from the tip of the endoscope to the eyepiece or video monitor.

In a fibrescope, the image is transmitted via a fibre-optic image bundle from the objective lens at the tip of the insertion tube to the ocular lens located in the eyepiece. Transmission of the image to a video monitor requires the attachment of an endoscopic video camera to the eyepiece of the fibrescope (see below).

A video-endoscope has no image fibre bundle and no eyepiece (Figure 2.7). The image is transmitted electronically through wires from a sensor located just behind the objective lens at the tip of the endoscope, along the length of the entire endoscope directly to the video processor, and finally to a display monitor. The sensor at the tip of the insertion tube is a semiconductor or 'chip', analogous to the one found in the camera head of endoscopic video

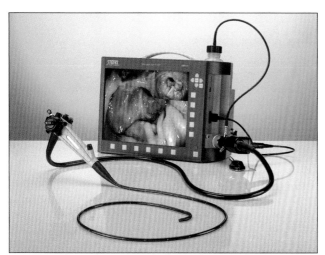

2.7 Video-endoscope attached to an all-in-one video system that includes a video processor, light source, monitor, digital capture system and insufflation/irrigation pump.
(© Karl Storz SE & Co. KG)

cameras that attach to the eyepiece of fibrescopes or rigid endoscopes. For this reason, video-endoscopes are sometimes referred to as 'distal chip' endoscopes or 'chip-in-the-tip' endoscopes.

The quality of the image obtained with a fibrescope is determined by a number of factors, including the number, size, quality and cladding of glass fibres in the image bundle, as well as the optical technology and quality of the lenses at the proximal and distal ends of the image bundle. When the image is displayed on a monitor, other critical factors determining image quality include the level of illumination and the endoscopic video camera and monitor technology.

Fibreoptic images may appear pixelated (i.e. a 'honeycomb' pattern is seen) to a greater or lesser degree, depending on the above-mentioned factors. It should also be noted that over time individual glass fibres in the image bundle will inevitably break, appearing as black spots in the image (Figure 2.8). These individual broken fibres cannot be repaired, and the only option is to replace the entire image bundle of the fibrescope when the image has degraded unacceptably; this typically costs as much as 50% or more of the price of a new endoscope.

Fibrescopes have one significant advantage over video-endoscopes in that they cost appreciably less in the first place; they are approximately half the cost of a video-endoscope. However, the higher cost of a video-endoscope is justified, in many cases, by the better image quality, reduced incidence of repair and longer lifespan of the endoscope compared with a fibrescope.

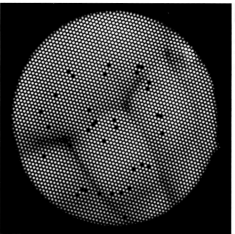

2.8 Fibreoptic image with broken fibres.
(© Karl Storz SE & Co. KG)

Selection

Selecting a flexible endoscope for small animal practice can be a daunting task, given the vast array of models and sizes of endoscope available, both new and used. Given the assumption that any consumer wants to get as much as possible for their money, the following factors are worthy of consideration.

- **Size:** Is the endoscope of an appropriate diameter and length to perform the desired procedures?
- **Optics:** Does the endoscope provide adequate image quality to perform the desired tasks with ease?
- **Dependability:** Does the endoscope supplier provide adequate warranty, service, and equipment loans in the case of instrument failure or lengthy repairs?
- **Ease of use:** Is the endoscope comfortable in the operator's hand and easy to set up, take down, clean and store?

- **Future integration:** Can the endoscope system be upgraded and/or integrated with other types of endoscopic equipment as the practice expands in the future?
- **Cost:** What is the endoscope system likely to cost over the next 5–10 years, including the cost of acquisition and any repairs not covered under warranty?

Size

The most versatile endoscopes for use in small animals are <10 mm in diameter, >125 cm in length and have four-way tip deflection. The small diameter and extended length enables the small animal practitioner to examine a wide range of patients, from cats and puppies to giant-breed dogs. Some veterinary gastroenterologists prefer an endoscope 9 mm or less in diameter and 140 cm in length. Attention should also be paid to the diameter of the instrument channel, which should be at least 2 mm in order to collect diagnostic biopsy samples. Smaller diameter fibre-scopes for respiratory and urinary endoscopy are also available in extended lengths for veterinary use, which is important to reach the bladder of large-breed dogs or the distal portions of the bronchial tree.

Optics

The optical quality of an endoscope is very difficult to judge from the specifications alone. Ideally, an objective and 'blinded' comparison of the endoscopes under consideration should be made side by side in a real patient. In addition to the optical resolution, particular attention should be paid to the illumination or brightness of the endoscopic image, especially when viewed on a video monitor, bearing in mind that brightness will be inversely proportional to the size of the viscus being examined. In other words, an endoscope system may produce a beautiful image of the palm of the operator's hand but be unacceptably dark in the stomach of a dog.

Dependability

In addition to the reputation of the manufacturer, the level of service expected from the vendor is critical. Any new endoscope should include at least a 1-year warranty. Occasional repairs of flexible endoscopes are inevitable. It is advisable to choose a vendor that will provide either reasonable repair turnaround times or loan instruments in the case of extended repairs.

Ease of use

The endoscope should be handled by the potential buyer; the deflection control knobs and focus rings should be turned and instruments should be passed through the channel. A thorough understanding of the set-up and the options for disinfection should also be obtained. For example, an endoscope that can be entirely immersed and gas sterilized may be much more desirable than one that cannot.

Future integration with other equipment

In the author's experience, one endoscope is never enough for the practice that seriously adopts this technology. The components of a system may or may not be compatible with other types of endoscopes. Particular consideration should be given upon initial investment to whether the light source, camera and other devices are compatible with future expansion.

Cost

The overall cost of owning an endoscope may not be directly related to the purchase price. For example, the income-generating potential of the endoscope, which may vary considerably between different models, must be taken into consideration. In addition, the cost of repairs, the longevity of the product and potential integration of the endoscope system with future products should be taken into account. For example, approximately half the cost of a flexible endoscope system lies with the light source and video camera. Ensuring that these items will function optimally with other endoscopes as the practice grows may be a significant factor in determining the overall cost of endoscopy.

There is a seemingly endless supply of used endoscopes available on the market, either online or through second-hand dealers. Most of these endoscopes come from the human medical field.

Buyer beware – there is a reason these endoscopes were retired. The prudent consumer should identify any shortcomings with such endoscopes before making such a purchase. In some cases, a second-hand endoscope in good working order can be purchased at a very reasonable price. In other cases, what appeared to be a good deal can turn out to be money wasted on a product that is unusable, unserviceable or not appropriate for the vast majority of procedures performed by veterinary surgeons.

In addition to noting the points mentioned above, when selecting a used endoscope, the purchaser should conduct a rigorous examination that includes leakage testing, passage of instruments through the channel, judgement of optical quality both through the eyepiece and on a video monitor, assessment of the integrity of the light bundle, deflection of the tip and examination of the rubber covering the bending section of the endoscope. If at all possible, a minimum 30-day money back guarantee should be negotiated with the vendor of a second-hand endoscope, which would allow time for several trials in patients.

While purchasing a new endoscope direct from the manufacturer requires more money up front than purchasing a second-hand endoscope, it may cost less in the long term. The value of product quality, full warranty, serviceability, veterinary-specific design and the relationship between buyer and seller should not be underestimated. Just as the veterinary profession needs medical instrument manufacturers to develop products specifically suited to veterinary medicine and surgery, the manufacturers need veterinary surgeons to invest in their products in order to fuel their development. Only through such collaboration will the veterinary profession be able to benefit, as medical doctors do, from highly advanced and cost-effective technology specifically suited to their patients.

Instrumentation

A wide variety of reusable and disposable instruments (Figure 2.9) is available for passing down the channel of flexible endoscopes. Some of those commonly used in veterinary practice include:

- Biopsy forceps
- Foreign body graspers
- Cytology brushes
- Bronchoalveolar lavage tubing
- Stone retrieval baskets (also used for foreign bodies)
- Polypectomy snares (also used for foreign bodies).

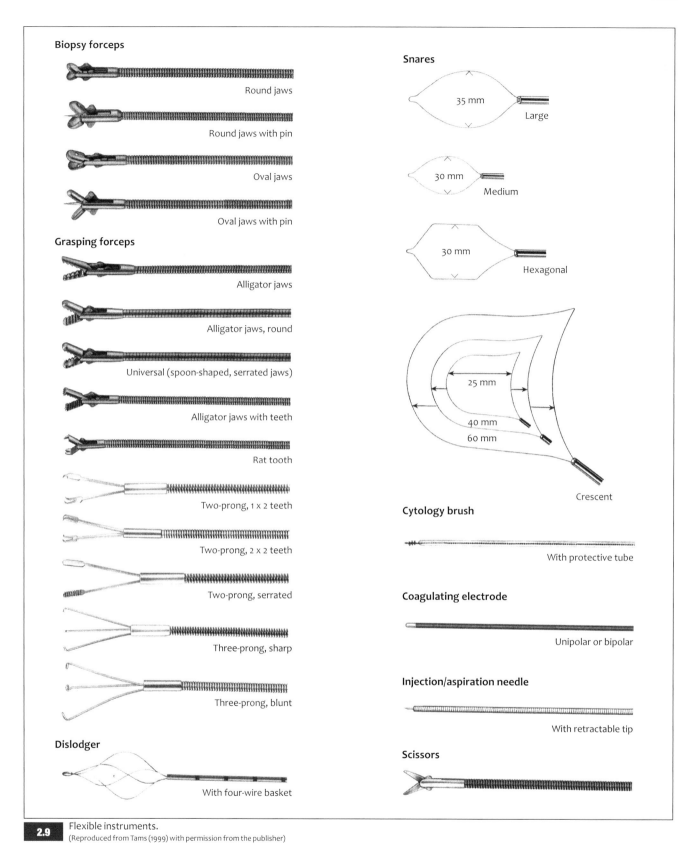

2.9 Flexible instruments.
(Reproduced from Tams (1999) with permission from the publisher)

Although reusable instruments cost more, they tend to last longer than disposable instruments and are designed for cleaning and multiple uses. After thorough cleaning, it is recommended that flexible instruments be oiled or soaked in instrument milk (a type of lubricant) to keep them well lubricated and functioning properly. Disposable instruments should be considered if they must remain sharp for optimal function, as in the case of biopsy forceps.

It is critical that the instruments selected are of an appropriate diameter and style for the endoscope being used. Instruments should always be passed carefully through the channel, in a closed position, and *never* forced against any resistance. If positioning an instrument for its use requires deflection of the endoscope tip, it is always best to pass the forceps through the *undeflected* tip until the instrument can be seen in the field of view, before deflecting the tip by using the control knobs. Tears of the instrument channel due to aggressive passage of instruments or the use of inappropriate instrumentation are among the most common causes of damage to flexible endoscopes.

Rigid endoscopes

Like flexible endoscopes, rigid endoscopes come in a variety of sizes (Figure 2.10), making them useful for a number of minimally invasive diagnostic and surgical procedures. Rigid endoscopes are simpler and less expensive than flexible endoscopes, and can last a lifetime if they are not dropped or knocked. Although they cannot manoeuvre around corners through a tubular structure as flexible endoscopes can, rigid endoscopes offer unsurpassed optics, and their rigidity allows them to be more easily manoeuvred inside non-tubular structures, such as the abdomen, thorax, urinary bladder and joints. Rigid endoscopes are therefore preferred for laparoscopy, thoracoscopy and arthroscopy, and for cystoscopy in female animals. They are also commonly used for otoscopy and rhinoscopy. For some veterinary surgeons they are the endoscope of choice for oesophagogastroscopy, tracheobronchoscopy and colonoscopy.

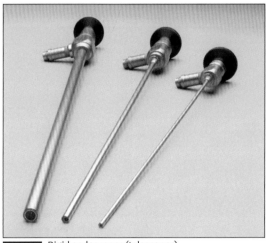

2.10 Rigid endoscopes (telescopes).
(© Karl Storz SE & Co. KG)

Structure

The highest quality rigid endoscopes are actually telescopes, consisting of a series of rod lenses arranged in a specific linear sequence to maximize light transmission, magnification and resolution. Figure 2.11 shows the HOPKINS® rod-lens system in comparison with a traditional optical system. Rod-lens telescopes are capable of transmitting considerably more light and producing a wider field of view than traditional telescopes. Surrounding the tube of lenses are numerous glass fibres, much like those found in a flexible endoscope, which transmit light from the light post of the telescope to its distal tip, where the subject is illuminated. One end of a fibreoptic light cable is connected to the light post of the telescope and the other end is connected to a remote light source. The image produced by a rigid endoscope can be viewed directly at the eyepiece of the endoscope or transmitted to a display monitor by attaching an endoscopic video camera to the eyepiece.

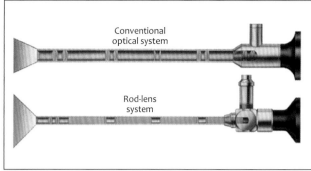

2.11 The HOPKINS® rod-lens system and a conventional optical system.
(© Karl Storz SE & Co. KG)

Since rigid endoscopes contain glass lenses and glass fibres, it is important to handle them with care. Knocking or dropping them could cause damage to the lenses or fibres, reducing the image quality and/or light transmission. A damaged rigid endoscope may contain one or more dislodged or cracked lenses, which do not completely obscure the image but reduce its quality.

Rigid endoscopes are available in a variety of viewing angles. The viewing angles of the telescopes most commonly used in veterinary practice are 0 and 30 degrees (Figure 2.12). A 0-degree or forward-viewing telescope has a field of view aligned with the long axis of the telescope. A telescope with a 30-degree viewing angle has a field of view where the centre is offset by 30 degrees from the axis of the telescope. Acute viewing angles enable the operator to visualize a greater area simply by rotating the telescope on its long axis. Although telescopes with larger angles of view enable examination of a wider area, they present a challenge to the novice endoscopist with regard to spatial orientation, particularly when using instrumentation through additional ports, such as during laparoscopic or arthroscopic surgery.

Most rigid endoscopes are relatively simple in structure (see Figure 2.10) and designed to be used with various sheaths or cannulae. However, some telescopes are more specialized and contain an integrated working channel (Figure 2.13). A telescope with an integrated channel may be more convenient for a dedicated purpose and less susceptible to damage than a telescope with individual sheaths. The advantages of these specialized designs

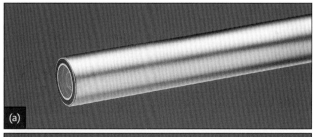

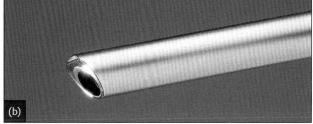

2.12 Telescope viewing angles. (a) 0 degrees. (b) 30 degrees.
(© Karl Storz SE & Co. KG)

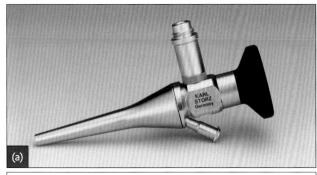

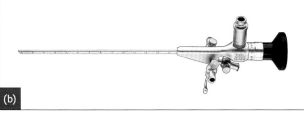

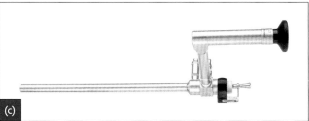

2.13 Rigid endoscopes with integrated working channels.
(a) Rod-lens otoscope (5 mm diameter with a 5 Fr integrated channel). (b) Cystoscope/rhinoscope (9.5 Fr diameter with a 3 Fr integrated channel). (c) Operating laparoscope (10 mm diameter with a 5 mm integrated channel).
(© Karl Storz SE & Co. KG)

must be weighed against the loss of versatility inherent in such a design.

The optical quality of rigid endoscopes varies greatly and is dependent upon the optical design and quality of lenses used in the manufacturing process. Telescopes also vary in terms of durability and their ability to be immersed, gas sterilized and autoclaved. Finally, it should be remembered that one manufacturer's rigid telescope will not necessarily be compatible with another manufacturer's light cable, video camera or sheath system.

A subclass of rigid endoscopes at the lower end of the size spectrum (<2 mm in diameter) is the semi-rigid endoscope (Figure 2.14). Rather than the rod-lens optical system of larger diameter telescopes, these fine-diameter semi-rigid endoscopes contain a fused silica bundle. Semi-rigid endoscopes are useful for examining anatomical areas that cannot be accessed with rod-lens telescopes or fibrescopes, such as the trachea of small birds and the urethra of male cats. They are also used by veterinary surgeons who wish to take a 'quick look' into a joint with the patient sedated but not under anaesthesia.

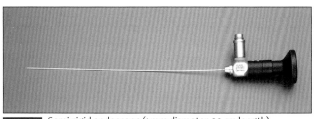

2.14 Semi-rigid endoscope (1 mm diameter, 20 cm length).
(© Karl Storz SE & Co. KG)

Selection

The dizzying array of rigid endoscopes available in the marketplace can be even more confusing than the choice of flexible endoscopes. The most versatile endoscope for small animal practice is the Multi-Purpose Rigid™ endoscope (Figure 2.15a). With a diameter of 2.7 mm, a working length of 18 cm and a 30-degree viewing angle, this endoscope is ideal for rhinoscopy, cystoscopy, otoscopy (in anaesthetized patients) and endoscopy of small exotic animals (coelioscopy and oral cavity examinations). It is also commonly used for arthroscopy in dogs, intubation in rabbits and laparoscopy (Figure 2.15b) or thoracoscopy in small mammals, kittens and puppies.

When seeking to identify the best size of endoscope for a given medical or surgical procedure, the following should be borne in mind:

- Larger diameter endoscopes produce larger images and transmit more light
- Smaller diameter endoscopes fit into smaller places but transmit less light
- Longer endoscopes will reach further, but excessive length increases the risk of breakage
- Specific sheaths and cannulae are required for most rigid endoscopic procedures and must fit properly in order to perform the desired examination or surgery with ease, and without causing damage to the telescope or injuring the patient.

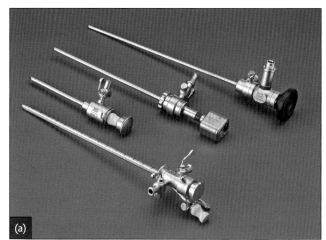

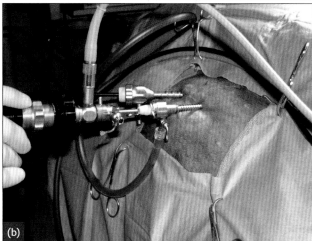

2.15 Multi-Purpose Rigid™ (MPR) endoscope. (a) Top to bottom: the MPR endoscope in an examination and protection sheath, an arthroscopy sheath, a laparoscopy trocar and an operating sheath.
(b) Laparoscopic ovariectomy in a puppy using the MPR endoscope.
(© Karl Storz SE & Co. KG)

The second most popular size of rigid endoscope (Figure 2.16) for small animal use is a 5 mm diameter, 0-degree laparoscope, typically with a working length of 33 cm. This telescope size is ideal for both laparoscopy and thoracoscopy in small animals. It is also the standard laparoscope used in many human surgical procedures, and therefore a wide range of ancillary instrumentation is available. Since most laparoscopic hand instruments are also 5 mm in diameter, this means that the telescope and instruments can be passed through the same cannula, without the need for reducers or different-sized cannulae.

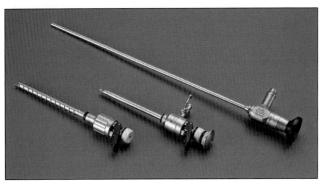

2.16 Laparoscope (5.0 mm diameter) (right) with a standard trocar/cannula (middle) and an ENDOTIP cannula (left).
(© Karl Storz SE & Co. KG)

Many other sizes of rigid and semi-rigid endoscopes are available and useful for small animal practice. For example, a short 1.9 mm or 2.4 mm diameter telescope (Figure 2.17a) is commonly used for arthroscopy in dogs. An extended-length 3.5 mm or 4 mm diameter cystoscope (Figure 2.17b) is commonly used for uroendoscopy in larger bitches, as well as transcervical endoscopic insemination. Long, narrow rigid endoscopes (Figure 2.17c) are used for obtaining biopsy samples and retrieving foreign bodies from the trachea, oesophagus and stomach. A 7 mm or 10 mm diameter telescope can also be used for laparoscopy and thoracoscopy (see Chapters 9 to 14 for recommendations of endoscope size for each organ system).

In addition to the critical factor of size in the choice of the appropriate rigid endoscope, the recommendations for the selection of a flexible endoscope described above also apply to rigid endoscopes. Of particular importance with rigid endoscopes is the need for compatibility with appropriate sheath systems, cannulae, and connections to light sources and video cameras.

When selecting a second-hand rigid endoscope, particular attention should be paid to the optical quality and light transmission. A simple inspection of light transmission can be performed by pointing the light post towards a window or light and examining the distal tip of the endoscope for black or grey areas in the light fibre transmission zone, which indicate broken fibres. Better still, the endoscope can be connected to the light source that will be used and the tip placed inside a dark container of similar size to that of the body cavity to be examined. If a video camera is to be used, it should be borne in mind that this may require considerably more light than viewing directly through the eyepiece.

The shaft of the telescope and its distal tip should be carefully inspected for any dents, cracks or other external damage that would be likely to cause damage to the optical system and thus affect image quality. An endoscope is only as good as the picture it can produce.

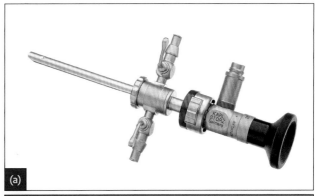

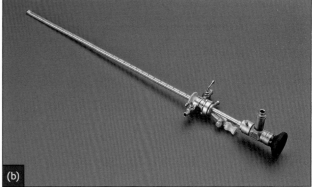

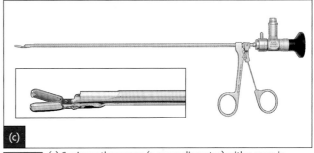

2.17 (a) Canine arthroscope (2.4 mm diameter) with a snap-in sheath with two stopcocks. (b) Extended-length cystoscope (17 Fr outer diameter, 29 cm working length). (c) Rigid endoscope (2.9 mm diameter, 36 cm length) with optical grasping forceps.
(© Karl Storz SE & Co. KG)

Instrumentation

A variety of ancillary instrumentation is required to perform rigid endoscopic procedures. In most cases, some sort of sheath or cannula is required to gain access to the anatomical region to be examined.

- The term 'sheath' usually refers to a tube that locks on to the telescope, providing not only anatomical access but also access for the passage of instrumentation, fluids or gas as needed for the given procedure.
- The term 'cannula' usually refers to a tube through which rigid endoscopes or instruments are placed and are freely movable within the cannula rather than being locked in place.

Sheaths

Operating sheaths serve a variety of functions. They protect the telescope, facilitate the ingress and egress of fluids via the side ports and allow the passage of flexible instruments (Figure 2.18) through the channel; the instrument comes into view as its tip exits the distal end of the sheath. This type of telescope and sheath system is

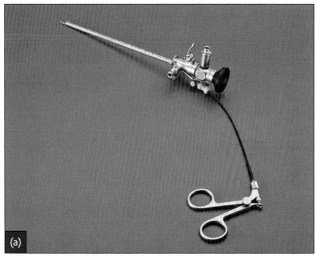

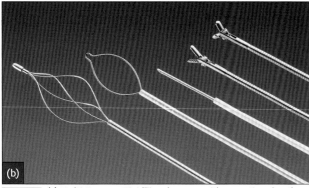

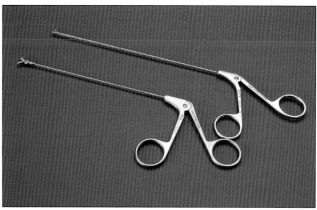

2.20 Biopsy forceps for use alongside a telescope.
(© Karl Storz SE & Co. KG)

2.18 (a) Multi-Purpose Rigid™ endoscope with operating sheath and biopsy forceps. (b) Tips of a variety of 5 Fr flexible instruments.
(© Karl Storz SE & Co. KG)

commonly used for cystoscopy, rhinoscopy and otoscopy. The same system is used without irrigation fluids for coelioscopic examination of small birds and reptiles.

Arthroscope sheaths (see Figures 2.15a and 2.17a) have no instrument channel but serve to protect the telescope and provide ingress of fluid around the telescope to distend the joint during arthroscopy. Arthroscope sheaths are also often used in rhinoscopy, cystoscopy and otoscopy, when the total diameter of an operating sheath is too large for the opening (Figure 2.19), for example, in a small cat's nose or urethra. When a biopsy sample is acquired via an arthroscope sheath, small rigid forceps (Figure 2.20) are used alongside the telescope. The use of a small-diameter telescope without a sheath should be avoided because the sheath protects the fragile telescope and provides a means for fluid ingress, which helps to maintain a clear field of view.

Since arthroscopy requires a small incision into the joint cavity, an arthroscope sheath system has optional sharp and blunt obturators (see Figure 2.17a), which can be used for initial creation of the portal. Once access to the joint is successfully achieved, the obturator is removed from the sheath and replaced by the arthroscope. Fluid egress and the insertion of operating instruments during arthroscopy requires accessory instruments to be placed through additional portals (for more information see Chapter 14).

Cannulae

A conventional laparoscopy trocar and cannula are shown in Figure 2.21. The trocar has a pyramidal tip with cutting edges, which facilitates piercing of the body wall to provide a port for the laparoscope and rigid instrumentation. The Luer lock valve is used for the attachment of insufflation tubing to establish a pneumoperitoneum during laparoscopy. The cannula contains an automatic valve, which snaps shut when an instrument or telescope is not in place, thus maintaining insufflation. A rubber washer provides a tight seal around the telescope or instrument when it is placed through the cannula (Figure 2.22).

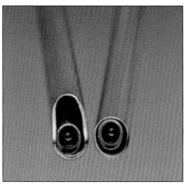

2.19 Multi-Purpose Rigid™ endoscopes (2.7 mm diameter) in an operating sheath (left) and an arthroscope sheath (right).
(© Karl Storz SE & Co. KG)

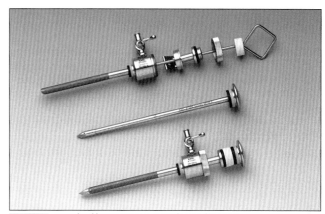

2.21 Standard laparoscopy cannulae and trocars.
(© Karl Storz SE & Co. KG)

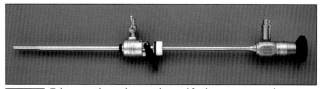

2.22 Telescope through cannula used for laparoscopy and thoracoscopy.
(© Karl Storz SE & Co. KG)

An ENDOTIP cannula (Figure 2.23) requires no trocar. Instead, the cannula is surgically placed by making a small stab incision through the body wall, placing the tip of the cannula in the incision and inserting the cannula with a twisting 'corkscrew'-like motion. By eliminating the need for a sharp trocar, these cannulae minimize the risk of inadvertent laceration of intra-abdominal organs.

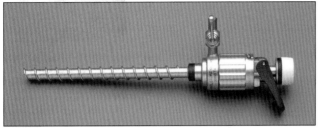

2.23 The ENDOTIP cannula requires no trocar for entry.
(© Karl Storz SE & Co. KG)

Single-incision ports

Inspired by the desire for ever-improving cosmesis in human surgery, manufacturers have developed several different styles of laparoscopy ports that accommodate the telescope as well as a number of instruments (Figure 2.24), such that only a single port is required to complete certain surgical interventions. While the concept of triangulation of instrumentation is certainly challenged with these devices, many veterinary surgeons experienced in minimally invasive surgery have moved to use these devices and find them to be faster and simpler to use than multiple traditional trocars. They are not, however, recommended for the novice laparoscopist.

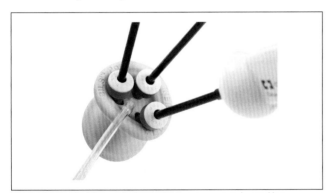

2.24 The SILS™ port is the device most commonly used by veterinary surgeons for single-port access.

Other instruments

Various styles of rigid instruments for laparoscopy and thoracoscopy are available in varying lengths and diameters (Figure 2.25a). The instruments most commonly used in small animal laparoscopy and thoracoscopy are palpation probes, grasping forceps and biopsy forceps (Figure 2.25b). As the surgeon becomes more skilled with endoscopic procedures, more advanced interventions can be performed, requiring more sophisticated instrumentation, such as retractors (Figure 2.26), vessel sealers, staplers and clips.

Ultrasonic dissectors and vessel-sealing devices (Figure 2.27) are very convenient to have. They improve the efficiency and safety of laparoscopic surgery because a single instrument coagulates and effectively transects vascular tissue. This is particularly useful in the most commonly performed surgery in small animals – ovariectomy or ovariohysterectomy – but has also been used successfully for

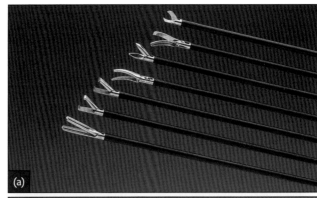

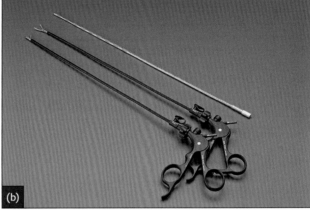

2.25 Rigid instruments used for laparoscopy and thoracoscopy. (a) A variety of 5 mm laparoscopy instruments with different tips. (b) Laparoscopic palpation probe, grasping forceps and biopsy forceps.
(© Karl Storz SE & Co. KG)

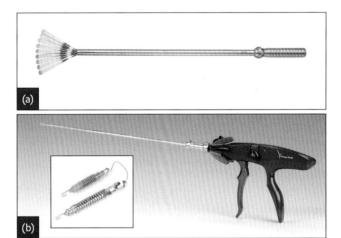

2.26 (a) A simple fan retractor used for holding tissue through a dedicated cannula. (b) The EndoGrab™ device facilitates retraction of organs without the need for additional ports.
(a, © Karl Storz SE & Co. KG; b, © STI Virtual Ports, Israel)

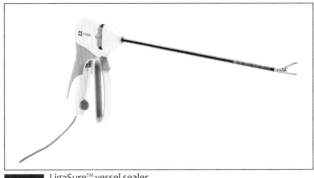

2.27 LigaSure™ vessel sealer.

splenectomy, nephrectomy, adrenalectomy and pericardiectomy. True vessel sealers and ultrasonic instruments are generally able to seal larger vessels (5–7 mm) than basic bipolar reusable instruments, but the latter have proven very dependable for small vessels (2–3 mm) and have the added advantage of generating minimal heat, and therefore very little lateral thermal spread, compared with bipolar vessel-sealing devices. Whether using an advanced bipolar device or an ultrasonic device, the reduced need to exchange instruments is a significant time saver for most surgeries.

Haemostasis can also be achieved with staples or clips, for which applicators are designed to fire rows of staples or individual clips, as needed. The laparoscopic stapling device most commonly used in veterinary surgery is the Endo Gia™ stapler, which is available in three lengths (30, 45 and 60 mm) with four staple sizes (2.0, 2.5, 3.5 and 4.8 mm). This device is ideal for procedures such as lung lobectomy: the disposable cartridges fire six staggered rows of staples and then cut in between, leaving three rows of staples on each side of the cut.

Clips are typically applied individually and are most commonly used to occlude the cystic duct during cholecystectomy, or to occlude the thoracic duct for the treatment of chylothorax (Figure 2.28). Commonly used clip appliers include the Endo Clip™ (Medtronic), LIGACLIP® (Ethicon) and M/L-10 (Microline Surgical).

Many rigid and flexible instruments, as well as trocars and cannulae, are available in both reusable and disposable forms. Although disposable instruments are designed and recommended for single use only, and therefore are not easily cleaned and sterilized, many of these instruments can be reused several times as long as sterility, lubrication and sharpness can be maintained. Reusable instrumentation is designed for longevity and repeated cleaning and sterilization, and therefore comes at a higher price than disposable instruments. It is important to determine which type of instruments will be more convenient and cost-effective in the long term.

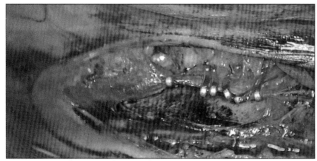

2.28 Six clips placed on the thoracic duct.
(© Dr Ameet Singh, University of Guelph)

The endoscope system

In addition to the endoscope and instruments, a complete endoscope system includes other devices such as:

- A light source
- A video camera and monitor
- A suction pump
- A digital documentation/storage device
- An insufflation pump (for gastrointestinal endoscopy; also drives irrigation of the gastroscope)
- Other optional devices, e.g. electrosurgical generators, arthroscopic shavers and irrigation pumps.

The most basic endoscope system must include a light source and fibreoptic light-transmitting cable (Figure 2.29) to deliver light through the endoscope and illuminate the site of examination. Depending on the particular endoscopic procedure and the model of endoscope being used, a video camera and monitor may or may not be necessary. However, in most cases a video camera system is highly desirable, as the image seen on a monitor is much larger than that seen through the eyepiece of an endoscope, and it is more comfortable for the endoscopist to accomplish the procedure while viewing a monitor rather than peering through the eyepiece (which may require the endoscopist to adopt an uncomfortable position). Furthermore, video imaging allows other members of the endoscopy team to view the procedure and also makes it possible to capture and store still images or video footage.

The final image produced on a display monitor originates at the endoscope tip, and its quality is dependent upon the optics of the endoscope, the power and colour temperature of the light source, the electronics and resolution of the endo-video camera and, finally, the quality of the monitor itself. Each of these devices is one part of the entire video chain (Figure 2.30). In order for a video system to function at its maximum potential, each item in the chain must be functioning properly. The quality of the final image viewed on the monitor can only be as good as the weakest link in the chain.

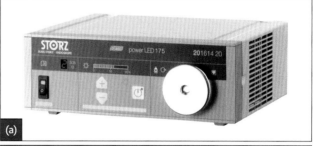

(a)

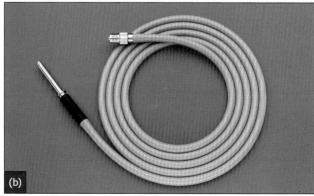

(b)

2.29 (a) LED light source. (b) Fibreoptic light-transmitting cable.
(© Karl Storz SE & Co. KG)

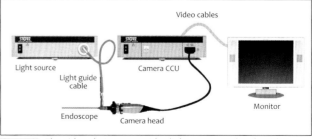

2.30 The video chain starts with a light source and ends with a video monitor.
(© Karl Storz SE & Co. KG)

Light sources

Light sources are available in several technology types, styles and wattages. The amount of light required for a given procedure depends upon a number of factors:

- The size of the cavity to be illuminated
- The type of endoscope being used
- The light sensitivity of the endo-video camera
- The condition and length of the light-transmitting cable.

The most common types of light source technology now used in endoscope light sources are LED and xenon. For decades, xenon has been the gold standard in endoscope systems. However, thanks to their small size, long lifespan and low energy consumption, LED sources are rapidly gaining favour as their illumination is almost comparable to xenon lamps and are they cheaper.

When comparing the output of light from sources of different technology types, simply comparing the wattages is not sufficient. Light output is measured in lumens, whereas electricity usage is measured in watts. The key specification indicating brightness is the total lumens produced by a given light source, rather than the wattage of the source. The foolproof test of light output is, of course, a procedure with a live patient.

Most light sources are fitted with an intensity adjustment control knob, and some include an integrated insufflation pump that may be used to drive the insufflation and irrigation functions of a gastroscope. When using higher quality endo-video cameras with an auto-exposure feature, manual adjustment of the light intensity is not critical, as the camera will automatically illuminate the subject properly, as long as enough light is provided by the source.

The light connector of a gastroscope is typically quite different from that of a simple rigid endoscope light cable (see Figure 2.29); hence, the gastroscope connector in a light source designed for that purpose must accommodate the inlet pipe for air that drives insufflation and irrigation (Figure 2.31).

As well as the technology type and versatility, the portability of a light source (Figure 2.32) might be important to practitioners for some situations, such as use in an examination room, mobile practice or emergencies.

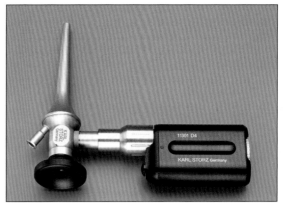

2.32 Hand-held light source attached to a rod-lens otoscope.
(© Karl Storz SE & Co. KG)

Pumps and insufflators

Various types of pumps and insufflators are available to aid in endoscopic imaging or therapeutic processes. It is very important to be aware of the different uses of room air and CO_2 for insufflation. Insufflation of the upper or lower GI tract during endoscopy is achieved using room air. The air pump may be integrated into the light source or contained within a stand-alone unit (Figure 2.33). Air distension of the viscus during GI endoscopy is controlled manually by depressing a valve on the gastroscope handpiece.

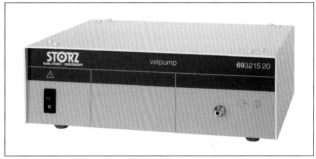

2.33 Air pump designed for insufflation during gastrointestinal endoscopy.
(© Karl Storz SE & Co. KG)

The insufflation required during laparoscopy is typically CO_2 (see also Chapters 8 and 12). The choice of CO_2 rather than room air eliminates the possibility of air embolism formation, which could, in rare instances, be fatal to the patient. An insufflator for laparoscopy (Figure 2.34) is a much more sophisticated and sensitive device than the air pump used in gastroscopy. This is because it must automatically regulate the gas flow and pressure in order

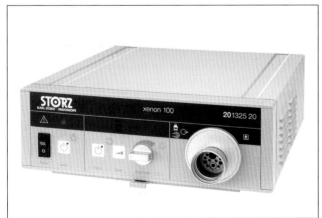

2.31 Light source with a built-in air pump and a connector for a gastroscope.
(© Karl Storz SE & Co. KG)

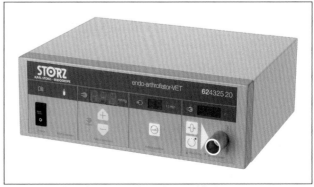

2.34 Carbon dioxide insufflator designed for laparoscopy.
(© Karl Storz SE & Co. KG)

to maintain appropriate pneumoperitoneum, while not exceeding values that could compromise venous return or ventilation of the patient. The source of gas is a pressurized tank of CO_2, which is regulated by the insufflator and connected to it by a high-pressure hose. The gas is then delivered to the patient via sterile tubing, which connects the outlet of the insufflator to a Veress needle or the Luer lock connector on a laparoscopy cannula.

A Veress needle (Figure 2.35) (or a modified Hasson (paediatric) technique; see Chapter 8) is used for initial insufflation of the patient, before the placement of any trocars, telescopes or instruments. The needle consists of a sharp outer cannula and a blunt hollow spring-loaded inner stylet, through which the gas passes.

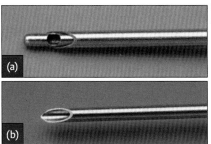

2.35 Veress needle. (a) The blunt hollow stylet protrudes through the sharp outer needle. (b) Sharp outer needle with the spring-loaded stylet retracted.
(© Karl Storz SE & Co. KG)

Pump systems for irrigation and suction are useful for a variety of endoscopic procedures, including otoscopy, laparoscopy and thoracoscopy. Lavage of the external or middle ear, abdomen or thorax under endoscopic guidance is a relatively new concept in veterinary medicine. The therapeutic value of powerful yet precise flushing and suctioning of contaminated or inflamed cavities is considerable. A versatile pump system (Figure 2.36) can be used for these procedures, as well as for insufflation, irrigation and suction in the GI tract in the course of endoscopic procedures.

Fluid pumps designed for arthroscopy (Figure 2.37) are also available and represent an advanced method of joint distension that allows accurate and rapid adjustment of flow rates and pressures. Joint distension can also be achieved by the gravitational flow of fluids hung above the level of the patient, or by inserting a fluid bag into a pressurized cuff (see also Chapter 14).

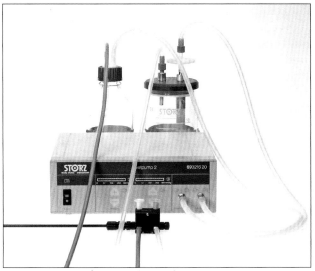

2.36 VETPUMP®2 suitable for insufflation, irrigation and suction.
(© Karl Storz SE & Co. KG)

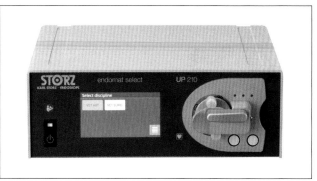

2.37 A fluid pump designed for arthroscopy regulates the flow rate and pressure of sterile fluids used to distend the joint space.
(© Karl Storz SE & Co. KG)

Video imaging systems

Although endoscopic images can be viewed directly through the eyepiece of a fibrescope or rigid telescope, most endoscopy systems now include a video camera or processor capable of transmitting the image to a display monitor. Not only does this capability make performing endoscopic procedures much more comfortable for the surgeon, it also enables all members of the team to view the procedure, and allows documentation of the findings with video clips or still images.

A basic endoscopic video system consists of a camera head with integrated cable, a camera control unit (CCU) or processor, and a video monitor (Figure 2.38a). The camera head contains a coupler, which attaches to the eyepiece of a flexible or rigid endoscope (Figure 2.38bc). The camera head itself contains an objective lens, a prism assembly and either one or three sensors. The sensor is responsible for sensing the image and converting it to a digital image and is one of two types, either a CCD (charge-coupled device) or CMOS (complementary metal oxide semiconductor). In three-chip cameras, each of the three primary colours (red, green and blue) is transmitted separately. Historically, this has resulted in more accurate colour reproduction and higher resolution than with single-chip cameras. However, single-chip cameras have improved dramatically in recent years, and are now even capable of producing high-definition (HD) images. Therefore, the broad categories of single-chip *versus* three-chip cameras are giving way to standard definition *versus* HD and even ultra-high definition (UHD), also known as 4K. This new generation of cameras represents a further step in terms of resolution, depth perception and colour contrast. In addition, the HD and 4K formats offer a 16:9 aspect ratio, giving the surgeon a wider lateral view than the 4:3 aspect ratio of standard definition cameras.

Modern high-quality single-chip cameras can produce perfectly acceptable results for endoscopic diagnosis and surgery. Camera heads should be lightweight, small, and easy to clean and sterilize. Some are soakable, gas sterilizable and even autoclavable. If the camera head is needed for surgery but cannot be sterilized in a timely manner, a disposable sterile camera sleeve may be used.

The endoscopic image is transmitted from the sensor in the camera head, along a series of wires in the cable, to a CCU or processor. Here, the video signal is processed for display on the monitor as well as for transfer to digital recording devices. Some newer CCUs are capable of connecting to video-endoscopes as well as endoscopic camera heads. These models eliminate the need for two different CCUs.

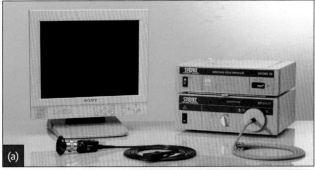

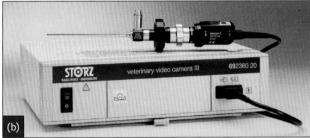

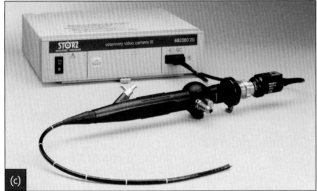

2.38 Endo-video cameras. (a) Clockwise from lower left: camera head, video monitor, camera control unit, xenon light source with fibreoptic cable. (b) Endo-video camera attached to a rigid endoscope. (c) Endo-video camera attached to a fibrescope.
(© Karl Storz SE & Co. KG)

Modern endoscopic video cameras may contain a wide variety of features, which are controllable via buttons either on the camera head or on the CCU. Some of the most useful features are white balance, freeze frame, zoom, gain, contrast enhancement and control of peripheral recording devices.

The video monitor displays the endoscopic image and is connected via a cable, either directly from the camera processor or from any number of various recording devices that may be placed between the camera processor and the monitor. The video chain should always terminate with the monitor. The resolution of the monitor must be properly matched to that of the camera head in order to take full advantage of the image quality capabilities of an endoscopic video camera; attaching a low-resolution consumer-grade monitor to a high-quality endoscopic video camera will not yield the best results. High-quality single-chip cameras typically produce about 450 lines of horizontal resolution, three-chip cameras 750 lines, HD cameras 1080 lines and 4K UHD cameras 2160 lines. It is important to note that the ultimate quality of the image produced by a camera is determined not only by pixel quantity (i.e. the number of lines of resolution) but also by pixel quality, which can vary substantially and contribute to light sensitivity, noise (random variation of brightness or colour, which reduces the quality of the viewed image),

and so on. It is therefore advisable to seek out a manufacturer with a reputation for good quality and, ideally, to view the image produced by a given camera before deciding to purchase it.

Digital capture and data storage

In the digital age, video printers and VHS recorders have been largely replaced by digital capture devices, which facilitate the capture, storage and archiving of still images and video footage on to a variety of digital media, including CDs, DVDs, flash drives (e.g. USB storage devices) and computer hard drives. The stored images can then be printed whenever a hard copy is needed, without concern for the deterioration of image quality over time. An advanced image and data archiving (AIDA®) system (Figure 2.39a) with a touch screen is also available, which enables the endoscopist or an assistant to capture digital still images and start or stop digital video sequences during an endoscopic procedure by simply tapping an icon. Other devices, such as the TELE PACK® (Figure 2.39b), combine a light source, air pump, camera processor, monitor, character generator (to enter patient data) and still image capture system into one compact unit. The images can be captured on to any of a number of approved USB storage devices.

Digital capture and storage of images has several advantages compared with hard copy prints and videotape:

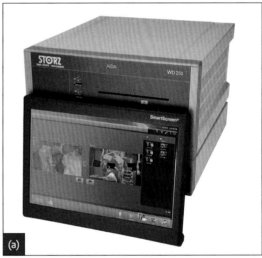

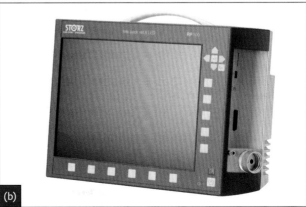

2.39 Digital image capture devices. (a) The AIDA® (advanced image and data archiving) system. (b) The TELE PACK® compact portable endoscopy system includes a camera, light source, keyboard, digital capture system and integrated flatscreen monitor.
(© Karl Storz SE & Co. KG)

- The storage devices take up less physical space
- There is no degradation of image quality over time
- Images and videos can easily be transmitted by email to colleagues
- It is easy and cost-effective to produce duplicates for colleagues, medical records or clients.

Energy sources

As veterinary surgeons move beyond diagnostic endoscopy into minimally invasive surgical procedures, there is an increasing need for energy sources that attach to hand instruments (both rigid and flexible) to provide haemostasis, cutting and other desired functions, such as lithotripsy in cystoscopy and tissue debridement or capsular shrinkage in arthroscopy. Electrosurgery units continue to be the standard in veterinary practice, although lasers and ultrasonic cutting and coagulation devices are gaining popularity (see Chapter 16).

Electrosurgical units (Figure 2.40) operate in either a monopolar or a bipolar mode. Insulated instruments designed for either monopolar or bipolar use are available. Monopolar settings generate a current that runs from the instrument tip to the target tissue, and through the body of the patient to a return electrode. Care must be taken to avoid lateral thermal damage to the tissues. Bipolar settings provide more discrete intraoperative haemorrhage control, require significantly less electrical voltage and current, and do not require a return electrode since the current is passed between the two electrodes located at the tip of the bipolar instrument (see also Chapter 8 for more details of monopolar and bipolar electrosurgical devices).

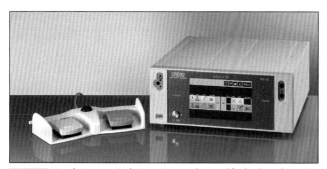

2.40 An electrosurgical generator can be used for both endoscopic and open surgery.
(© Karl Storz SE & Co. KG)

Care must be taken to apply the appropriate amount of electrical energy to provide adequate haemorrhage control, while preventing tissue damage resulting from carbonization. A bipolar device that is popular among veterinary surgeons, and which addresses these concerns, is the LigaSure™ vessel-sealing device (Figure 2.41). With this device, the electrical energy applied and its duration of application are determined by virtue of 'smart technology' within the generator, which produces an audible signal when appropriate vessel sealing has been achieved.

Electrosurgery is particularly advantageous for the more complex abdominal and thoracic surgeries that are now being performed via laparoscopy and thoracoscopy. By reducing the need to exchange instruments or introduce suture material, a single instrument capable of both coagulation and cutting, such as the LigaSure™ or ROBI® plus (Figure 2.42), can significantly reduce surgical time.

When choosing a unit for electrosurgery or laser surgery, attention should be paid to whether the instrumentation will be used in a fluid or gas medium, because

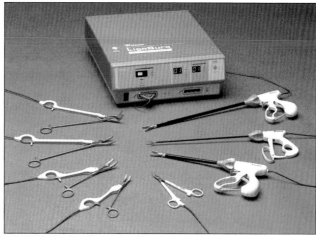

2.41 LigaSure™ vessel-sealing device,

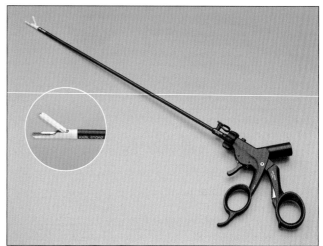

2.42 ROBI® plus: a reusable, easily sterilized bipolar cutting and coagulation instrument. Only the blade needs to be replaced when dull.
(© Karl Storz SE & Co. KG)

certain devices and instrument tips are designed to be effective in different media. In most cases, a single unit may be useful for both endoscopic and open surgery.

Power shavers

Power shavers are used in arthroscopy for the rapid debridement of tissues within the elbow, shoulder and stifle joints (see Chapter 14). The system consists of an electronic control box, a handpiece and a variety of tips, including blades and burrs (Figure 2.43). The handpiece connects to the control box and also has a connector for suction tubing, through which debrided material is removed along with irrigation fluids, which are continually replaced through the arthroscope cannula ingress.

One of the primary indications for a power shaver in canine arthroscopy is debridement of the fat pad in the stifle joint to improve visibility; an aggressive cutting blade is most useful for this purpose. Burrs are used for debridement of bone. Blades and burrs are available in a variety of sizes and styles, in both reusable and disposable designs. Each instrument consists of two parts: a rotating inner cutting blade or burr, and a hollow outer cannula. The most useful sizes for canine arthroscopy are in the range of 2.0–4.0 mm.

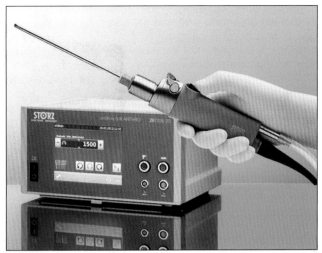

2.43 Arthroscopic power shaver system with handpiece and blade.
(© Karl Storz SE & Co. KG)

The endoscopy team and theatre set-up

The successful establishment of an efficient and cost-effective endoscopy service requires a dedicated team that is thoroughly familiar with equipment set-up, procedures and troubleshooting. Since a substantial financial investment is required when starting to use endoscopy in the practice, it is recommended that only a limited number of well trained staff are authorized to use and handle the instrumentation. One of the best sources of information regarding equipment care and set-up is a knowledgeable vendor who is experienced in all aspects of the care and use of endoscopy instrumentation.

During each endoscopic procedure it is advisable to have a veterinary nurse or surgeon dedicated to anaesthesia, so that the endoscopist is free to focus on the procedure itself. Although many diagnostic procedures and some simple surgeries can be performed by a single person, there are times when an additional pair of hands will make the procedure much easier to perform and more time-efficient. For example, it may be helpful to have a camera operator during laparoscopic surgery, or an assistant to operate the biopsy forceps and prepare the samples for submission to the laboratory during GI endoscopy or bronchoscopy.

It is most convenient if the endoscopy system is stored on a ready-to-use cart or in a dedicated room, so procedures can be initiated with a minimum of set-up time. Figure 2.44 shows an example of a complete endoscopy system on a mobile cart, which can be easily moved to the most convenient location in the practice as needed. If the equipment is stored in this way, practitioners will be more inclined to use the system often, and for applications that might otherwise be overlooked or considered too cumbersome. It is recommended that spares of certain critical items be kept on hand, such as light bulbs and flexible biopsy forceps. This prevents the need to abort a procedure once the patient is under anaesthesia if one of these items fails.

Large or busy practices that perform a lot of endoscopic procedures often have multiple systems for use in different locations in the practice, depending on the frequency and types of cases seen. For example, a

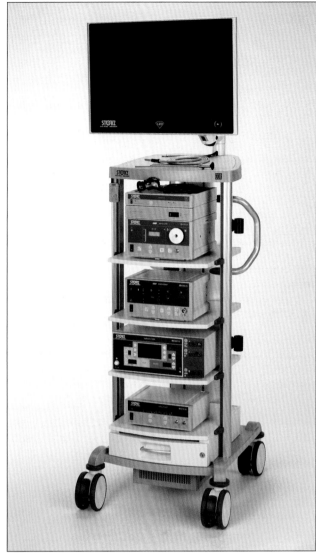

2.44 Mobile endoscopy cart. Top to bottom: monitor, telescope and light cable, modular camera units, light source, CO_2 insufflator, electrosurgical generator and VETPUMP®2 insufflation, irrigation and suction pump.
(© Karl Storz SE & Co. KG)

surgery tower would be stored in the operating theatre, where sterility is a constant concern; another system for non-sterile procedures, such as gastrointestinal endoscopy or otoscopy, might be kept in another room where these procedures are performed; and finally, a portable system can be available in the consulting room for, for example, performing otoscopy in the non-anaesthetized patient and sharing initial findings with the owner.

An efficient, ergonomic set-up of the cart or operating theatre is also vital for making endoscopy attractive and minimizing operator fatigue. At all times the monitor should be adjusted to the eye level of the surgeon and positioned in such a way as to minimize neck strain. The ideal positioning of the monitor is directly across from the endoscopist (Figure 2.45ab). In cases where an assistant is involved, the monitor should be placed so that it is easily viewed by both parties (Figure 2.45c). Relatively inexpensive flatscreen monitors can be mounted on the walls of the endoscopy room to aid the surgeon(s) and/or assistant; these will be useful even if they are not of the same quality as the primary viewing monitor stored permanently on the endoscopy tower.

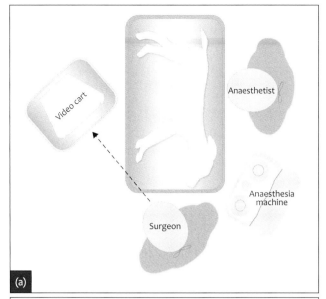

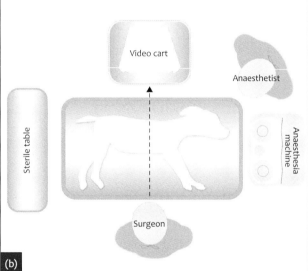

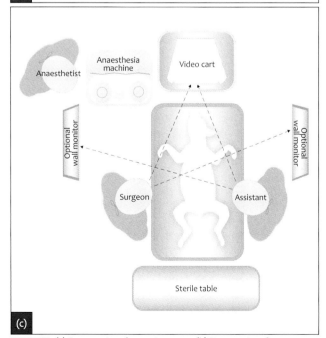

2.45 (a) Room set-up for gastroscopy. (b) Room set-up for laparoscopy with the patient in left lateral recumbency. (c) Room set-up for laparoscopy with the patient in dorsal recumbency.
(© Karl Storz SE & Co. KG)

Before the procedure, all electronic devices and non-sterile instrumentation should be tested by the assistant or the endoscopist, in order to minimize the procedure time once the patient has been anaesthetized. Before introducing the endoscope into the patient, a clear, focused, white-balanced image should be obtained on the monitor. Care should always be taken before, during and after the procedure to protect the endoscope and the camera head, as these two items represent a substantial portion of the cost of an endoscope system.

Care, cleaning, storage and maintenance

Proper care, cleaning and sterilization of endoscopes and instruments will prolong the life of the equipment and prevent iatrogenic infection of the patient. All individuals using the equipment should be trained in its proper care and handling to prevent unnecessary damage and costly repairs. The following recommendations are general guidelines only. The manufacturer's specific recommendations for care, cleaning and sterilization of the instrumentation purchased should always be consulted.

- Endoscopic instrumentation should be cleaned immediately after use. This prevents proteinaceous matter and bodily fluids from drying and adhering to the surface of the instruments, which would make them more difficult to clean.
- Hand instruments and trocars should be disassembled before cleaning, disinfecting and sterilizing, so that all surfaces and crevices come into adequate contact with cleaning and disinfecting agents.
- A neutral pH enzymatic cleaning solution should be used for initial cleaning of endoscopes and instrumentation.
- Only distilled or demineralized water should be used for diluting cleaning solutions and rinsing instrumentation, to avoid mineral deposits that may damage instruments, clog channels and prevent smooth operation of moving parts.
- Items containing optics, such as the endoscope, camera head and light cable, should be handled with particular care to prevent damage to the glass lenses or fibres. It should also be noted whether the particular items are completely immersible in fluids, gas sterilizable or autoclavable before proceeding.

Cleaning

Various brushes (Figure 2.46) are available to aid in cleaning endoscopic equipment. Brushes for instrument channels or the lumen of sheaths and cannulae should be of the appropriate diameter and length for the equipment in question, to avoid causing damage to the instrument channel and to ensure thorough cleaning. The length of a flexible endoscope channel cleaning brush is important because back-and-forth motion of the bristles inside the channel can cause micropunctures, which may lead to leakage of fluids into the inner workings of the endoscope. A flexible endoscope channel cleaning brush should be long enough to pass all the way through the channel and exit the other end, and should be smoothly withdrawn, avoiding a back-and-forth 'scrubbing' motion inside the channel.

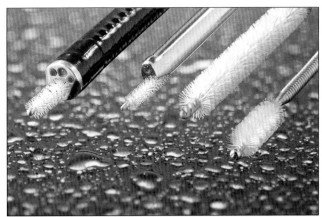

2.46 Cleaning brushes for endoscopes and instruments.
(© Karl Storz SE & Co. KG)

Ultrasonic cleaners are an excellent alternative to manual cleaning of both rigid and flexible hand instruments. Ultrasonic cleaning is helpful for cleaning hard-to-reach areas of instruments, such as hinges and locking mechanisms, but should not be used for any equipment that has lenses or fibreoptic bundles.

Enzymatic cleaning solution should be disposed of once cleaning is complete, and all equipment should be rinsed thoroughly. A clean, lint-free soft cloth should be used to dry the equipment completely. Alternatively, compressed air can be used for drying instruments; this is particularly helpful for instrument channels, cannula/sheath lumens and hinged areas. To maintain the working parts of the instruments, all joints, hinges, locks and stopcocks should be lubricated using the manufacturer's recommended lubricants or instrument milk. Opening and closing joints, hinges, locks and stopcocks repeatedly will work the lubricant into the intended area. Any excess lubricant should be removed.

Once cleaning is complete, the equipment can be disinfected or sterilized according to the manufacturer's recommendations. More and more endoscopy instruments and devices are autoclavable, but many are still not. For soakable instrumentation, high-level disinfection can be achieved using a manufacturer-approved disinfectant solution, such as glutaraldehyde or MEDDIS (Medichem International Ltd). Glutaraldehyde-containing disinfectant solutions are still used quite commonly in the USA and other countries. However, as glutaraldehyde is a known carcinogen, its use in the UK and other EU countries has been replaced by safer alternatives, such as MEDDIS. It is imperative to consult with the relevant authorities to determine the safe and legal use of glutaraldehyde in veterinary facilities. Proper staff training, use of personal protective equipment and adequate ventilation are important to ensure that these products are used in a safe and efficacious manner. These solutions usually have a shelf-life of 14 or 28 days from the time they are activated. It is important to follow the instructions on the label of the chosen product, as soaking times and the recommendations for reuse and disposal of the solution may vary. It is recommended not to soak instruments containing optics (i.e. endoscopes, light cables and camera heads) in any solution for longer than 45 minutes. Sterile water should be used to rinse equipment thoroughly, as disinfectant residues that come into contact with a patient can cause irritation. Instruments should then be dried completely with sterile soft cloths or sterile (filtered) compressed air. Lenses, light posts and the glass surfaces of light cables

can be cleaned with alcohol wipes to thoroughly dry them and remove any remaining residue. Disinfected instruments should either be used immediately or stored in a manner that avoids recontamination.

Sterilization

There are several methods of sterilization for endoscopic equipment. It is important to check with the equipment manufacturer which methods are authorized for the instrumentation in question before proceeding. Equipment that is to be sterilized will need to be packaged properly, depending on the method of sterilization. There are a variety of storage/sterilization trays available that are designed for specific instrumentation (Figure 2.47). The correct tray should be chosen, based on the type of instrumentation and the method of sterilization.

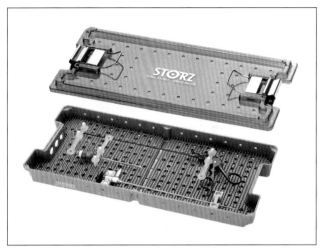

2.47 Sterilization and storage tray for a rigid endoscope and instruments.
(© Karl Storz SE & Co. KG)

A common method for sterilizing rigid endoscopes, flexible endoscopes and instruments is ethylene oxide gas sterilization. A pressure compensation cap must be attached to flexible endoscopes during gas sterilization. Steam sterilization or autoclaving is another common method of sterilization for some instruments and rigid endoscopes. Telescopes and camera heads that are autoclavable may be authorized only for specific cycles and temperatures. Flexible endoscopes are usually not steam sterilizable due to the high temperatures involved in this process.

Two additional sterilization methods, STERRAD® and STERIS, are relatively uncommon in private veterinary practice due to their cost. STERRAD® is a type of hydrogen peroxide gas plasma sterilization. The STERIS system uses peracetic acid for the sterilization process.

Storage

Endoscopes and instruments should be stored in a convenient and safe place so that damage is prevented yet the equipment is readily available for use without undue set-up time. Flexible endoscopes are best stored in a hanging position (Figure 2.48) to allow any residual fluid to drain and to minimize stress on the fibres, which would otherwise occur if they were left coiled for extended periods of time in their transportation case.

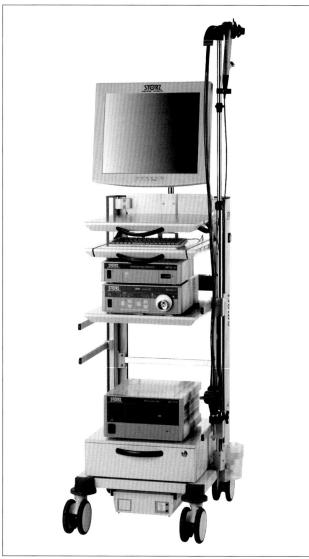

2.48 Mobile cart with a video-endoscope stored in the hanging position to maximize drainage and reduce stress on the glass fibres.
(© Karl Storz SE & Co. KG)

References and further reading

Baron JK and Runge JJ (2015) Miscellaneous surgical instrumentation. In: *Small Animal Laparoscopy and Thoracoscopy*, ed. BA Fransson and PD Mayhew, pp. 53–57. Wiley-Blackwell, Chichester

Brandao F and Chamness CJ (2015) Imaging equipment and operating room setup. In: *Small Animal Laparoscopy and Thoracoscopy*, ed. BA Fransson and PD Mayhew, pp. 31—40. Wiley-Blackwell, Chichester

Buote NJ (2015) Trocars and cannulas. In: *Small Animal Laparoscopy and Thoracoscopy*, ed. BA Fransson and PD Mayhew, pp. 49-52. Wiley-Blackwell, Chichester

Chamness CJ (2011) Endoscopic instrumentation. In: *Small Animal Endoscopy, 3rd edn*, ed. TR Tams, pp. 3–26. Mosby, St. Louis

Hotston Moore A and Ragni RA (2012) Rigid endoscopy. In: *Clinical Manual of Small Animal Endosurgery*, ed. A Hotston Moore, pp. 1–29. Wiley-Blackwell, Chichester

Marvel S and Monnet E (2015) Energy devices and stapling equipment. In: *Small Animal Laparoscopy and Thoracoscopy*, ed. BA Fransson and PD Mayhew, pp. 58–64. Wiley-Blackwell, Chichester

Runge, JJ (2015) Single-incision laparoscopic surgery devices. In: *Small Animal Laparoscopy and Thoracoscopy*, ed. BA Fransson and PD Mayhew, pp. 65–72. Wiley-Blackwell, Chichester

Swanson EA and Towle Millard HA (2015) Surgical instrumentation. In: *Small Animal Laparoscopy and Thoracoscopy*, ed. BA Fransson and PD Mayhew, pp. 42–48. Wiley-Blackwell, Chichester

Tams TR (1999) *Small Animal Endoscopy, 2nd edn*, Mosby, St. Louis

Chapter 3

Flexible endoscopy: basic technique

Edward J. Hall

Introduction

Since the previous edition of this Manual, flexible endoscopy has advanced dramatically in human medicine, with the introduction of high-definition (HD) imaging quality with dual-focus magnification, and new imaging modalities (Figure 3.1) such as narrowband imaging, chromoendoscopy, autofluorescence, endomicroscopy and endoscopic ultrasonography. The addition of carbon dioxide (CO_2) insufflation capability, a flushing pump and disposable suction pump liners enables safer and more effective endoscopy (Figure 3.2). Variable-stiffness insertion tubes, virtual positioning guides using remote tracking of the endoscope (e.g. ScopeGuide, Olympus) and a wider range of endotherapeutic instruments are now available. Some of these enhancements are filtering through to veterinary medicine, although the indications for therapeutic interventions remain fewer than in human medicine. Yet, the basic principles for using flexible endoscopes remain unchanged, and are detailed in this chapter.

The development of flexible video-endoscopy has made endoscopic examinations easier and more enjoyable compared with using a fibreoptic endoscope, and the ability to examine the gastrointestinal (GI), respiratory and urogenital tracts without surgery means that pet owners often expect such minimally invasive techniques to be used. Consequently, the use of flexible endoscopy to examine these organ systems is becoming more commonplace in

veterinary practice. Indeed, the Royal College of Veterinary Surgeons (RCVS) Day One Competences states that new graduates are expected to be competent to *'Use basic imaging equipment and carry out an examination effectively as appropriate to the case, in accordance with good health and safety practice and equipment change to current regulations,'* and clarifies that *'Basic equipment includes, for example, x-ray, ultrasound and endoscopes...'* (RCVS, 2014).

While simple rigid endoscopic procedures such as otoscopy and laryngoscopy are clearly within the capabilities of new graduates, the proficient use of steerable, flexible endoscopes can be achieved only with practice. Although the basics may now be taught in veterinary schools, competence in the required techniques can, for the most part, be obtained only by repeatedly undertaking procedures in live patients. There is some, but limited, expertise to be gained by using models or cadavers. For example, the ability to manipulate the tip of the endoscope so that the view remains centred in the lumen of the viscus as the endoscope is advanced can be acquired by passing the endoscope within a model or a fresh cadaver, although the colour, movement and feel are not realistic. Training on healthy animals in wet labs is not permitted in the UK except under the Animals (Scientific Procedures) Act 1986; such classes may be available in other countries but are ethically questionable. Therefore, in the UK, veterinary surgeons seeking to become proficient in endoscopy should ideally train under an experienced endoscopist. Yet, such

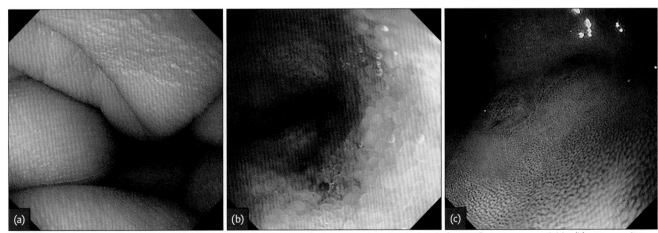

3.1 Advances in imaging quality. (a) HD-quality image of human fingerprints, showing the level of magnification now available. (b) HDTV-quality image of normal canine duodenal mucosa. Note that the individual villi are visible. (c) Narrowband endoscopic image of the stomach of a dog. Removal of red light from the illumination makes red objects (blood and blood vessels) appear black. The distortion of normal blood vessel patterns in the mucosa is suggestive of dysplasia or neoplasia.

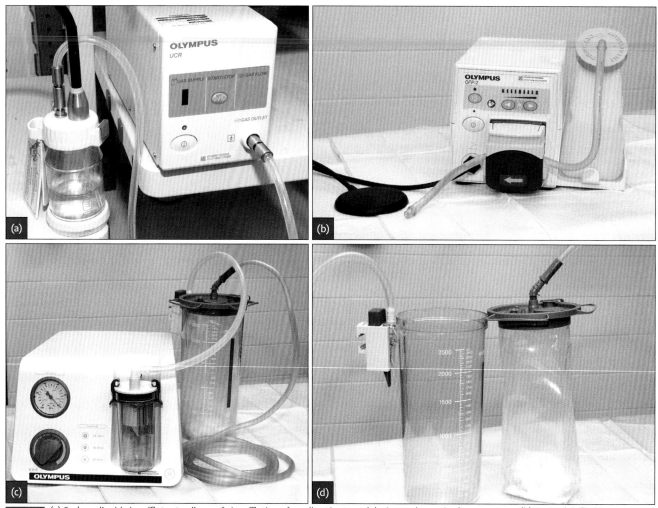

3.2 (a) Carbon dioxide insufflator to allow safe insufflation of small patients and during endoscopic electrosurgery. (b) Peristaltic flushing pump, operated by foot pedal, allows food and faecal material to be cleared from the field of view. (c) Suction pump with collecting reservoir. (d) Disposable liners for suction pump reservoirs contain a gel that solidifies liquid waste, allowing safe disposal in a clinical waste bin.

opportunities are limited, and therefore continuing professional development courses, extensive reading, use of models, viewing recorded endoscopy procedures and observing experienced endoscopists should be undertaken before contemplating performing endoscopy. Regular and frequent participation in endoscopic examinations is then needed to develop and maintain proficiency.

Equipment costs have declined relatively since the previous edition of this Manual, although endoscopes are still not cheap. Dedicated veterinary endoscopes are now available and affordable for many practices, and good-quality second-hand endoscopes designed for use in humans are available for purchase more often. Consequently, with the right equipment and skill, veterinary surgeons (veterinarians) can now access most parts of the GI tract, major airways and lower urogenital tract endoscopically, and many patients have benefited from such investigations. However, in some cases endoscopy may be unhelpful, and both indications and contraindications for various procedures can be found in specific chapters in this Manual. Endoscopy can result in serious complications, such as hypoxia during respiratory endoscopy and perforation during GI endoscopy. Thus, as in human endoscopy, *'The goal must be to maximize the benefits and minimize the risks. We need competent endoscopists, working for good indications on patients who are fully prepared and protected, with skilled assistants, and using optimum equipment. The basic principles are similar for all areas of gastrointestinal endoscopy, recognizing that there are specific circumstances where the risks are greater'* (Haycock *et al.*, 2014). Minimum standards are applied to endoscopic proficiency in human medicine, and the veterinary profession should aspire to the same level. As yet there are no regulated training programmes for veterinary endoscopists but, ultimately, they will be required.

Safe use of the endoscope

Before explaining the generic skills needed to use an endoscope, it is important to emphasize the need for safe practice to protect the patient, the equipment and the endoscopist. In particular, rigorous compliance with methods for cleaning and disinfecting endoscopes (see Chapter 2) is critical to minimize the risk of transmitting infection – not only from patient to patient, but also from patient to operator. Only fully immersible endoscopes should be used, as only they can be completely disinfected.

Protecting the patient

Endoscopy should be performed only when indicated, and not simply because the equipment is available. Thorough investigation by blood tests, radiography and ultrasound examination should generally precede endoscopy, to help the veterinary surgeon decide on the most appropriate course of action. Endoscopy to investigate vomiting in a patient with end-stage renal disease would be inappropriate, for example. Large gastric foreign bodies often cannot be retrieved endoscopically, despite being swallowed, because of the limited size of retrieval instruments, and a gastrotomy is indicated in such cases. Localization of an ingested foreign body by imaging may also indicate that it is already beyond the reach of an endoscope.

The place of endoscopy in the investigation of different organ systems is put into context in the following chapters, but it must be remembered that endoscopy is not without risk and may not be the best approach. The risks and benefits to the patient must be considered: how likely is endoscopy to give a diagnosis that alters the patient's management, and does the potential benefit justify the risk of the anaesthetic and the procedure? Standard procedures using a flexible endoscope are minimally invasive and atraumatic, with low morbidity and very low mortality compared with their traditional 'open' counterparts, although the risks are not negligible. For all types of GI endoscopic examinations, perforation has been reported in 0.08% (1/1240) of dogs and 1.6% (6/377) of cats (Irom *et al.*, 2014). However, with colonoscopy, major complications – consisting of fatal aspiration of polyethylene glycol laxative solutions, colonic perforation, and excessive haemorrhage after biopsy with rigid forceps – occurred in 0.85% of dogs (Leib *et al.*, 2004). The risks of bronchoscopy largely relate to difficulty maintaining oxygenation, but barotrauma and (tension) pneumothorax can occur.

Attainment of a certain level of proficiency, as described above, is necessary before any endoscopy should be attempted without supervision, and an understanding of the place of endoscopy in the whole diagnostic effort as well as its indications, relative merits and dangers must be appreciated. Inappropriate use (e.g. mishandling, overly aggressive or forceful use) can result in significant injury to the patient. Therefore, adequate equipment, and not necessarily the cheapest, is needed for maximum benefit. Factors influencing the choice of equipment are discussed in Chapter 2 and in the chapters describing the application of endoscopy in specific organ systems. It must also be recognized that the wide range of patient sizes in veterinary medicine means that it may not be possible to examine all patients with a single flexible endoscope.

Except perhaps for proctoscopy, veterinary patients must be anaesthetized to permit endoscopy without compromising the safety of the patient and endoscopist and risking damage to the endoscope. The requirement for general anaesthesia necessitates the presence of an assistant to monitor the patient, as the endoscopist may be too engrossed in the procedure to recognize significant changes in vital signs before it is too late. The 'assistant' must be in control and be able to intervene if the endoscopist is endangering the patient, perhaps by overinflating the stomach. Indeed, *'Endoscopy is a team activity... It is difficult to overstate the importance of appropriate facilities and adequate professional support staff, to maintain patient comfort and safety, and to optimize clinical outcomes'* (Haycock *et al.*, 2014). Thus, although the endoscope may be manipulated by a single operator, it is essential to have at least one assistant present to monitor the patient.

Protecting the endoscope

A flexible endoscope is a very effective tool if used properly. However, inappropriate use can result in not only injury to the patient but also expensive damage to the endoscope. As endoscope technology has advanced, instrument durability has improved, but endoscopes remain expensive investments and must be handled carefully and well maintained. An understanding of the strengths and limitations of endoscopic equipment and its care is essential for its longevity. With care, the working life of a flexible endoscope should exceed 10 years, and some 20-year-old endoscopes are still in service today.

As detailed in Chapter 2, both fibreoptic endoscopes and video-endoscopes contain light/illumination 'guides', that is, bundles of glass fibres that transmit light to illuminate the patient. Fibreoptic endoscopes also contain an image bundle of similar diameter glass fibres arranged in a coherent pattern. Both of these glass fibre bundles are flexible (hence the endoscope is flexible) but very fragile; they are susceptible to damage by compression and sudden shocks. If the insertion tube is bitten by the patient, or trapped in a door or the hinge of its carrying case, this is very likely to result in damage (Figure 3.3). However, even merely tapping the end of the endoscope on the edge of a table once may be sufficient to shatter fibres, or dislodge the objective lens, or damage the video chip.

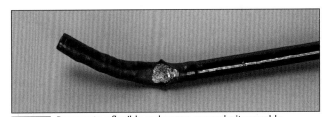

3.3 Damage to a flexible endoscope can make it unusable. Compression damage to the bending section of this gastroscope was caused by a trolley being wheeled over the tip as it trailed on the floor.

Illumination by the light guide will gradually diminish as more fibres in it are broken, and so minor damage may not be instantly apparent. However, the breakage of a single fibre among the coherent fibres of the image bundle immediately results in a black spot in the viewed image of a fibreoptic endoscope. The presence of too many broken fibres impairs viewing (see Figure 2.8) and ultimately can render the endoscope unusable. The endoscope must then be repaired by replacement of the whole bundle, which can cost thousands of pounds. Similarly, perforation of the insertion tube or biopsy channel causes leakage and allows ingress of water, which loosens the glue securing the ends of the fibres and ultimately leads to fibre breakage. Thus, leakage testing should be performed after every procedure to avoid the need for expensive repairs (Video 3.1). Heat sterilization irreversibly damages the whole endoscope and must *never* be used. Information on how to test for leakage and clean and disinfect flexible endoscopes is provided in Chapter 2.

For the reasons given above, it is imperative that the endoscopist takes care to ensure secure handling of the endoscope. When the endoscope is being held outside the patient, all ends of the endoscope should be secure, with no part being allowed to dangle or swing freely because of the risk that it might knock against a solid surface. The endoscope can be held securely in one or both hands (Figure 3.4).

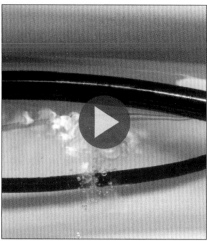

Video 3.1   Escape of air bubbles during a leakage test of an endoscope.

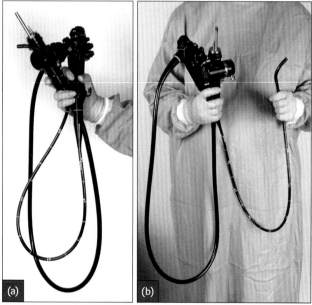

(a)

(b)

3.4   Endoscopes should be carried securely in (a) one or (b) both hands to avoid accidental damage.

When the umbilical cord is attached to the light source and the insertion tube is within the patient, only the handpiece (control body) needs to be held. However, care should be taken when withdrawing the insertion tube from the patient, as its tip may unexpectedly exit the patient, pulled by the weight of the unsupported insertion tube, and drop, potentially striking the examination table or floor and causing damage. This is more likely when using veterinary gastroscopes, which are typically 1.4 m in length compared with a 1.0 m medical gastroscope; the extra length and weight of any loop of insertion tube outside the patient can pull the endoscope out unexpectedly. Having an assistant making sure the endoscope does not suddenly exit the patient is a sensible precaution.

Demonstrating the flexibility of an endoscope by tightly coiling it should be avoided, and the bending section should not be manipulated by the fingers; only the control knobs should be used to check the range of bending. The umbilical cord should be connected and disconnected from the light source by pushing/pulling in a straight line, with twisting or rocking motions avoided. After use, especially if cleaning of the endoscope is likely to be delayed, the channels should be flushed and clean water suctioned to remove gross debris and prevent the development of a blockage when the channels dry out.

When the endoscope is not in use it must be stored securely and not left unattended on a work surface. It may be transported safely within its carrying case but should not be stored there in the long term, as it will ultimately take on a permanent curve. Furthermore, storage in the carrying case is likely to encourage microbial growth, especially if the endoscope channels are not dried thoroughly before it is put away. Storage on a secure wall hanger that allows the insertion tube to hang vertically and air to circulate freely is ideal.

Rules for handling flexible endoscopes

The following operations should *never* be performed:
- Manipulating the tip by hand; only the steering wheels should be used
- Inserting biopsy forceps when the bending section at the endoscope tip is retroflexed
- Heat sterilization of the endoscope.

A flexible endoscope should be used gently, and excessive force should be avoided when:
- Passing the insertion tube into the patient
- Rotating the endoscope on its long axis (applying torque), especially when it is looped within a viscus
- Turning the steering wheels to deflect the tip.

After the procedure, the endoscopist should flush all channels to remove gross debris before hanging up the endoscope ready for cleaning and disinfection by trained personnel.

Protecting the endoscopist

Although the risk of a veterinary endoscopist contracting an infection from a patient is small compared with that faced by their counterparts in human medicine, contact with potentially zoonotic material (e.g. GI contents, faeces, respiratory secretions), either directly, by splashing or via aerosolization, is still possible. Appropriate precautions should always be adopted, making the assumption that all patients are potentially infectious, even if there is no objective evidence of infection. Protective clothing should always be worn, and gowns, gloves and eye protection are all recommended.

Bronchoscopy of patients suspected of having tuberculosis should be undertaken only by trained personnel wearing appropriate personal protective equipment (PPE). Any faecal material aspirated from the colon also represents a significant potential hazard, and the use of a suction pump with a disposable liner containing a gel to solidify liquid waste is recommended (see Figure 3.2cd).

Measures to reduce infection recommended in human endoscopy (Haycock *et al.*, 2014) include:

- Wearing appropriate PPE – gloves, gowns and eye protection (glasses or visor)
- Good general hygienic practice in the endoscopy room:
  - Frequent hand-washing
  - Covering all skin breaks with waterproof dressings
  - Use of paper towels when handling soiled accessories
  - Putting soiled items directly into a sink and not on to clean surfaces
- Appropriate disposal of hazardous waste, needles and syringes.

Preparation for endoscopy

Preparation of the patient for endoscopy varies depending on the procedure being performed, and is detailed in the relevant chapters. Every time an endoscope is used, the equipment should be checked to ensure it works. An image should be visible, and the following components and functions should be checked before the patient is anaesthetized:

- Air pump
- Suction
- Air/water valve
- Suction valve
- Disposable cap on biopsy/accessory channel
- Tip deflection.

To maximize its lifespan, the light source should be switched on just before the induction of anaesthesia or placed in 'standby' if that option is available. All necessary ancillary equipment required for the specific procedure should be made available; this includes some or all of the following:

- Protective clothing
- Mouth gag if performing upper GI or respiratory endoscopy
- Biopsy forceps
- Formalin pots with or without tissue biopsy cassettes
- Wash tube and sterile saline
- Cytology brush and slides
- Grasping forceps, basket forceps and other retrieval devices
- Injection/aspiration needles
- Recording equipment (PC and image capture software, DVD recorder, USB capture, etc.).

Handling a flexible gastroscope or colonoscope

There are certain endoscopic techniques and 'tricks' that are applicable in specific circumstances in the upper or lower GI tract, and these are detailed in the relevant chapters. However, the way to hold and use flexible endoscopes is generic, and this information follows. With practice, manoeuvring becomes second nature, and the length of the procedure becomes shorter, permitting the skilled endoscopist to examine more carefully and consider the findings in relation to the clinical problem and previous experience. However, endoscopy is not a race, and adequate time should be taken to minimize trauma and maximize the value of any investigation.

Holding the handpiece

When performing flexible endoscopy, the umbilical cord is plugged into the air/water pump and light source, and the endoscopist and patient are positioned (see Figure 2.45) in an arrangement that permits efficient technique. The endoscopist holds the handpiece in their left hand, while guiding the insertion tube into the patient with their right hand (Figure 3.5).

All flexible endoscopes are designed for the handpiece to be held in the left hand, and are grasped most securely by placing the control head in the palm of the hand with the

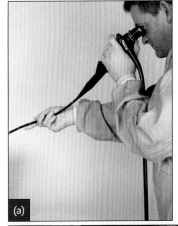

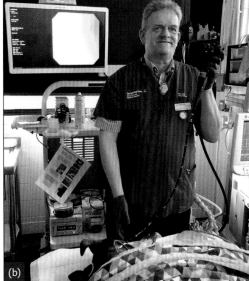

3.5 (a) Holding a fibreoptic gastroscope correctly in the left hand while guiding the insertion tube with the right. Fibreoptic endoscopes must be held to the eye to view unless a charge-coupled device (CCD) camera attachment is available. (b) Holding a video-gastroscope. Without the need to hold a eyepiece to the eye, the endoscopist can stand in a more relaxed position and view the monitor in front of them. In this image, the monitor behind the endoscopist is for teaching purposes and the monitor viewed by the endoscopist is connected by Wi-Fi.

umbilical cord running down the back of the hand between the thumb and index finger (Figure 3.6). This positioning allows easy placement of the fingers on the valves and steering controls and, with fibreoptic endoscopes, is necessary to keep the endoscope correctly oriented to the eye.

When the handpiece is held in the palm, with the umbilical cord running between the thumb and index finger, the index and middle fingers can be used to operate the valves, while the fourth and fifth fingers provide stability through a 'two-finger' grip (Figure 3.7a). Alternatively, the middle, fourth and fifth fingers can be used to hold the body of the handpiece (Figure 3.7b). This 'three-finger' grip requires the left index finger to operate both valves, but there is rarely a time when both would be operated simultaneously, and it offers easier control of the steering wheels by the left thumb. Ultimately, the choice between using the two- or three-finger grip is based on the comfort of the grip, which is dependent on the shape of the handpiece body, the distance between the control wheels and the accessory/biopsy channel opening, and personal preference.

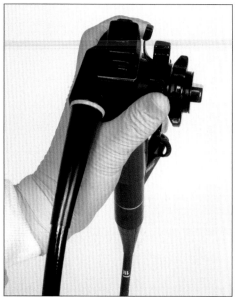

3.6 Holding the handpiece. The handpiece is held in the palm of the left hand with the umbilical cord running down the back of the hand between the thumb and index finger, allowing the fingers to reach the buttons and control wheels.

Rotation of the handpiece

The handpiece of a video-endoscope can be rotated on its long axis in order to help steer (see below). Such movement is more limited if a fibreoptic endoscope is used because this type of endoscope is held to the eye; in these cases, the operator tends to alter their head and/or body position as the endoscope is rotated. However, if a fibreoptic endoscope with a camera attachment or a video-endoscope is being used for gastroscopy, when almost full insertion has been achieved, some endoscopists prefer to rotate the handpiece 90 degrees anticlockwise so that it lies flat in the palm of their left hand. The left thumb can then manipulate the valves, while the right hand operates the steering wheels (Figure 3.7c), and forward and backward movement of the insertion tube is imparted directly by movement of the handpiece. This reduces the strain on the endoscopist, who can remain standing upright. However, this variation is not possible in smaller patients when significant lengths of insertion tube remain outside the patient, or with a fibreoptic endoscope held to the eye as the endoscopist's eye must be at the level of the patient when the insertion tube is almost fully inserted. This position is uncomfortable unless the endoscopist sits or kneels, and it places their head in a position of risk relative to the patient and any material that may leak out during the procedure.

Using the controls
The valves/buttons

The top of the gastroscope handpiece houses two valves activated by buttons: air/water and suction. The forward button (normally colour-coded blue) controls the air/water channel, and the rear button (normally colour-coded red) controls suction (Figure 3.8, and see Figure 2.1).

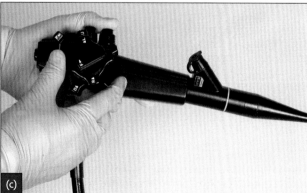

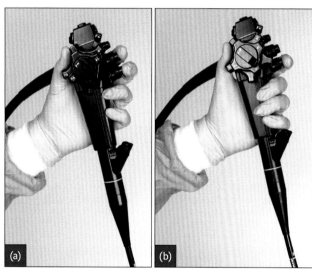

3.7 Gripping the endoscope handpiece. (a) Using the fourth and fifth fingers to stabilize the endoscope handpiece, the left index and middle fingers are free to operate the air/water and suction buttons, respectively. (b) Using a three-finger grip to stabilize the handpiece, the left index finger is used to operate the buttons, while the thumb controls the up/down steering wheel. (c) Rotation of the handpiece of a video-endoscope once almost full insertion has been achieved allows the left thumb to operate the suction and air/water buttons, and the right thumb and fingers to manipulate the steering wheels.

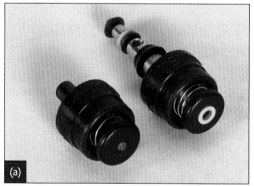

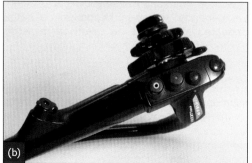

3.8 The suction valve/button (red) and air/water valve/button (blue). Covering the hole in the air/water button deflects air and insufflates the viscus. Depression of the red and blue buttons causes suction and water flushing, respectively. (a) Suction (red) and air/water (blue) valves before insertion in the handpiece. (b) Position of the suction (red) and air/water (blue) buttons on the handpiece.

Insufflation/washing: Air from the air pump passes continuously along the umbilical cord and out through a hole in the centre of the air/water button. Coverage of the hole by a finger deflects the airflow along the insertion tube and into the patient, to enable insufflation of the viscus. Leakage of air back up the biopsy channel is prevented by a disposable rubber valve (Figure 3.9). Depression of the air/water button allows water to flow down the channel, and the water is then deflected across the tip of the endoscope to flush mucus, blood or debris from the objective lens at the tip when the view is obscured.

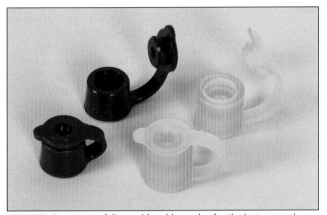

3.9 Two types of disposable rubber valve for the instrument/accessory/biopsy channel. These valves provide a seal around biopsy forceps, preventing the escape of air after insufflation.

The ability to instil air into the GI tract and to wash the lens is essential to be able to obtain a clear view. The rate of air insufflation should be varied depending on the size of the patient, the size of the viscus and its ability to expand, and the rate of any air escape. The rate of insufflation can be controlled by adjusting either the setting on the air pump or the length of time the air hole is covered. The novice endoscopist often forgets that their finger is covering the air hole, and the resulting inadvertent continuous insufflation leads to overinflation of the viscus. Overinflation of the stomach is poor technique because, as well as making pyloric intubation difficult (see Chapter 5), the gastric dilation impairs venous return to the heart and splints the diaphragm, threatening the anaesthetized patient's life. The anaesthetic assistant should always be aware of the possibility of overinflation and inform the endoscopist whenever they feel air should be withdrawn.

If a viscus will not inflate, the first things to check are that the air pump is on and working, and that the water bottle is attached properly: it must be attached to the port on the umbilical cord, the 'O' ring on the connector must not be worn or missing and the bottle's screw lid must be firmly closed to prevent air leakage. If the endoscope is then shown to be capable of insufflation and the channel is not blocked (this can be checked by placing the tip under water and operating the air/water button to see that air bubbles are produced), failure of the viscus to expand must be because of air escaping. This can occur when the rubber seal on the accessory/biopsy channel valve is not closed or is leaking because it is worn. Use of a new disposable valve for each procedure precludes air leakage and is also considered best practice for infection control. Air escaping up the oesophagus may also prevent insufflation of the stomach, and can be stopped by an assistant gently constricting the oesophagus in the neck. Similarly, during colonoscopy an assistant can squeeze the anus shut to aid insufflation. Finally, neoplastic infiltration may

make the GI tract wall rigid, so an inability to insufflate the tract can be a sign of pathology, assuming that the other causes of failure to insufflate have been ruled out.

In almost all endoscopy systems currently used in veterinary practice, air is used for insufflation. However, this can lead to uncontrolled inflation of the stomach if colonoscopy is performed in a patient immediately after gastroscopy, particularly in cats and small dogs. Air tracks up the small intestine and causes overinflation of the stomach, sometimes necessitating decompression by placement of a stomach tube during the colonoscopy. This problem is minimized if CO_2 is used for insufflation and a dedicated regulator is added to the system to control the flow of CO_2 via the air/water channel (see Figure 3.2a), as CO_2 is much more rapidly absorbed than air. It is also safer to use CO_2 when performing electrosurgery in the colon, although this is a rare event in veterinary endoscopy, as a spark can ignite the mixture of air and volatile colonic gases and cause an explosion.

Suction: After insufflation, suction is used to remove the air. This can correct overinflation of the stomach and should be undertaken before withdrawal of an endoscope from the GI tract to make the patient more comfortable on recovery.

To enable suction of liquids, the tip of the endoscope is deflected into any pools of liquid and submerged, and the suction button is depressed. Suction is generally not possible when instruments have been inserted through the accessory channel. Particulate matter may clog the orifice of the channel, and if this occurs alternate flushing and suction may facilitate removal of the liquid. A flushing pump, if available, helps liquidize any retained material and clear the view if there is food or faeces in the GI tract. Alternatively, and more cheaply, water can be forced down the working channel with a large syringe to flush the channel. As liquid is removed via suction, it is not uncommon for the GI mucosa eventually to be sucked into the channel. When released, a small red dot on the mucosa, a suction artefact, may be seen (Figure 3.10). This is not a serious problem, but the mark must not be mistaken for a lesion.

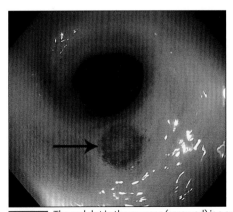

3.10 The red dot in the mucosa (arrowed) is a suction artefact caused by tissue being sucked up accidentally, and must not be mistaken for a lesion.

The steering wheels

Gastroscopes and colonoscopes have two wheels on the handpiece to control the deflection of the tip. The smaller diameter 'outer' wheel (i.e. the wheel further from the body of the handpiece) deflects the tip left/right, while the larger diameter 'inner' wheel rotates it up/down. The ability to retroflex the bending section at least 180 degrees in at least one plane is essential for gastroscopy, and 210–90 degrees up/down is the norm for gastroscopes (see Chapter 2). Paediatric and veterinary gastroscopes that have a tight radius of curvature of the bending section, to enable manoeuvring in the stomach of smaller patients, are preferred.

The conventional orientation when holding the gastroscope handpiece in the left hand (see Figure 3.6) permits manipulation of both steering wheels with the left hand alone. Steering 210–90 degrees up/down is achieved by turning the inner wheel anticlockwise/clockwise (forwards/backwards), respectively. This should always be achieved by using the left thumb to move the wheel, with the middle finger acting as a ratchet to stabilize the position of the wheel as the thumb is repositioned on the next notch on the wheel. Moving the left thumb towards the palm when controlling the up/down wheel (i.e. the wheel moves anticlockwise) will result in retroflexion (upwards movement) of the tip; all other wheel movements cause only a maximum of 90-degree deflection in the other directions.

Deflection 90–90 degrees in the orthogonal (left/right) plane is achieved by turning the outer wheel anticlockwise/clockwise (forwards/backwards), respectively. With much practice this can be achieved using the tip of the left thumb, while the knuckle of the thumb is used to turn the inner (up/down) wheel. However, fine control is more easily achieved by using the left hand on the inner wheel and the right hand on the outer wheel (Video 3.2).

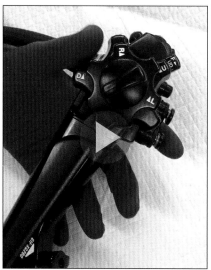

Video 3.2

Single- and two-handed manipulation of steering wheels.

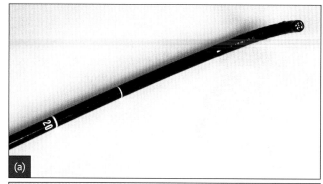

(a)

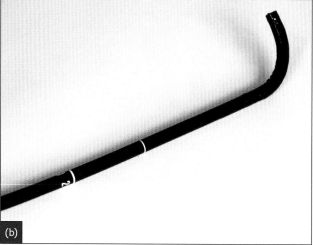

(b)

3.11 (a) Upward deflection of the endoscope tip and (b) longitudinal rotation effectively allow the endoscopist to look to the left or right without having to manipulate the left/right steering wheel.

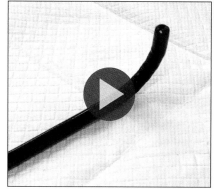

Video 3.3 Steering by tip deflection and torquing.

Single-handed control of steering is possible with practice, and is necessary when the right hand is manipulating the insertion tube or inserting biopsy forceps. In reality, a major part of steering can be achieved simply through deflecting the tip up/down by the left thumb manipulating the inner wheel, and then flexing/extending the left wrist so that the endoscope rotates on its long axis. This has the effect of making the tip 'look' to the left and right (Figure 3.11; Video 3.3) without the need to turn the outer wheel at all. Only when fine control is needed (e.g. when intubating the pylorus) is it necessary to use the right hand to operate a steering wheel, although inexperienced endoscopists usually find it easier to use both right and left hands to steer. At nearly full insertion of a video-gastroscope, when trying to intubate the pylorus, rotation of the handpiece in the palm of the hand (see Figure 3.7c) allows fine control of both wheels with the right hand.

Friction brakes

Friction brakes (Figure 3.12) are operated by levers or knobs labelled 'F' or 'B', depending on the manufacturer. They permit the position of any tip deflection to be maintained without holding the steering wheels in position manually, although it is still possible to move the steering wheels by applying increased pressure to them. Friction brakes were devised to help maintain deflection during certain phases of endoscopy in humans, and the experienced veterinary endoscopist may not need to use them. Nevertheless, the ability to fix the endoscope tip may help the novice endoscopist maintain the tip position at times when the right hand is undertaking other functions such as inserting biopsy forceps. It should be noted that on some makes of endoscope, the brake on the outer (left/right) wheel is applied progressively as the wheel is turned, and

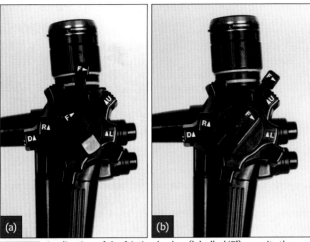

3.12 Application of the friction brakes (labelled 'F') permits the endoscope tip to be held in a deflected position without the need to control the steering wheels. (a) Friction brakes 'off'. (b) Friction brakes 'on'. With the brakes 'off', the small arrows indicate the direction of turn of the lever and knob to put the brakes 'on' for the up/down and left/right wheels, respectively.

the brake must be 'clicked off' completely or it will be gradually applied inadvertently as the wheel is turned for steering. The brake on the inner (up/down) wheel is always a simple on/off lever.

Handling a flexible bronchoscope

Dedicated bronchoscopes need to deflect only 90–90 degrees in one plane in order to examine the bronchi, but full retroflexion (180–210 degrees) upwards is needed for examining the nasopharynx. This deflection is often controlled by a simple lever, which is operated by the left thumb (Figure 3.13). Bronchoscopes also do not have an air/water button as there is no need to insufflate the respiratory tract to gain a view. These modifications allow bronchoscopes to have narrower insertion tubes than gastroscopes. Some, but not all, bronchoscopes have a suction channel, which, if the bronchoscope has been disinfected properly, can be used to aspirate

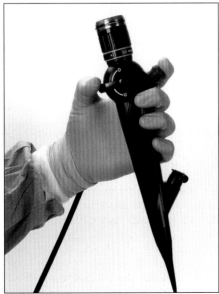

3.13 Holding the handpiece of a fibreoptic bronchoscope, with a lever for two-way tip deflection being operated by the left thumb, and the suction button by a finger. There is no air/water channel in bronchoscopes.

bronchoalveolar lavage fluid into a trap container placed in the suction line. A small (~1.8 mm) biopsy channel may also be present.

Video-endoscope controls

Most video-endoscopes and video camera attachments for fibreoptic endoscopes have a number of buttons on the handpiece or camera, which toggle on/off. They can be programmed to control a number of functions related to the image depending on user preference and the availability of accessory equipment:

*   White balance (see Chapter 2)
*   Freeze-frame – often a small live image will appear in the corner of the screen while the main image is frozen
*   Open/close iris – to alter the level of illumination directly or to change the sensor to respond to 'peak' or 'averaged' illumination
*   Zoom in/out – to magnify the image
*   Image recorder on/off/pause – to control recording to DVD, USB or PC
*   Video print – to control printing of images as hard copies.

Using the endoscope in a patient

Operator position

The endoscopist should either try to stand upright (to avoid back strain) or be seated. This is much easier with a video-endoscope. With a fibreoptic endoscope, the requirement to look through the eyepiece can necessitate the endoscopist being in a contorted position and, during endoscopy of large dogs, their face may be very close to the patient when the endoscope is at full insertion.

Controlling the insertion tube
Endoscope position

The insertion tube outside the patient should be kept in as straight a line as possible. Leaning over the patient loops the insertion tube outside the patient, leading to operator strain, tension on the endoscope and difficulty in steering: as soon as the tip is deflected, any bending of the insertion tube outside the patient will result in movement of the endoscope tip and a change in the view. This problem is exacerbated if using a long endoscope in a small patient. While a 1.4 m gastroscope is required to intubate the pylorus of a giant-breed dog, it may be cumbersome to use in cats and small dogs, as the majority of the insertion tube is outside the patient and almost inevitably does not remain straight. A 1.0 m gastroscope is preferred but, as most practices will have only one gastroscope, a longer one is a necessary compromise to be able to examine large/giant-breed dogs.

Endoscope insertion

To insert the endoscope into the patient, the insertion tube is supported and guided with the right hand. Support is not necessary when the endoscope is at nearly full insertion during gastroscopy or colonoscopy; insertion and withdrawal are simply accomplished by pushing the handpiece in and out, because the insertion tube is being held in a relatively straight line within the oesophagus or descending colon and cannot loop.

Looping of the insertion tube within the patient, especially in the stomach, makes advancing the endoscope more difficult: the loop grows larger as the endoscope is inserted further, and the tip does not advance. Indeed, in the stomach the pylorus may actually move away from the endoscope (so-called paradoxical motion) as the greater curvature stretches (see Chapter 5). This problem is countered by withdrawing the endoscope until the loop is flattened and deflating the viscus if there has been overzealous inflation so that the endoscope can be inserted further in a straighter line.

Some endoscopists use an assistant to stabilize the insertion tube and to advance or withdraw it. This may be helpful during colonoscopy because the endoscopist's right hand remains clean as it does not have to touch faecal contamination on the insertion tube (see Chapter 6). However, having to instruct an assistant to move the insertion tube forwards and backwards adds a layer of complexity to the process and is not generally recommended. It can be useful to have an assistant to manually close the anus to stop air escaping during colonoscopy, making insufflation more efficient. An assistant also can be invaluable in controlling the insertion tube on withdrawal of the endoscope, to prevent it unexpectedly falling out, pulled by the weight of an external insertion tube loop, and hitting the floor.

Longitudinal rotation

Rotating the insertion tube on its long axis (sometimes referred to as 'torquing') is facilitated by the endoscopist holding the insertion tube with the right hand and rotating it while turning the handpiece with the left hand in the same direction. This function of the right hand used to be essential with older fibreoptic endoscopes, when the construction of the insertion tube was inadequate to prevent twisting and possible damage to the fibreoptics during rotation. In modern endoscopes, the more robust construction means that this role for the right hand is not essential, and the insertion tube can be rotated simply by rotating the handpiece. Nevertheless, longitudinal rotation should not be performed if the endoscope is looped within a viscus, as the distal tip may be constrained within a length of intestine and be unable to rotate; rotation of the handpiece while the tip is fixed will simply strain the endoscope.

Steering the endoscope

Steering is accomplished by a combination of:

- Insertion and withdrawal
- Longitudinal rotation (torquing)
- Up/down tip deflection
- Left/right tip deflection
- Passive movement as the endoscope follows the wall of a viscus.

The novice endoscopist often struggles to steer the endoscope, not only because they are not proficient in the use of the steering wheels and rotating the endoscope, but because they over-think about which way to turn the endoscope tip. The direction of tip deflection is written on the steering wheels, but that is of little help when trying to see where to go, and when it is not obvious which direction is which. Indeed, unless there are distinct visible landmarks, such as the incisura angularis in the stomach (see Chapter 5), the orientation of the endoscope within a tube (such as the oesophagus or intestine) is not particularly relevant, as the true orientation of the image depends on the relative rotational position of both the patient and the

endoscope. It can be impossible to determine which direction is up/down or left/right except by noting:

- Pooling of liquid in the most dependent part of the viscus, although this may be confusing if the patient is in lateral recumbency
- A black triangular notch in the uppermost part of a fibreoptic image
- The top of the screen for a video-endoscope image relates to the 'up' (retroflexed) direction of the up/down steering wheel.

The experienced endoscopist does not think in terms of turning left/right and up/down, but almost intuitively knows which way to turn by observing the direction in which the image moves as they start to move a steering wheel, and when to insufflate in order to be able to see where the tip is going. Unfortunately, this skill can be acquired only through practice, although prior proficiency with video games may impart some advantage. The thought process involved is similar to that of reversing a car around a corner; initially one has to think which way to turn the steering wheel to direct the car in the correct direction, but with practice it becomes second nature. However, just as there are good and bad drivers, some operators find endoscopy easier than others. Nevertheless, with adequate practice, most should be able to perform a satisfactory endoscopic examination.

Red-out

Although the focal length of the objective lens in endoscopes is very short, usually being able to focus at distances as near as 2–3 mm, if the lens is too close or even in contact with tissue, it is impossible to see more than an out-of-focus red blur. This is called 'red-out' (Figure 3.14). Novice endoscopists often feel they have done something wrong when red-out occurs. However, it happens to all endoscopists; it is just that more experienced operators know how to correct the image quickly so that it is not a problem. To get rid of red-out, some or all of the following manoeuvres are undertaken:

- Slight withdrawal of the endoscope – this moves the tip back from the mucosa
- Insufflation with air – inflation of the viscus moves the mucosa away from the lens
- Deflection of the tip – a slight deflection combined with the above techniques will allow the endoscopist to obtain a view of the lumen. Movement towards the darkest part of the blur is generally in the direction of the lumen (Figure 3.14b), unless the tip is up against food or faecal matter.

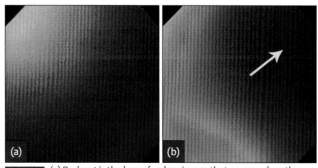

3.14 (a) Red-out is the loss of a clear image that occurs when the endoscope lens is too close to the mucosa. (b) Red-out is corrected by withdrawing the endoscope, deflecting the tip slightly and insufflating. In general, the lumen is towards the darker region of the image; in this image, the direction of the lumen is denoted by the arrow.

Clearing the view

During GI endoscopy, it is not uncommon for the lens to be obscured by blood, mucus or GI contents. This material can be cleared by depressing the air/water button and flushing the lens with water. After flushing, a drop of clear water on the tip may interfere with the view, and should be removed by repeatedly using suction and blowing air. Failure to flush properly if air insufflation is working may be due to:

- The water bottle being empty, or lid not closed
- The channel being blocked
- Loss of the 'O' ring sealing the connection between the water bottle and endoscope
- Adherent material covering the lens, e.g. lubricant, solid faeces.

Whenever pools of liquid are found during endoscopy, it is important to use suction to remove them as the fluid may obscure a lesion. If there is solid matter present, simple flushing with water may be enough to clear it. Where there is considerable food or faecal material, a large-bore syringe inserted through the rubber valve of the biopsy channel can be used to force larger volumes of warm water down the channel (Figure 3.15a), although

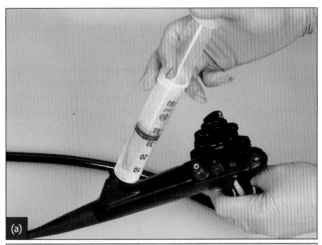

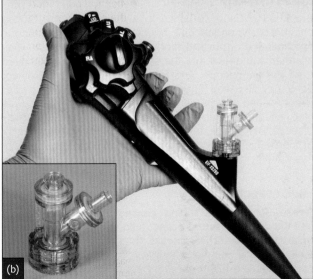

3.15 (a) Flushing using a large-bore syringe attached to the biopsy channel valve. (b) Adapter for the biopsy channel to allow flushing by syringe or flushing pump while still permitting biopsy.

blowback of some of the water may happen. If this fails to clear the material, repeat endoscopy after adequate preparation of the patient may be necessary unless a flushing pump (see Figure 3.2b), which allows gross debris and faecal material to be washed away from the field of view, is available. Some modern endoscopes have a separate channel in the insertion tube to which the pump is attached, but if there is no channel, an adaptor can be used to allow flushing through the biopsy channel while still permitting biopsy forceps to be inserted (Figure 3.15b).

Occasionally during gastroscopy and duodenoscopy, insufflation causes bilious fluid to foam, obscuring the view. In minor cases, flushing with water and suctioning the fluid is effective in clearing the view. In more severe cases, it is possible to instil a dilute solution of the anti-foaming agent simethicone (see Chapter 5), or simethicone can be added to the water bottle.

Advancing through sphincters

It is generally recommended that the endoscope should be advanced only under direct vision in order to avoid iatrogenic damage. Within the GI tract, if the way forward cannot be seen, the endoscope should be withdrawn and more air insufflated until the lumen is visible. However, this general principle may have to be modified to traverse sphincters, such as the oesophageal sphincters, pylorus and ileocolic valve.

Occasionally, the sphincter is open and the lumen can be visualized as the endoscope is advanced through, but in many cases the sphincter remains closed. In such situations, red-out will occur until the endoscope tip reaches the far side of the sphincter. To pass closed sphincters, gentle pressure is applied while constantly readjusting the tip to engage it in the opening of the sphincter. As red-out occurs, there is usually the impression of aiming for the darkest area of red-out, which represents the lumen. It is also usually possible to recognize that the endoscope tip is advancing as the red-out is seen to be moving.

In the stomach, after engagement with the pylorus, suctioning air out of the stomach may collapse it over the endoscope tip, forcing the tip through the sphincter into the duodenum (see Chapter 5).

Advancing around flexures

Red-out may also occur as the endoscope advances around a flexure (e.g. proximal duodenal flexure, colonic flexures) as the tip impinges on the outer curvature of the intestinal bend. If the red-out is seen to be moving, it is generally safe to keep advancing the endoscope until it enters the next straight length of intestine and the lumen can be seen again (Figure 3.16). With this 'slide-by' technique, it is important to realize that the manoeuvre may have caused some mucosal damage, and any linear streaks of hyperaemia or haemorrhage on the mucosa of the outer curvature of the flexure that are seen as the endoscope is withdrawn back around the flexure should be recognized as artefacts (Figure 3.17).

One method that may help to avoid such artefacts is to pre-deflect the tip before the flexure is reached and rotate the endoscope on its long axis so that the next length of intestine can be entered atraumatically (Figure 3.18).

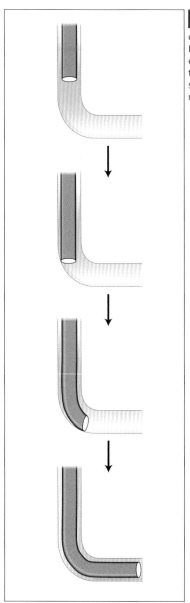

3.16 Slide-by technique for advancing the endoscope around a flexure. Red-out occurs as the endoscope tip passes along the wall until the next straight length of intestine is reached.

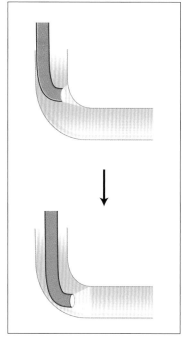

3.18 Pre-deflection of the endoscope tip before reaching a flexure allows visualization along the next length of intestine, and avoids slide-by induced artefacts.

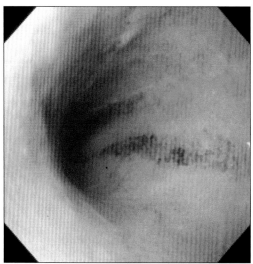

3.17 Artefactual linear haemorrhages at a small intestinal flexure caused by the tip of the endoscope scraping the mucosa of the outer curvature of the flexure.

Biopsy techniques, handling and preparation

Originally, endoscopes were devised merely to view the inside of various organ systems. Advances in technology now mean that it is also possible to collect fluid, cytology samples and biopsy specimens. Therapeutic procedures are also increasingly undertaken and are discussed in the relevant chapters.

Collection of fluid and cytology samples

Instruments used for collecting samples via the endoscope are shown in Figure 2.9.

Brush cytology

Sheathed cytology brushes are inserted via the biopsy channel of the endoscope, opened beyond the endoscope tip within the organ and rubbed against the mucosa. They are then withdrawn into the sheath before being removed from the endoscope, and smears are made and stained. They may be useful in the detection of gastric *Helicobacter* infection and for differentiation of neoplastic masses, as well as for the identification of inflammatory airway disease. Disposable brushes are preferred to avoid the risk of 'carry-over' of cells when sampling more than one site in a patient.

Fluid collection

Sterile polyethylene tubing passed through the biopsy channel can be used to collect fluid samples; for example, mucus and pus from airways or duodenal aspirates for culture. These samples should be collected before biopsy specimens are taken, to avoid contamination with blood. Bronchoalveolar lavage can also be performed using this tube, or through the biopsy channel if it has been sterilized (see Chapter 7).

Fine-needle aspiration

Fine-needle aspirates are occasionally taken with sheathed injector needles to obtain cytological samples from mucosal masses, and transbronchially for lung samples, but pinch biopsy specimens for histological and other laboratory examinations are more valuable.

Biopsy

When to perform a biopsy

Specimens should always be obtained during endoscopy, even if the mucosa appears grossly normal. The exceptions to this rule are that biopsy samples are taken from the lower respiratory tract and the oesophagus only if there are visible lesions. The risk of bleeding within the airway means that biopsy is justified only if a mass or unusual lesion is seen; brush cytology and/or broncho-alveolar lavage are usually performed instead. Biopsy of grossly normal oesophageal mucosa is not usually undertaken, as the mucosa is very tough and inadequate tissue samples are typically obtained. Oesophagitis is usually recognizable grossly, and so oesophageal biopsy is mostly reserved for rare cases of oesophageal neoplasia.

Collecting biopsy specimens

Before beginning endoscopy, biopsy forceps should be made ready and checked to ensure that the cups open easily. It is difficult to steer the endoscope and operate the forceps simultaneously, so usually the forceps are operated by an assistant, who should be familiar with the opening/closing mechanism before commencing the procedure. The thumb is inserted through the ring and the fingers operate the mechanism (Figure 3.19): opening the hand opens the cups, and closing the hand closes them. If the endoscope has passed around a number of flexures, opening the cups may be difficult as the wire is bent; straightening the insertion tube as much as possible, especially the bending section (by making sure both inner and outer wheels are in the neutral position), or extending the end of the forceps in a straight line beyond the end of the endoscope helps with opening. The operator should not squeeze too hard when closing the cups, as this does not improve the grip on the tissue but merely stretches the wire, and it may break. Reusable forceps should be well maintained and lubricated, as they are expensive to purchase. Disposable biopsy forceps need no maintenance and can be more cost-effective (although they may have to be purchased in bulk), and allow the practice to ensure a pair is always available.

When the endoscopist is taking a biopsy sample, the forceps are inserted through the cap on the disposable rubber valve on the biopsy channel (see Figure 3.9). This maintains a seal, preventing insufflated air from escaping. The forceps are inserted in repeated short lengths to avoid kinking. Similarly, forceps are removed in short lengths after biopsy, as too rapid removal can damage the biopsy channel due to the heat generated by friction. A cardinal rule to maintain the condition of the endoscope is that biopsy forceps should not be inserted while the endoscope tip is retroflexed. If the forceps are forced forward with the tip in a retroflexed position, there is a real danger of perforating the biopsy channel. This is disastrous, as a hole in the biopsy channel allows ingress of water inside the insertion tube (as much as a hole in the outer sleeve) and, importantly, may not be detected until a leakage test is performed, by which time damage will already have been caused to the fibreoptics and electronics.

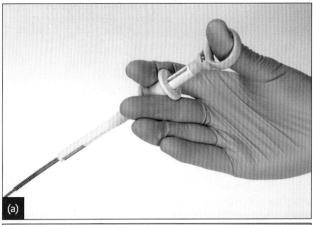

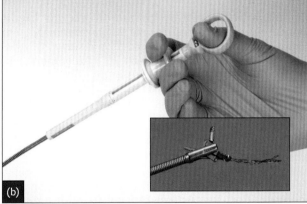

3.19 Correct (a) opening and (b) closing of biopsy forceps. The thumb is inserted in the handle and the fingers clasp the slider. As the palm of the hand is clenched, the cups close. Insert: Breakage of reusable biopsy forceps due to over-vigorous closure of the cups. Excessive pressure on the handles does not improve the quality of the biopsy specimen, but stretches and ultimately breaks the internal operating wire or the hinge mechanism.

When the endoscopist is ready to take a biopsy sample, having inserted the forceps so that they can be seen exiting the endoscope tip, they should instruct the assistant to 'open' the forceps cups and then 'close' them once the biopsy site is impacted by the open cups. The tissue is grasped by the cups, but unless it is very friable it is not actually cut off; tissue has to be avulsed by pulling the forceps sharply. With GI tissue, a tug can often be felt as the tissue is avulsed, indicating that a deep enough specimen has been obtained. If the tissue pulls away easily, either it is too superficial or it is severely diseased.

Choosing biopsy forceps

There is a vast array of types of biopsy forceps available (see Chapter 2) and it is not always clear when a particular type is preferable. *In vitro* tests suggest that forceps with a spike are better for taking samples of canine intestinal tissue (Dahan *et al.*, 2017), but experience *in vivo* does not support this conclusion.

- Oval/ellipsoid cups tend to collect more tissue than round cups, as they open wider, and the presence of a fenestration in the cup potentially reduces crush artefacts by allowing the tissue to bulge through the holes.
- The choice of smooth or serrated/alligator edges to the cups depends on the toughness of the tissue being sampled. If the tissue is very tough and the forceps tend to slip off, serrated forceps are preferred.

- Forceps containing a pin or spike can also help when sampling tough tissue, especially the oesophagus, although they may reduce the volume of tissue that is sampled.
- Rotatable forceps, where turning the handle turns the cups, can be helpful when trying to biopsy on the edge of a fold and the cups open in the wrong plane; these forceps are more robust but more expensive.

The major factors influencing the size and quality of any biopsy specimen, apart from the nature of the tissue, are the cup shape (see above), the size of the biopsy forceps (as dictated by the diameter of the biopsy channel) and the pressure exerted by the operator. There is always a compromise between the diameter of the biopsy channel (and hence the size of the biopsy specimen that can be obtained) and the external diameter of the endoscope (which is dependent on the size of the patient), but the largest channel possible in a gastroscope that is small enough to pass through the pylorus is desirable (see Chapter 2).

The harder the forceps are pushed against the tissue, the bigger the tissue sample obtained (Danesh *et al.*, 1985), and it is here that experience pays dividends. The most pressure can be exerted if the open biopsy cups are perpendicular to the tissue, and the experienced endoscopist knows how to achieve this position, and how hard to push safely. When taking biopsy specimens along a tube (e.g. the descending duodenum), 'swing-jaw' forceps help turn the open cups in towards the tissue to get a bigger bite (Figure 3.20). Techniques for taking biopsy specimens from specific areas are detailed in the relevant chapters, but in general deflation of a GI viscus before biopsy can increase the size of the sample, by reducing stretching of the mucosa and drawing the tissue closer to the biopsy cups.

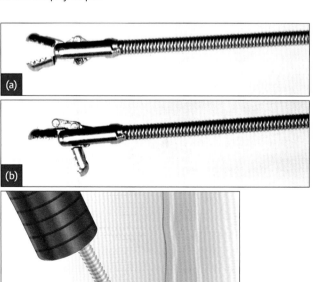

3.20 (a) As swing-jaw biopsy forceps are opened, (b) the cups tilt towards the tissue. This aids taking biopsy samples when the forceps are not perpendicular to the tissue surface. (c) Illustration showing swing-jaw forceps in use.
(c, Redrawn after Haycock *et al.* (2014))

Processing biopsy specimens

There are several ways of dealing with the biopsy specimen when the forceps have been withdrawn from the endoscope. The cups can simply be immersed in 10% formalin, opened and agitated, releasing the tissue into the pot; the forceps are then rinsed in water before being reinserted into the endoscope to take another specimen. Alternatively, the biopsy forceps can be agitated in saline, and the specimens decanted into formalin later; while this is quicker, as the forceps do not need to be rinsed, autolysis of the biopsy samples may occur. As a third option, the specimen can be carefully removed from the cups with a fine needle and oriented before fixation. The tissue can then be laid on card or even slices of dehydrated cucumber, but tissue cassettes with a foam insert (Figure 3.21) are easiest to use (Ruiz *et al.*, 2016).

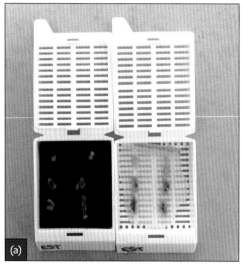

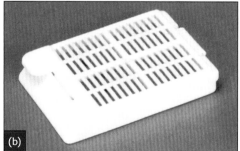

3.21 Tissue cassette with a foam insert for collecting biopsy specimens before fixation in formalin and processing. (a) Open cassette with foam insert (left) and dehydrated cucumber slice (right) each with six biopsy samples. (b) The cassette is closed before being placed in 10% formalin.
(a, courtesy of Guillaume Ruiz)

The needle-and-cassette method has the advantage that histological processing is more efficient; samples are not lost and tissue is not sectioned in the wrong plane. However, the method is tedious and the sample can become macerated as it is manipulated by the needle. Proponents of the immersion method argue that it is much quicker and that many more specimens can be collected in the same time, so that it does not matter if some are lost or wasted in processing.

It is rare to take more than two or three specimens from the respiratory tract, but at least six and preferably nearer 12 samples should be collected from each region of the GI tract examined (Willard *et al.*, 2008), with the exception of the oesophagus unless there are visible lesions (see above). This number is necessary because some specimens may be too small, some may fragment or be lost in processing, and some may be sectioned in the wrong plane (Figure 3.22).

Biopsy specimens are usually processed for routine histology, but specimens can also be used for electron microscopy, immunohistochemistry, fluorescence *in situ* hybridization (FISH), PCR for antigen receptor rearrangement (PARR) and biochemical analysis. Cytological examination of squash preparations may be worthwhile if trying to reach an early presumptive diagnosis of lymphoma (Maeda *et al.*, 2017).

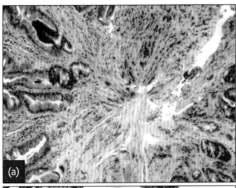
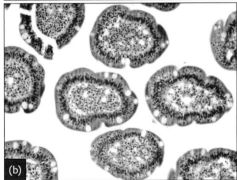
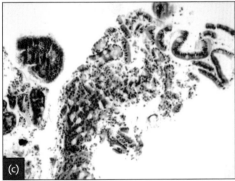

3.22 Sections of endoscopic biopsy samples demonstrating common artefacts. (a) Crush artefact with loss of discernible tissue and cellular structure. (b) Cross-sections of isolated villi when tissue is not oriented in a perpendicular fashion. (c) Fragmentation of a small tissue biopsy sample. Haematoxylin and eosin-stained sections. (Reproduced from the BSAVA *Manual of Canine and Feline Gastroenterology, 3rd edn*)

Fine-needle techniques

Injector needles can be passed atraumatically down the accessory/biopsy channel of the endoscope when sheathed, and then unsheathed at the endoscope tip. These needles are used primarily in human endoscopy to inject sclerosant into oesophageal varices (acquired shunts in individuals with portal hypertension) to stop bleeding. In veterinary endoscopy, they are occasionally

used to inject adrenaline into bleeding ulcers, or triamcinolone into oesophageal strictures before balloon dilation, to try to prevent re-stricturing (see Chapter 4). They can also be used to take fine-needle aspirates from mass lesions. In addition, they may be used to inject saline into the submucosa of the GI tract below a small lesion to elevate it, allowing an excisional biopsy to be taken with a polypectomy snare.

Endoscopic procedures

Details of how to perform various endoscopic procedures are described in the relevant chapters. These procedures include:

- Foreign body removal
- Feeding tube placement
- Stricture dilation
- Needle injection
- Polypectomy.

For all of these procedures, the technique depends on being able to operate the endoscope as described above, and having a large enough biopsy/accessory channel to accommodate the necessary instruments. More complex endoscopic procedures performed in human patients often require dual-channel interventional endoscopes, which are too large in diameter to be used in dogs and cats.

Image recording and reporting

There are a variety of ways of recording the endoscopic image, as detailed in Chapter 2. For good medical records it is advisable to try to record any lesions found during endoscopy, in addition to taking biopsy specimens. It is also sometimes suggested that either the whole procedure or at least images of all landmarks be recorded, to be able to prove that a full examination was performed in case of future litigation. When using a video-endoscope, the simplest and cheapest option is to connect a standard commercial digital recorder/player, such as a hard disc/DVD recorder or smartphone, to the video output of the endoscopy processor to record the whole procedure.

All endoscopic investigations should be accompanied by a written report. Standardized proforma reports have been produced by the World Small Animal Veterinary Association GI Standardization Group and can be downloaded free of charge (see also Chapter 5). Alternatively, there are software packages, such as iCAP® (ESS Inc.), that can produce a written report incorporating recorded images.

References and further reading

Dahan J, Semin MO, Monton C *et al.* (2017) Comparison of routinely used intestinal biopsy forceps in dogs: an *ex vivo* histopathological approach. *Journal of Small Animal Practice* **58**, 162–167

Danesh BJZ, Burke M, Newman J *et al.* (1985) Comparison of weight, depth, and diagnostic adequacy of specimens obtained with 16 different biopsy forceps designed for upper gastrointestinal endoscopy. *Gut* **26**, 227–231

Hall EJ, Williams DA and Kathrani A (2020) BSAVA Manual of Canine and Feline Gastroenterology, 3rd edn. BSAVA Publications, Gloucester

Haycock A, Cohen J, Saunders B, Cotton PB and Williams CB (2014) *Cotton and Williams' Practical Gastrointestinal Endoscopy: The Fundamentals, 7th edn.* Wiley Blackwell, Oxford

Irom S, Sherding R, Johnson S and Stromberg P (2014) Gastrointestinal perforation associated with endoscopy in cats and dogs. *Journal of the American Animal Hospital Association* **50**, 322–329

Leib MS, Baechtel MS and Monroe WE (2004) Complications associated with 355 flexible colonoscopic procedures in dogs. *Journal of Veterinary Internal Medicine* **18**, 642–646

Maeda S, Tsuboi M, Sakai K *et al.* (2017) Endoscopic cytology for the diagnosis of chronic enteritis and intestinal lymphoma in dogs. *Veterinary Pathology* **54**, 595–604

RCVS (2014) Day One Competences; updated March 2014. Available from https://www.rcvs.org.uk/document-library/day-one-competences/

Ruiz G, Reyes-Gomez E, Hall EJ and Freiche V (2016) Comparison of 3 handling techniques for endoscopic gastric and duodenal biopsies: a prospective study in dogs. *Journal of Veterinary Internal Medicine* **30**, 1014–1021

Tams T and Rawlings C (2010) *Small Animal Endoscopy, 3rd edn.* Mosby, St. Louis

Willard M (2020) Endoscopy. In: *BSAVA Manual of Canine and Feline Gastroenterology, 3rd edn.*, ed. EJ Hall, DA Williams and AA Kathrani, pp. 25–30. BSAVA Publications, Gloucester

Willard MD, Mansell J, Fosgate GT *et al.* (2008) Effect of sample quality on the sensitivity of endoscopic biopsy for detecting gastric and duodenal lesions in dogs and cats. *Journal of Veterinary Internal Medicine* **22**, 1084–1089

Video extras

- **Video 3.1** **Escape of air bubbles during a leakage test of an endoscope**
- **Video 3.2** **Single- and two-handed manipulation of steering wheels**
- **Video 3.3** **Steering by tip deflection and torquing**

Access via QR code or: bsavalibrary.com/endoscopy2e_3

Chapter 4

Flexible endoscopy: oesophagoscopy

David Twedt

Introduction

Oesophagoscopy refers to the examination of the lumen and mucosal lining of the oesophagus using an endoscope. Oesophagoscopy usually involves the use of flexible gastro-intestinal (GI) endoscopes; however, rigid oesophageal endoscopes are sometimes used for foreign body removal. Endoscopy is the best minimally invasive method for evaluating the oesophagus for inflammatory disease, strictures, foreign bodies and neoplasia, while contrast fluoroscopy provides the best means for evaluating oesophageal motility disorders. Oesophagoscopy also facilitates various thera-peutic interventions, such as dilation of oesophageal stric-tures and removal of foreign bodies.

Instrumentation

Flexible endoscopes

Oesophagoscopy is performed primarily using flexible GI endoscopes. Endoscopes are discussed in detail in Chapter 2. The newer flexible video-endoscopes, whether designed for veterinary or human medicine, are ideal for oesophageal evaluation because of their excellent optics and distal tip manoeuvrability. GI endoscopes between 5.5 and 9 mm in diameter with an insertion tube length of 110 cm are a suitable size for evaluating the oesophagus of most dogs and cats. Longer endoscopes up to 140 cm are required for endoscopic evaluation of the duodenum in large-breed dogs. Ideally, the endoscope should have four-way distal tip deflection, a water/air channel and a suction/biopsy channel. Biopsy channels range from 2 to 2.8 mm in diameter and larger diameter biopsy channels are optimal for accommodating larger instruments. The endoscope should have a distal tip deflection in one plane to 210 degrees to permit examination of the lower oesophageal sphincter (LOS), also termed the gastro-oesophageal sphincter, from the gastric lumen.

Accessory instruments that are passed through the biopsy channel include biopsy forceps, cytology brushes, various types of foreign body retrieval instruments, baskets, snares, suction tubes, balloon catheters and injection needles (see Chapter 2). A number of different types of biopsy forceps are available, but the author pre-fers the serrated-edge 'alligator-type' forceps for mucosal biopsy. Various electrocautery and laser fibres can also be used in conjunction with flexible endoscopy.

Rigid endoscopes

Rigid endoscopes are either solid rods containing a series of lenses and fibreoptics or simply rigid hollow tubes of various lengths and diameters. The rigid tubes are useful for the removal of large oesophageal foreign bodies (discussed below). Human rigid sigmoidoscopes used for colonoscopy in both humans and dogs, can also be used for oesophagoscopy. Paediatric sigmoidoscopes are approximately 12 mm in diameter, while adult sigmoido-scopes are approximately 25 mm in diameter; both are equipped with a light source and the means for insufflation of the oesophageal lumen. They also come with a remov-able internal obturator to ease passage into the proximal oesophagus. Vintage human rigid hollow oesophageal endoscopes, if available, can also be used. The limiting factor on the diameter of a rigid endoscope is the ability to pass the endoscope through the pharynx into the proximal oesophagus. Once entry into the cervical oesophagus is achieved, the oesophagus will dilate to accommodate the rigid endoscope.

Hollow rigid endoscopes can also be fabricated from plastic or polypropylene plumbing pipes of various dia-meters for use in oesophagoscopy. When using these, either a flexible endoscope can be passed through the centre of the tube or an external light source used for illu-mination. The rigid endoscope can also serve as a protec-tive 'overtube' guard when removing large sharp foreign bodies. Large rigid grasping forceps can be passed through the centre of the tube to grasp and retrieve oesophageal foreign bodies by pulling them up to or into the tube (see Foreign bodies, below).

Indications

Oesophagoscopy is used for evaluating patients sus-pected of having oesophageal disease. Clinical signs relat-ing to the oesophagus, such as regurgitation, dysphagia, odontophagia (painful swallowing), salivation or anorexia, and/or abnormal radiographic findings involving the oeso-phagus are the primary indications for endoscopy. Often, signs associated with upper GI disease overlap and could reflect disease involving more than one region of the upper GI tract. Endoscopy makes it possible to evaluate not only the oesophagus but also the stomach and proxi-mal small intestine, thus helping to localize the cause of clinical signs.

Oesophagoscopy is indicated when a patient has a suspected oesophageal foreign body, to confirm its location, assess the extent of oesophageal damage and facilitate endoscopic removal. Oesophagoscopy is also the best means for evaluation, diagnosis and biopsy of suspected inflammatory oesophageal disease. In most cases reflux oesophagitis is diagnosed by observing distal oesophageal inflammation, often in conjunction with an open LOS or the presence of a sliding hiatal hernia. Radiographic evidence of oesophageal neoplasia, perioesophageal mass, diverticulum or hiatal hernia are indications for endoscopy to confirm the diagnosis. Oesophagoscopy, however, has limited usefulness for the diagnosis of oesophageal motility disorders.

Contraindications

The major contraindication of oesophagoscopy is the unstable patient that is unable to undergo general anaesthesia. Patients with severe aspiration pneumonia or a pneumothorax secondary to oesophageal perforation would also not be suitable for endoscopy. Since insufflation is required during endoscopy, oesophageal perforation could result in a serious tension pneumothorax, and so an animal with any evidence of oesophageal perforation should not undergo oesophagoscopy. Animals with megaoesophagus are always at risk for secondary aspiration pneumonia, and the value of the information to be gained from oesophagoscopy should be seriously considered before performing the procedure in patients with oesophageal motility disorders.

Patient preparation

Usually, food is withheld from the patient for 12 hours before oesophagoscopy because of the potential for aspiration while the patient is under anaesthesia for the procedure. In patients with oesophageal motility disorders it may take considerable time for the oesophagus to empty (or it may not empty fully), and the risk associated with the procedure must be carefully weighed against the information likely to be obtained. If a barium contrast study of the oesophagus has been performed the endoscopy should be delayed for 6–24 hours to allow the barium to leave the oesophagus. Repeat radiographs are advised before the endoscopic procedure to check that the oesophagus is clear of contrast agent. Barium will hinder mucosal evaluation and tends to plug the suction channel of the endoscope.

One exception to the rule to allow sufficient time for the oesophagus to clear is an oesophageal foreign body. Foreign bodies are considered emergency conditions and should be removed as soon as possible because of the risk of severe mucosal damage or oesophageal perforation. Routine thoracic radiographs should be taken before anaesthesia to confirm the location of a previously identified foreign body.

Premedication and anaesthesia

Premedication is used to improve induction of anaesthesia and recovery. However, some narcotics increase pyloric tone and inhibit intubation. In dogs, acepromazine alone, or in combination with butorphanol, has minimal effect on pyloric tone. For cats, acepropazine may be supplemented with low dose midazolam or ketamine. The author will also administer the antiemetic maropitant to prevent vomiting during the pre- and post-anaesthetic period. Following induction, an endotracheal tube is placed and volatile anaesthesia administered. Patients with oesophageal disease should always have an endotracheal tube placed to prevent aspiration during anaesthesia and endoscopy. The endotracheal tube should be secured to the mandible using roller gauze. The endotracheal tube should not be tied to the maxilla as this will hinder passage of the endoscope into the pharynx. A mouth speculum/gag should always be placed before endoscopy to prevent damage to the endoscope. Care should be taken not to over-expand the mouth with excessive pressure from the mouth speculum/gag. In cats, over-expansion of the speculum/gag can result in compression of the maxillary artery, leading to cerebral ischaemia and blindness.

Patient positioning

For routine oesophagoscopy the patient is placed in left lateral recumbency. This is the position used for all routine upper GI endoscopy for ease of pyloric entry. However, the patient can be moved into other positions to facilitate proper examination of the oesophagus.

Procedure

Before beginning oesophagoscopy, the endoscopist should ensure that the endoscope is in working order, with light, air/water and suction functioning properly. All anticipated endoscopic instruments to be used should also be readily available and in good working order. When the patient is at an adequate level of anaesthesia, the endotracheal tube is in place with the cuff inflated and a mouth speculum/gag is in place, endoscopy can begin.

The endoscope tip is lubricated with a water-based lubricant. With the animal's head and neck extended, the insertion tube of the endoscope is placed into the pharynx and directed dorsal to the larynx. The endoscope will generally pass easily through the upper oesophageal sphincter into the proximal cervical oesophagus. Usually the sphincter is not visualized upon entry, and is best evaluated by slowly withdrawing the endoscope back from the cervical oesophagus and through the sphincter. If the endoscope meets resistance during passage through the pharynx it is likely that the tip is lodged in the piriform recesses located on either side of the larynx. If this occurs, simply withdrawing and re-advancing the endoscope tip generally allows it to enter the cervical oesophagus.

Once within the cervical oesophagus, either the lumen is visualized or, more likely, the view is totally white (called a 'white-out'), resulting from the endoscope tip being in direct contact with the oesophageal mucosa. At this point, insufflation of the oesophagus with air should begin, and the oesophageal lumen should soon come into view. Occasionally, following adequate insufflation, the oesophageal lumen still cannot be identified because the insufflated air is leaking back around the endoscope into the pharynx. If this occurs, an assistant should apply hand pressure around the patient's neck caudal to the larynx to form an external seal between the endoscope and the oesophagus. As the oesophageal lumen becomes insufflated with air the endoscopist should begin to see the imprint of the trachea against the wall of the cervical oesophagus. Once the lumen is in view, the endoscope is slowly advanced, adjusting the distal tip to visualize the entire lumen. Usually there is a slight dip in the lumen as the endoscope passes through the thoracic inlet. Occasionally the brachiocephalic artery or one of its branches can be observed pulsating against the oesophagus at the level of the thoracic inlet. Moving distally into the thoracic oesophagus, imprints of the trachea and its rings are observed extending to the level of the tracheal bifurcation. At the heart base, pulsations of the aorta against the oesophageal wall are observed.

Beyond the heart base is the caudal oesophagus. With the oesophagus insufflated, the lumen ends at the LOS. The distal end of the oesophagus passes obliquely through the diaphragm in an opening referred to as the oesophageal hiatus. The LOS is usually closed and appears as a slightly bulging slit located at the end of the oesophageal lumen. The sphincter is a confluence of many small radial folds configured in a rosette pattern. It is not located in the centre of the oesophageal lumen, but rather is slightly offset to the side. Occasionally the LOS may be open, and this is not necessarily considered abnormal. Due to the offset position of the LOS, passage through the sphincter can sometimes be difficult for the novice endoscopist. To advance the endoscope tip through a closed sphincter with the patient in left lateral recumbency, the endoscope tip is directed approximately 30 degrees to the left and slightly upward, and then slowly advanced forward through the lumen. If resistance is met, then the endoscope tip is most likely adjacent to the sphincter opening, and should be withdrawn and re-advanced.

As the endoscope enters the stomach, the mucosa is much redder than the oesophageal mucosa and rugal folds of the stomach can often be observed. Sometimes the endoscopist encounters a complete 'red-out' resulting from the endoscope tip being in direct contact with the fundic mucosa. If this occurs, the endoscope tip should be withdrawn back away from the mucosa and the gastric lumen insufflated. Then, on directing the endoscope tip to the right, the lumen should come into view. It is advisable to examine the stomach and the proximal duodenum, since upper GI signs can often overlap. See Chapter 5 for a description of endoscopy of the upper GI tract.

Before withdrawing the endoscope back into the oesophagus, the LOS should be examined from the gastric side. The gastric lumen is insufflated and when the rugal folds are almost flattened a 'J' manoeuvre is performed to visualize the LOS. This manoeuvre involves rotating the up/down lever to maximal upward deflection, putting the distal tip into a 'J' configuration, enabling the operator to look back at the LOS from the gastric side. The sphincter is generally fairly snug around the insertion tube. After the sphincter has been evaluated, the distal tip is returned to the 'neutral' (straight) position and the endoscope is withdrawn. As the endoscope is withdrawn through the oesophagus the entire luminal mucosa should be re-examined.

At this point biopsies can be performed if indicated. Oesophageal biopsies are not generally required for the investigation of most oesophageal disorders, and the diagnosis of oesophagitis is often made on the basis of visual inspection of the mucosa. It is difficult to obtain endoscopic mucosal biopsy samples, particularly if the mucosa is normal. This is because the mucosa, consisting of stratified squamous epithelium, is very tough and the forceps tend to slide down the mucosa. It is easier to obtain biopsy samples from mass lesions protruding into the lumen or areas of erosion. The operator should try to avoid

sampling in the middle of ulcerated or necrotic areas. Generally, 6–12 samples should be obtained. Brush cytology may be helpful to diagnose neoplasia or mucosal abnormalities such as yeast (candidiasis) or fungal infections. A guarded cytology brush is generally used for this purpose.

Before the endoscope is fully withdrawn, excess air should be removed from the oesophagus. It is not unusual to identify fluid in the oesophagus from gastric reflux, even in normal patients. All luminal fluid should be removed using suction because refluxed gastric acid or bile can damage the oesophageal mucosa. Following aspiration of any oesophageal fluid, the author will often lavage the oesophagus through the suction channel of the endoscope using a 2% sodium bicarbonate solution to neutralize acid reflux. Usually 20–60 ml are infused into the lumen and then suctioned out. Following a routine diagnostic oesophagoscopy there are generally no specific post-endoscopic medications or pain management required.

Normal findings

The canine oesophagus consists of striated muscle and the mucosa consists of stratified squamous epithelium. Endoscopically, the mucosa appears as a seashell-white or pale pink colour with linear longitudinal folds that will flatten as the lumen is insufflated with air. The mucosa glistens from swallowed saliva and mucus (Figure 4.1). There should be little fluid within the lumen other than a small amount of swallowed saliva. The presence of food, considerable fluid or bile is abnormal. Occasionally a peristaltic contraction can be observed coursing the length of the oesophagus, especially if the patient is at a light plane of anaesthesia. In heavily pigmented dogs (i.e. those with black tongues) there may also be patches of black-pigmented oesophageal mucosa. The normal mucosa is very tough and resistant to trauma from the endoscope.

The proximal two-thirds of the feline oesophagus is skeletal muscle and the distal third consists of smooth muscle. The superficial submucosal blood vessels are normally very prominent throughout the length of the oesophagus in the cat (Figure 4.2); in contrast, in the dog there are few if any such vessels present. Distal to the base of the heart, where the skeletal muscle transitions to smooth muscle in the cat, there are many circumferential mucosal folds forming prominent annular ridges, described by radiologists as a 'herringbone' pattern observed on contrast oesophagograms.

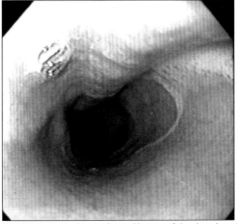

4.1 Normal oesophageal lumen of the dog showing imprints of the trachea in the 12 o'clock position.

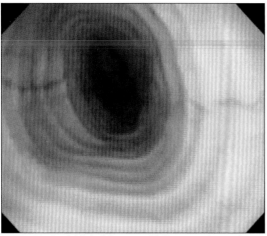

4.2 Distal third of the normal feline oesophagus showing linear striations and submucosal blood vessels.

Within the LOS is the demarcation between the pale pink oesophageal mucosa and the red gastric mucosa. In humans, this demarcation is called the Z-line. When the sphincter is open the gastric mucosa can be seen within the sphincter lumen (Figure 4.3). In some patients the Z-line is very obvious and gastric mucosa can be seen in the closed sphincter; this should not be confused with inflammation of the LOS or oesophagitis.

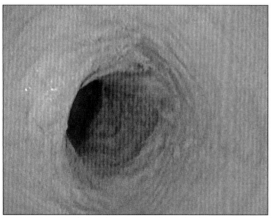

4.3 Normal open lower oesophageal sphincter showing the Z-line, a demarcation between the oesophageal mucosa and the redder gastric mucosa.

Pathological conditions

Figure 4.4 lists the more common oesophageal conditions that can be identified with endoscopy. The endoscopic diagnosis is aided by clinical findings, routine thoracic radiographs and contrast fluoroscopy. The following sections will describe specific oesophageal abnormalities and their characteristic endoscopic findings.

- Oesophagitis/reflux oesophagitis
- Hiatal hernia
- Gastro-oesophageal intussusception
- Motility disorders
- Vascular ring anomalies
- External oesophageal compression
- Neoplasia/granuloma
- Oesophageal diverticula
- Foreign bodies
- Strictures

4.4 Common oesophageal abnormalities.

Oesophagitis/reflux oesophagitis

The diagnosis of oesophagitis is made endoscopically based on the visual appearance of the mucosa. Oesophageal mucosal biopsies are rarely performed due to the difficulty in collecting samples using endoscopic biopsy forceps. The mucosa in oesophagitis may appear reddened, have an irregular surface or be haemorrhagic, with erosions or ulceration (Figure 4.5). The mucosa is often quite friable and contact with the endoscope can cause iatrogenic superficial erosions or ulceration. Oesophagitis can involve the entire length of the oesophagus, as may be seen in animals that have ingested a caustic substance, or can be more focal, as can occur secondary to an oesophageal foreign body. If the cause of the oesophagitis is not readily apparent, attempts to perform mucosal biopsies or brush cytology should be made to rule out infectious or neoplastic aetiologies.

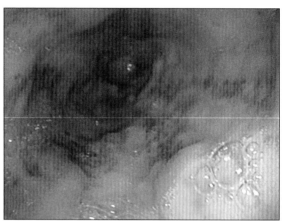

4.5 Dog with severe erosive oesophagitis of unknown aetiology. Examination of oesophageal biopsy samples showed acute inflammation.

Reflux oesophagitis is quite common. It is characterized by oesophagitis localized to the distal oesophagus extending cranial from the LOS, due to reflux of gastric contents (Figure 4.6). The severity of the oesophagitis depends on the frequency, character and duration of contact of the refluxed gastric material. Frequently, the LOS is open and the endoscopist might observe gastric fluid or food within the oesophageal lumen. Luminal fluid should always be aspirated, followed by lavage, as retention of refluxed acid will worsen the oesophagitis. The endoscopist should not misinterpret the normal red gastric mucosa located within

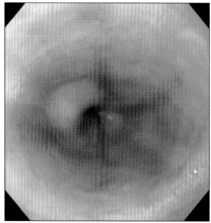

4.6 Reflux oesophagitis in a young French Bulldog showing inflammatory streaks extending up the oesophagus from the open lower oesophageal sphincter. Oesophagitis resolved following management of the dog's upper airway disease.

the LOS abutting the oesophageal mucosa (the Z-line) as oesophageal mucosal ulceration or oesophagitis. If distal oesophagitis suggestive of reflux oesophagitis is observed, the patient should always be evaluated for a hiatal hernia, a frequent cause of reflux oesophagitis (see below). Both reflux oesophagitis and hiatal hernias commonly occur in brachycephalic breeds of dog.

Hiatal hernia

A hiatal hernia is the herniation of a portion of the stomach through an abnormally large oesophageal hiatus in the diaphragm. There are two basic types of hiatal hernias: sliding and paraoesophageal. Sliding hiatal hernias are by far the more common, and occur when the LOS and proximal stomach slide through the diaphragm into the thoracic mediastinum. With loss of sphincter competence, reflux oesophagitis occurs. A paraoesophageal hernia occurs when a portion of the stomach invaginates through the oesophageal hiatus adjacent to the oesophagus. In this situation the LOS remains in the abdominal cavity and the endoscopist may note extrinsic compression on the distal oesophagus. With both types of hiatal hernia the stomach may intermittently slide through the oesophageal hiatus and so the herniation is not always observed on routine or contrast radiographs.

The first endoscopic evidence of a sliding hiatal hernia is reflux oesophagitis with an open LOS. Just distal to the sphincter the endoscopist may observe imprints of the oesophageal hiatus encircling the very proximal cardia portion of the stomach where it passes through the diaphragm. The endoscope should be passed into the stomach and, with the gastric lumen maximally insufflated, the endoscope tip is retroflexed ('J' manoeuvre) to examine the appearance of the LOS from the gastric side (Figure 4.7). This manoeuvre allows evaluation of the

oesophageal hiatus of the diaphragm along with assessment of whether there is axial displacement of the stomach through the diaphragm. The endoscopist should be able to see imprints of the oesophageal hiatus against the fundic gastric mucosa (Video 4.1).

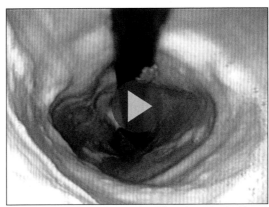

Video 4.1 The endoscope in a j-flexed position looking at the lower oesophageal sphincter (abnormally dilated) in a patient presenting with chronic vomiting. A case of sliding hiatal hernia.

Gastro-oesophageal intussusception

Gastro-oesophageal intussusception is a rare condition described in young larger breed dogs. Affected animals show acute vomiting and are usually presented in acute distress from oesophageal obstruction. Radiographically, there is a caudal mediastinal mass and dilatation of the oesophageal lumen with gas and fluid. On endoscopic examination, characteristic findings are hyperaemic gastric rugal folds filling the distal oesophageal lumen (Figure 4.8). It is usually not possible to pass the endoscope around the rugal folds or identify the LOS. On rare occasions it may be possible to pass a gastric tube adjacent to the endoscope to manually push the stomach back into the abdominal cavity. The endoscope itself should not be used to attempt to reduce the intussusception because of the risk of causing damage to the endoscope. Generally, abdominal surgery is required to reduce the intussuscepted stomach.

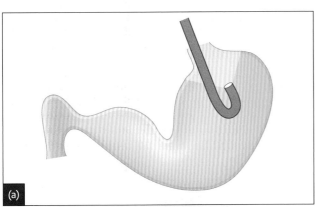
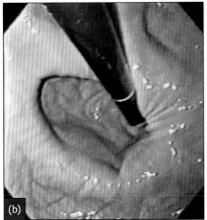

4.7 (a) Withdrawal of the retroflexed endoscope in the 'J' position within the stomach allows visualization of the cardia. (b) When the stomach is distended with air and the endoscope is in the 'J' position, the imprint of the oesophageal hiatus is observed, with the fundic portion of the stomach protruding through the oesophageal hiatus.

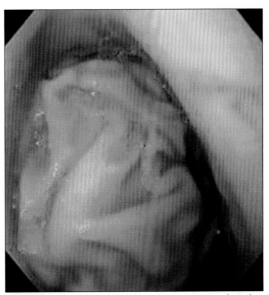

4.8 Gastro-oesophageal intussusception in a dog, showing the rugal folds of the stomach obstructing the oesophageal lumen. The dog required abdominal surgery to reduce the intussusception.

Motility disorders

Oesophageal motility disorders such as idiopathic mega-oesophagus, myasthenia gravis, hypoadrenocorticism and myopathies are generally diagnosed using radiography and/or fluoroscopy. There is rarely a need for endoscopy except to rule out inflammatory or obstructive disorders. In dogs, megaoesophagus is characterized by a large dilated aperistaltic oesophagus. Since insufflation is required during endoscopy, it is often difficult to determine whether the oesophagus is dilated as a result of endoscopic insufflation or secondary to a primary motility disorder. Characteristic endoscopic findings of mega-oesophagus include abnormal retention of food and fluid within the lumen of the oesophagus. The oesophageal lumen may also be obviously quite dilated compared with the appearance of a normal oesophagus following insufflation. Attempts should be made to aspirate the oesophageal contents, followed by lavage. Care should be taken if there is a considerable amount of food, sand or grit, because of the risk of clogging the suction channel of the endoscope. It may be better to use a larger diameter suction tube, if available, to remove the material. The greatest danger in endoscopy of a patient with mega-oesophagus is aspiration. There is often a secondary oesophagitis with hyperaemia and erosions of the mucosa resulting from retention of ingesta. The mucosa may appear thin and submucosal blood vessels may be prominent. The LOS is normal in almost all cases.

Oesophageal achalasia, a very rare condition described in dogs, refers to a disorder in which the LOS fails to relax for the passage of a food bolus into the stomach, resulting in an obstructive oesophageal dilatation. Diagnosis requires a barium swallow study coupled with high-resolution oesophageal manometry. On endoscopic examination, it may be difficult to pass the endoscope through the LOS. The two most commonly used endoscopic interventions for achalasia are balloon dilation of the LOS or injection of botulinum toxin directly into the sphincter to paralyse the muscle. However, the treatment of choice is surgical myotomy of the sphincter.

Vascular ring anomalies

A vascular ring anomaly results from malformation of one of the great vessels that entraps the oesophagus at the level of the base of the heart and causes clinical signs of oesophageal obstruction. The diagnosis of a vascular ring anomaly is generally made in young animals that show chronic regurgitation shortly following weaning. Barium contrast radiographs typically demonstrate oesophageal dilatation cranial to the heart base and narrowing at the level of the heart base. Endoscopy is helpful in confirming the diagnosis of extraluminal compression of the oesophagus by large blood vessels (Figure 4.9). At the level of the oesophageal entrapment, pulsation of the aorta against the oesophageal wall can be seen. Cranial to the vascular ring anomaly, the oesophagus is often quite dilated, with retention of food or fluid, and there is often a secondary oesophagitis. In some cases, it may be difficult to pass the endoscope through the constriction into the distal oesophagus. Endoscopy may also help the surgeon to determine the best surgical approach for a particular case, and to evaluate the oesophagus postoperatively.

Neoplasia

Oesophageal neoplasia is uncommon, accounting for less than 0.5% of all cancers diagnosed in dogs and cats.

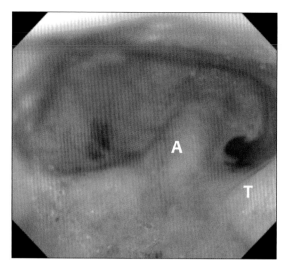

4.9 Endoscopic view of a persistent right aortic arch entrapping the oesophagus at the base of the heart between the trachea (T) and the aorta (A). The oesophagus is dilated cranial to the entrapment.

Neoplasia may arise either as primarily oesophageal in origin or as a perioesophageal mass or metastatic oesophageal disease. Leiomyomas are the most common benign tumours of the oesophagus. They arise from smooth muscle located in the LOS and may be an incidental finding unless they are large enough to obstruct the oesophageal lumen (Figure 4.10). Oesophageal leiomyomas are characterized as smooth round protrusions into the oesophageal lumen. Leiomyomas are submucosal and if the mucosa over the mass is grasped with biopsy forceps the mucosa will easily slide over the mass, confirming its submucosal location. Due to the submucosal location of these tumours, it is not possible to perform endoscopic biopsies. In some cases, it may be easier to delineate a leiomyoma from the gastric side using the 'J' manoeuvre.

Squamous cell carcinoma is the most common primary malignant oesophageal neoplasm in cats and can also occur in dogs. Most are located in the thoracic oesophagus. Carcinomas are usually multilobulated and occasionally ulcerated (Figure 4.11). Endoscopic biopsies are generally diagnostic. Other primary tumours and metastatic neoplasia may also occur.

Granulomas associated with the nematode parasite *Spirocerca lupi* appear as variably sized broad-based smooth mucosal protrusions into the lumen in the distal oesophagus. There is usually a small opening through the

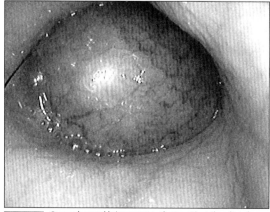

4.10 Oesophageal leiomyoma obstructing the distal oesophagus in a dog. Leiomyomas are characterized as a smooth submucosal mass protruding into the oesophageal lumen.

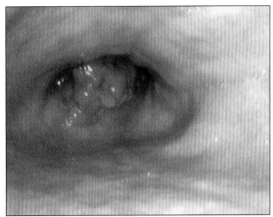

4.11 A multilobed oesophageal carcinoma in the distal oesophagus, obstructing the oesophageal lumen.

mucosa and sometimes the parasite can be seen projecting into the lumen. The granulomas can transform into malignant neoplasia.

Oesophageal diverticula

Pulsion diverticula are rare sac-like dilatations or outpouchings of tissues below the mucosa through one or more layers of the oesophageal wall (Figure 4.12). They generally result from damage to the mucosal wall caused by a foreign body or associated with oesophageal stricture formation, or may develop following stricture dilation. Constant luminal pulsion forces are responsible for the development of the diverticulum. Small diverticula may not cause clinical signs, while large ones usually result in significant clinical signs associated with eating, with accumulation of food or liquid within the diverticulum causing postprandial dyspepsia, regurgitation or anorexia. In some cases, the opening into the diverticulum can be small but the diverticulum itself may be quite large. If the diverticular opening is large enough, the endoscope can sometimes enter the pouch. Some diverticula may progress to severe oesophageal food impaction and even perforation, so care should be taken when endoscopically evaluating a diverticulum. Traction diverticula are rare and occur secondary to perioesophageal inflammation and fibrous contraction pulling out the oesophageal wall. All layers of the oesophagus are involved in the diverticulum.

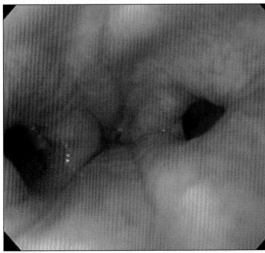

4.12 Endoscopic view of two oesophageal diverticula at 3 and 9 o'clock in the distal oesophagus that developed secondary to an oesophageal foreign body (a bone). The diverticula were closed surgically.

Foreign bodies

Oesophageal foreign bodies are one of the most common oesophageal disorders in dogs and cats. In dogs, the most common foreign bodies are bones. Pins, needles, plastic objects, balls, toys, fishhooks and trichobezoars are examples of other types of foreign body that are sometimes encountered.

The key to endoscopic removal of an oesophageal foreign body is having the proper endoscopic equipment and attempting prompt removal as soon as the foreign body is identified. It is said that 'the sun should never set on an oesophageal foreign body', as delay in removal may lead to serious oesophageal wall damage or even perforation. With time, foreign bodies can cause pressure necrosis at contact points within the oesophagus, seating them tightly in the wall and making them more difficult to remove. Routine thoracic radiographs should always be taken before endoscopy to confirm the position of the foreign body and to look for evidence of oesophageal wall perforation.

The basic equipment required for endoscopic foreign body removal includes various endoscopic grasping forceps (three- or four-pronged, rat-toothed or alligator-type), baskets or snares. The various endoscopic grasping forceps are often too small and fragile to remove large foreign bodies seated in the oesophagus. Baskets or snares will often get a stronger hold on the foreign body, but it can be difficult to snare the foreign body. The author frequently uses a rigid hollow endoscope in conjunction with large rigid graspers to remove large bones and other large foreign bodies (Figure 4.13).

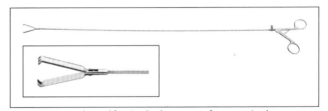

4.13 Oesophageal foreign body graspers for removing large bone-type foreign bodies. The graspers can be passed either adjacent to the endoscope or through a large overtube.
(© Karl Storz SE & Co. KG)

With a tight endotracheal tube cuff and mouth speculum/gag in place, the endoscope is advanced into the cervical oesophagus and passed to the level of the foreign body. If the foreign body is obstructing the oesophageal lumen, there is often considerable saliva and sometimes ingesta proximal to the obstruction; this material must be suctioned, followed by lavage, to allow assessment of the foreign body and the amount of oesophageal wall trauma. Care should be taken not to over-insufflate the oesophagus because of the risk of oesophageal perforation or over-distension of the stomach if the endoscope cannot be advanced past the foreign body to deflate stomach distended with air. The clinician should always be prepared to deal with a tension pneumothorax if one should occur during insufflation as the result of oesophageal perforation.

Once the foreign body has been assessed, a decision can be made on the method of removal. The small diameter of the instrument port in most flexible gastroscopes limits the size of the grasping instruments that can be used. Removal of large foreign bodies, such as bones, often requires a large rigid hollow endoscope along with large pronged grasping forceps. The advantage of using a rigid endoscope is that it mechanically dilates the oesophagus, and the endoscopist can pass larger sized grasping forceps through the centre of the endoscope to retrieve the foreign body. If a rigid tube of sufficient diameter is used, the endoscopist may be able to pass an endoscope through it along with the grasping forceps, to allow better visualization. It is possible to construct a rigid endoscope using appropriately-sized plastic or polypropylene plumbing pipes for use in removing large foreign bodies.

Bones that have remained in the oesophagus for a considerable time will erode into the wall and become difficult to move. If this occurs, the endoscopist should first try to rotate the foreign body out of the erosion before attempting to pull it out. Some large bones or other foreign bodies cannot be retrieved orally, and the endoscopist may instead attempt to push the foreign body into the stomach; it is much safer to surgically remove foreign bodies from the stomach than from the oesophagus. Bones delivered into the stomach can be left, as they will be dissolved by gastric acid and digested.

Following endoscopic removal of a foreign body, the oesophagus should be carefully evaluated; the stomach should also be examined for additional foreign material. Lacerations that do not extend through the oesophageal wall or small perforations usually heal without complications. Circumferential mucosal ulcerations may result in stricture formation (see below) and the owner should be warned of this potential complication. Full-thickness tears or large areas of necrosis often require surgical intervention. Oesophageal surgery always carries the risk of postoperative stricture formation. Following foreign body removal, the author usually treats the patient with a proton pump inhibitor (e.g. omeprazole) and a gastric prokinetic agent (cisapride or metoclopramide) to prevent further damage from acid reflux.

Removing oesophageal fishhooks can also pose problems. They are almost always attached to fishing line and the barb is usually seated through the mucosa by the time of presentation. Owners should be told not to cut the line before bringing their pet to the surgery, as the attached line will aid in removal of the hook. Endoscopic foreign body grasping forceps can be used to remove the hook by pulling it out of the mucosa. The hook is then grasped so that the barb is facing caudally before it is retrieved. There should be little concern in tearing the hook out of the oesophageal wall, as the defect caused usually heals rapidly without problems. Fishhooks attached to a line can sometimes be removed by simply stringing the line through a small hollow rigid oesophageal endoscope. The endoscope is then advanced down the line to the hook. Once in contact with the fishhook, the endoscope is then used to displace the hook from the oesophageal wall. The line can then be gently tugged to pull the hook into the tube, and everything is then removed.

Oesophageal strictures

Benign oesophageal strictures are acquired consequences of severe mucosal and underlying submucosal and muscularis ulceration and inflammation, causing fibrous scarring of the oesophageal wall resulting in luminal narrowing. In the author's experience the ulcerations must be deep and extend more than 180 degrees circumferentially to result in a clinically apparent stricture. Inflammatory oesophageal strictures may be either simple or complex. Simple strictures are single and narrow (less than 1 cm in length) (Figure 4.14). They are usually located within the thoracic cavity, most commonly just proximal to the LOS, and next most commonly at the heart base. Simple strictures often appear as a thin circumferential

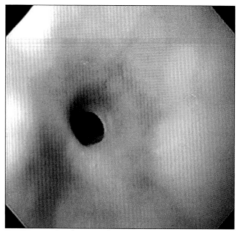

4.14 Simple oesophageal stricture in a cat secondary to oesophagitis caused by a doxycycline tablet being lodged in the oesophagus. The stricture, which had a lumen diameter of 3 mm, was successfully managed with balloon dilation.

band of fibrous tissue narrowing the oesophageal luminal diameter. Some strictures may almost completely obstruct the lumen. The first endoscopic indication of a stricture is when the luminal diameter does not expand during insufflation of the lumen. Strictures with a luminal diameter less than 9 mm will hinder or prevent passage of the endoscope beyond the stricture. The stricture may have smooth mucosal edges or may be ulcerated. There is often secondary oesophagitis proximal to the stricture resulting from chronic retention of food and liquids.

Complex oesophageal strictures consist of a long stricture or multiple narrower strictures. They may be associated with severe ulceration, fibrous bands or webs of tissue across the stricture opening, or even pulsion-type diverticulum formation within the oesophageal wall. In some strictures, fibrotic ridges may take on a spiral configuration extending along the length of the stricture. Complex strictures are much more difficult to manage than simple strictures and have a poorer outcome.

The most common cause of stricture formation is gastric acid reflux, frequently following an episode of anaesthesia. Strictures secondary to acid reflux are most often located just cranial to the LOS. Other common causes of stricture formation include oesophageal trauma from a foreign body, retention of tablets or capsules (e.g. doxycycline) or ingestion of other corrosive substances. Contrast studies may not always delineate an oesophageal stricture, especially if only liquid barium is used. A barium–food mixture is the best way to delineate a stricture radiographically. Endoscopy is the best method to determine the location and characteristics of the stricture. Other conditions causing oesophageal narrowing include vascular ring anomalies, extrinsic perioesophageal masses and oesophageal neoplasia (see above). If there is any question whether the oesophageal narrowing is secondary to neoplasia or granuloma formation, oesophageal biopsies should be performed. Sometimes a very distal oesophageal stricture just proximal to the LOS can be misidentified as oesophageal achalasia. Cases of achalasia will usually be dilated easily with a balloon catheter.

Oesophageal strictures are best treated with dilating devices, using either direct endoscopic visualization or fluoroscopic guidance. Stricture dilation can be accomplished using either balloon catheters or bougie dilators. There is as yet no consensus in veterinary medicine as to which type of dilator is better; however, most authors prefer to use balloon dilators because of their safety and ease of use. When the deflated balloon is placed in the stricture lumen and then expanded it delivers a uniform radial force on the stricture, breaking the fibrous connective tissue. Bougies are tapered rigid dilators that, when passed through the stricture lumen, exert both longitudinal and radial forces. Some clinicians believe that there is a higher chance of oesophageal trauma and even perforation with rigid bougies, especially when they are used without a guidewire. The use of rigid dilators should generally be restricted to simple rather than complex strictures. The following section will briefly describe the balloon dilation technique. The reader should refer to other texts for comprehensive descriptions of stricture management.

Balloon dilation requires a set of balloon dilators of increasing diameter and an inflation device that also measures the pressure within the balloon. There are a number of types of balloons, including single-use balloons that can be passed through a 2.8 mm biopsy channel, passed adjacent to the endoscope or passed using a preplaced guidewire through the stricture lumen. The author prefers to place a guidewire down the endoscope biopsy channel and direct it through the stricture and run it on into the stomach. The endoscope is removed, leaving the guidewire in place. The endoscope is then placed back into the oesophagus to allow the operator to view the stricture. Next, the deflated balloon is lubricated and passed down the guidewire and into the stricture so that it straddles both sides of the stricture. The inflated diameter of the first balloon to be used should be approximately 4–5 mm greater than the stricture diameter. The author inflates the balloon to the manufacturer's maximum pressure and holds it for a minute. The balloon is deflated, repositioned and inflated a second and then a third time. The stricture is then evaluated endoscopically and, if necessary, progressively larger balloons are used until the desired diameter is achieved. There is no consensus as to the maximum diameter to which a stricture should be dilated. The author generally attempts to dilate the stricture to the estimated normal oesophageal diameter, based on endoscopic observation and the amount of trauma caused by the balloon.

Re-stricture formation is common, and many endoscopists will automatically repeat the dilation procedure at prescribed intervals (often fortnightly or weekly). In one study, the average number of dilation episodes was three. Several studies in humans have reported the benefit of triamcinolone injections in four quadrants around the stricture before the stricture is dilated. Use of a corticosteroid is thought to decrease inflammation and allow healing to occur in a less fibrotic fashion, potentially decreasing the need for repeat dilation. A specialized injection needle is passed through the biopsy channel and up to 0.6 mg of triamcinolone is injected into each site, separated by 0.5–2.5 cm, around the periphery of the lesion to provide a total dose of 1.2–1.8 mg. Dilution of the triamcinolone 1:1 with sterile saline may be required to provide sufficient volume. Some simple strictures can be improved before dilation by making three or four radial cuts through the mucosa and the fibrotic bands using an endoscopic laser fibre or electrocoagulation wire.

Complications of stricture dilation include mucosal tearing, diverticulum formation or oesophageal perforation. The endoscopist should always be prepared to deal with a tension pneumothorax if perforation occurs (see the *BSAVA Manual of Canine and Feline Head, Neck and Thoracic Surgery*). Surgical resection of oesophageal strictures is often complicated by re-stricture formation at the surgical site.

Complications

The complications of oesophagoscopy are few and most are usually related to the nature of the underlying disease. In addition to the obvious anaesthesia-related complications there are several complications associated with endoscopy itself. Pre- and postoperative aspiration are always a concern for patients with oesophageal motility disorders and oesophageal obstruction. Oesophageal perforation during endoscopy can result in mediastinitis and pneumothorax, which are serious complications. The operator should always be aware that during insufflation a tension pneumothorax could occur in patients with foreign bodies, strictures, tumours, diverticula or severe erosive disease. Iatrogenic mucosal damage during endoscopy is uncommon due to the resilience of the normal oesophageal mucosa.

References and further reading

Adamama-Moraitou KK, Rallis TS, Prassinos NN *et al.* (2002) Benign esophageal stricture in the dog and cat: a retrospective study of 20 cases. *Canadian Journal of Veterinary Research* **66**, 55–59

Bissett SA, Davis J, Subler K and Degernes LA (2009) Risk factors and outcome of bougienage for treatment of benign esophageal strictures in dogs and cats: 28 cases (1995–2004). *Journal of the American Veterinary Medical Association* **235**, 844–850

Brockman D, Holt D and ter Haar G (2018) *BSAVA Manual of Canine and Feline Head, Neck and Thoracic Surgery, 2nd edn.* BSAVA Publications, Gloucester

Burton AG, Talbot CT and Kent MS (2017) Risk factors for death in dogs treated for esophageal foreign body obstruction: a retrospective cohort study of 222 cases (1998–2017) *Journal of Veterinary Internal Medicine* **31**, 1686–1690

Gianella P, Pfammatter NS and Burgener IA (2009) Oesophageal and gastric endoscopic foreign body removal: complications and follow-up of 102 dogs. *Journal of Small Animal Practice* **50**, 649–654

Gualtieri M (2001) Esophagoscopy. *Veterinary Clinics of North America: Small Animal Practice* **31**, 605–630

Hall EJ (2008) Flexible endoscopy: upper gastrointestinal tract. In: *BSAVA Manual of Canine and Feline Endoscopy and Endosurgery, 1st edn*, ed. P Lhermette and D Sobel, pp. 196–326. BSAVA Publications, Gloucester

Leib MS, Dinnel H, Ward DL *et al.* (2001) Endoscopic balloon dilation of benign esophageal strictures in dogs and cats. *Journal of Veterinary Internal Medicine* **15**, 547–552

Muenster M, Hoerauf A and Vieth M (2017) Gastro-oesophageal reflux disease in 20 dogs (2012–2014). *Journal of Small Animal Practice* **58**, 276–283

Rousseau A, Prittie J, Broussard JD *et al.* (2007) Incidence and characterization of esophagitis following esophageal foreign body removal in dogs: 60 cases (1999–2003). *Journal of Veterinary Emergency and Critical Care* **17**, 159–163

Sherding RG and Johnson SE (2011) Esophagoscopy. In: *Small Animal Endoscopy, 3rd edn*, ed. TR Tams and CA Rawlings, pp. 41–96. Elsevier, St. Louis

Washabau RJ (2013) Esophageal endoscopy. In: *Canine and Feline Gastroenterology, 1st edn*, ed. RJ Washabau and MJ Day, pp. 272–275. Elsevier, St. Louis

 Video extra

● **Video 4.1** The endoscope in a j-flexed position looking at the lower oesophageal sphincter (abnormally dilated) in a patient presenting with chronic vomiting. A case of sliding hiatal hernia

Access via QR code or: bsavalibrary.com/endoscopy2e_4

Chapter 5

Flexible endoscopy: upper gastrointestinal tract

Edward J. Hall

Introduction

Upper gastrointestinal (GI) endoscopy is one of the most common flexible endoscopic procedures performed in companion animal practice, and encompasses examination of the oesophagus (see Chapter 4), stomach and proximal small intestine. Only a flexible endoscope is able to allow complete examination of the stomach and intubation of the small intestine. While older flexible endoscopes were able to permit only observation of the GI tract, modern gastroscopes can now also be used for sampling tissues and liquids and even for some therapeutic procedures.

Gastroduodenoscopy is minimally invasive and atraumatic, with low morbidity and very low mortality. Hence, its popularity as a way of investigating GI disease is increasing almost exponentially. However, it should be used only in cases where a diagnosis has not been achieved by conventional non-invasive investigations. Furthermore, to perform this procedure effectively and safely takes much practice, and it is sensible to use the endoscope initially only to carry out simple procedures, such as oesophagoscopy, to avoid the disappointment of failure while developing skill and confidence. Success with the more advanced manoeuvres, such as passage of the endoscope through the pylorus into the duodenum, should not be expected every time during the first few attempts; even the most experienced endoscopist finds this process difficult sometimes and occasionally impossible.

Role of endoscopy in investigating gastrointestinal disease

Complete information on the investigation of GI disease is available in the *BSAVA Manual of Canine and Feline Gastroenterology,* but it is important to emphasize here that endoscopy and GI biopsy are only part of the investigative process. Before endoscopy, routine investigations should be performed to confirm that the procedure is indicated. A complete history and full physical examination are mandatory, and a faecal examination is important if the patient has diarrhoea. Routine laboratory tests may determine first whether systemic disease is causing the GI signs, and second, whether it is safe to anaesthetize the patient.

Plain abdominal radiographs and an abdominal ultrasound examination should also always be performed before endoscopy to ensure there are no unexpected foreign bodies present or masses/lesions beyond the reach of the endoscope, and to confirm that a foreign body is still within the stomach if endoscopic retrieval is planned. The utility of contrast radiography has changed since endoscopy has become available, although it should be considered a complementary procedure and not necessarily redundant. Contrast procedures do not require anaesthesia and provide a better estimation of oesophageal diameter and function, and gastric motility and emptying. Radiographs and ultrasonography can also detect extramural diseases. However, endoscopy is more sensitive for the detection of mucosal disease and has the clear advantage of a potential definitive diagnosis through biopsy. Yet, the limitations of endoscopy should be recognized (Figure 5.1).

Endoscopy cannot assess:
- Functional disease
  - Motility disorders
  - Hypersecretory disorders (e.g. associated with enterotoxigenic bacteria)
  - Brush border enzyme deficiencies
- The whole GI tract
- Submucosal lesions
- Intraperitoneal lesions

5.1 Limitations of endoscopy in investigating GI disease.

Indications

Endoscopy is often indicated in the investigation of suspected gastric and small intestinal disease if the lesion can reasonably be expected to be accessible from the GI tract lumen. Exploratory surgery is realistically the only other alternative in general practice for reaching a definitive diagnosis, but carries more risk. Dehiscence rates of between 2.5% and 12% are reported following full-thickness intestinal biopsy (Shales *et al.*, 2005; Swinbourne *et al.*, 2017), and there is an inevitable convalescence period while wounds heal. In addition, patients with protein-losing enteropathies or neoplasms often have impaired healing, and endoscopy provides the safest method of obtaining a definitive diagnosis in most cases. Thus, the clinical advantages of endoscopy to the patient are:

- The patient can be discharged on the same day as the procedure
- There is no convalescence period or wound healing
- The patient can be immediately treated with steroids if indicated.

The recommended best practice for intestinal biopsy (Figure 5.2) is to perform endoscopy first and reserve surgery for focal disease or where endoscopy fails to provide an answer (Elwood, 2005). Yet, it is important to emphasize that with some diseases (e.g. lymphangiectasia, alimentary lymphoma) endoscopic biopsy samples may not be diagnostic, and full-thickness biopsy specimens obtained by laparoscopy or exploratory laparotomy may be required. Exploratory surgery has a higher diagnostic sensitivity, as the whole GI tract can be examined, full-thickness biopsy specimens can be obtained from all levels of the GI tract and intraperitoneal disease can be investigated. Even if ileoscopy (via colonoscopy; see Chapter 6) is performed in addition to upper GI endoscopy, there is a significant length of intestine that cannot be examined by standard flexible endoscopes, and views of the pancreas, liver and other abdominal organs are, hopefully, never seen on endoscopy of the GI tract.

It should again be stressed that upper GI endoscopy is only part of the investigation of suspected GI disease, and that it is inappropriate to perform the procedure before less invasive and less risky investigations have been carried out. The value of routine laboratory tests to rule out non-GI disease and diagnostic imaging to localize disease and identify surgical conditions must never be forgotten, and they should precede endoscopy routinely.

Endoscopic intestinal biopsy:
- Is preferred
- Is adequate for diagnosis in most cases
- Carries a significantly lower risk than surgery

Effective endoscopic intestinal biopsy requires:
- A competent endoscopist using adequate technique
- The endoscopist to have clinical responsibility and to work with an experienced pathologist

Surgical biopsy should be reserved for those cases where:
- Diseased tissue is known to be beyond the reach of an experienced endoscopist
- Endoscopic biopsy has failed to produce a diagnosis
- Non-mucosal disease is suspected or full-thickness biopsy is required

5.2 Best practice in intestinal biopsy.
(Elwood, 2005)

Full upper gastrointestinal tract endoscopy

In patients where clinical signs or other investigations do not localize the disease, a full endoscopic examination (i.e. oesophago-gastro-duodenoscopy) should always be performed; colonoscopy and ileoscopy may also be indicated (see Chapter 6). However, if oesophageal disease is suspected on the basis of the clinical signs and/or radiographs, there is usually no need to advance beyond any significant lesion that is found (see Chapter 4). In contrast, when performing gastroscopy, it is likely that it will be necessary to examine the small intestine as well as the stomach, and therefore it is standard practice to do so. For example, an animal presenting with vomiting due to gastric ulceration may also have intestinal disease, which can cause vomiting in its own right, and duodenal biopsy samples are necessary to rule this in or out. Thus, endoscopists need to be able to intubate the duodenum if they are to perform an adequate examination, and inexperienced endoscopists should not investigate such cases until they are proficient.

It is not possible to be prescriptive about how an individual veterinary surgeon (veterinarian) performs gastroduodenoscopy, and the method described in this chapter is the author's personal preference. As long as the endoscopist examines all areas safely, the endoscopic examination will be adequate.

The examination needs to be documented to demonstrate that the procedure was performed fully. This can be achieved using either recording equipment (see Chapter 2) or a reporting form that requires a complete endoscopic examination to have been performed in order for it to be filled in properly. The WSAVA GI Standardization Group (Washabau et al., 2010) has produced a standardized reporting proforma (Figure 5.3), which endoscopists can download free of charge and personalize for their own practice.

Gastroscopy

Gastroscopy is indicated in patients presenting with chronic vomiting for diagnostic and specific therapeutic purposes (Figure 5.4). It is rarely indicated in cases of acute vomiting unless it is required to:

- Confirm the presence of a gastric foreign body following diagnostic imaging
- Remove selected foreign bodies
- Investigate significant haematemesis that is not responding to symptomatic treatment.

In chronically vomiting patients, routine investigations should be performed before considering endoscopy, as non-gastric diseases frequently cause vomiting. Plain radiographs and an ultrasound examination are performed first to guide the endoscopist as to what to look for and to find any unexpected chronic gastric foreign bodies. Gastroscopy can be used to confirm the likely presence of an ulcer or a tumour suspected on the basis of imaging by allowing inspection of the tissues and the collection of biopsy specimens. Gastritis is a common cause of chronic vomiting but specific changes are rarely found on laboratory tests or imaging. Endoscopic examination and biopsy collection are therefore required to reach a definitive diagnosis.

Duodenoscopy

Intubation of the small intestine (duodenoscopy with or without jejunoscopy) is indicated in patients presenting with vomiting or other GI signs, and for diagnostic and specific therapeutic purposes (Figure 5.5). Except in the smallest patients, only duodenoscopy is likely to be possible because of the limited length of gastroscopes designed for use in human patients; even with a 1.4 m veterinary gastroscope it becomes more difficult to pass the insertion tube around flexures in the jejunum, as rotation of the gastroscope on its long axis becomes impossible.

Duodenoscopy is indicated in cases of chronic small intestinal diarrhoea when a diet trial has failed and/or chronic vomiting, and especially when the patient exhibits haematemesis, melaena or panhypoproteinaemia. The results of preliminary investigations (including abnormalities of serum folate and cobalamin concentrations) are used to provide evidence to suggest small intestinal disease. Cats with small intestinal disease often present with chronic vomiting rather than chronic diarrhoea, and some cats with recurring hairballs have chronic inflammatory enteropathy, indicating the need for intestinal biopsy samples in cases of chronic vomiting even when a hairball has been found. Thus, in all cases where the stomach is

Endoscopic examination report: upper GI endoscopy

Date of procedure:.. Case number: ....

Patient and client information: *(card or stamp)*

Procedures(s):

Indication(s) for procedure: ....

Endoscope(s) used: ....

Forceps/retrieval device(s) used: ....

Problems/complications: None ☐

Perforation ☐   Excessive bleeding ☐   Anesthetic complications ☐   Excessive time ☐   Other ☐

Comments:...

☐ Unable to complete full examination: Why?...

☐ Unable to obtain adequate biopsies: Why?...

☐ Unable to retrieve foreign object: Why?...

☐ Visualization obscured   Why?...

Sampling: Biopsy ☐   Brush cytology ☐   Washing ☐   Aspiration ☐   Foreign body retrieved ☐

Documentation: Video ☐   Photographs ☐

Esophagus   Normal ☐   Foreign body ☐   Mass ☐   Stricture ☐   Hiatal hernia ☐

Lesion	Code	Comments (include location)	Code:
Hyperemia/vascularity			Normal = 0
Discoloration			Mild = 1
Friability			Moderate = 2
Hemorrhage			Severe = 3
Erosion/ulcer			
Contents (mucus/bile/food)			
Dilation			
Gastroesophageal sphincter			
Other			

Stomach   Normal ☐   Foreign body ☐   Mass ☐   Polyp(s) ☐   Parasite(s) ☐

Site(s) of lesions: Fundus ☐   Body ☐   Incisura ☐   Antrum ☐   Pylorus ☐

Site(s) of biopsies: Fundus ☐   Body ☐   Incisura ☐   Antrum ☐   Pylorus ☐

Lesion	Code	Comments (include location)	Code:
Unable to inflate lumen			Normal = 0
Hyperemia/vascularity			Mild = 1
Edema			Moderate = 2
Discoloration		▶	Severe = 3

5.3 Upper GI endoscopy reporting proforma. This standardized form was developed by the WSAVA Gastrointestinal Standardization Group, with sponsorship from Hill's Pet Nutrition. (continues) ▶

(Washabau *et al.*, 2010)

Endoscopic examination report: upper GI endoscopy *continued*

Stomach *(continued)*   Normal ☐   Foreign body ☐   Mass ☐   Polyp(s) ☐   Parasite(s) ☐

Site(s) of lesions: Fundus ☐   Body ☐   Incisura ☐   Antrum ☐   Pylorus ☐

Site(s) of biopsies: Fundus ☐   Body ☐   Incisura ☐   Antrum ☐   Pylorus ☐

Lesion	Code	Comments (include location)
Friability		
Hemorrhage		
Erosion/ulcer		
Contents (mucus/bile/food)		
Gastroesophageal sphincter		
Passing scope through pylorus		
Other		

Code:
Normal = 0
Mild = 1
Moderate = 2
Severe = 3

Duodenum/jejunum   Normal ☐   Foreign body ☐   Mass ☐   Polyp(s) ☐   Parasite(s) ☐

How far was the tip of the scope advanced?

Was/were the papilla(e) seen?   Yes ☐ (which? ....)   No ☐

Lesion	Code	Comments (include location)
Unable to inflate lumen		
Hyperemia/vascularity		
Edema		
Discoloration		
Friability		
Texture		
Hemorrhage		
Erosion/ulcer		
Lacteal dilatation		
Contents (mucus/bile/food)		
Other		

Code:
Normal = 0
Mild = 1
Moderate = 2
Severe = 3

Comments and recommendations: ....

....

Endoscopist signature: ....

5.3 (continued) Upper GI endoscopy reporting proforma. This standardized form was developed by the WSAVA Gastrointestinal Standardization Group, with sponsorship from Hill's Pet Nutrition.
(Washabau *et al.*, 2010)

Diagnostic gastroscopy

Investigation of signs of gastric disease
- Nausea and salivation
- Chronic vomiting
- Haematemesis and/or melaena
- Unexplained anorexia

Investigation of imaging abnormalities
- Plain radiographs:
  - Radiodense foreign body
  - Suspected neoplasia
- Contrast radiographs:
  - Radiolucent foreign body
  - Ulcers
  - Suspected neoplasia
- Ultrasonography:
  - Foreign body
  - Ulcer
  - Suspected neoplasia (mass, thickened gastric wall, loss of layering, ulceration)

Therapeutic gastroscopy

- Removal of selected foreign bodies
- Percutaneous endoscopic gastrostomy tube placement (± removal)
- Polypectomy

5.4 Indications for gastroscopy.

Diagnostic duodenoscopy

Investigation of signs of intestinal disease [a]
- Chronic vomiting
- Chronic diarrhoea
- Melaena (and haematemesis if no gastric lesions are present)
- Change in appetite
- Unexplained weight loss
- Abdominal pain (although investigation by laparoscopy or laparotomy may be more useful)

Investigation of imaging abnormalities
- Radiographs:
  - No radiographic abnormalities despite clinical signs
  - Diffusely thickened intestinal wall
  - Loss of intestinal wall layering in proximal intestine
- Ultrasonography:
  - Diffusely thickened intestinal wall
  - Loss of normal wall layering in proximal intestine

Therapeutic duodenoscopy

Endoscopic placement of a jejunostomy tube

5.5 Indications for duodenoscopy. [a] Preferably combined with ileoscopy (see Chapter 6).

being examined, it is usual to examine the duodenum at the same time. Contemporaneous examination and biopsy of the ileum (approached via a colonoscopy; see Chapter 6) increases the chances of reaching a diagnosis in cases of chronic small intestinal diarrhoea (Casamian-Sorrosal et al., 2010). However, in stable patients with chronic diarrhoea but no concerning signs (i.e. no anorexia, severe weight loss, GI bleeding, hypoalbuminaemia, abnormal abdominal palpation and/or imaging), empirical treatment with parasiticides and an exclusion or hydrolysed diet are usually indicated before considering endoscopic biopsy.

Jejunoscopy

Although it may be possible to reach the proximal jejunum in smaller patients, one of the significant limitations of gastroscopy is that the intestinal tract is much longer than a standard gastroscope, and thus large sections cannot be examined. Jejunoscopy (also known as enteroscopy), in addition to duodenoscopy, may be indicated for the investigation of specific small intestinal problems (Figure 5.6). However, the availability of dedicated enteroscopes (at least 2 m in length) is very limited in veterinary medicine, and an exploratory laparotomy is usually performed if the whole small intestine requires examination. Surgical exploration does not allow direct visualization of mucosal lesions; however, it is possible to pass a flexible endoscope through a gastrotomy incision and then feed it along the small intestine to inspect the mucosa. In this situation, it is imperative that the endoscope has been completely sterilized with ethylene oxide gas (see Chapter 2) to reduce the risks of this procedure. Capsule endoscopy (see below) also allows visualization of all the small intestinal mucosa, but biopsy is not possible with this method.

- Focal causes of haemorrhage
- Focal neoplasia
- Patchy disease (if duodenoscopy is not diagnostic):
  - Chronic inflammatory enteropathy
  - Lymphangiectasia
  - Alimentary lymphoma

5.6 Indications for jejunoscopy or capsule endoscopy. Note that neither technique allows biopsy samples to be obtained.

Contraindications

Endoscopy may be an inappropriate way to reach a diagnosis in some patients with suspected GI disease; for example, gastroduodenoscopy cannot diagnose pancreatitis as a cause of vomiting and diarrhoea. Endoscopy also requires general anaesthesia and in some instances this may be too dangerous to perform. If a patient is too sick to be anaesthetized for surgery, it is also too sick for endoscopy. Specific contraindications to endoscopy are listed in Figure 5.7.

Poor anaesthetic risk
- Relative:
  - Poor cardiopulmonary reserve
  - Uraemia
- Absolute:
  - Uncorrected bleeding disorder
  - Non-reversible hypoxaemia
  - Unstable cardiac arrhythmia
  - Cardiac failure
Poorly prepared patient
- Food not withheld (stomach full)
- Known coprophagia not prevented by muzzling
- Inadequate investigations before endoscopy

5.7 Contraindications to endoscopy.

Instrumentation

The technological advances in endoscope design and construction have made gastroscopes narrow enough to pass the pylorus in dogs and cats and yet be steerable. However, the skill needed to intubate the duodenum through the pylorus can be acquired only by practice, although an understanding of what one is trying to achieve and how to manipulate the endoscope helps (see Chapter 3).

The components of a flexible endoscopy system are discussed in detail in Chapter 2. The features specifically needed for an endoscope capable of performing upper GI endoscopy are listed in Figure 5.8. The greater the tip deflection and the smaller the radius of the bending section, the greater the manoeuvrability of the endoscope, but it is the capability to be retroflexed that is essential for complete examination of the stomach (see Figure 2.3).

- Insertion tube of at least 1 m working length
- Tip diameter <9.5 mm
- Minimum 2.2 mm accessory/biopsy channel
- Four-way tip deflection:
  - Ability to retroflex tip (turn ≥180 degrees) in one plane
  - Small radius of curvature of the bending section
- Ability to insufflate with air
- Ability to wash lens remotely

5.8 Features of a flexible endoscope suitable for gastroscopy.

The distance along the GI tract that can actually be reached depends on the size of the patient and the length of the gastroscope. Human paediatric gastroscopes have a bending section with a small radius of curvature, making them manoeuvrable, but have a working length of only 1 m. With skill, the duodenum of dogs up to approximately 40 kg bodyweight can be routinely intubated, while in cats and small dogs, it may be possible to reach the jejunum. However, pyloric intubation in an adult Great Dane, for example, would be impossible with these gastroscopes, as the insertion tube would not reach. Thus, a 1 m insertion tube is of adequate length to perform duodenoscopy in most patients but will be too short in some adult large-breed dogs and all adult giant-breed dogs. Dedicated veterinary gastroscopes have a longer working length (up to 1.4 m) and are therefore useful for larger dogs. However, they are more difficult to manoeuvre, especially in smaller animals, as a large part of the insertion tube remains outside the patient and tends to loop. Alternatively, a colonoscope designed for human use with an insertion tube of 1.4–1.7 m would be of adequate length for duodenoscopy in giant-breed dogs, but such endoscopes have too large a tip diameter (10–13 mm) to pass the pylorus of small patients.

The diameter of the tip of the insertion tube is critical in dictating the size of patient that can be examined. A tip diameter >9.5 mm cannot easily be inserted into puppies and cats, and is likely to preclude pyloric intubation in cats and dogs <10 kg. Thus, the diameter of the endoscope used is typically a compromise: a narrower endoscope will allow passage through the pylorus in smaller patients, but wider endoscopes have a bigger accessory/biopsy channel, allowing larger biopsy specimens (which are likely to be of better diagnostic quality) to be harvested. Both 2.2 mm and 2.8 mm biopsy channels will permit the collection of adequate biopsy samples, but those from the 2.8 mm channel will inevitably be bigger. Biopsy channels smaller than 2.2 mm are inadequate for intestinal biopsies, as the samples collected will be so small that they are likely to fragment (see Chapter 3); these small biopsy specimens will be so superficial that they do not contain the connective tissue necessary to hold them together. For most patients, a gastroscope with a tip diameter between 7 mm and 9 mm is appropriate. In a gastroscope with a tip diameter <9.5 mm, the largest biopsy channel available is 2.8 mm. However, even the narrowest gastroscope currently available (designed for transnasal gastroscopy in human patients), with a tip diameter of 5.4 mm, can still accommodate 2.0 mm biopsy forceps by combining the biopsy channel with the air/water channel.

Only forward-viewing endoscopes are used routinely for veterinary gastroscopy. Side-viewing endoscopes (duodenoscopes) are used in human gastroenterology for endoscopic retrograde cholangiopancreatography (i.e. catheterization of the bile and pancreatic ducts and injection of radiographic contrast medium) and endoscopic procedures such as cholelith removal, bile duct sphincterotomy and stent placement. These procedures are not routine in veterinary endoscopy yet. The purchase of a second-hand duodenoscope is not recommended, even though they are often available cheaply, as steering is difficult because of the direction of view. A wide field of view (90–120 degrees) in forward-viewing gastroscopes facilitates orientation and a panoramic examination, thereby decreasing the likelihood of missing a lesion or foreign body in the stomach. A depth of focus of 3–100 mm is usually adequate; a minimum visible distance of >5 mm prevents detailed examination of the mucosa.

Insufflation capability is essential as the stomach and small intestine must be inflated to enable visualization. A xenon light source is preferred because the greater illumination permits a panoramic view across the distended stomach. Suction is necessary to remove GI secretions and air (see Chapters 2 and 3 for more details about equipment).

Finally, a range of endoscopic accessories may be required for therapeutic purposes (see below). It is essential that biopsy forceps are available for diagnostic purposes. Biopsy samples from the stomach and intestine should always be taken, even if the tissue appears grossly normal.

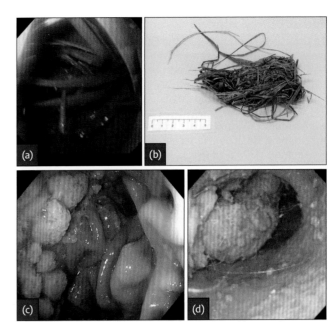

5.9 Inadequate preparation for gastroscopy. (a) Mass of grass in the stomach of a poorly prepared dog obscuring visualization of the gastric mucosa. (b) Mat of grass removed from the stomach of a dog before gastroscopy could proceed. (c) Food in the stomach of a dog that had inadvertently been fed. (d) Partially digested food retained in the stomach of a dog due to delayed gastric emptying secondary to chronic inflammatory enteropathy.

Normally, the stomach will be empty within 12 hours of withholding food. So, assuming that the animal has not inadvertently eaten (Figure 5.9c), finding food in the stomach on endoscopic examination can give useful information about an anatomical outflow obstruction or a functional delay in gastric emptying. It is not unusual to find food in the stomach of animals with intestinal malabsorption even if there is no gastric pathology (Figure 5.9d), as the delay in digesting food slows the rate of gastric emptying via neurohormonal feedback.

If a barium contrast radiographic study has been performed, endoscopy should be delayed for 24 hours if possible: aspiration of barium into the endoscope could cause a serious blockage. Any residual barium found during endoscopy should be aspirated only through a tube and not directly via the suction channel.

Patient preparation

Preparation of the patient for upper GI endoscopy requires nothing more than the withdrawal of food for at least 12 hours before the procedure so that the stomach is empty. Water does not need to be withheld before the procedure. Endoscopy too soon after a meal should be avoided because:

- Visualization is difficult; lesions and foreign bodies may be missed
- Pyloric intubation is difficult or impossible
- The endoscope may become clogged
- There is a danger of aspiration during recovery.

Day-case endoscopy is more likely to result in gastric contents being found because, even if the client does withhold food, they do not realize that their pet may scavenge or eat grass (Figure 5.9ab). It is preferable to hospitalize the patient overnight before gastroscopy; this allows time for preliminary investigations and ensures that the patient does not eat before the procedure.

Patient management

Premedication

Premedication should be used to smooth induction and recovery. If dogs are very agitated before induction it is common to find foamy swallowed saliva in the oesophagus, and this can interfere with the endoscopic view (see below). A mixture of dexmedetomidine and an opioid is a suitable premedication for dogs and cats. However, a recent pilot study showed that the combination of butorphanol and dexmedetomidine made pyloric intubation faster than in patients premedicated with methadone and dexmedetomidine (McFadzean *et al.*, 2017) Acepromazine maleate with buprenorphine is another suitable combination for dogs. In cats, ketamine or midazolam may be preferred. Atropine is not necessary and some clinicians believe that, by drying secretions, it actually makes the procedure more difficult. Others, however, claim that it makes pyloric intubation easier, whereas narcotic premedications may increase pyloric tone.

Antifoaming agents

To try to prevent foaming in the GI tract from obscuring the view, pre-emptive treatment with antifoaming agents may be used. A mixture of one part acetylcysteine to five parts simethicone is given orally at least 30 minutes before induction at the following doses:

- Animals <10 kg: 6 ml of mixture
- Animals 10–20 kg: 12 ml
- Animals >20kg: 18 ml.

Alternatively, simethicone can be added to the bottle supplying the water for irrigation during endoscopy.

Anaesthesia

General anaesthesia is essential for upper GI endoscopy, and intubation with an endotracheal tube tied securely in place is mandatory. Tying or taping the endotracheal tube around the mandible or maxilla is most secure but passage of the endoscope into the pharynx may be easier when the tube is tied to the mandible. Passing the tie around the back of the head is less secure, as the repeated movements of the endoscope tend to dislodge the endotracheal tube, but is a necessity in cats and brachycephalic dogs. In dogs, a cuffed endotracheal tube is preferred because of the increased risk of reflux resulting from the gastroscope acting as a wick as it passes forwards and backwards through the lower oesophageal sphincter. In cats, a non-cuffed endotracheal tube is preferred because of the risk of tracheal damage from an overinflated cuff; fortunately, the frequency and volume of reflux is much lower in cats than in dogs. An elbow connector may be used to keep the anaesthetic circuit away from the insertion tube of the endoscope.

The safest anaesthetic regime is the one with which the operator is most familiar; for example, induction with intravenous alfaxalone or propofol and maintenance with isoflurane or sevoflurane with oxygen are suitable options. The anaesthetic circuit used (from T-piece to circle) depends on the size of the patient. Nitrous oxide is not used because insufflation of the stomach will permit the diffusion of nitrous oxide (the 'third space effect') and cause overdistension of the stomach. However, with the analgesic properties of nitrous oxide being absent, some patients show signs of discomfort (e.g. tachypnoea) even when apparently fully anaesthetized, especially when the pylorus is intubated or the GI tract is inflamed. This temporary problem can be overcome by the tactical use of intermittent intravenous diazepam.

Air insufflation is essential during upper GI endoscopy to open the lumen and move the wall away from the tip of the endoscope so that an image can be obtained. However, the assistant monitoring the anaesthetic should be alert to overinflation of the stomach, as it may cause cardiorespiratory compromise through compression of the diaphragm and caudal vena cava.

Patient positioning

After induction and intubation, the patient is placed in left lateral recumbency for routine upper GI endoscopy (Figure 5.10). This position places the gastric antrum uppermost (i.e. right side up) so that air will fill it and make the pylorus more visible. However, retroflexion of the endoscope to examine the cardia and fundus is essential, especially as foreign bodies tend to fall into the fundus and would

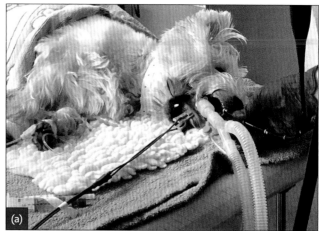

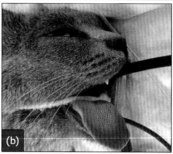

5.10 Patient positioning. (a) The anaesthetized dog is placed in left lateral recumbency for routine upper GI endoscopy; air fills the antrum, making pyloric intubation possible. A pulse oximeter is placed on the tongue. (b) The anaesthetized cat is also placed in left lateral recumbency for routine upper GI endoscopy. Note that the endotracheal tube is fastened around the back of the head, and a chopped down needle cap is being used to maintain safe access into the oral cavity. A spring-loaded gag should not be used in cats as it may cause ischaemic brain damage and cortical blindness post procedure.

otherwise be missed. For gastrostomy tube placement right lateral recumbency is used, as the tube is placed through the left flank (see below).

A mouth gag (speculum) **must** always be inserted to prevent damage to the endoscope, but this should be done with care in cats as excessive opening of the jaw can occlude blood flow to the brain, with deleterious neurological consequences.

Monitoring

An intravenous catheter should be placed before induction to ensure intravenous access at all times. Electrocardiographic monitoring, pulse oximetry and capnography are recommended. Throughout the procedure, the anaesthetist should be in control and be ready to instruct the endoscopist to deflate the stomach if overinflation is affecting the patient's cardiorespiratory status.

Recovery

Recovery tends to be smoother if the stomach is deflated before the gastroscope is removed. If gastric contents are observed in the oesophagus and/or pharynx during withdrawal of the endoscope, they should be suctioned and, if necessary, the oesophagus lavaged. Leaving gastric acid, bile and digestive enzymes in the oesophagus of a patient recovering from anaesthesia (and therefore having a depressed swallowing reflex) can predispose to inhalation pneumonia, oesophagitis and even oesophageal stricture formation.

On recovery, the patient usually shows no ill effects and can usually be discharged the same day to await biopsy results. As the biopsy sites are so small and bleeding is minimal, there is no need to prescribe gastroprotectants. It is advisable to feed the patient only a small meal that evening, but there is no need for a prolonged convalescence.

Endoscopic procedure

The patient should be prepared as described above. Contrast studies should not be performed immediately before endoscopy. The endoscopy equipment should be checked before the patient is anaesthetized (see Chapter 3). When anaesthesia has been induced and the endotracheal tube has been placed and secured, the patient is positioned in left lateral recumbency for the procedure. As soon as the swallowing reflex has been abolished, the procedure can begin. Lubrication of the endoscope tip with a sterile lubricant gel or silicone spray can ease insertion as long as this material is kept off the lens, but is rarely necessary. **A mouth gag must always be inserted.** The procedure should then be carried out as quickly as possible, but without rushing, and so it is important that all ancillary equipment (e.g. biopsy forceps, formalin pots) are made ready beforehand.

It is usual to perform a full upper GI tract examination, but with only a quick initial inspection of the oesophagus and stomach on the way to the duodenum. It is recommended to try to intubate the pylorus as soon as possible. Overinflation of the stomach stimulates peristalsis and also introduces a bulge in the greater curvature that makes advancement of the endoscope into the antrum and through the pylorus more difficult; it also compromises the patient's respiration and venous return. Therefore, the stomach is examined fully and the required biopsy samples are collected on withdrawal from the duodenum. Nevertheless, it is important to make a brief initial inspection of the stomach to ensure that, when viewed after duodenoscopy, any artefacts caused by the endoscope are correctly identified and not misinterpreted as lesions.

The following notes describe the procedure in order of anatomical location following oesophagoscopy (described in Chapter 4).

Gastroscopy
Initial examination

In the distal oesophagus the lower oesophageal sphincter will be seen, usually as a star- or slit-like opening and occasionally bulging slightly cranially (see Chapter 4). Anatomically this is not a true sphincter, but endoscopically it usually acts as one. Depending on the depth of anaesthesia, it may be open rather than closed. Abnormalities of the lower oesophageal sphincter (e.g. hiatal hernia) are discussed in Chapter 4.

If the lower oesophageal sphincter is closed, slight angulation (~30 degrees) of the endoscope tip and continued insufflation are needed to pass into the stomach. Red-out, resulting from the lens being in contact with the mucosa, may occur until the gastric lumen is reached, at which point there will be a sudden loss of resistance to forward motion. If resistance is not overcome when trying to enter the stomach, it is usually because the endoscope tip has missed the opening of the sphincter and has impacted the wall lateral to it. Excessive force should not be applied; the endoscope should be withdrawn slightly and redirected before trying to pass through the sphincter again.

Once in the stomach, it is necessary to orientate so that a quick inspection can be performed to identify any lesions to be examined more closely later, and so that the antrum and pylorus can be located. The initial examination of the stomach will detect foreign material, food, fluid, bile and blood. Such findings can be important indicators of underlying pathology but may hinder further endoscopic examination of the stomach, as they may impair visualization and make passage of the endoscope into the duodenum difficult. If there are significant amounts of gastric contents, they may need to be flushed and aspirated to allow the initial examination and then pyloric intubation; any mats of grass should be removed with grasping forceps (see Figure 5.9b).

Orientation

In order to navigate around the stomach, it is helpful to have a mental image of the gastric anatomy (Figure 5.11). On entering the stomach, once any red-out has been corrected, the initial view is of the greater curvature at the junction of the fundus and body. If there is red-out, slight withdrawal of the tip and more insufflation will enable a view of the lumen. Slight deviation of the tip will then give a panoramic view of the body of the stomach towards the antrum, with rugal folds tending to run parallel to the long axis of the stomach (Figure 5.12).

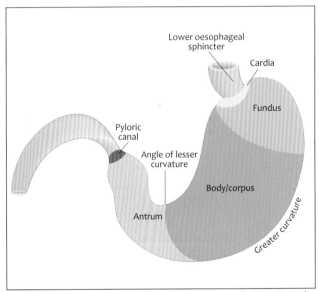

5.11 Ventrodorsal diagrammatic representation of the regions of the stomach.

To find the pylorus, there are a number of landmarks that can be used (Figure 5.13). If one is 'hopelessly lost', retroflexion of the endoscope tip and further insertion of the tube with insufflation is probably the best technique to help establish orientation. Once the cardia has been identified, by observing the point where the insertion tube enters the stomach, relaxation of the tip deflection (i.e. reducing retroflexion) brings the lesser curvature into view, and below the angle of the lesser curvature (angularis incisura) will be the antrum with the pylorus at its base (Figure 5.14). The angularis incisura is the most important landmark, with the cardia above and the antrum below.

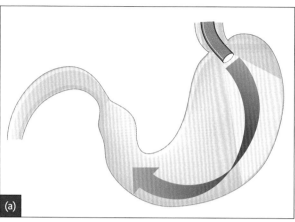

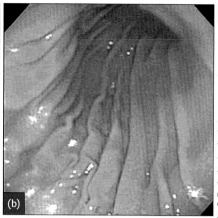

5.12 Passage of the endoscope into the stomach. (a) On entering the stomach, the view is of the greater curvature at the junction of the fundus and body. Slight redirection of the endoscope tip (in the direction of the arrow) produces a view along the gastric body towards the antrum. (b) Parallel rugal folds running along the greater curvature. The entrance to the antrum is visible at the far end of the gastric body.
(b, Reproduced from the *BSAVA Manual of Canine and Feline Gastroenterology*, 3rd edn)

- Rugal folds on the greater curvature are roughly parallel and run towards the antrum (see Figure 5.12b)
- On retroflexion of the endoscope and inflation of the stomach, the endoscope entering through the cardia is visible (see Figure 5.14a)
- The lesser curvature divides the fundus and body from the antrum (see Figure 5.14)
- The antrum has fewer rugal folds (see Figure 5.14c)
- Waves of peristalsis may be seen rolling along the antrum towards the pylorus (see Figure 5.15)
- The pylorus may be visible at the end of the antrum, or its position may be identified by:
  - Bile and foam being refluxed though it (see Figure 5.14a)
  - Waves of peristalsis encircling it (see Figure 5.15)
  - A group of rugal folds (see Figure 5.17)

5.13 Landmarks used to provide orientation in the stomach.

Examination of the antrum

Once orientation has been achieved, the endoscope can be advanced along the rugal folds of the greater curvature into the antrum. The antrum can be recognized by its smaller number of rugal folds, and sometimes a periodic wave or ring of peristalsis is observed passing towards the pylorus (Figure 5.15). In cats, the angle into the antrum at the lesser curvature is quite acute, and the slide-by technique or pre-deflection of the endoscope tip (see Chapter 3) may be needed to pass into the antrum.

In larger dogs, as the endoscope approaches the antrum, there may be a tendency for the tip to get stuck in the greater curvature, and slight tip deflection may be

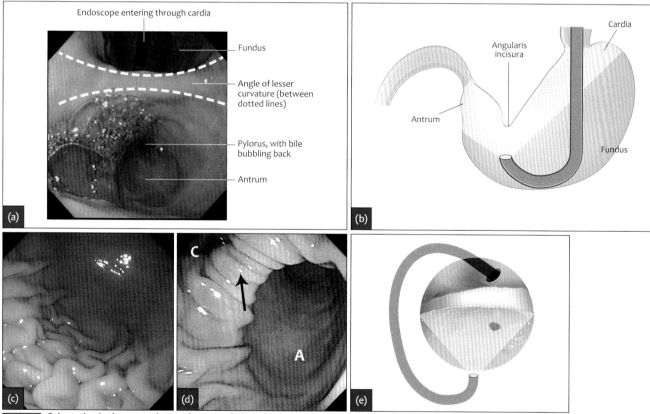

5.14 Orientation in the stomach. In order to reach the pylorus there are a number of landmarks that can be used. (a) The angle of the lesser curvature (angularis incisura) divides the antrum (below) from the fundus and cardia (above), through which the insertion tube can be seen entering the stomach. In this image, bile can be seen bubbling back from through the pylorus. (b) Diagram showing the position of the endoscope tip in the stomach in order to achieve a view of the angularis incisura with the cardia above and antrum below. (c) Entrance below the lesser curvature into the antrum, which has no rugal folds. (d) The insertion tube has been passed along the greater curvature and retroflexed to view the angularis incisura (arrowed) dividing the antrum (A) from the fundus and cardia (C). (e) Diagram showing the insertion tube entering at the cardia, passing along the greater curvature into the antrum showing the pylorus in the distance.

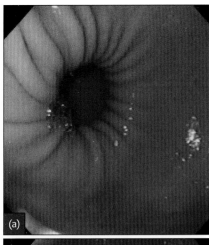

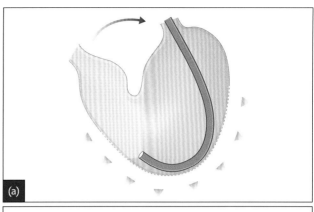

5.15 (a) Circular wave of peristalsis migrating down the antrum towards the pylorus. (b) As the circular wave of peristalsis reaches the end of the antrum, the pylorus (arrowed) comes into view.

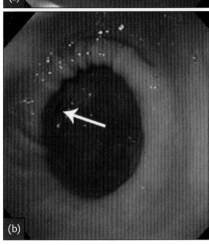

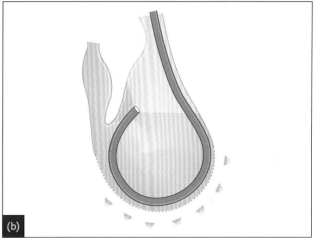

5.16 (a) Diagram demonstrating the effects of overinflation of the stomach during gastroscopy. Distension of the gastric body and fundus allows the insertion tube to form an expanding loop, which tends to direct the tip up towards the cardia. Attempts to advance the gastroscope distend the greater curvature further, compounding the problem. (b) This stomach has been overinflated and, in the retroflexed view, the angularis incisura is narrowed compared with the appearance in Figure 5.14a, and the pylorus is no longer directly visible, such that the insertion tube turns back towards the cardia.

needed to allow further advancement. Alternatively, and more commonly, as the insertion tube is advanced, the tip appears to move backwards – that is, away from the pylorus. This so-called 'paradoxical movement' tends to happen when the stomach is overinflated. It occurs because when forward pressure is applied to the insertion tube to try to advance the tip it actually stretches the greater curvature even more, such that the tip does not move forward and may even appear to move backwards. Overinflation makes the greater curvature so rounded that the endoscope tip cannot enter the antrum because the angle of the lesser curvature and the entrance to the antrum have become too narrow (Figure 5.16a). The extent to which the lesser curvature has narrowed is an indicator of how much the stomach has been inflated (Figure 5.16b). With continuing pressure on the insertion tube, the distortion of the stomach results in the tip swinging past the angularis incisura and back into the fundus, towards the cardia. This problem can be prevented by deflating the stomach as much as possible while still maintaining a view, or by turning the tip slightly into the greater curvature so that it advances into the antrum, or by rotating the endoscope slightly on its long axis as it is advanced. Finally, if all else fails, applying external compression to the lower right body wall will flatten the greater curvature and may assist entry into the antrum.

The pylorus is found at the end of the antrum and duodenal intubation is attempted (see below). The pylorus may demonstrate rhythmic opening and closing. Occasionally, bile or foam will reflux from the duodenum (see Figure 5.14a). The pylorus can have a wide variety of appearances. There may be a few mucosal folds, but is should not be obscured by excessive folds (Figure 5.17).

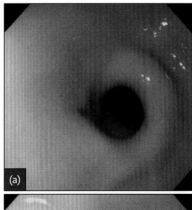

5.17 (a) The normal pylorus of a cat. (b) The normal pylorus of a dog; a few mucosal folds are slightly obscuring the entrance to the pylorus.

Examination of the body of the stomach

After pyloric intubation and duodenoscopy (see below), a more complete examination of the whole stomach is made. Fluid may pool in the stomach, particularly in the left side of the fundus, and should be suctioned to ensure that no submerged lesions are missed. Rugal folds on the greater curvature will be seen to flatten as the stomach is inflated and reappear as it is deflated. At some point during the examination, the stomach should be briefly overinflated to almost completely flatten the rugal folds, so that no lesions remain hidden between the folds (Figure 5.18).

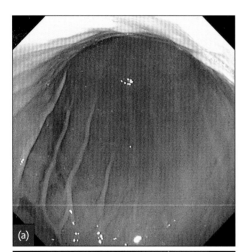

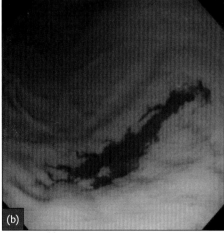

5.18 (a) Insufflation of the stomach to flatten all the rugal folds ensures that no lesions remain hidden. (b) Complete flattening of the rugae enables a small gastric ulcer to be found or, as here, the full extent of a larger lesion to be seen.

Examination of the cardia and fundus

Complete anticlockwise rotation of the inner, up/down wheel (i.e. downward movement with the left thumb towards the palm) will move the gastroscope tip upwards into full retroflexion (see Chapter 3). Inserting the gastroscope further while it is retroflexed will allow visualization of the lesser curvature, with the cardia and fundus above it and the antrum below (see Figure 5.14). The degree of narrowing of the lesser curvature is an indication of the degree of inflation of the stomach; a sharp 'edge' to the angularis incisura and complete flattening of rugal folds is an indication of overinflation, and if this is seen air should be suctioned out of the stomach.

Partial withdrawal of the gastroscope while it is retroflexed (the so-called 'J' manoeuvre (Figure 5.19); see also Chapter 4) will bring the view of either the cardia and

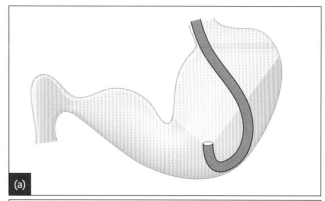

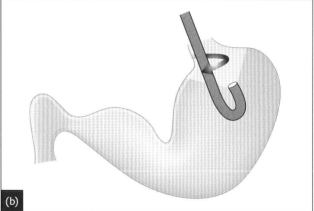

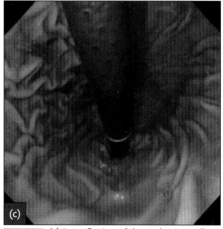

5.19 (a) Retroflexion of the endoscope allows visualization of the cardia and fundus, and (b) simultaneous rotation about the long axis of the endoscope allows examination of the whole area. (c) The 'J' manoeuvre, showing the retroflexed insertion tube entering at the cardia with the blind-ended fundus beyond; the lesser curvature lies at the bottom of the image.

fundus or the antrum closer, depending on which way the tip is pointing. Although the tip can be moved towards the pylorus, it cannot be intubated by this approach. When viewing the fundus and cardia, withdrawing the endoscope will draw the tip towards the cardia for a closer view, and rotating the retroflexed insertion tube on its long axis ('torquing') makes it possible to view the whole cardia (Figure 5.19). Care must be taken when performing this manoeuvre because if the tip becomes trapped, the rotational force could damage the insertion tube.

Gastric biopsy

Before taking biopsy samples, brush cytology is a simple and sensitive technique for identifying spiral bacteria. A small amount of gastric mucus is collected from the mucosa with a sleeved cytology brush, retrieved and smeared on to a slide; when stained with Diff-Quik®, spiral bacteria are readily seen by light microscopy (Figure 5.20). However, the significance of gastric *Helicobacter* organisms is still uncertain, and biopsy specimens should always be collected.

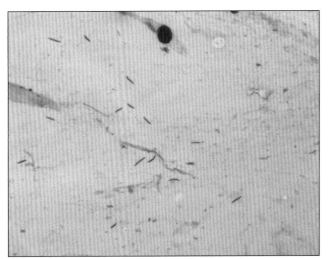

5.20 Brush cytology showing gastric spiral organisms.
(Reproduced from the BSAVA Manual of Canine and Feline Gastroenterology, 2nd edn)

The general technique for taking and handling biopsy specimens is described in Chapter 3. Where gross lesions are detected during gastroscopy, multiple biopsy samples should be collected from the lesion and the surrounding, apparently normal, tissue. Even if no macroscopic lesions are observed, chronic inflammatory disease may still exist, and so samples should always be collected from all regions of the stomach (cardia, fundus, greater and lesser curvature, and antrum). At least two biopsy samples should be collected from the fundus, four from the body (lesser and greater curvature) and two from the antral canal. Alternatively, a total of 10–12 samples from different areas can be pooled. Samples may be placed in different formalin pots, although if grossly normal there is an inclination to pool them (and a cost saving from doing so). However, if a specific lesion is seen and biopsied, the tissue should be fixed and submitted separately.

The gastroscope naturally tends to turn the biopsy forceps towards the lesser curvature, which will be easier to biopsy if the stomach is deflated. Overinflation of the stomach stretches the mucosa, meaning that smaller amounts of tissue will be sampled. If insufflation is needed to see the area from which the biopsy sample is being taken, it is worth deflating the stomach after positioning the open cups of the forceps so that when the cups are closed more tissue is grasped. Taking samples from the edge of a rugal fold also increases the yield (Figure 5.21).

Biopsy specimens from the fundus and cardia should be collected by inserting the forceps through the biopsy channel when the endoscope is in a neutral position and then retroflexing the tip. This is critical for avoiding damage to the biopsy channel within the bending section. When the endoscope is retroflexed, care must also be taken to avoid taking biopsy samples of the insertion tube itself as it enters at the cardia, and so a clear view should be obtained before attempting to take samples. The antral mucosa is tougher than the other areas and biopsy specimens are consequently small; taking two biopsy samples during the same pass of the forceps will give an increased yield.

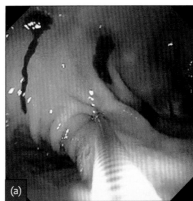

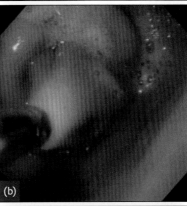

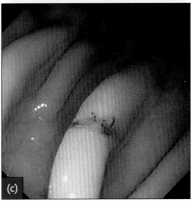

5.21 Gastric biopsy. (a) Biopsy of the lesser curvature. The sites of previous biopsies are indicated by the small areas of bleeding, with blood trickling down. (b) The edge of a rugal fold is grasped by biopsy forceps and a sample of tissue is avulsed. (c) Site of a gastric biopsy.
(c, Reproduced from the *BSAVA Manual of Canine and Feline Gastroenterology, 2nd edn*)

Biopsy samples should be collected from the periphery of any ulcer and not the centre of the lesion. This is because sampling the centre of the ulcer may result in perforation and is usually not diagnostic, collecting only fibrinous or necrotic tissue and inflammatory cells. When malignancy is suspected, repeated sampling from the same site may reveal neoplastic cells deeper in the lesion, while superficial layers contain only non-specific necrotic tissue. However, it is important to remember that it may not be possible to distinguish between benign and malignant gastric ulcers on the basis of their appearance.

Once all the gastric biopsy specimens have been collected, as much air as possible should be suctioned from the stomach before the endoscope is withdrawn into the oesophagus, to reduce any respiratory embarrassment and the risk of reflux.

Duodenoscopy

Entering the duodenum through the pylorus is the hardest part of upper GI endoscopy, and has been likened to trying to push a metre-long piece of stiff rope through a small hole in a strong wind! Pharmacological intervention with metoclopramide has not been shown to help experienced endoscopists, and its augmentation of peristalsis may even make the procedure more difficult. Premedication with butorphanol appears to make pyloric intubation in dogs easier than premedication with methadone (McFadzean *et al.*, 2017).

Engaging the pylorus

Overinflation of the stomach is the biggest mistake made when trying to intubate the pylorus (see Figure 5.16). The inflation and stretching of the greater curvature closes off the antral canal. The stomach assumes a bloated 'U' shape with the antral opening flattened and the pylorus moved out of view; antral contractions are also stimulated. In this situation it is difficult to enter the antrum and virtually impossible to reach the pylorus, let alone intubate the duodenum, and paradoxical motion (see above) may occur if the stomach is overinflated even more.

When this occurs, the endoscope tip must be moved back and air suctioned out before repeating the forward manoeuvre. When repeated, it is important to ensure that the stomach is not continually being insufflated – novice endoscopists, in particular, tend to forget that their finger is covering the hole in the air/water button on the handpiece. The insertion tube should be kept lying along the greater curvature so that the tip is more likely to move into the antral canal successfully. Particularly in cats, slight rotation of the insertion tube on its long axis may assist the process. However, the inexperienced endoscopist may have to attempt this manoeuvre several times before the endoscope passes into the antrum and on to the pylorus, and this can be frustrating.

Pyloric intubation

The pylorus is visualized at the end of the antrum. By advancing the endoscope along the greater curvature of the stomach, the tip engages with the pyloric canal and passes through into the duodenum. This manoeuvre may fail, especially if the stomach is overinflated, with the tip moving up towards the cardia (as described above). The tip needs to be continually realigned because as the endoscope is advanced it distorts the greater curvature and moves the relative position of the pylorus.

Once the endoscope tip is engaged with the pylorus and centred in the lumen, the aim is to move the endoscope forward while continually readjusting the tip to keep it in the centre of the pyloric canal. With video-endoscopes in large dogs, it may be easier to rotate the endoscope through 90 degrees so that the handpiece lies flat in the palm of the hand (see Chapter 3). Red-out often occurs as the pylorus is passed, and so the endoscopist may simply aim at the darkest area; there is often an impression of the mucosa sliding by. Intermittent puffs of air may assist the passage of the tip, but continual insufflation will probably cause overinflation. Although it seems logical to keep pushing the endoscope forward to pass the pylorus, because of paradoxical movement, it can actually help to withdraw the endoscope slightly to straighten it before proceeding forward. It may also help to suction air out of the stomach; the deflation of the stomach will force the endoscope tip forward as the stomach collapses over it, and if it has been steered to the right position the tip may exit the pyloric canal automatically.

The keys to success in pyloric intubation are:

- The insertion tube of the endoscope must be long enough to reach the pylorus

- The endoscope tip diameter should not be too large for the patient
- Intubation should be performed as soon as possible after orienting the endoscope in the stomach, but patience is required
- The stomach should not be overinflated
- The position of the endoscope tip should be constantly readjusted by steering manoeuvres to keep the pylorus in the centre of the field of view.

If the tip keeps slipping out of the pylorus or cannot even reach the pylorus, the endoscope should be withdrawn, air suctioned to partially deflate the stomach and the process started again. Repeated attempts at intubation may be needed, and patience is important. However, making too many repeated attempts will ultimately cause mechanical trauma to the pyloric canal, making intubation more difficult or even impossible (Video 5.1).

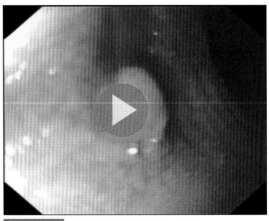

Video 5.1 Upper GI endoscopy.

Entering the duodenum

As the pyloric canal is passed, the mucosal colour changes to red, or to orange if it is stained with bile. However, red-out may continue as the cranial duodenal flexure is negotiated. If the endoscope is moving freely there will be an impression of the red-out sliding by as forward pressure is exerted. Turning the control wheels and/or rotating the gastroscope in the direction of the flexure assists slide-by. After 3–5 cm of the insertion tube has passed into the duodenum, intermittent tip deflection and insufflation will usually achieve a view of the lumen of the descending duodenum. The area obscured during intubation must be examined during withdrawal of the gastroscope.

Consolidating small intestinal intubation

Once the proximal duodenal flexure has been passed and the lumen is visualized, it is relatively easy to advance the endoscope along the small intestine. The duodenum should not be overinflated as air may reflux into the stomach and distend it excessively. In most dogs, intubation of the descending duodenum to the distal duodenal flexure should be possible. In small dogs and cats, it may even be possible to reach the proximal jejunum with a 1 m insertion tube. However, in larger dogs, it is often impossible to advance the endoscope further than the proximal duodenum by further insertion because the handpiece of a video-endoscope is already entering the patient's mouth or, if using a fibreoptic endoscope, the endoscopist's face (at the eyepiece) is adjacent to the patient's mouth.

Paradoxically, further movement along the duodenum can often be achieved by slightly withdrawing the endoscope while observing that the image does not change (i.e. the tip remains stationary); this reduces any looping of the insertion tube in the stomach and then allows it to be pushed further into the duodenum. Further insertion may also be achieved by external compression of the abdomen to slide the duodenum over the insertion tube. A slide-by technique may help to pass around further flexures, but rotational 'torquing' of the insertion tube becomes more difficult as loops of intestine form and the insertion tube tip passes through 360 degrees.

Failure to intubate

As discussed above, intubation of the duodenum is the most difficult procedure in upper GI endoscopy, especially when the pylorus is closed. Even experienced endoscopists can occasionally find it impossible to achieve in some patients. Brachycephalic dogs can be particularly challenging to intubate because of the shape of their stomach and the presence of redundant mucosal folds around the pylorus. It is therefore important not to persist for too long, as injury or even perforation can occur. Undue force should not be used to try to enter the duodenum as it increases the risk of perforation.

Occasionally, if intubation is difficult, rotating the patient to dorsal or right lateral recumbency may be helpful. Another trick is to blindly pass biopsy forceps through the pylorus and then pass the endoscope along this temporary 'guidewire', as in a Seldinger catheterization technique. However, this technique is often not successful for intubating the pylorus, as the proximal duodenal flexure prevents any more than minimal entry of the forceps; it is more useful when trying to intubate the ileum from the colon (see Chapter 6). A few biopsy specimens may be obtained blindly from the duodenum, but it is unsafe to take repeated samples from the same site without being able to view it.

Duodenal fluid collection

Before harvesting biopsy specimens, duodenal fluid can be collected to examine for *Giardia* and for qualitative and quantitative culture. A sterile polyethylene tube is passed down the biopsy channel and any liquid in the duodenal lumen is collected. However, fluid is often sparse and frequently becomes contaminated with blood and tissue. It may be more productive to insert the tube as far as possible, deflate the duodenum and then slowly withdraw the tube while applying very gentle suction to retrieve the fluid that has pooled between the mucosal folds. It is often recommended that the first 1 ml of fluid be discarded, as it is likely to be contaminated, but, in reality, it is often difficult to collect even this volume in total. Consequently, fluid collection is not done routinely. Faecal analysis is a more sensitive technique when looking for *Giardia*, and the results of culture often reflect the bacteria the patient has recently swallowed rather than those that are resident in the intestine, while quantification is labour-intensive and unreliable (Leib *et al.*, 1999). A diagnosis of small intestinal bacterial overgrowth may be spurious, as many organisms are not culturable; in any case, the problem is typically dysbiosis rather than overgrowth.

Duodenal biopsy

It is important to note that many forms of small intestinal disease are not apparent macroscopically and can be detected only after histological examination of biopsy samples. It is also not possible to distinguish between intestinal inflammation and alimentary lymphoma by their gross endoscopic appearance. Therefore, in all cases, multiple mucosal biopsy samples should be collected from different regions of the small intestine.

For the collection of optimal biopsy specimens, the biopsy forceps cups should be positioned perpendicular to the intestinal mucosa. A number of techniques can be used to achieve this (Figure 5.22; see also Video 5.1). Increased pressure will increase the size of the specimen (Danesh *et al.*, 1985); perforation of the intestinal wall is unlikely if the cups are opened before pushing. If the biopsy forceps are used parallel to the duodenal mucosa only villus tips will be sampled. The use of swing-jaw biopsy forceps improves the ability to obtain good samples in the descending duodenum.

If the jejunum is reached, more flexures will have been passed, and it not only becomes harder to rotate and steer the endoscope but it is also more difficult to collect biopsy specimens. Indeed, the mechanism of old reusable forceps that have not been lubricated adequately may be so 'sticky' that the cups will not open because of the strain of excessive twisting, even though they opened when tested before insertion. Failure of the forceps to open within the small intestine is frustrating, but sometimes the cups will eventually open if the forceps can be advanced out of the endoscope sufficiently far to be relatively straight. Alternatively, brand new forceps may be robust enough to open, and the use of new disposable forceps should prevent this problem.

After examination and biopsy of the duodenum, the endoscope is withdrawn into the stomach for a more careful examination (see above). It is important to observe the proximal duodenal flexure during withdrawal, as any lesions that were missed as the endoscope entered the duodenum may now be seen.

Jejunoscopy

So-called 'push enteroscopy' to examine the jejunum uses an endoscope with an insertion tube 2–3 m in length. Such an endoscope is usually narrow and may not have a biopsy channel, and so is used only for viewing without biopsy. Typically, this type of endoscope is difficult to steer and may need to be guided through the stomach by passage through an oversleeve or by being 'piggy-backed' on a standard gastroscope.

Complete examination of the whole length of the small intestine using a flexible endoscope can be guaranteed only by using a double-balloon enteroscope. This specialized endoscope has an oversleeve with an inflatable balloon, in addition to an inflatable balloon behind the endoscope tip. By repeated cycles of inflating and deflating each balloon alternately, while advancing the insertion tube and then the oversleeve, the intestine can be shortened like a concertina so that its whole length is eventually seen. This process is complex and slow and, although it has been reported in dogs (Sarria *et al.*, 2013), it has not been adopted by most specialist veterinary practices, as it is technically difficult, time-consuming and expensive. Similar visualization can be achieved more easily by capsule endoscopy (see below).

Ending the examination

After a full duodenal and gastric examination and biopsy, as much air as possible is suctioned from the stomach. Further investigation of any oesophageal lesions can be performed as the endoscope is withdrawn (see Chapter 4).

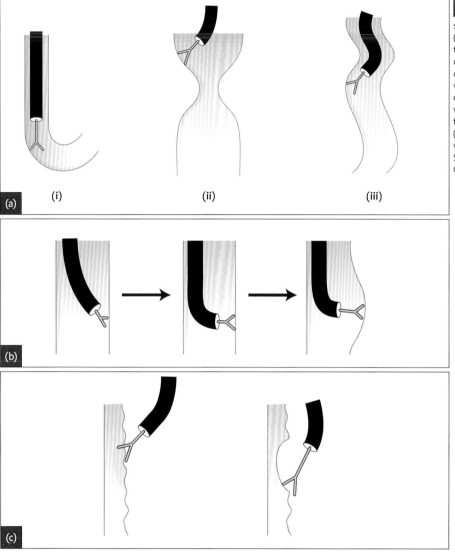

5.22 Techniques to enhance the size and quality of duodenal biopsy specimens. (a) Samples should be taken (i) from the distal duodenal flexure, (ii) from the 'back' of a peristaltic wave and (iii) after deflation of the duodenum so that folds develop. (b) The forceps are placed on the wall of the descending duodenum and the endoscope tip is then deflected into the wall while pushing the mucosa away with the forceps to allow the biopsy site to be viewed. (c) The open cups should be pushed along the wall to scoop up a larger piece of mucosa. Swing-jaw forceps should be used (see Chapter 3, Figure 3.20).

Capsule endoscopy

Conventional flexible gastroscopes are unable to examine the whole small intestine, even if intubation of the ileum via colonoscopy (see Chapter 6) is achieved, and double-balloon enteroscopy is not generally available. Capsule endoscopy is a method that makes it possible to observe the whole small intestine. It is not a form of flexible endoscopy, and is unable to obtain biopsy samples, but it is useful for observing mucosal lesions, particularly if there is focal bleeding in the small intestine. The capsule is swallowed by the patient and a light source and camera in the capsule, powered by an internal battery, capture repeated images as the capsule passes through the GI tract.

Medical capsule endoscopy systems (ENDOCAPSULE (Olympus) and PillCam™ (Medtronic)) use real-time telemetry via body surface detectors in a waistcoat worn by the patient to capture and record images taken by the capsule. The use of the ENDOCAPSULE system in dogs to monitor the efficacy of anthelmintics (Lee *et al.*, 2011) and to detect bleeding GI lesions (Davignon *et al.*, 2016) has been reported. Reviewing the whole recording can be tedious, and sophisticated image analysis software can now eliminate duplicate images to shorten the time taken to review

the passage of the capsule. Obstruction is a recognized but quite rare complication in humans, but a capsule should not be used when a benign or malignant stricture is suspected. The transit time of the capsule may exceed its battery life and so lesions in the distal intestine may not be visualized, particularly if the capsule gets stuck in the stomach for a period. This can be avoided by using an endoscopic device (AdvanCE® Delivery Device, US Endoscopy Inc.) to place the capsule directly in the duodenum.

The Alicam® (Infiniti Medical) is a veterinary capsule endoscopy system designed for use in dogs. The capsule has four cameras to capture a 360-degree view and, rather than exporting the images by telemetry, the recorded images are stored within the device (Figure 5.23). Once the capsule has been passed in the faeces, it is retrieved, cleaned and returned to the supplier (Infiniti Medical) for the images to be downloaded. Image analysis is performed by specialists using dedicated software that detects changes in the image pixelation suggestive of a lesion (Video 5.2). If the capsule is bitten during peroral administration, it must not be used. No food, treats or chews should be given for 24 hours before the capsule is swallowed and for 8 hours after, as the image could be obscured. The size of the capsule means that it should not

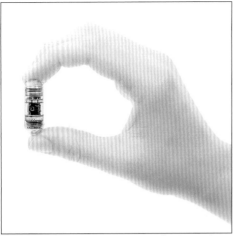

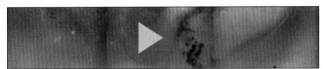

5.23 Capsule endoscopy. Alicam® video-endoscopy capsule (see Video 5.2 for a detailed video sequence).
(Courtesy of Infiniti Medical LLC, Redwood City, CA, USA)

Video 5.2 Video sequence recorded from an Alicam® video-endoscopy capsule, showing a bleeding gastric polyp.

be used in dogs <8 kg or in cats, as it may cause an obstruction. Passage of the capsule from the stomach into the duodenum may be facilitated by the administration of a prokinetic such as metoclopramide.

The indications for capsule endoscopy in veterinary medicine are limited, as focal GI bleeding is less common in dogs than in humans, but it is a method available to practitioners who cannot afford a flexible endoscopy system to examine even the stomach. The cost of capsule endoscopy is similar to that of a single gastroscopic procedure under anaesthesia, but does not require any capital investment in equipment.

Normal findings

Stomach

The gastric mucosa (Figure 5.24) should be pink and glistening. Patches of hyperaemia are sometimes seen and are thought to be due to local variations in blood flow. They often disappear as the examination proceeds and are not considered to be pathological. Submucosal vessels are seen in the cardia and fundus only when the stomach is fully inflated. There may be a few strands of mucus crossing the lumen as opposing mucosae are separated by insufflation. In some dogs, dark spots within the mucosa are seen; these seem to correspond to the lymphoid follicles induced by *Helicobacter* infection, but it is not clear whether they are actually abnormal.

The rugal folds are generally smooth and tend to run in straight lines along the long axis of the stomach. They flatten on insufflation and re-form as the stomach is deflated. The antrum has few folds except around the pylorus, where a few folds are expected. The normal pylorus may be open or closed but should not be obscured by mucosal folds. Waves of peristalsis may be seen migrating concentrically towards the pylorus (see Figure 5.15). These waves are more common in dogs

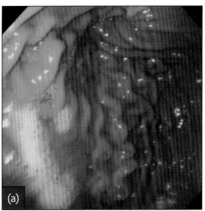

(a)

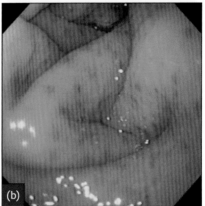

(b)

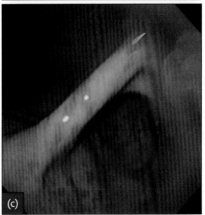

(c)

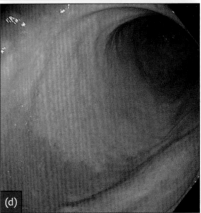

(d)

5.24 Endoscopic appearance of the normal stomach. (a) Rugal folds on the greater curvature. A small amount of bile-stained fluid is present and should be aspirated during examination of the stomach. (b) Lymphoid follicles may be seen in the mucosa as darker spots; these have been associated with *Helicobacter* infection. (c) Transient patches of hyperaemia are sometimes seen as here on the angularis incisura. (d) In this image, there is a sharp line of demarcation of redness between the gastric body and antrum; the significance of this finding is unknown.

than cats, occurring three to four times per minute, and seem to be stimulated by overdistension of the stomach. They also become more frequent the longer the procedure takes.

Duodenum

The duodenal mucosa (Figure 5.25) is pink and has the appearance of crushed velvet or good-quality terry towelling, although the granularity depends to a certain extent on the degree of distension, the species and the magnification of the endoscopy system (see Chapter 3); the texture is slightly grainier and the mucosa slightly pinker in dogs compared with cats. Submucosal vessels are not visible.

One landmark in the duodenum of dogs is the major duodenal papilla, where the common bile duct and major pancreatic duct enter (Figure 5.26a); it is not always readily visible in cats. In some dogs (but not in cats) there is also a minor duodenal papilla where a second pancreatic duct enters (Figure 5.26b). The minor papilla (if present) is slightly clockwise to the position of the major papilla. These papillae appear as small, white, fairly flat protuberances and may be overlooked until the endoscope is being withdrawn. It is important to recognize these as normal anatomy rather than pathology, so as not to biopsy them and cause iatrogenic trauma, which carries the risk of resultant stenosis. In dogs, Peyer's patches (lymphoid aggregates) are usually visible as 1–3 cm pale oval depressions along the antimesenteric border of the descending duodenum (Figure 5.26c); these are not seen in cats.

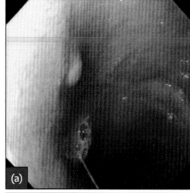

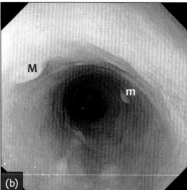

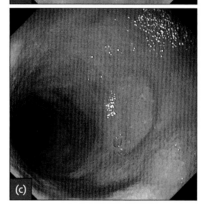

5.26 Landmarks in the normal canine duodenum. (a) The major duodenal papilla in the duodenum of the dog is the site of entry of the common bile duct and major pancreatic duct. (b) A minor duodenal papilla (m) is seen in some but not all dogs distal to the major papilla (M) and approximately 90 degrees clockwise from it. The distal duodenal flexure is seen in the distance. (c) Peyer's patches (lymphoid tissue) in the canine duodenum appear as a line of pale oval depressions along the antimesenteric border of the descending duodenum. White spots probably represent follicles within the lymphoid tissue.

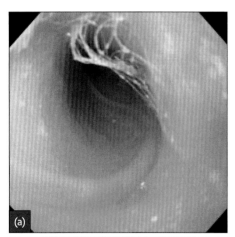

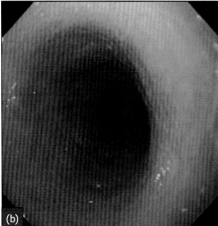

5.25 Endoscopic appearance of the normal descending duodenum in (a) a cat and (b) a dog. Note the paler duodenal mucosa in the cat and the presence of hair and an incidental roundworm.

Pathological conditions

The aetiopathogenesis, diagnosis and treatment of various GI conditions are discussed in the *BSAVA Manual of Canine and Feline Gastroenterology*. The endoscopic appearance of the more common diseases is described here.

Stomach

Irregularity, friability, ulceration and overt masses in the gastric mucosa are all abnormal. Patches of hyperaemia are not necessarily considered pathological and the significance of lymphoid follicles is uncertain. Fresh or changed blood (with an appearance like coffee grounds) is abnormal, and if it is observed a bleeding ulcer or tumour should be sought. The presence of food is abnormal if the patient has truly had food withheld for 12 hours, and may reflect an outflow obstruction or abnormal motility, which is most frequently associated with gastritis, gastric ulceration or chronic inflammatory enteropathy.

The more common pathological conditions that can be recognized endoscopically in the stomach are listed in Figure 5.27, with examples shown in Figures 5.28–5.31.

Condition	Appearance
Gastritis (Figure 5.28ab)	• May appear grossly normal • Increased mucus • Increased number of lymphoid follicles • Mucosal thickening, granularity and friability • Superficial and/or deep ulcers • Subepithelial ('paintbrush') and frank haemorrhage • Reduced size and number of rugal folds and prominent submucosal vessels in atrophic gastritis
Superficial ulcers (Figures 5.28c and 5.29a)	• Shallow areas of mucosal disruption (sometimes incorrectly termed erosions) • Brown discoloration of luminal blood • Causes: inflammatory disease, NSAIDs, 'stress'
Deep ulcers (Figures 5.28d and 5.29b)	• Mucosal disruptions penetrating the submucosa • Raised and thickened border • Dark brown ulcer bed due to bleeding • Yellow/white necrotic tissue • Changed (oxidized) brown blood in gastric fluid in the fundus • Causes: inflammatory disease, NSAIDs, neoplasia
Pyloric stenosis	• Enlarged, protuberant pylorus • Narrowed pyloric canal • Retained food sometimes observed • Erythema/erosions around pylorus sometimes observed
Benign mucosal antral polyps (Figure 5.30a–c)	• Commonly seen in old dogs • Of no clinical significance unless bleeding
Hypertrophic pylorogastropathy (Figure 5.30d)	• Thickened rugae, not completely flattened by insufflation • Prominent light reflectivity suggestive of oedema • May occlude the pylorus
Neoplasia (Figure 5.31)	• Mass lesion • Gastric haemorrhage • Ulcerated tissue • Thickening/stiffening of mucosa; rigid when biopsied • Carcinoma often on the lesser curvature extending to the cardia or antrum • Ulcers on the greater curvature are rarely carcinomas and are either non-malignant (e.g. leiomyoma) or malignant (e.g. leiomyosarcoma, lymphoma, or rarely histiocytic sarcoma, mast cell tumour)
Parasites	• *Physaloptera* spp. worms (not in the UK) • *Ollulanus tricuspis* in cats is a microscopic cause of gastritis

5.27 Endoscopic appearance of gastric lesions. NSAIDs = non-steroidal anti-inflammatory drugs.

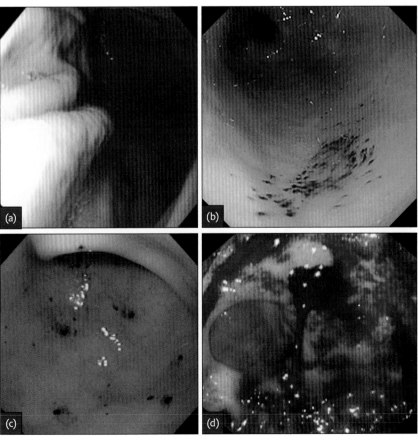

5.28 Endoscopic appearance of gastritis.
(a) Subtle irregularities in the mucosa of the rugal folds, consistent with chronic gastritis.
(b) 'Paintbrush' haemorrhages in the antrum.
(c) Multiple superficial gastric ulcers associated with chronic gastritis, showing small amounts of changed (brown) blood. (d) Severe diffuse ulceration with significant bleeding in chronic gastritis; fresh blood is dripping down.
(a, b, d, Reproduced from the *BSAVA Manual of Canine and Feline Gastroenterology*, 3rd edn)

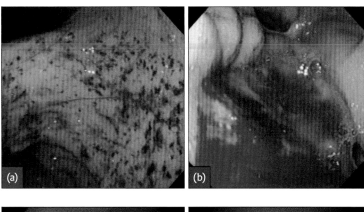

5.29 Endoscopic appearance of NSAID-induced gastric ulcers. (a) Multiple ulcers following NSAID administration. (b) A single large ulcer. NSAIDs = non-steroidal anti-inflammatory drugs.

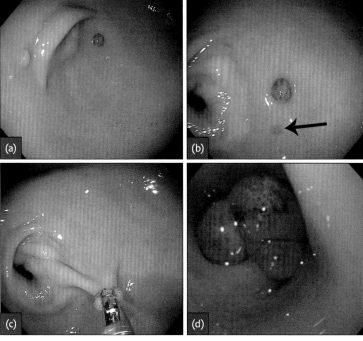

5.30 Endoscopic appearance of antral lesions. Polypoid lesions sometimes bleed and are biopsied as a precaution, but are usually benign, whereas hypertrophic mucosa may obstruct the pylorus. (a) Two small polyps in the antrum of a dog either side of the pylorus. (b) One of these polyps appears very vascular, and another, very small polyp is just below it (arrowed). (c) Biopsy sample being taken from the vascular polyp shown in (b). (d) Hypertrophic pylorogastropathy.

(d, Reproduced from the *BSAVA Manual of Canine and Feline Gastroenterology, 3rd edn*)

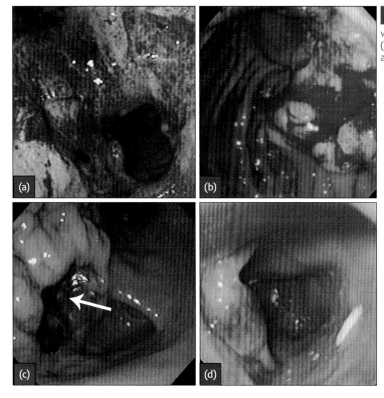

5.31 Endoscopic appearance of mass lesions in the canine stomach. (a) Diffuse gastric carcinoma infiltrating the whole of the lesser curvature, which is completely ulcerated. (b) Bleeding from a gastric carcinoma. (c) Gastric carcinoma with a large deep ulcer (arrowed). (d) Gastric leiomyoma in the antrum.

Gastritis

Gastritis is indicated by irregularity and friability of the mucosa (see Figure 5.28). There may be small areas of haemorrhage associated with superficial ulcers (often incorrectly termed erosions) in gastritis. Biopsy specimens should always be collected even if there is no macroscopic evidence of gastritis, as microscopic inflammation may be detected.

Benign ulcers

Benign ulcers are seen in chronic gastritis and following non-steroidal anti-inflammatory drug (NSAID) adminis-tration. NSAID-induced ulcers may be multiple or single, and tend to have smooth edges and form a depression in the mucosa (see Figure 5.29b). By contrast, neoplastic ulcers are often proliferative, raised and feel rigid on biopsy.

Pyloric stenosis

This may be caused by a congenital excess of mucosal folds around the pylorus, but more often is due to musc-ular hypertrophy, especially in brachycephalic dogs; in these cases the only endoscopic abnormality is an inability to pass an endoscope of appropriate size for the animal. A technique using olives (blunt-ended probes) to assess the diameter of the pylorus endoscopically has been described (Lamoureux *et al.*, 2019). Functional dyssynergia between antral contraction and pyloric relaxation can pro-duce similar signs, but in such cases the pylorus has a normal endoscopic appearance.

Antral polyps

Benign polyps (see Figure 5.30a–c) are quite common in the antrum of older dogs. Occasionally, they bleed a little. It is debatable whether they should always be biopsied, but biopsy is advisable if they are bleeding or have an atypical appearance.

Hypertrophic pylorogastropathy

Excessive folds around the pylorus are typical of hyper-trophy (Figure 5.30d) and can be the cause of an outflow obstruction.

Gastric neoplasia

Gastric adenocarcinoma (see Figure 5.31a–c and Video 5.3) is most commonly seen on the lesser curvature and may be suspected if more than three of the following six observations are made (Simpson, 2005):

- Change in the colour of the mucosa to a mottled purple instead of pink
- Deep pigmentation of the mucosa
- An obvious mucosal mass
- Ulceration
- Loss of normal gastric landmarks
- Rigidity of the gastric mucosa.

Gastric lymphoma can affect some or all of the stomach and the mucosa is often lumpy and friable. However, in all cases the observation must be confirmed by histopathological examination. Deep biopsy specimens may be required to make the diagnosis, as the superficial tissue is often necrotic.

Leiomyoma (see Figure 5.31d) and leiomyosarcoma can occur in the stomach; although these tumours are

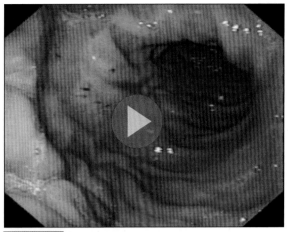

Video 5.3 Upper GI endoscopy of a dog with a gastric carcinoma.

derived from the muscle layers, they may protrude into the gastric lumen and may be ulcerated. They can be mistaken for gastric carcinoma, so biopsy is essential, but they may not occur at the typical site of carcinoma on the lesser curvature.

Gastric parasites

Physaloptera spp. worms in the stomach are not seen in the UK, and *Ollulanus tricuspis* is too small to be recog-nized grossly by endoscopy.

Duodenum

Deep duodenal ulceration is rare in the dog and cat and is most commonly associated with malignancy, but inflam-mation and erosions are common, leading to friability of the mucosa, increased granularity and sometimes bleed-ing. However, there is a well recognized disparity between the gross and histological appearance, and so intestinal biopsy specimens should always be taken.

The more common pathological conditions that can be recognized endoscopically in the duodenum are listed in Figure 5.32, with examples shown in Figures 5.33–5.35.

Condition	Appearance

Inflammatory disease (Figures 5.33 and 5.34a)	• Increased granularity
	• Increased friability
	• Ulcers
	• Haemorrhage
	• Linear haemorrhage:
	  • Artefact caused by trauma
	  • Eosinophilic inflammatory disease

Neoplasia (Figure 5.34b–d)	• Thickening and irregularity if lymphosarcoma • Mass or annular obstruction with adenocarcinoma • Adenomatous polyps occasionally seen in cats
Lymphangiectasia and crypt abscessation (Figure 5.35ab)	• Multiple white spots indicating dilated lipid-filled lymphatics • Similar appearance may be seen in postprandial state
Parasites (Figure 5.35cd)	• *Toxocara* spp. – motile, photophobic • *Uncinaria* spp. – small (1–2 cm), white, embedded in mucosa • *Taenia* spp. – recognizable by segmentation

5.32 Endoscopic appearance of duodenal lesions.

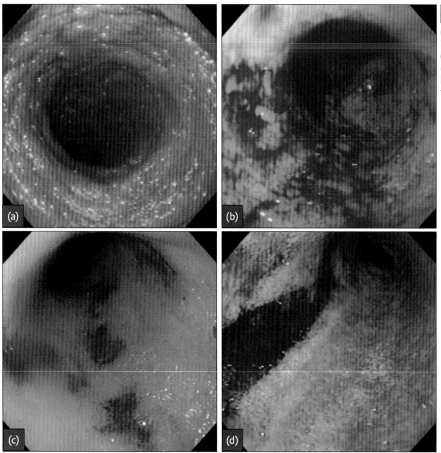

5.33 Endoscopic appearance of inflammatory duodenal lesions. (a) Lymphoplasmacytic enteritis. (b) Spontaneous bleeding associated with eosinophilic enteritis. (c) Ulceration associated with eosinophilic enteritis. (d) Stripping of the mucosa during insertion of the endoscope, suggestive of very friable, inflamed tissue.

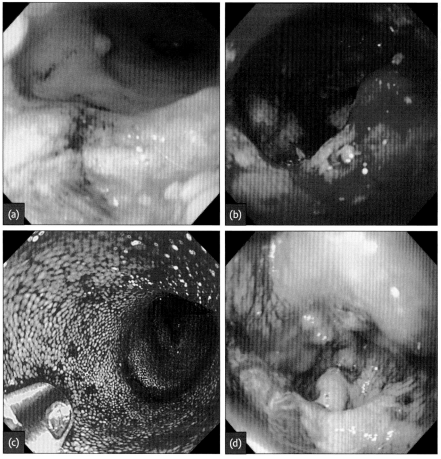

5.34 Endoscopic appearance of ulcerative duodenal lesions. (a) Benign chronic deep ulcer in the proximal duodenum of a dog caused by treatment with NSAIDs. The major duodenal papilla is seen distal to the ulcer. (b) Alimentary lymphoma in a dog. (c) Small cell alimentary lymphoma in a cat with spontaneous bleeding highlighting the preserved villous structure. (d) Intestinal adenocarcinoma in a dog. NSAIDs = non-steroidal anti-inflammatory drugs.

(c, Courtesy of Claudia Gil Morales)

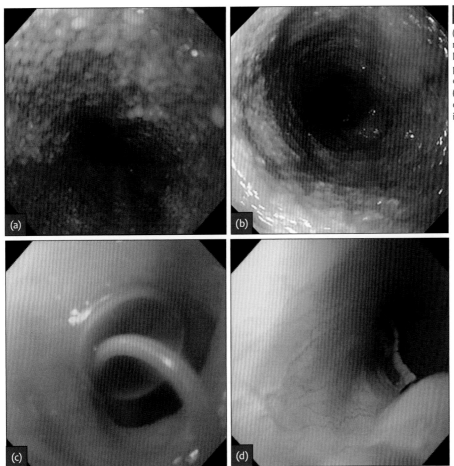

5.35 Endoscopic appearance of miscellaneous duodenal lesions. (a) Lymphangiectasia in a dog. Note the multiple dilated lacteals containing white lymph. (b) Crypt abscessation in a dog with a protein-losing enteropathy; the white spots could be mistaken for lymphangiectasia. (c) Isolated *Toxocara* roundworm in the duodenum of a dog. (d) Segmented tapeworm in the duodenum of a cat.

Chronic inflammatory enteropathy

In intestinal inflammation, the mucosa is often irregular and may be ulcerated and even bleeding (see Figure 5.33). The tissue is usually friable: bleeding often occurs when the mucosa is traumatized by the endoscope merely touching it, and large pieces may be avulsed when biopsy is performed. Spontaneous bleeding is more typical of eosinophilic inflammation rather than lymphoplasmacytic enteritis.

Duodenal ulceration

Spontaneous duodenal (peptic) ulcers are rare and are most commonly caused by NSAID administration. They are typically seen just distal to the pyloric canal (see Figure 5.34a) and are most easily observed during slow withdrawal of the endoscope from the duodenum, as they may be missed when advancing the endoscope past the proximal duodenal flexure.

Alimentary lymphosarcoma

There is no pathognomonic gross appearance for alimentary lymphosarcoma (see Figure 5.34b), and biopsy should always be performed. However, mucosal biopsy may be inadequate in some cases, with a full-thickness biopsy being required for a definitive diagnosis. The mucosal surface may appear very smooth because of effacement of the villi, or very irregular and friable, and there may be patchy, lumpy infiltration. Small cell alimentary lymphoma in cats may be grossly indistinguishable from intestinal inflammation (see Figure 5.34c), and biopsies must be performed.

Intestinal adenocarcinoma

Carcinomas are more common in the stomach (see above) and colon (see Chapter 6), although gastric carcinomas can extend to involve the duodenum. Primary intestinal adenocarcinomas (see Figure 5.34d) are seen most commonly in the ileum of older cats, and are occasionally found endoscopically in the canine duodenum, where they typically are ulcerated.

Lymphangiectasia

Lymphangiectasia may be identified in the duodenum by its gross appearance, but it can be patchy, and full-thickness biopsy of other parts of the small intestine may be needed to reach a diagnosis. The appearance of multiple small white spots, which are fat-filled lacteals, is characteristic (see Figure 5.35a). Typically, the lymphatics are markedly dilated with fat and appear as multiple white globules in the mucosa. However, a similar but less severe appearance can occur postprandially, and so biopsy confirmation is essential. Furthermore, similar scattered white spots may be seen with crypt abscessation (see Figure 5.35b) and in some inflammatory diseases (Garcia-Sancho *et al.*, 2011).

Intestinal parasites

Occasionally, roundworms (see Figure 5.35c) and tapeworms (see Figure 5.35d) are seen endoscopically. They are rarely of clinical significance. Single roundworms can be retrieved endoscopically for identification, although they are photophobic and migrate away from the endoscope light if they are not caught quite quickly. *Uncinaria* spp. hookworms (small white worms) are occasionally found in the duodenum embedded in the mucosa. *Trichuris* spp. whipworms are typically found in the caecum (see Chapter 6).

Complications of upper gastrointestinal tract endoscopy

Although endoscopy is minimally invasive, there is the potential to do harm to the patient (this is fortunately rare) or to damage the equipment (see Chapter 3).

Gastrointestinal perforation

Perforation of the GI tract can result from forceful insertion of the endoscope without adequate visualization of the lumen, or from poor biopsy technique. It is most likely to occur when trying to intubate the duodenum. However, most perforations occur when the tissue is diseased, and sometimes even just vigorous insufflation is sufficient to rupture an ulcerated area. The perforation (and even intraperitoneal organs) may be visible endoscopically, but as the viscus is likely to collapse, observing this cannot be relied upon. Air escaping into the peritoneal cavity will cause abdominal distension that cannot be relieved by endoscopic suction, and can be verified by abdominal radiography or abdominocentesis. Although this is a rare complication, the endoscopist should always be prepared to take a patient to emergency laparotomy if perforation occurs.

Mucosal haemorrhage

Significant haemorrhage is a rare event in GI endoscopy, and intervention is rarely needed. It is usually associated with malignancy. Haemorrhage following the collection of biopsy samples is rarely significant, and it is not routine practice to prescribe acid blockers or sucralfate after biopsy. Where a significant bleed does occur (see Figure 5.28d), the application of ice-cold water through an endoscopic catheter will usually halt it. If this fails, a 1:10,000 adrenaline solution may be applied in a similar manner.

Gastric dilatation

Gastric dilatation can occur during recovery if air is not adequately removed after gastroscopy. Theoretically, a volvulus could follow, and it is wise to deflate the stomach before withdrawing the endoscope. Very occasionally, gastric instability and partial torsion without dilatation is identified endoscopically, but requires a familiarity with the normal gastric position to be recognized.

Decreased venous return from gastric overdistension

Overdistension of the stomach during upper GI endoscopy is a much more common problem than volvulus. As well as making pyloric intubation difficult or impossible, it has significant haemodynamic and cardiorespiratory effects similar to those seen in a spontaneous volvulus:

- Compression of the caudal vena cava, causing a rapid drop in venous return and blood pressure
- Compression of the diaphragm and decreased tidal volume: splinting of the diaphragm prevents adequate respiratory function.

Acute bradycardia

A slowing heart rate is sometimes encountered, especially when the small intestine is entered, and occurs particularly in toy-breed dogs and patients with severe GI disease. This appears to be a vagal reflex and can be abolished by atropine. However, there may also be increased respiratory and skeletal movements, and tactical intravenous diazepam can be helpful.

Bacteraemia

Transient bacteraemia occurs in about 5% of humans undergoing colonoscopy. The incidence of bacteraemia in dogs and cats undergoing any form of GI endoscopy is unknown, and perioperative antibiotics are not routinely used. However, it may be sensible to use them in 'at-risk' patients, such as patients with diffuse GI bleeding or valvular heart disease and immunosuppressed patients.

Transmission of infection

Poorly disinfected endoscopes can transmit enteropathogenic organisms, and even within the same patient, it is common sense to perform upper **before** lower GI endoscopy. Adequate disinfection of a gastroscope is an essential part of the process and starts as soon as the endoscopic procedure finishes, with the endoscopist flushing the channels to remove gross material before thorough cleaning (see Chapter 2).

Therapeutic procedures
Foreign body removal

Foreign bodies in the GI tract are quite a common problem in dogs, and range from soft objects (e.g. socks) to bones, stones, balls and fishhooks, and even bizarre objects such as toys (Figure 5.36). Cats are more fastidious and more typically swallow needles and thread, elastic bands and baby feeding teats. Foreign bodies can be managed conservatively (e.g. bones dissolve in gastric acid, or some foreign bodies may pass through the GI tract naturally) or by surgical or endoscopic removal. The method chosen for removal will depend on the:

- Clinical state of the patient
- Anatomical location of the foreign body
- Size of the foreign body
- Type of foreign body:
  - Sharp or smooth
  - Containing caustic agents, lead or zinc (e.g. batteries, coins)
- Radiological evidence of:
  - Obstruction
  - Perforation.

Instrumentation

A number of instruments that fit through a 2.8 mm accessory channel are available for grasping foreign bodies

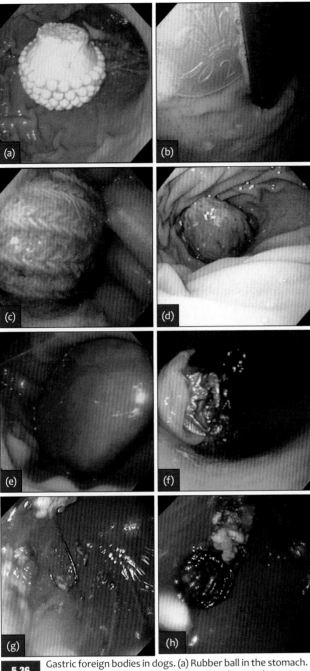

5.36 Gastric foreign bodies in dogs. (a) Rubber ball in the stomach. Despite being swallowed, the ball was too large to be retrieved endoscopically and a gastrotomy was performed. (b) Coin. Note that it has fallen down to the cardia. (c) Sock. (d) Peach stone. (e) Stone. (f) Gold ring with paper tissue stuck to it. (g) Fishhook and (h) peach stone in the stomach of the same dog.

The instruments available include:

- Wire baskets
- Roth basket (wire loop with a net)
- Snares
- Rat-toothed or alligator jaw grasping forceps
- Multi-pronged forceps (two-, three-, four- and five-pronged, W-shaped)
- Magnets.

Of these, large grasping forceps and both types of basket forceps are the most versatile and useful. Basket forceps and snares, when opened, spring to a 'memorized' shape and can be manipulated by steering the endoscope over the foreign body before being closed tightly around it. Similar instruments can be used to retrieve oesophageal and pulmonary foreign bodies (see Chapters 4 and 7).

Gastric foreign bodies

Endoscopic removal of gastric foreign bodies can be very rewarding if it obviates the need for surgery, but it can be frustrating if it is attempted when inappropriate and the attempt is unsuccessful. It is sensible to put a time limit on attempts to remove objects, and move to surgery if one is failing. When attempting to grasp objects, they tend to fall into the fundus as the stomach is insufflated if the patient is in left lateral recumbency. Manipulating the object back into the antrum either with the endoscope or by turning the patient on to the right side can help.

Once the foreign body has been securely grasped, the endoscope, grasping instrument and foreign body are removed as a whole until they are outside the mouth, when the foreign body can be released; this is done as the foreign body is obviously too large to be pulled up the biopsy channel. When doing this, the biggest difficulty is manoeuvring out past the lower oesophageal sphincter. It may help to hold the cervical oesophagus closed and insufflate to the maximum while deflecting the endoscope tip obliquely.

Sharp-pointed foreign bodies, such as pins and needles, should be grasped at their point (ideally with rubber-tipped forceps) so that they do not cause trauma on withdrawal. Alternatively, the object should be held so that the sharp point is trailing as the object is pulled up the oesophagus; for example, grasping a fishhook in the middle of the curve so that the barbed tip is pointing backwards as it is removed. It can be helpful to insert a rigid hollow colonoscope or oversleeve into the oesophagus when using a flexible endoscope to remove multiple or sharp gastric foreign bodies, as this will reduce the risk of trauma to the oesophagus by repeated intubation or by sharp foreign bodies, and allows simple passage through the upper oesophageal sphincter.

Soft foreign bodies such as items of clothing (most often socks) can be grabbed by almost any instrument (e.g. grasping or pronged forceps, basket forceps), but reusable biopsy forceps should not be used as they will be blunted.

Ring-shaped foreign bodies can sometimes be removed by entrapment with suture material when they are too large for biopsy forceps and grasping forceps are not available. Biopsy forceps are pre-placed through the endoscope and used to grasp one end of a long length of strong suture material before the endoscope is inserted. Once in the stomach, the suture material is passed through a hole in the foreign body and let go. It is then picked up on the far side and withdrawn through the

(see Chapter 2). There are fewer instruments small enough to pass through a 2.2 mm channel. However, some dogs can swallow remarkably large foreign bodies, and when deciding whether a foreign body can be removed endoscopically, its size, shape and nature, and whether adequate grasping instruments are available, must be considered. For example, balls bigger than squash balls are typically impossible to retrieve endoscopically even though the patient managed to swallow them. It must be remembered that even with instruments that can be inserted through a 2.8 mm accessory channel, some objects may never be retrievable endoscopically. A quick exploratory laparotomy is preferable to spending an extended period of time 'fishing' in the stomach and failing.

oesophagus and the mouth. The foreign body can then be withdrawn on the loop produced by pulling on both ends of the suture material.

The presence of a stone or bone in the stomach should not immediately be assumed to be the cause of any vomiting. Bones will dissolve in gastric acid, and stones are frequently passed. Hairballs in cats are better treated conservatively (e.g. with laxatives) or removed surgically depending on the likelihood that they will be passed. Hairballs often shred when endoscopic removal is attempted and become very frustrating to remove.

Duodenal foreign bodies

Foreign bodies that are stuck in the pylorus and only partly in the duodenum are removed as above unless they represent the start of a linear foreign body, which should be removed surgically. It is rare for foreign bodies that are wholly within the duodenum to be amenable to endoscopic removal, and surgical intervention is indicated if there is evidence of obstruction or perforation.

Contraindications

Endoscopic retrieval is the safest and preferred method of removing gastric foreign bodies, but a number of objects cannot or should not be removed this way because they are:

- Sharp
- Stuck
- Causing perforation
- Too large to grasp
- Too large to be pulled up through the lower oesophageal sphincter.

Complications

Trauma to the oesophagus can be caused during removal of a gastric foreign body, but is much more common with oesophageal foreign bodies (see Chapter 4). Sharp gastric foreign bodies such as bottle caps and pointed or sharp-edged stones may cause gastric ulceration. This should be treated symptomatically with sucralfate and acid blockers once the foreign body has been removed.

Percutaneous endoscopic gastrostomy tube placement

Indications

The principle of assisted feeding is to place a feeding tube as high up in the GI tract as is anatomically possible and to use a tube that can be left in place for as long as is necessary. Although other methods of tube feeding are used more commonly (see the *BSAVA Manual of Canine and Feline Emergency and Critical Care*), gastrostomy tubes are very useful for maintaining nutrition in chronically ill animals where naso-oesophageal tube feeding is too short-term and oesophagostomy tube feeding is not possible. Naso-oesophageal tubes are suited only to short-term liquid feeding. Oesophagostomy tubes are used when there is anorexia and where any structural disease is confined to the oronasopharynx. Percutaneous endoscopic gastrostomy (PEG) tubes do not need to be used in patients for which these other options are appropriate.

However, patients that have suffered severe head trauma tend to tolerate a PEG tube better than an oesophagostomy tube.

PEG tubes can be used for:

- Prolonged anorexia (e.g. feline hepatic lipidosis)
- Severe, painful oropharyngeal disease (e.g. facial fractures)
- Oesophageal disease:
  - Severe oesophagitis
  - During serial dilations of a stricture
  - Incurable obstruction (e.g. recurrent/refractory stricture, neoplasia)
  - Megaoesophagus. However, the use of permanent gastrostomy tubes in animals with megaoesophagus is controversial; some patients do well but others continue to inhale saliva and ultimately die of pneumonia.

Gastrostomy tubes can be placed:

- Surgically:
  - This is a logical option if the patient is undergoing a laparotomy, e.g. after gastric dilatation–volvulus
  - This is often too invasive in a potentially debilitated patient if other surgery is not required
- Blindly (e.g. with an ELD device):
  - This method is rarely if ever used because of the risk of splenic laceration
- Endoscopically:
  - This method is safer and quicker
  - It is also more convenient.

Only endoscopically placed feeding tubes are true PEG tubes.

Principle

The principle of endoscopic placement of a gastrostomy feeding tube is that an endoscope is used to snare a line inserted through the body wall into the stomach and to pull it out through the mouth. The line is then fixed to the end of the gastrostomy tube and pulled back out through the body wall, with the feeding tube attached, until only the mushroom tip of the tube remains in the stomach. After fixation of the tube on the outside of the body, food can be introduced directly into the stomach through the PEG tube (Figure 5.37).

The earliest descriptions of this technique (Armstrong, 1992; Bright, 1993) described quite complex methods for securing the tube before pulling it into the stomach and out through the body wall. Today, the process is much simpler with the development of PEG tube kits, which contain all the equipment needed. The PEG tube has an integral dilator at one end with a wire loop attachment swaged on, allowing a knotless connection (see below). Only the kit method is described here, as kits are now readily available (Figure 5.38) and their ease of use makes this method achievable by any veterinary surgeon with a gastroscope. The original method is described in the first edition of the *BSAVA Manual of Canine and Feline Endoscopy and Endosurgery*.

Contraindications

A PEG tube should not be placed if there is:

- Persistent vomiting
- Persistent aspiration of saliva in patients with megaoesophagus
- Very temporary anorexia.

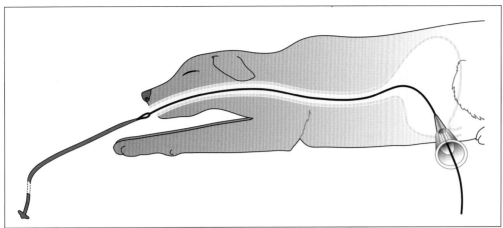

5.37 The principle of placing a PEG tube. A wire loop is passed through a large-bore needle inserted into the stomach after endoscopic insufflation. Endoscopic forceps are used to snare the wire and pull it out through the mouth, where it is then attached to the gastrostomy tube. The wire and gastrostomy tube are then pulled back into the stomach and out through the body wall until the mushroom tip of the gastrostomy tube lies against the gastric mucosa. PEG = percutaneous endoscopic gastrostomy.

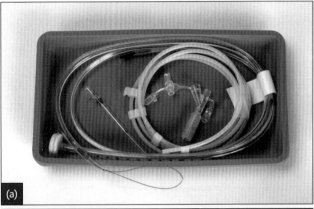

- Mushroom-tipped catheter
  - The tip is large and rigid enough to be self-retaining
  - The other end is tapered to act as a dilator
  - A swaged-on wire loop at the dilator end is used for attachment to the wire pulled through endoscopically
- Large-bore needle or over-the-needle catheter
- Wire loop long enough to reach from the flank to the mouth
- Syringe port adaptor
- Scalpel
- Suture material with needle

Note: Some PEG tube kits designed for use in humans also contain drapes and disposable basket forceps as standard.

5.39 Equipment needed for placement of a PEG tube by the kit method. PEG = percutaneous endoscopic gastrostomy.

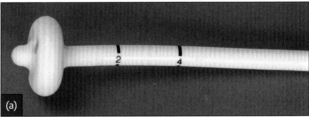

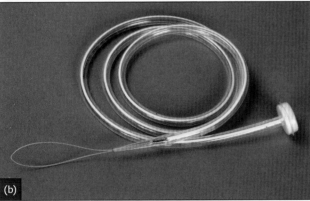

5.38 (a) PEG tube kit (Mila International Inc.) (b) PEG tube. A wire loop is swaged on to the hard conical end of the tube, which acts as a dilator as it is pulled through the body wall; the mushroom tip is at the other end. PEG = percutaneous endoscopic gastrostomy.

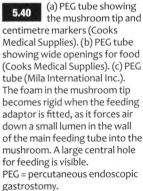

5.40 (a) PEG tube showing the mushroom tip and centimetre markers (Cooks Medical Supplies). (b) PEG tube showing wide openings for food (Cooks Medical Supplies). (c) PEG tube (Mila International Inc.). The foam in the mushroom tip becomes rigid when the feeding adaptor is fitted, as it forces air down a small lumen in the wall of the main feeding tube into the mushroom. A large central hole for feeding is visible. PEG = percutaneous endoscopic gastrostomy.

Instrumentation

The equipment needed for the kit method of placement is listed in Figure 5.39. A siliconized mushroom-tipped gastrostomy tube is used (Figure 5.40). The mushroom tip is necessary to keep the tube in place in the stomach. An 18–20 Fr tube is suitable for cats, and an 18–24 Fr tube for dogs. A large-bore needle or over-the-needle catheter and a strong wire loop are needed to pull the tube into position. An endoscope is needed to grasp the wire with grasping forceps or a snare. An integral conical dilator on the other end of the tube from the mushroom tip is used to ease the passage of the tube through the stomach and body walls. Finally, suture material is needed to fix the tube in place.

Method

The patient is anaesthetized and placed in right lateral recumbency as the tube will be inserted through the left flank. A site on the left flank, from behind the costal arch to just ventral to the end of the 13th rib, is clipped and surgically prepared (Figure 5.41a). The endoscope is inserted into the stomach, which is then inflated as much as possible; this pushes the spleen away from the space between the stomach and body wall so that it cannot be traumatized. It also allows identification of the site into which the tube will be inserted.

- The endoscope light may be seen shining through the body wall (transillumination); some light sources can produce a burst of very bright light to aid transillumination (Figure 5.41a).
- A gloved finger pushed into the prepared site will produce an indentation in the stomach that is visible endoscopically (Figure 5.41bc).

Ideally, the insertion site should be at the junction of the gastric body and the antrum; if it is too near the pylorus, the mushroom tip may cause an obstruction. It can be difficult or even impossible to access this optimum site in deep-chested breeds of dog. Once the optimum site has been determined, the endoscope is withdrawn back to the cardia for safety, and a large-bore needle or over-the-needle catheter is pushed through the body wall into the lumen of the stomach (Figure 5.41de).

The wire loop is threaded through the needle or catheter into the stomach and grasped using the endoscope (Figure 5.41f). Biopsy forceps are not recommended for grasping the line, as they will be blunted, but grasping or basket forceps or a snare can be used. It is easiest to pre-place open basket forceps or a snare over the needle once it has entered the stomach, so that when the wire is threaded through it is instantly entrapped. Once the wire has been grasped, the needle is withdrawn from the stomach to prevent accidental trauma, and the wire is fed through as it is pulled out through the mouth with the endoscope (Figure 5.41g; Video 5.4). It is important to remember that the distal end of the wire needs to be anchored to stop it being pulled completely through by accident.

The wire loop exiting the mouth is then attached to the dilator end of the gastrostomy tube. The simplicity of the method becomes apparent when attaching the line to the tube, as the swaged-on loop can be attached without the need for knotting (Figure 5.42).

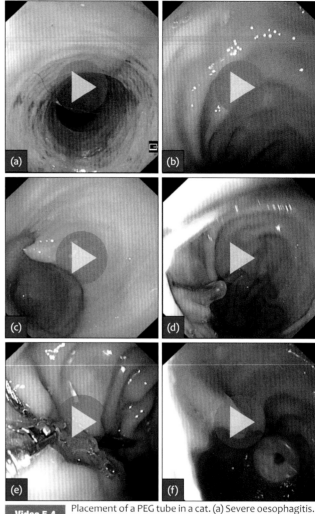

Video 5.4 Placement of a PEG tube in a cat. (a) Severe oesophagitis. (b) Identifying the PEG tube site. (c) Insertion of a needle into the stomach. (d) Passage of a wire loop into the stomach. (e) Grabbing and pulling the wire loop out of the mouth. (f) Positioning of the PEG tube mushroom. PEG = percutaneous endoscopic gastrostomy.

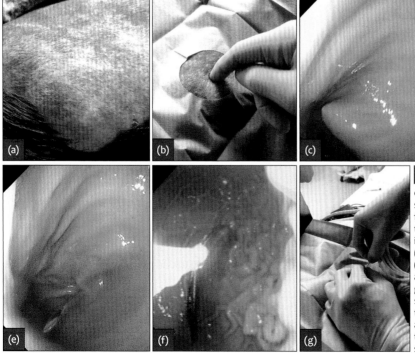

5.41 (a) A site on the left flank has been clipped and surgically prepared. The light from the endoscope in the inflated stomach transilluminates the site where the PEG tube will be placed. (b) A gloved finger is pushed into the prepared site to indicate where the PEG tube will be inserted. (c) Endoscopic view of the indentation caused by the gloved finger in Figure 5.41b. (d) A large-bore needle is pushed through the body wall. (e) The needle is seen emerging into the gastric lumen and a wire loop is then passed through it. (f) The wire is grasped by basket forceps as it emerges into the stomach through the needle. (g) As it is pulled out through the mouth by withdrawal of the endoscope and basket forceps, the wire is fed into the stomach through the body and gastric walls via the needle from a spool. PEG = percutaneous endoscopic gastrostomy.

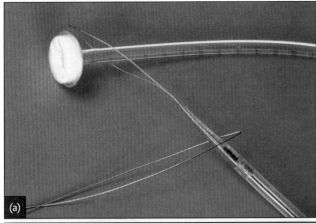
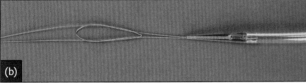
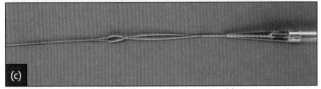

5.42 Attaching the wire loop to the PEG tube. (a) The swaged-on wire loop is passed through the wire loop that has been pulled out of the mouth, and then the mushroom tip of the PEG tube is passed through it. (b) The wire loops are interlocked as the PEG tube is straightened. (c) Pulling the wire loops tight produces a knotless connection. PEG = percutaneous endoscopic gastrostomy.

Once the dilator end of the PEG tube has been attached to the wire loop exiting the mouth, the end of the wire exiting the flank is pulled out through the body wall (Figure 5.43ab), pulling the PEG tube with it. As the dilator tip emerges, a small skin incision may be needed to ease its passage. Buttressing the skin surrounding the incision by hand will stop the body wall stretching (Figure 5.43c). Once the tube has begun to exit the body wall, it is pulled until the mushroom tip lies snugly against the mucosal surface of the stomach wall. The position of the mushroom tip should be checked endoscopically (Figure 5.43d); if there is blanching of the mucosa, the tube has been pulled too tight.

Fixing the PEG tube

The most secure way to fix the tube to the skin is with a Chinese finger-trap suture (Figure 5.44a). The position of the tube is noted against centimetre markers on the tube in case of future migration (see Figure 5.40a). The end of the tube is cut off, discarding the swaged-on wire loop, and a syringe adaptor port or 'Christmas tree' adaptor is fitted so that the tube can be capped (Figure 5.44b).

Maintenance

Patients generally tolerate PEG tubes well unless the suture is too tight or the site is wrapped in an occlusive dressing. A stretch netting dressing (e.g. Surgifix®; Figure 5.44c) is sufficient protection and an Elizabethan collar is not usually needed. The stoma site is cleaned daily and antibiotic cream applied if necessary.

Use

The PEG tube is not used for the first 24 hours, and then initially sterile water is inserted just in case the tube has migrated. If there is any doubt as to its position, an iodine-based liquid contrast medium (e.g. Conray®) is instilled and the abdomen is radiographed.

Once water can be given without problems, liquid feeding is introduced gradually, increasing from one-third to two-thirds to the whole of the calorific requirement over 3 days. The food is warmed before feeding. Usually, four divided meals a day are tolerated, but if that provokes vomiting, more frequent smaller feeds or even trickle feeding by syringe pump can be introduced. Before every feed or after 6 hours of trickle feeding, the residual volume in the stomach should be checked by aspirating the gastric contents through the tube. If the food is not being cleared from the stomach, the feeding rate should be reduced and prokinetics (e.g. metoclopramide) considered.

The tube should be flushed with water before each feed to ensure patency, and then again after feeding to try to keep it patent, as well as to give the patient its daily water requirement. If the tube becomes blocked it can be cleared either with a probe or by instilling a cola drink and leaving the tube capped; the acid and effervescence in the cola will usually resolve the obstruction. Blockages are most frequently caused by failure to flush the tube adequately or by including medication in the feed. Liquid medications are preferred and any tablets must be crushed finely before administration via the tube.

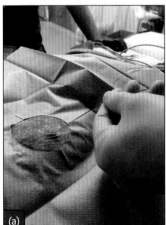
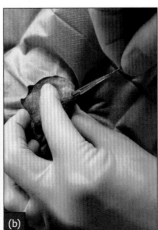
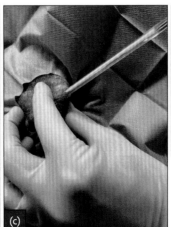
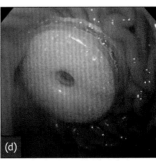

5.43 PEG tube placement. (a) As the wire is pulled back the conical tip of the gastrostomy tube reaches the body wall. (b) With the aid of a very small skin incision the conical tip of the tube is pulled through the body wall. (c) The tube is pulled through the body wall until the mushroom lies in the stomach adjacent to the gastric mucosa. (d) Endoscopic appearance of fitted PEG tube. PEG = percutaneous endoscopic gastrostomy.
(d, Courtesy of Mila International Inc.)

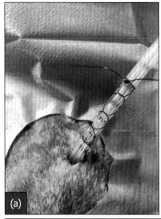

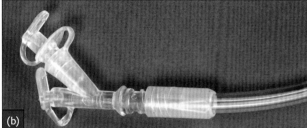

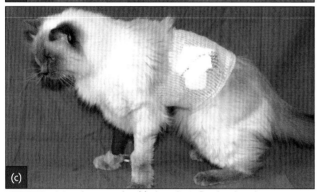

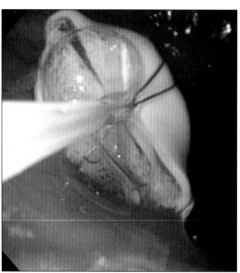

5.44 Fixing the PEG tube. (a) The tube is fixed with a Chinese finger-trap suture. (b) A feeding adaptor is placed on the end of the PEG tube. (c) The PEG tube is covered lightly with a stretch netting dressing. PEG = percutaneous endoscopic gastrostomy.
(c, Courtesy of A Harvey)

Long-term use

The first PEG tube can be left in for at least 6 months without problems in many patients, and owners are generally willing to manage tube feeding and maintenance at home. The tube is removed either when there are complications (e.g. wound infection), or when it is no longer needed as the patient is taking its full calorific requirement orally, or when a permanent device is going to be inserted. If or when the tube needs need replacing, a low-profile device (gastrostomy button) can be fitted without the use of an endoscope.

Removal

The PEG tube should not be removed for at least 7 days after insertion to allow adhesions to form and prevent leakage. This is why this method of feeding is not appropriate for patients that are considered likely to need assisted feeding for only a few days. There are several ways to remove the tube:

- The mushroom tip can be stretched with a stylet and the tube pulled out

- The tube can be cut off against the body wall:
  - It will pass naturally if the patient is >20 kg
  - It can be retrieved endoscopically; this also allows inspection of the stoma. The process can be speeded up by grasping the mushroom tip endoscopically before it is cut off (Figure 5.45).

Once the tube has been removed, the gastric mucosa will seal the hole within minutes and leakage should not be a problem.

5.45 Removal of a PEG tube. Basket forceps are used to grasp the mushroom tip of the PEG tube as it is cut off outside the patient; the mushroom tip is then retrieved endoscopically. PEG = percutaneous endoscopic gastrostomy.

Problems and failures

Although well tolerated, PEG tubes can cause problems:

- If a rubber Foley tube is used it will rapidly disintegrate in the gastric acid and fall out, leading to intra-peritoneal leakage of gastric contents
- If the mushroom is too small/soft, the tube may migrate out
- If the tube is too tight, it may cause tissue necrosis and the patient will chew the tube
- If the tube is not capped when not in use, gastric contents can leak and cause acid burns on the skin (Figure 5.46).

If the patient also has a chest drain in place, **the tubes must be labelled**. Accidental feeding through the chest tube into the pleural space has killed patients.

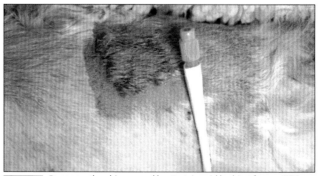

5.46 Burns on the skin caused by gastric acid leaking from a PEG tube when the owner left it uncapped. PEG = percutaneous endoscopic gastrostomy.

Jejunostomy tube placement

These are rarely of use and are employed only when feeding into the stomach is contraindicated. They are more commonly inserted surgically, but they can be inserted endoscopically if the patient already has a PEG tube (Whittmore and Bartges, 2010). The endoscope is advanced into the stomach and grasping forceps are placed through the accessory channel and then steered so that they exit via the PEG tube. The forceps are then used to grasp the tip of the jejunostomy tube, pull it into the stomach through the PEG tube and then carry it through the pylorus as far down the small intestine as possible. The tube must be long enough that the other end protrudes from the PEG tube in order that a syringe can be attached. Maintenance of these tubes is problematic, and they are frequently repulsed into the stomach.

Polyp removal

Pathological polyps in the upper GI tract (i.e. not benign antral polyps) are very rare compared with polyps in the large intestine (see Chapter 6), and their removal is not discussed here. Laser surgery can be performed with a compatible endoscope (see Chapter 16).

References and further reading

Armstrong JP (1992) Enteral feeding of critically ill pets. *Veterinary Medicine* **87**, 900–907

Bright RM (1993) Percutaneous endoscopic gastrostomy. *Veterinary Clinics of North America* **23**, 531–545

Casamian-Sorrosal D, Willard MD, Murray JK *et al.* (2010) Comparison of histopathologic findings in biopsies from the duodenum and ileum of dogs with enteropathy. *Journal of Veterinary Internal Medicine* **24**, 80–83

Danesh BJZ, Burke M, Newman J *et al.* (1985) Comparison of weight, depth, and diagnostic adequacy of specimens obtained with 16 different biopsy forceps designed for upper gastrointestinal endoscopy. *Gut* **26**, 227–231

Davignon DL, Lee ACY, Johnston AN *et al.* (2016) Evaluation of capsule endoscopy to detect mucosal lesions associated with gastrointestinal bleeding in dogs. *Journal of Small Animal Practice* **57**, 148–158

Elwood C (2005) Best practice for small intestinal biopsy. *Journal of Small Animal Practice* **46**, 315–316

Garcia-Sancho M, Sainz A, Villaescusa A *et al.* (2011) White spots on the mucosal surface of the duodenum in dogs with lymphocytic plasmacytic enteritis. *Journal of Veterinary Science* **12**, 165–169

Hall EJ, Simpson JW and Williams DA (2005) *BSAVA Manual of Canine and Feline Gastroenterology, 2nd edn.* BSAVA Publications, Gloucester

Hall EJ, Williams DA and Kathrani A (2020) *BSAVA Manual of Canine and Feline Gastroenterology, 3rd edn.* BSAVA Publications, Gloucester

King LG and Boag A (2018) *BSAVA Manual of Canine and Feline Emergency and Critical Care.* BSAVA Publications, Gloucester

Lamoureux A, Benchekroun G, German J *et al.* (2019) An endoscopic method for semi-quantitatively measuring internal pyloric diameter in healthy cats: a prospective study of 24 cats. *Research in Veterinary Science* **122**, 165–169

Lee ACY, Epe C, Simpson KW and Bowman DD (2011) Utility of capsule endoscopy for evaluating anthelmintic efficacy in fully conscious dogs. *International Journal for Parasitology* **41**, 1377–1383

Leib MS, Dalton MN, King SE and Zajac AM (1999) Endoscopic aspiration of intestinal contents in dogs and cats: 394 cases. *Journal of Veterinary Internal Medicine* **13**, 191–193

Lhermette P and Sobel D (2008) *BSAVA Manual of Canine and Feline Endoscopy and Endosurgery, 1st edn.* BSAVA Publications, Gloucester

McFadzean WJM, Hall EJ and van Oostrom H (2017) The effect of premedication with butorphanol or methadone on ease of endoscopic duodenal intubation in dogs. *Veterinary Anaesthesia and Analgesia* **44**, 1296–1302

Sarria R, Albors OL, Soria F *et al.* (2013) Characterization of oral double balloon endoscopy in the dog. *The Veterinary Journal* **195**, 331–336

Shales CJ, Warren J, Anderson DM *et al.* (2005) Complications following full-thickness small intestinal biopsy in 66 dogs: a retrospective study. *Journal of Small Animal Practice* **46**, 317–321

Simpson KW (2005) Diseases of the stomach. In: *BSAVA Manual of Canine and Feline Gastroenterology, 2nd edn.* eds: EJ Hall, JW Simpson and DA Williams, pp151–175. BSAVA Publications, Gloucester

Swinbourne F, Jeffery N, Tivers MS *et al.* (2017) The incidence of surgical site dehiscence following full-thickness gastrointestinal biopsy in dogs and cats and associated risk factors. *Journal of Small Animal Practice* **58**, 495–503

Washabau RW, Willard MD, Hall J *et al.* (2010) Gastrointestinal guidelines. WSAVA GI Standardization Group. Available from https://wsava.org/global-guidelines/gastrointestinal-guidelines/

Whittmore J and Bartges JW (2010) Endoscopic placement of gastrostomy and jejunostomy tubes. In: *Small Animal Endoscopy, 3rd edn*, ed. TR Tams and CA Rawlings, pp 311–330. Mosby, St. Louis

Willard M (2020) Endoscopy. In: *BSAVA Manual of Canine and Feline Gastroenterology, 3rd edn*, ed. EJ Hall, DA Williams and A Kathrani, pp. 25–30. BSAVA Publications, Gloucester

Video extras

- **Video 5.1 Upper GI endoscopy**
- **Video 5.2 Video sequence recorded from an Alicam® video-endoscopy capsule, showing a bleeding gastric polyp**
- **Video 5.3 Upper GI endoscopy of a dog with a gastric carcinoma**
- **Video 5.4 Placement of a percutaneous endoscopic gastrostomy (PEG) tube in a cat:**
  - **(a) Severe oesophagitis**
  - **(b) Identifying the PEG tube site**
  - **(c) Insertion of a needle into the stomach**
  - **(d) Passage of a wire loop into the stomach**
  - **(e) Grabbing and pulling the wire loop out of the mouth**
  - **(f) Positioning of the PEG tube mushroom**

Access via QR code or: bsavalibrary.com/endoscopy2e_5

Chapter 6

Flexible endoscopy: lower gastrointestinal tract

James W. Simpson

Introduction

The lower gastrointestinal (GI) tract of the dog and cat is a relatively simple anatomical structure compared with many other species. The tract is divided into four main components: the caecum, colon, rectum and anus (Figure 6.1). The colon can be further usefully divided into the ascending (hepatic flexure), transverse (splenic flexure) and descending colon. These divisions are recognizable during radiography and endoscopy. The ascending colon houses the caecocolic pouch and the ileocolic sphincter, which collectively are known as the ileocaecocolic junction (ICCJ). This is an important endoscopic landmark where the ileum enters the colon next to the opening into the caecum.

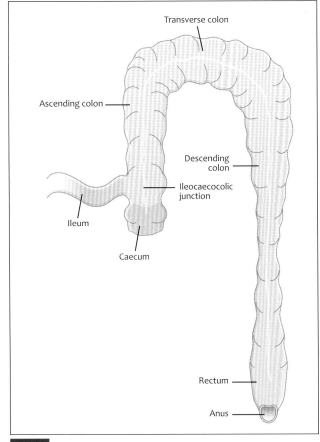

6.1 Anatomical structure of the large intestine.

Clinical signs of large intestinal disease can be investigated by radiography, barium studies, ultrasonography or, ultimately, laparotomy. However, flexible endoscopy is particularly useful for detailed examination of the large intestine because of the simple structure of the lower GI tract, the ease of patient preparation and the ability of relatively inexperienced endoscopists to carry out the procedure. The entire mucosal surface of the large intestine can be visualized, biopsy samples collected and, in many cases, a definitive diagnosis achieved.

Instrumentation

Flexible endoscopes

In small animal practice patients range in size from kittens to Great Danes. Consequently, the size of the large intestine varies considerably in length. In large breeds of dog, the entire length of a 1 m insertion tube may be required to reach the ICCJ; in small dogs and cats less than half this length may be required. The diameter of the insertion tube for colonoscopy is less important than for examination of the upper GI tract. This is because the colon has no powerful sphincters to negotiate (unlike the upper GI tract with the lower oesophageal sphincter and pylorus) and the diameter of the lumen is greater than that of the duodenum.

As there is no 'universal' endoscope available to examine the GI tract of all dogs and cats, a compromise is normally made in selecting an endoscope that will be suitable for the majority of patients. This normally means selecting an endoscope that is best suited to examination of the upper GI tract, as it will usually perform equally well in the lower GI tract.

The specifications for a colonoscope are an end-viewing flexible endoscope with an outside diameter of less than 9 mm (ideally 7 mm), with an insertion tube length of at least 1 m but ideally 1.4 m. The biopsy channel of such an endoscope will normally have a diameter of 2 mm but in some cases up to 2.8 mm. The endoscope must have an air and water (wash) facility and four-way tip deflection (Figure 6.2).

In addition to the endoscope, the equipment required for a colonoscopy includes a suitable light source with an air pump/wash facility and biopsy forceps of appropriate size for the endoscope selected. A suction unit is useful but is not essential for carrying out the procedure in a well prepared patient.

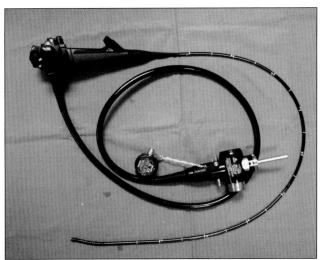

6.2 For carrying out an endoscopic examination of the large intestine in both dogs and cats a forward-viewing endoscope should be selected, with an insertion tube length of at least 1 m (ideally 1.4 m) and an outside diameter of 7–9 mm. There must be a wash and air facility, and a biopsy channel of at least 2 mm diameter.

Comments	Disorder/infection
Bacterial infections	• *Salmonella* spp. • *Campylobacter* spp. • *Clostridium* spp. • *Yersinia* spp.
Parasitic infections	• *Giardia* spp. • *Uncinaria* spp. • *Trichuris vulpis* • *Tritrichomonas foetus*
Colitis	• Lymphocytic–plasmacytic • Eosinophilic • Histiocytic • Granulomatous
Neoplasia	• Lymphoma • Adenocarcinoma • Leiomyosarcoma
Intussusception	• Ileocolic • Caecocolic • Colocolic
Caecal disorders	• Typhlitis • Abscessation • Neoplasia
Rectal disorders	• Adenomatous polyps • Stricture • Diverticulum

6.3 Disorders of the large intestine.

Rigid endoscopes

Although flexible endoscopes are now routinely used for examination of the large intestine, there is a place for use of a rigid endoscope or proctoscope for examination of the rectum. It can be difficult to inflate the rectum adequately to permit good visualization of the mucosa when using a flexible endoscope because the insufflated air tends to escape through the anus. Rigid endoscopes allow the rectal mucosa to be examined without the need for air insufflation, although in some cases this is still required. Biopsy samples can also be collected through a rigid endoscope. Care should be taken to select a rigid endoscope of the correct diameter for this procedure to ensure adequate visualization without causing tissue damage. Illumination can also be a problem in some cases, as the light beam in these units tends to be small. In general, larger biopsy samples can be collected when using a rigid endoscope because there is less restriction in the size of biopsy forceps that can be used than with flexible endoscopes.

Indications

The clinical signs of lower GI disease are generally diarrhoea, haematochezia, excess mucus, tenesmus, dyschezia and/or constipation. Occasionally, vomiting may be reported in patients with inflammation of the large intestine. These clinical signs carry a large differential diagnosis and none is pathognomonic of any individual disorder (Figure 6.3) and so an investigation must be carried out in order to reach a definitive diagnosis. In all cases, the investigation should start with collection of a detailed history, followed by a thorough physical examination. The physical examination should always include a rectal examination to assess sphincter function, check for disease of the anal sacs and look for evidence of rectal stricture, obstruction, masses or perineal herniation (see Figures 6.20 to 6.22). The clinical examination should help to determine whether systemic disease is present or the problem is localized to the large intestine.

Tenesmus and dyschezia resulting in the passage of formed or ribbon-like faeces as a primary clinical sign, suggest partial obstruction in the distal colon, rectum or anus. A rectal examination will help to determine whether anal sac disease or an anal sphincter problem is implicated, while flexible endoscopy will permit visualization of the rectal and distal colonic mucosa and may determine the cause of the signs. Where a mass is found, biopsy samples should be collected to determine whether benign or malignant disease is present. Similarly, where a stricture is found, biopsy samples should be collected, as these lesions can be associated with underlying neoplastic disease.

Many patients with lower GI tract disease present with chronic diarrhoea (often containing fresh blood and/or mucus), tenesmus and/or dyschezia. The starting point in the investigation of these patients should be faecal analysis to look for pathogenic bacteria and parasites. Nematodes are usually detected using flotation methods, while *Giardia* is best detected using an antigen SNAP test and *Tritrichomonas* species by polymerase chain reaction (PCR) testing (see the *BSAVA Manual of Canine and Feline Gastroenterology*). Where infection is detected, appropriate treatment should be provided and the patient reassessed at a later date. In addition, the patient's diet should be carefully considered, and where it is found to be inappropriate, dietary corrections should be made. A dietary trial using either a hydrolysed soya-based diet or a high-fibre diet may be worth considering.

In patients where systemic disease, dietary factors and infections have been ruled out and the clinical signs have persisted, the most likely cause of the GI signs is colitis. Endoscopic examination of the entire large intestine should then be considered. If there is significant haematochezia, then a clotting profile should be carried out first, including a manual platelet count, prothrombin time, activated partial thromboplastin time and buccal mucosal bleeding time. Pre-anaesthetic blood tests are not required as a specific pre-requisite to the procedure but may be appropriate as part of the complete diagnostic work-up.

Colitis is generally a diffuse disease that affects the entire colon; however, on occasion only part of the colon may be affected. It is therefore wise to examine the entire colon from rectum to ICCJ and also examine the caecum.

Where the patient presents with vomiting and diarrhoea, and the clinical signs and initial investigations indicate upper GI disease, being able to biopsy the duodenum and ileum has distinct diagnostic advantages. In particular, lymphoma often involves the more distal regions of the small intestine, and protein-losing enteropathy can involve only sections of the small intestine, so being able to obtain biopsy samples from the proximal small intestine (see Chapter 5) and the distal small intestine (via the lower GI tract) can be helpful in reaching a definitive diagnosis.

Irritable bowel syndrome (IBS) is a condition that has been identified in the dog but not the cat. The clinical signs can be identical to those seen with colitis. As there is no definitive diagnostic test for IBS the only method of obtaining a definitive diagnosis is by ruling out other causes of the clinical signs. Endoscopic examination of the lower GI tract should be used as part of the investigation; a hyperactive colon, which is difficult to dilate with air and contains large plaques of mucus attached to the mucosa, will often be observed in patients with IBS. Biopsy samples from these patients will reveal no evidence of inflammatory or neoplastic disease.

Disease of the caecum is rare in dogs and cats. Typhlitis is the most common disease and is usually the result of whipworm infection or extension of inflammation from the colon. Endoscopy and biopsy of the caecum will assist in the diagnosis of typhlitis and other caecal diseases, including caecal inversion, abscessation and neoplasia.

Endoscopy of the lower GI tract is also useful for follow-up evaluation of the response to treatment. As no surgical intervention is involved and anaesthesia is required for only a short period of time, many owners will permit a follow-up endoscopy where they would decline if a surgical intervention were required.

Patient preparation

It cannot be overemphasized how important patient preparation is to carrying out lower GI endoscopy. It is simply not possible to adequately examine the colon of a patient with solid or liquid faecal material present (Figure 6.4). When the tip of the endoscope and the objective lens come into contact with fluid or faeces, light is refracted and a 'red-out' occurs, making it impossible to view the mucosa. The presence of faecal material may also prevent the endoscope from being passed sufficiently far enough into the colon to reach the ileocaecocolic junction. Cleaning the bowel

properly is not easy, but is essential to be able to complete and full endoscopic examination of the lower GI tract.

A variety of protocols for colonic preparation in advance of colonoscopy can be employed and may largely be dictated by the operator's experience and preference. The author has tried many methods of cleansing the large intestine in dogs and has found that the best option is a sodium phosphate enema (saline laxative). Alternatively, a standardized protocol such as the one described below can be employed.

Withholding food for a prolonged period is advised – 36 hours without food is helpful, although the patient's nutritional status and GI transit times should be considered. The patient should be admitted for preparation before noon on the day prior to the procedure. A variety of oral preparation solutions are available (e.g. OCL solution, GoLytely, NuLytely, CoLyte, Kleenprep) but all are essentially variants of a polyethylene glycol 3350 solution, an iso-osmotic solution of polyethylene glycol and electrolytes that induces an osmotic diarrhoea to wash out the contents of the gut. The solution should be reconstituted as per the manufacturer's instructions.

Dogs should be given 2–4 doses of 30 ml/kg of the oral solution at least 2 hours apart, with the final dose being administered approximately 12 hours before the endoscopic procedure. The majority of dogs will not take this solution voluntarily and it is difficult to administer adequate volumes via an oral drench. An orogastric tube is therefore generally required for administration. The solution can be given with the dog conscious, but mild sedation with acepromazine is required in some cases. It is not unusual for patients to vomit shortly after administration of the solution and premedication with metoclopramide and/or acepromazine can help to prevent this. If vomiting occurs, it is advisable to wait for 30 minutes and then repeat the process; dividing the volume of solution administered should be considered.

Following administration of the final dose of the oral solution, a warm water enema should be given. Enemas alone can be used, but rarely provide adequate cleansing and will certainly not clear the ileum if ileoscopy is contemplated. A well lubricated soft enema tube should be inserted per rectum to the level of the last rib and approximately 15 ml/kg of warm water instilled under gravity, whilst the tube is gently agitated back and forth. It is important not to add soap or other irritants to the enema water as this may inflame the lining of the bowel and influence subsequent interpretation of biopsy results. Plain water is sufficient. The morning of the endoscopic procedure, further warm water enemas should be administered until the effluent runs clear.

A slightly different procedure is required for cats. The oral preparation solution should be administered through a nasogastric tube slowly at a rate of 20 ml/kg/hr for 4 hours. In addition, the volume of the enema should not exceed 20 ml/kg, as it can induce vomiting, and should be administered slowly via a soft urinary catheter attached to a syringe.

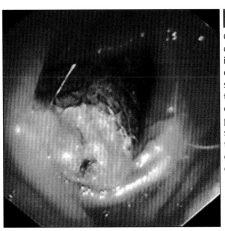

6.4 Careful preparation of the large intestine is essential if the entire mucosal surface is to be thoroughly examined. The presence of faeces severely restricts the ability to carry out this examination.

> **Editors' note**
>
> One editor [ER] has achieved excellent results using the following protocol to prepare cats for colonoscopy: a low-fibre diet for 48 hours before the procedure with ¼ teaspoon of polyethylene glycol 3350 (Miralax) twice daily, plus a beef-flavoured electrolyte broth (Oralade). Food is then withheld for 12 hours prior to the procedure and a Higginson's syringe enema with plain water administered once the patient is under general anaesthesia

Premedication and anaesthesia

Although colonoscopy is frequently carried out without anaesthesia in humans, this is rarely the case in canine and feline practice. It is usual to carry out the procedure under general anaesthesia, although in patients considered to be a very high anaesthetic risk it is possible to use deep sedation. General anaesthesia is essential if an upper GI endoscopy is to be carried out at the same time. There are no specific anaesthetic agents that are essential or that must be avoided for endoscopy; the choice of anaesthetic protocol is at the clinician's discretion. As the procedure is not considered particularly painful, a deep level of anaesthesia is not needed. The author generally uses a combination of acepromazine and buprenorphine for premedication and propofol for induction before intubating the patient and maintaining anaesthesia with isoflurane in oxygen.

Patient positioning

The patient should always be placed in left lateral recumbency for flexible endoscopy (Figure 6.5). This position ensures that the descending colon lies ventrally, which aids passage of the endoscope through the transverse and ascending colon; it also elevates the ileocolic sphincter, facilitating its identification and intubation. This position also assists in drainage of any faecal fluid from the transverse and ascending colon, which will pool at the proximal end of the descending colon. Where this occurs, the endoscope should be advanced through the fluid; the endoscopist will see a 'red-out' until the transverse colon is reached, when the image will be restored. Where rigid endoscopy is being used to examine the rectum, the patient should be placed in right lateral recumbency. It is useful to lightly tie a linen bandage around the tail from its base to the tip, as this prevents soiling and aids visualization of the anus, especially in long-haired breeds.

Procedure

The distal 20 cm of the insertion tube should be lightly coated with water-based lubricant (e.g. K-Y® jelly), taking care to avoid the lens. This will reduce friction and aid forward movement of the endoscope along the colon. The tip of the endoscope should then be inserted through the anus and into the rectum for about 10 cm, so long as there is no resistance to forward movement. The image will 'red out' during this procedure and the rectum should then be insufflated with air. Only once the mucosa of the rectum and descending colon can clearly be seen should the endoscope be advanced further. While trying to inflate the rectum, air may escape through the anus; if this occurs an assistant can gently pinch the anus around the endoscope to create a seal, reducing the volume of air escaping and preventing the lumen from collapsing on itself, so that the rectum inflates.

The mucosa of the descending colon should then be clearly visible directly in front of the endoscope tip (Figure 6.6). The mucosa should normally appear smooth and pale pink in colour, with submucosal blood vessels clearly seen through the thin mucosa (Figure 6.7). These blood vessels should not be interpreted as indicating inflammation. In fact, failure to see these blood vessels suggests thickening of the mucosa, which may be due to either inflammation or neoplasia.

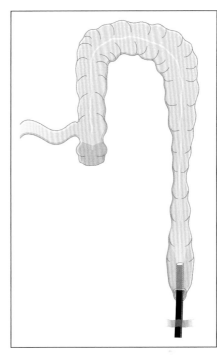

6.6 Once the endoscope has been advanced into the rectum, the lumen should be inflated with air. It should then be possible to visualize the descending colon extending in front of the endoscope.

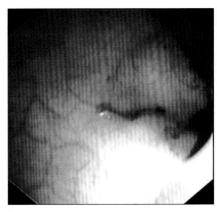

6.7 The mucosa of the colon should appear pale pink in colour and the submucosal blood vessels should be clearly visible through the thin mucosal layer.

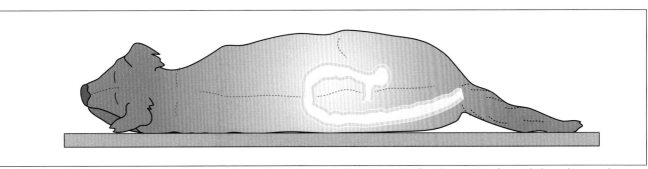

6.5 To aid intubation of the transverse and ascending colon, and to ensure that any residual fluid does not interfere with the endoscopy, the patient should be placed in left lateral recumbency.

Once the lumen of the descending colon has been visualized, the endoscope should be gently advanced while carefully examining the entire circumference for evidence of pathological change. If this is not done, iatrogenic damage caused by the endoscope may later be misdiagnosed as indicating pathology. As the endoscope reaches the end of the descending colon, an obvious bend (the splenic flexure, in which a shadow of the spleen can sometimes be seen as a darkened area in leaner animals) will be seen, marking the start of the transverse colon (Figure 6.8). The tip of the endoscope should be moved in the direction of the bend and advanced slowly. It is not uncommon for a red-out to occur during this manoeuvre and for the endoscopist to feel a slightly increased resistance to forward movement, as the endoscope tip slides along the mucosa. Once the tip of the endoscope enters the transverse colon, the lumen should be inflated with air to re-establish a clear image. There is little danger of overinflation of the colon, so long as the anus is not continually occluded; it acts as a 'safety valve' to relieve pressure.

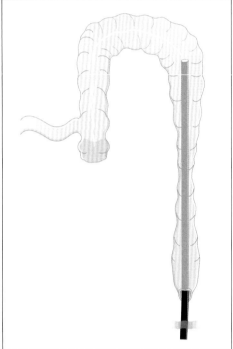

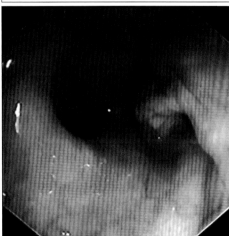

6.8 As the endoscope is advanced along the descending colon, eventually a 'bend' will be observed, which represents the flexure between the descending and transverse colon. This is a normal anatomical landmark, which will be observed on a second occasion as the endoscope reaches the flexure separating the transverse and ascending colon.

The transverse colon is relatively short, and a second bend (the hepatic flexure, which is less obvious in cats than in dogs) will quickly be visualized, marking the start of the ascending colon. The endoscope tip should be manoeuvred as before to enter the ascending colon. Again, visualization of the entire luminal circumference should be established before advancing the endoscope further.

The ascending colon is the shortest section of the colon and ends at the ICCJ (Figure 6.9). This important endoscopic landmark is readily identified by the opening into the blind-ended caecum and the raised prominent red-coloured ileocolic sphincter.

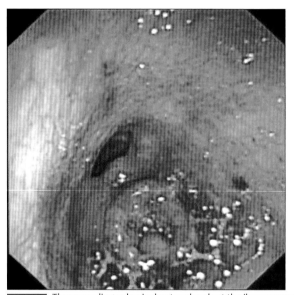

6.9 The ascending colon is short and ends at the ileocaecocolic junction. The ileum appears as a raised red button-shaped structure while the caecum is a blind-ended sac.

The caecum should be carefully examined as it can become inflamed (typhlitis) or may contain the nematode *Trichuris vulpis*. If the ileum is to be examined, the tip of the endoscope should be directed towards the ileocolic sphincter and slowly advanced. The ability to advance the endoscope into the ileum will depend on the size of the patient and the diameter of the endoscope insertion tube. If it is not possible to intubate the ileum for visual examination, it is permissible to advance the biopsy forceps 'blindly' into the ileum to collect biopsy samples. This must be done with care, and where any resistance to forward movement is detected, the procedure should be stopped.

Following examination of the entire large intestine, the endoscope should be withdrawn slowly while biopsy samples are collected. Even if no gross lesions have been found, it is still essential to collect biopsy samples because there is a poor correlation between visual assessment of the mucosa and the findings on histopathology. Biopsy samples should be collected from normal-appearing mucosa from at least three separate locations, and from any obvious lesions (Leib, 2011). This will provide a good representative sample for the pathologist to judge the health of the colon. Where a specific abnormality is detected, biopsy samples should be collected from the lesion and from the surrounding apparently normal tissue. The specimens from the 'lesion' and 'normal' areas should be placed in separate sample pots; this will allow the pathologist to compare tissue samples and make a better judgement regarding the type and extent of the changes identified. The exact location of any abnormality should be noted by recording the distance (in centimetres) marked on the insertion tube at the anus. This will be useful in any follow-up endoscopy so the location of the abnormality can be quickly found.

It is difficult to examine the rectum as the endoscope is being inserted through the anus. As previously described, air often leaks out through the anus, making inflation of the rectum difficult. Even quite large tumours can be missed if the rectum is examined as the endoscope is being inserted, due to the folds in the rectal mucosa. The author has found that inserting the endoscope through the rectum and into the descending colon, then inflating the colon with a continuous stream of air while slowly withdrawing the endoscope, provides better visualization of the rectal mucosa. Retroflexing the endoscope is another method of examining the rectum but is possible only in large breeds of dog or where a narrow diameter insertion tube with a long bending section is available.

Where a stricture is detected within the large intestine it is normally very difficult to advance the endoscope further. This is because the stricture forms a 'lip' around the circumference of the lumen, which catches the endoscope and prevents further forward movement. Although most strictures are associated with inflammatory changes, some are due to neoplasia, and so biopsy samples should always be collected from strictures before deciding on appropriate treatment.

Biopsy collection

When first starting to collect biopsy samples, it is not uncommon to receive reports from the pathologist indicating that the samples were not diagnostic due to inadequate size or crush artefact. To reduce crush artefact when collecting biopsy samples from the large intestine, forceps with fenestrated cups and no central spike should be used (Figure 6.10). The fenestrated cups allow the biopsy sample to expand through the fenestrations, thus reducing damage during collection.

According to the World Small Animal Veterinary Association guidelines for reporting endoscopic biopsies, the pathologist will require good-sized and deep biopsy samples in order to conduct a pathological investigation and produce a comprehensive report. To ensure that a biopsy sample of adequate size is collected, it is very important to ensure that the colon is not overinflated, as

overinflation will stretch the mucosa, making it difficult to grasp. To aid the collection of good-sized samples, it is important to direct the biopsy forceps so they open perpendicular to the mucosa (see also Chapter 3). If the biopsy forceps are used parallel to the mucosa, only superficial samples will be collected with no crypt tissue included (Figure 6.11), and these samples are unlikely to be diagnostic. The colonic mucosa extends inward from the surface epithelia to the deep crypt tissue (Figure 6.12).

It is relatively easy to obtain a perpendicular biopsy sample at the junction between the transverse and ascending colon, but more difficult in the descending colon. When collecting biopsy samples in the descending colon, the endoscopist should tilt the tip of the endoscope so that the forceps are as near perpendicular to the mucosa as possible. In all cases, the forceps should be advanced on to relaxed mucosal tissue with the cups open, until the

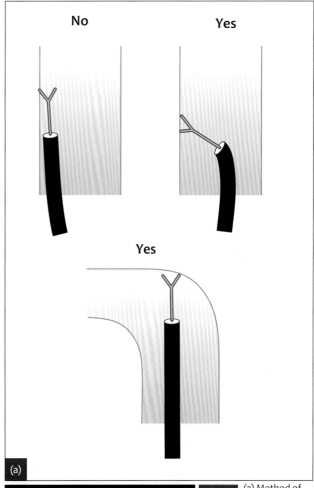

6.11 (a) Method of collecting biopsy samples from the colon. (b) The forceps should be advanced as near perpendicular to the mucosa as possible. This will ensure that a sample of good depth is collected.

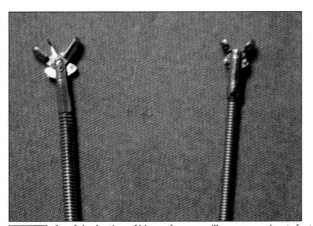

6.10 Careful selection of biopsy forceps will ensure crush artefact is reduced to a minimum. Forceps with a central spike (left) should not be used; forceps with fenestrated biopsy cups (right) should be selected.

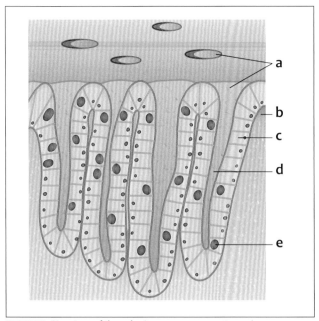

6.12 Structure of the colonic mucosa. **a** = crypt openings; **b** = lamina propria; **c** = columnar epithelium; **d** = crypt; **e** = goblet cell.

mucosa 'tents'; the forceps should then be closed and pulled directly backwards. This will effectively 'tear' off the biopsy sample – a process that will help to ensure haemostasis (see Figure 6.11).

When examining the large intestine endoscopically it is important not only to look for surface erosion and ulceration, cellular infiltration and fibrosis, but also to examine the crypts for evidence of loss, hyperplasia or abscessation. Biopsy samples should be collected from all lesions observed and from the surrounding apparently healthy tissue (see above).

Pathological conditions

Colitis

Colitis is the most common form of large intestinal disease seen in the dog and cat. It is generally a diffuse disease involving the entire colon, and may occur in conjunction with similar changes in the small intestine. These changes come under the umbrella of chronic inflammatory enteropathies. The aetiology of colitis is often not determined, and these cases are classified according to the predominant inflammatory cells present, namely, as lymphocytic–plasmacytic, eosinophilic, histiocytic or granulomatous colitis.

It has long been observed that certain breeds of dog seem to be predisposed to colitis, and genetic factors have now been identified to account for this predisposition. Similarly, intracellular bacteria are now known to cause colitis in Boxers and French Bulldogs. The causative bacteria can be identified by using fluorescent *in situ* hybridization (FISH) assays, and these cases respond well to antibiotic treatment. Pathogenic bacteria and parasites may also be an underlying cause of colitis in individual cases. Finally, some forms of colitis appear to be fibre responsive. It is therefore important to carry out a faecal analysis and review the patient's dietary history as part of the investigation of large intestinal disease, before performing an endoscopy.

Lymphocytic–plasmacytic colitis

Lymphocytic–plasmacytic colitis is the most common form of colitis seen in the dog and the cat. It is characterized by an infiltration of the mucosa with lymphocytes and plasma cells. In some cases, crypt abscessation with changes to goblet cell numbers and the presence of fibrosis may be detected, especially in chronic cases. Rarely, the fibrosis may be severe enough to result in the formation of a colonic stricture. On endoscopic examination, this form of colitis may be suspected on the basis of visualization of the presence of hyperplastic lymphoid tissue, which appears as multiple small 'doughnut'-shaped structures on the surface of the mucosa (Figure 6.13). It is very unusual for ulceration to be observed with this form of colitis. In some cases, especially those with a long history of clinical signs, the mucosa may be grossly thickened, with an appearance that may be suggestive of neoplasia (Figure 6.14). In particular, lymphocytic–plasmacytic colitis and lymphoma may appear very similar both macroscopically and microscopically. Where a uniform population of lymphocytes is detected by histopathology on biopsy samples, immunohistochemistry and/or PCR for antigen receptor rearrangement (PARR) should be used to differentiate the two conditions. A high incidence of colitis has been observed in dogs presented with anal furunculosis.

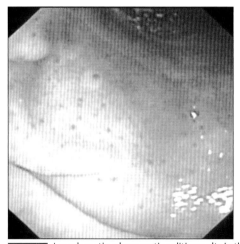

6.13 Lymphocytic–plasmacytic colitis results in thickening of the mucosa so submucosal blood vessels can no longer be seen. In many cases lymphoid hyperplasia will be observed as raised 'doughnut'-shaped structures.

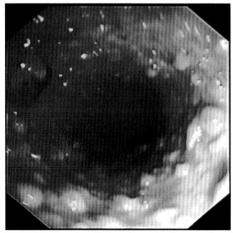

6.14 Occasionally, lymphocytic–plasmacytic colitis may be severe. In such cases proliferative changes may be seen suggesting the possible presence of neoplasia. It is essential to collect biopsy samples for histopathology and not to overinterpret the visual changes.

Colonoscopy should be carried out as part of the investigation and subsequent treatment of anal furunculosis. In cats, colitis has been associated with *Tritrichomonas foetus* infection. Cases are usually seen in young adult cats presenting with watery diarrhoea, tenesmus, haematochezia and occasionally faecal incontinence. Bengal cats appear to be predisposed to *T. foetus* infection. It would be wise to carry out a faecal PCR test for this organism before considering endoscopy. However, it is sometimes possible to detect the organism in biopsy samples of colonic mucosa collected endoscopically.

Eosinophilic colitis

Eosinophilic colitis is less common than lymphocytic–plasmacytic colitis and is mainly seen in the dog. Cats rarely develop this form of colitis. Colonoscopy often reveals evidence of mucosal ulceration and erosion. The remaining mucosa may be very friable and bleed easily on manipulation. In severe cases submucosal haemorrhage may occur, giving the mucosa a purple coloration (Figure 6.15). Histologically, it is usual for there to be a mixed cell population, with lymphocytes, plasma cells and a significant number of eosinophils present. Where there is mucosal ulceration, neutrophils may also be detected histologically.

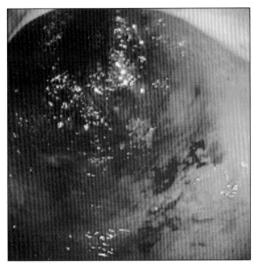

6.15 Eosinophilic colitis usually results in erosions and ulceration of the mucosa, which will also be friable and bleed readily. Submucosal bleeding may give the mucosa a red to purple coloration.

Histiocytic colitis

Histiocytic colitis is an uncommon form of colitis in dogs and is not seen in cats. The Boxer and French Bulldog appear to be predisposed to the disease. Clinical cases are usually seen in young adult dogs. These cases present with severe diarrhoea, which is usually liquid in nature and contains significant amounts of fresh blood. Tenesmus and faecal mucus are also commonly seen. At colonoscopy, the mucosa is usually observed to be inflamed and friable, with multiple small ulcers throughout the colon. Histopathology of biopsy samples reveals a mixed population of inflammatory cells, including periodic acid–Schiff (PAS)-positive macrophages, neutrophils, lymphocytes and plasma cells. There is often extensive mucosal erosion and ulceration. Further investigation using FISH assays has identified the presence of intramucosal *Escherichia coli* in cases of histiocytic colitis. Although this form of colitis was previously considered to be refractory to treatment, it responds well to antibiotic treatment, further supporting the role of intramucosal bacteria in the aetiology of the disease.

Granulomatous colitis

Granulomatous colitis is the rarest form of colitis seen in the dog; it is not seen in the cat. This form of colitis often affects only a small region of the colon. The majority of the colonic mucosa will appear normal on endoscopy, but an area of marked mucosal thickening, to the point of obstructing the lumen, may be seen, often in the transverse or ascending colon. These changes may be accompanied by ulceration and bleeding (Figure 6.16). It is not usually possible to advance the endoscope past the lesion. The main differential diagnosis for these mucosal changes is neoplasia. Therefore, it is essential to collect biopsy samples for histopathology to make a definitive diagnosis.

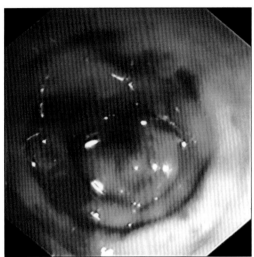

6.16 Where granulomatous colitis is found, the majority of the colon will usually appear normal and only a small section of the colon will be affected. The lumen of the intestine may appear obstructed by marked mucosal thickening, and bleeding is not uncommon. The changes must be differentiated from neoplasia by examination of biopsy samples.

Irritable bowel syndrome

IBS is well recognized in humans and giant pandas. In the author's opinion, IBS also occurs in the dog but not the cat. Working dogs under stress and dogs of a nervous disposition are more likely to be affected, and present with clinical signs similar to those of colitis. Typical clinical signs are episodes of diarrhoea with excess mucus production and tenesmus. Haematochezia is not a feature of IBS. Some dogs may show signs of abdominal pain, which is thought to be associated with colonic spasm.

Unfortunately, there is no definitive diagnostic test for IBS, so the only way in which a diagnosis can be made is by ruling out all other causes of large intestinal disease. A full clinical examination should be performed to rule out systemic disease, and faecal analysis should be undertaken to rule out pathogenic bacteria and parasites. At endoscopy, no gross mucosal changes will be observed, and examination of biopsy samples will reveal no pathological change. The endoscopist may observe large amounts of mucus within the colon (Figure 6.17), and the colon may be difficult to dilate with air due to colonic spasm.

Neoplasia

Colonic neoplasia is most often associated with lymphoma or adenocarcinoma in the dog and the cat. Lymphoma is usually a diffuse condition that affects the entire colon and

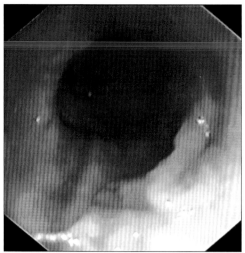

6.17 Irritable bowel syndrome is difficult to diagnose as there are no visual or pathological changes present. However, at endoscopy the colon may be difficult to dilate and excessive amounts of mucus may be observed.

may appear very similar to lymphocytic–plasmacytic colitis. As discussed above, differentiating the two conditions normally requires immunohistochemistry; in cats, if the immunohistochemical findings are suggestive of T-cell behaviour, PARR is used to confirm clonal expansion. Occasionally patients diagnosed with lymphocytic–plasmacytic colitis may fail to respond to treatment; follow-up endoscopy in these cases may provide evidence of progression of disease to lymphoma. With lymphoma, the lumen of the large intestine is rarely occluded, and ulceration of the mucosa is rarely observed. Even when a mass is detected at endoscopy, it is important not to rely on visual assessment alone; biopsy samples should always be collected to confirm the diagnosis.

Adenocarcinoma is normally a more focal disease of the colon and may appear similar to granulomatous colitis (discussed above). The majority of the colon may appear visually normal at endoscopy, but a focal area of proliferation, which often occludes the lumen of the colon, with mucosal ulceration and bleeding will be found with adenocarcinoma. The mass may be friable and may appear irregular in outline (Figure 6.18). Secondary inflammation and infection are common. Consequently, superficial

biopsy samples often reveal only inflammation, fibrosis and infection. In order to reach a definitive diagnosis, biopsy samples should be collected from the base of the mass and deeper tissues. This is achieved by carefully taking multiple samples from the same site within the mass. Great care is required when 'mining' for tissue in this way to ensure the intestinal wall is not perforated.

Caecal disorders

Typhlitis is rare and may occur on its own or be associated with colitis. It is sometimes associated with whipworm (*Trichuris vulpis*) infection. If present, these worms may be observed during endoscopic examination of the caecum. Alternatively, a faecal analysis for parasitic eggs will detect the presence of whipworm.

When a mass is found within the caecum it is usually due to abscessation or neoplasia. Great care should be exercised in collecting biopsy samples in this situation, and surgery may be considered the safer option for obtaining a definitive diagnosis.

Intussusception

Both ileocolic and ileocaecal intussusception occur in the dog and cat, although the former is more common. With both types of intussusception, the patient may present with chronic diarrhoea with or without haematochezia. It is therefore not unreasonable for endoscopy to be used to investigate the cause of the clinical signs. Intussusception is readily recognized at endoscopy (Figure 6.19) and when found, the endoscopic procedure should be halted and the patient referred for surgery.

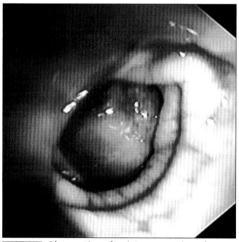

6.19 Observation of an intussusception when carrying out large intestinal endoscopy is rare. However, when one is present, the ileum will appear as a normal pink colour filling the lumen of the colon, with no bleeding or ulceration in the majority of cases.

Constipation

Colonoscopy is rarely performed in animals with constipation, as it is not possible to view the colonic lumen and mucosa properly in the presence of faecal material. Constipation has a large differential diagnosis list, which includes IBS, megacolon, stricture formation and obstructive tumours, which are often located in the descending colon, rectum or anus. A rectal examination followed by careful removal of the faecal material may allow endoscopy to be carried out in cases where an obstruction is suspected and biopsy samples are required for diagnostic pathology.

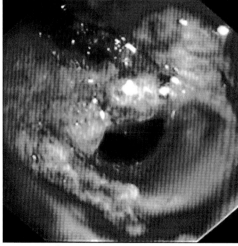

6.18 Adenocarcinoma is an aggressive tumour that invades the lumen of the colon. The tumour will appear irregular and proliferative in appearance, may bleed easily and may appear very friable to touch. The remainder of the colon may be unaffected.

Rectal tumours

Rectal polyps are a common cause of rectal tenesmus, haematochezia and malformed faeces. They are particularly common in older dogs and the smaller breeds, especially the West Highland White Terrier. A rectal examination may detect a mass but because these adenomatous polyps are soft and friable in consistency, they can sometimes be difficult to palpate. Where a polyp is suspected, endoscopic examination of the rectum to assess the extent of any changes present and collect biopsy samples is essential, to determine whether the mass is benign or malignant.

Enema administration before endoscopy should be carried out with great care, and in some cases should be avoided due to the risk of tissue damage and haemorrhage. Each case must be individually assessed for risk before endoscopy.

To examine the rectum endoscopically, the distal end of the endoscope should be lubricated (as described above) and gently inserted into the rectum to a distance of about 10–20 cm. If resistance is felt, the procedure should be halted; in some cases a gloved finger may assist in directing the endoscope through the rectum. Once the endoscope tip is in the descending colon, forward motion should be stopped and air should be insufflated to dilate the colon until its lumen can be viewed. The endoscope should then be withdrawn slowly while maintaining air insufflation to ensure that the rectal mucosa can be clearly visualized. The polyp will come into view during this procedure, and its size and exact location can be determined (Figure 6.20). The mass is usually proliferative, partially obstructs the lumen of the rectum, appears soft and friable and bleeds readily. Biopsy samples taken from the proliferative mass are likely to yield only inflammatory cells. The best location for obtaining diagnostic biopsy samples is the base of the mass where it attaches to the rectal wall. Samples from this location will allow the pathologist to determine whether the mass is benign or malignant. It is important to note that benign and malignant rectal masses may appear macroscopically very similar and cannot be differentiated on the basis of visual assessment. It is therefore essential to obtain good diagnostic biopsy samples.

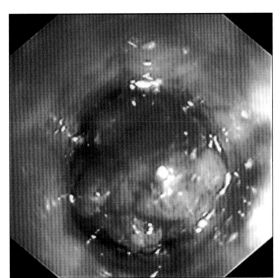

6.20 Rectal adenomatous polyps can be diagnosed easily with the aid of endoscopy. They appear very similar to adenocarcinoma and must be differentiated by collecting and examining biopsy samples.

Rectal strictures

Rectal strictures occur rarely in dogs and cats, and may occur concurrently with strictures in the descending colon. Although the aetiology may not be determined, the majority are associated with either trauma or chronic inflammation, and a minority are associated with neoplasia. So, where a rectal stricture is detected on rectal examination, it is wise to carry out an endoscopic examination of the rectum and colon to assess the extent of mucosal changes and collect biopsy samples (Figure 6.21). This will allow the clinician to reach a definitive diagnosis and establish the most appropriate treatment plan.

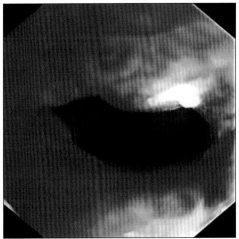

6.21 Rectal strictures often appear as an obvious narrowing of the lumen, and a circumferential lip may prevent forward movement of the endoscope.

Rectal diverticulum

Rectal diverticulum is a rare condition that is seen more often in dogs than in cats. It is most often associated with a perineal hernia, where persistent tenesmus may result in the rectal wall bulging into the weakened pelvic diaphragm. Dogs with a rectal diverticulum usually present with dyschezia and tenesmus, and occasionally constipation; diarrhoea is rarely associated with this condition. Following suitable preparation of the large intestine, endoscopic examination will reveal a large pocket in the wall of the rectum (Figure 6.22). Biopsy samples are not usually collected in these cases unless there is suspicion that the tenesmus that has led to perineal herniation is due to colitis.

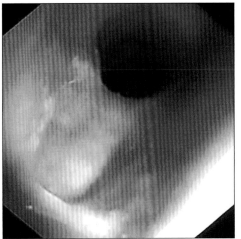

6.22 A diverticulum can be seen at the 7 o'clock position in this view of the rectal mucosa in a dog.

Postoperative care

Following endoscopy of the large intestine, the patient should be carefully monitored during recovery from anaesthesia. If analgesia has been provided as part of the premedication it is rarely necessary to provide further analgesia postoperatively, as the procedure is rarely painful. However, careful pain assessment should be carried out with all patients and analgesia provided as required. Once the patient has fully recovered from the anaesthetic, food and water should be offered as normal. Unless a serious problem requiring immediate treatment has been detected at endoscopy, it is better to await the pathology results before starting any specific treatment.

Complications

Endoscopy of the large intestine is generally a safe procedure if carried out correctly, and in the author's experience complications are rare. Perforation of the colonic wall, which is much thinner than the small intestinal wall, can occur. Perforation is more likely if excessive force has been applied when advancing the endoscope, or following aggressive use of the biopsy forceps. Iatrogenic trauma to the mucosa may occur as the endoscope is advanced along the colon. The risk of trauma or perforation may be greater if the large intestine is diseased. Haemorrhage at biopsy collection sites has also been recorded, but is rare.

References and further reading

Davies DR, O'Hara AJ, Irwin PJ and Guilford WG (2004) Successful management of histiocytic ulcerative colitis with enrofloxacin in two Boxer dogs. *Australian Veterinary Journal* **82**, 58–61

Day MJ, Blizer T, Mansell J et al. (2008) Histopathological standards for the diagnosis of gastrointestinal inflammation in endoscopic biopsy samples from the dog and cat: a report from the World Small Animal Veterinary Association Gastrointestinal Standardization group. *Journal of Comparative Pathology* **138**, S1–S43

Hall EJ, Williams DA and Kathrani A (2019) *BSAVA Manual of Canine and Feline Gastroenterology, 3rd edn.* BSAVA Publications, Gloucester

Jamieson PM, Simpson JW, Kirby BM and Else RW (2002) Association between anal furunculosis and colitis in the dog; Preliminary observations. *Journal of Small Animal Practice* **43**, 109–114

Knottenbelt CM, Simpson JW, Tasker S et al. (2000) Preliminary clinical observations on the use of piroxicam in the management of rectal tubulopapillary polyps. *Journal of Small Animal Practice* **41**, 393–397

Mansfield CS, James FE, Craven M et al. (2009) Remission of histiocytic colitis in Boxer dogs correlates with eradication of invasive intramucosal *Escherichia coli*. *Journal of Veterinary Internal Medicine* **23**, 964–969

Leib M (2011) Colonoscopy. In: *Small Animal Endoscopy, 3rd edn*, ed. T Tams and CA Rawlings, pp. 217–244. Mosby, St. Louis

Ohmi A, Tsukamoto A, Ohno K et al. (2012) A retrospective study of inflammatory colorectal polyps in Miniature Dachshunds. *Journal of Veterinary Medical Science* **74**, 59–64

Willard M, Moore G, Denton B et al. (2009) Effect of tissue processing on assessment of endoscopic intestinal biopsies in dogs and cats. *Journal of Veterinary Internal Medicine* **24**, 84–89

Xenoulis PG, Lopinski DJ, Reed SA et al. (2013) Intestinal *Tritrichomonas foetus* infection in cats: a retrospective study of 104 cases. *Journal of Feline Medicine and Surgery* **15**, 1098–1103

Useful websites

World Small Animal Veterinary Association gastrointestinal guidelines: https://www.wsava.org/Global-Guidelines/Gastrointestinal-Guidelines

Chapter 7

Flexible endoscopy: respiratory tract

Diane M. Levitan and Susan Kimmel

Introduction

Flexible endoscopy of the respiratory tract can be a valuable therapeutic, diagnostic and prognostic tool for most patients with respiratory disease. Endoscopy can be used for diagnostic evaluation of the airways, including the nasal passages, nasopharynx, dorsal soft palate, pharynx, larynx, trachea and pulmonary tree, and to assess laryngeal function. Tissue and fluid samples can be collected for microbiological or histopathological evaluation. The bronchoscope is also a valuable therapeutic tool and can be used to remove foreign objects from the nose, nasopharynx, pharynx, trachea and bronchi. It can also be used to place and evaluate airway stents. Visualization of airway injury or chronic airway changes can be monitored over time and will aid in determining the prognosis of conditions. Bronchoscopy is most rewarding when the veterinary surgeon (veterinarian) has a good understanding of airway anatomy, use of the endoscope and other instruments, anaesthetic protocols and techniques. As with any skill, practice is essential.

Dogs and cats with chronic unilateral or bilateral nasal discharge, chronic sneezing or reverse sneezing, chronic stridor or stertor are seen regularly by veterinary surgeons. Evaluation of these problems often includes imaging techniques such as radiography, computed tomography and magnetic resonance imaging. These modalities are useful for evaluation of the location and extent of lesions in the upper respiratory tract; however, tissue biopsy, cytology and culture are essential for definitive diagnosis of most disease processes. Rhinoscopy is often an essential diagnostic procedure, and is discussed in detail in Chapter 9.

Indications

The indications for flexible endoscopy of the respiratory tract are listed in Figure 7.1.

A thorough evaluation of the oral cavity, oropharynx, nasopharynx, posterior nasal cavity, larynx, trachea and lower airway can be performed in one quick procedure using a flexible endoscope. Foreign objects can be identified and possibly removed. Tracheobronchial collapse can be definitively diagnosed, as the dynamics of the airway lumen can be directly observed.

Bronchoscopy, combined with bronchoalveolar lavage (BAL) and airway brush cytology, is used to aid in the diagnosis and identification of the aetiology of many disorders,

Posterior nasal passages, pharynx, nasopharynx and larynx

- Chronic nasal discharge, sneezing or reverse sneezing
- Dysphagia
- Respiratory stertor or stridor
- Laryngeal function
- Developmental abnormalities
- Chronic gagging
- Excessive salivation

Trachea and lower airways

- Acute cough
- Assessment of airway integrity
- Chronic bronchitis
- Chronic cough
- Chronic halitosis
- Tracheobronchial collapse
- Pulmonary infiltrative disease
- Recurrent pneumonia
- Neoplastic conditions
- Haemoptysis
- Ciliary dyskinesia
- Intratracheal device monitoring
- Placement of airway stents
- Airway stricture, lung lobe torsion or bronchiectasis
- Foreign body evaluation/retrieval
- Tracheal/airway trauma

7.1 Indications for flexible endoscopy of the respiratory tract.

such as eosinophilic airway disease, lungworm infection, toxoplasmosis, bacterial or fungal infection and neoplastic infiltrates. Other conditions can be diagnosed by examination of samples collected from sites within specific lung lobes and from areas deep in the respiratory tract. Tumours can be visualized and biopsy samples taken. Extrapulmonary masses can also be aspirated or biopsied through the respiratory tract.

Technological advances in the field of interventional airway endoscopy are made frequently in human medicine, and are becoming commonplace in veterinary medicine. Applications include surgical laser therapy, brachytherapy, electrocautery, cryotherapy, placement of airway stents for the management of tracheal collapse and balloon dilation to relieve airway obstruction caused by lesions. The use of fluoroscopy with bronchoscopy allows specific interventional procedures to be performed with greater precision. Such tools allow improved characterization of lesions, accurate biopsy of the airways and treatment of various conditions.

Bronchoscopy is generally a very safe procedure with few contraindications (Figure 7.2). Using a flexible endoscope, the procedure is quick and practical, and can also

Absolute contraindications
• Severe hypoxaemia • Known bleeding disorder/platelet dysfunction • Severe cardiac arrhythmia • Cardiac failure or severe dysfunction
Significant increased risk of complications
• Partial tracheal obstruction • Marked hypoxaemia • Uraemia/severe hepatic dysfunction • Pulmonary hypertension • Lung abscessation • Immunosuppression • Unstable asthma

7.2 Contraindications to flexible endoscopy of the respiratory tract.

be used to follow progress, treat and aid the management of many conditions of the upper respiratory tract. The benefits of bronchoscopic evaluation must be weighed against the potential risk of complications based on the individual patient's condition.

Instrumentation

Flexible and rigid endoscopes have both been used to visualize the airways. However, the flexible endoscope provides more advantages, especially for the lower airways, due to its length and manoeuvrability.

Flexible endoscopes range in size. The ideal size for a small airway ranges from 2.5 to 5 mm in diameter, with a length of 25–85 cm; however, larger endoscopes may be used depending on the size of the patient's airway (Figure 7.3). A limitation for procedures in large dogs is the length of the endoscope; however, a 4–5 mm diameter, 85 cm long endoscope is suitable for cats and large dogs. In giant-breed dogs, a paediatric gastroscope is an excellent tool, as its 7.8–8 mm diameter is tolerated and the length of 107–160 cm permits diagnostic procedures deep in the airways.

There must be a channel within the endoscope to allow the passage of instruments as well as oxygen. The use of a video-endoscope or the attachment of a video camera system makes visualization and manoeuvring easier, but is not necessary. Cytology brushes (Figure 7.4) can be placed through the lumen of the bronchoscope or used alongside the endoscope to obtain samples for cytology

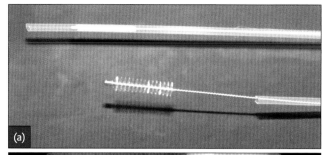
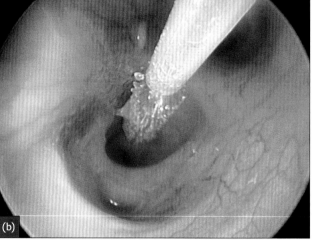

7.4 (a) Cytology brush in its sheath (top) and in the extended position (bottom). (b) Use of a cytology brush in an airway.

from the airway surfaces. Aspiration catheters (Figure 7.5) are thin tubes with Luer lock tips used for fluid collection and suction during procedures. These can also be placed adjacent to the endoscope or through the instrument channel for collection of sterile samples. Transbronchial aspiration or biopsy can be performed using aspiration needles (Figure 7.6). Aspiration or biopsy of paratracheal, carinal, hilar or peripheral lung lesions can be performed through the bronchoscope, with or without concurrent use of fluoroscopy.

A swivel-tip T-adaptor attached to the endotracheal tube allows anaesthetic gas to be continuously delivered while the bronchoscope is passed through the endotracheal tube (Figure 7.7). Use of an endotracheal tube depends on the size of the patient's airway relative to the size of the endoscope; in small patients, intubation may not be possible.

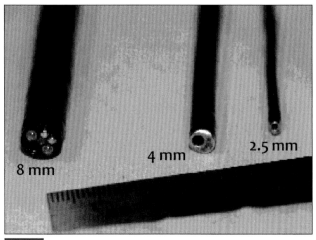

7.3 Flexible endoscopes in several different sizes are available.

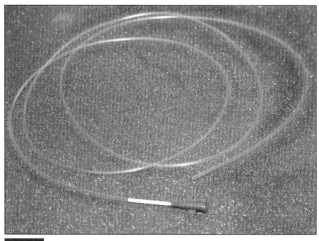

7.5 Aspiration/lavage catheter.

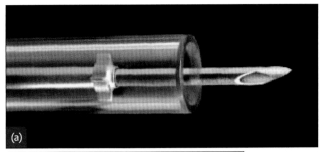

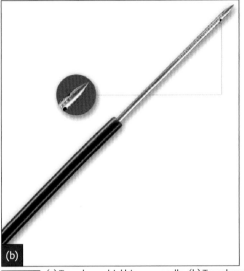

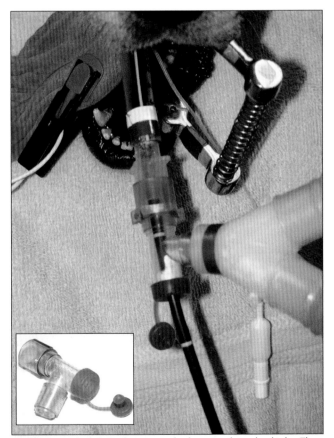

7.6 (a) Transbronchial biopsy needle. (b) Transbronchial aspiration needle.

7.7 A swivel-tip T-adaptor attached to an endotracheal tube. The adaptor has a rubber valve at the top of the port, which opens enough to allow the endoscope to pass into the airway without allowing gas to escape into the environment. This allows maintenance of oxygen and anaesthetic gas flow to the patient.

Cleaning

The endoscope must be sterilized before each instance of use according to the manufacturer's recommendations (see Chapter 2). Care must be taken when disinfecting the channels and storing the endoscope to avoid moisture build-up, which can lead to bacterial or fungal growth in the channels that could result in iatrogenic airway infections.

Handling

Bronchoscopes are very delicate and should be handled with the utmost care to avoid damage (see Chapters 2 and 3).

Premedication and anaesthesia

Evaluation of the respiratory tract with any endoscope must be performed under deep sedation or general anaesthesia. Without deep sedation, elicitation of reflexes causing laryngospasm, coughing, sneezing and gagging will result in trauma to the patient and will likely cause damage to the endoscope. Administration of a narcotic premedication, such as butorphanol, can reduce gagging and coughing during airway endoscopy. Additionally, infiltration of 1 ml of 2% lidocaine to achieve a maxillary nerve block can be used in dogs to reduce adverse reactions during posterior rhinoscopy.

Use of a protective intraoral device (mouth speculum/gag) or even a roll of tape (avoiding types that may cause disease/damage to the dentition) will prevent trauma to the endoscopic equipment from accidental biting. Each patient should be assessed to ensure suitability for anaesthesia, and an anaesthetic protocol that is suitable for the individual patient and the planned procedure should be selected. Patient risk increases greatly with general anaesthesia if there is pre-existing hypoxia, cardiac disease or cardiac arrhythmia. Coagulopathy, severe arrhythmia, heart failure or severe hypoxia are contraindications to bronchoscopy (see Figure 7.2).

All patients should have their electrocardiogram, pulse oximetry and cardiovascular parameters monitored before, during and for a period after anaesthesia. End-tidal capnography can be very helpful in prolonged procedures. Pre-oxygenation for 10 minutes is advised, especially when the patient's oxygenation is compromised. Pre-oxygenation can be provided by nasal oxygen delivery or via a mask. Topical 2% lidocaine will help to prevent laryngospasm upon introduction of the endoscope and endotracheal tube in both dogs and cats.

Inhalation anaesthesia is recommended for most procedures; however, if the patient is too small to have an endoscope passed through an endotracheal tube, intravenous anaesthesia must be used. Intubation should be performed only if the endoscope can fit easily through the endotracheal tube, allowing movement of air and the endoscope at the same time. This is dependent on the size of the patient's trachea and the luminal diameter of the endotracheal tube. The ability of the endoscope to move easily in the endotracheal tube should be tested before beginning the procedure. A swivel-tip T-adaptor (see Figure 7.7) can be used to allow continuous administration of anaesthetic agent in oxygen while the endoscope is passed through the endotracheal tube. A sterile endotracheal tube should be used.

The endoscope should not remain in any airway for longer than 30–50 seconds as it will interfere with ventilation and could result in hypercarbia, overinflation of the lungs, trauma or bronchospasm. It is useful to have an assistant or anaesthetist monitoring this time period, as it is sometimes difficult for the endoscopist to appreciate the passage of time when concentrating on operating the endoscope or performing a procedure. It should be remembered that if oxygen is being constantly delivered through the channel, carbon dioxide cannot escape through the same channel. Oxygen should therefore be delivered through an endotracheal tube if possible, or through one of the ports on the endoscope during procedures. Oxygen can also be delivered nasally or through a red rubber catheter or dog urinary catheter placed into the trachea alongside the endoscope. Flow volumes of 1–3 litres per minute can be safely used; higher flows have been associated with overinflation of the small airways, ruptured alveoli and pneumothorax. Adequate ventilation during endoscopic procedures is imperative.

An anaesthetic protocol that minimizes cardiopulmonary depression should be used. The anaesthetist should be alert to the possibility of an emergency before, during or after a procedure, as rapid respiratory or cardiovascular decompensation can occur in these patients. The anaesthetist should be prepared to intubate the patient in case of respiratory difficulty during the procedure or for the delivery of oxygen after the procedure. Anaesthetic reversal agents (if applicable) should be readily available in case of an emergency.

An evaluation of the patient's laryngeal function should be performed before other diagnostic examinations, or during recovery, as it requires a lighter plane of anaesthesia than bronchoscopy. Small amounts of ultra-short-acting barbiturates, acepromazine, narcotics or propofol can be used to provide a suitable level of anaesthesia. The dose of anaesthetic agent must be titrated carefully, as moderate or deep levels of anaesthesia will result in the complete absence of laryngeal motion. Doxopram at 2.2 mg/kg i.v. is useful to stimulate respiration and increase intrinsic laryngeal motion; its effect occurs within 15–30 seconds and can last approximately 2 minutes. Examination of the oropharynx, larynx and proximal trachea should be undertaken before intubation in order to visualize these structures adequately; intubation can take place after examination of these structures, if indicated. Visualization of the dorsal soft palate, nasopharynx and nasal cavity require intubation and should be performed after bronchoscopy to avoid contamination of the bronchoscope.

Before anaesthetizing a patient for any procedure, all necessary instruments should be set up and inspected to be certain they are in perfect working condition.

Patient positioning

For most airway evaluations, the patient is placed in sternal recumbency with the head elevated and the neck extended. For oropharyngeal and nasopharyngeal examination and biopsy procedures, the patient should be intubated with a cuffed endotracheal tube. Packing the back of the throat with gauze (Figure 7.8) is useful to catch blood, secretions and potential biopsy samples or fungal plaques that may drop into the pharynx. On completion of the procedure, the gauze can be used to remove blood and blood clots from the throat. The material collected in the gauze should be examined for tissue or particulate matter that may be valuable for diagnostic pathology.

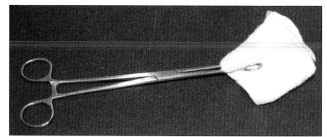

7.8 Babcock forceps with gauze squares are used to protect the airway from aspiration of blood or particulate matter during posterior rhinoscopy.

Procedures

Retropharyngeal posterior rhinoscopy

Retropharyngeal posterior rhinoscopy allows examination of the choana for strictures, stenosis, foreign material, polyps or masses. The endoscope is advanced just beyond the soft palate and then deflected dorsally so that the tip of the endoscope sits in the nasopharynx above the soft palate. In larger dogs, the endoscope can be flexed before advancement and then hooked over the edge of the soft palate. Insufflation of air during retropharyngeal posterior rhinoscopy will improve visualization by preventing the tissues of the nasopharynx and soft palate from collapsing around the endoscope. It is advisable to advance biopsy or foreign body retrieval instruments into the biopsy channel before deflecting the endoscope tip, because damage can be caused to a flexible endoscope if instruments are forced through the channel while the tip is maximally deflected.

An additional technique often performed following retropharyngeal posterior rhinoscopy is nasal hydropulsion, during which foreign material or pieces of soft tissue masses can be retrieved for therapeutic and diagnostic purposes. To avoid aspiration into the lower airway, a suction tip and/or several gauze sponges (held within the tip of clamped blunt sponge forceps) can be placed into the common pharynx after ensuring there is a tight seal on the endotracheal cuff. Warm saline (20–60 ml) is injected rapidly under high pressure into one nostril while holding the other closed. The pharynx should be examined and the gauze replaced after each injection, which can be repeated once or twice via each nostril. When present, fragments of tumour tissue or foreign material can be retrieved from the pharynx or the gauze upon removal.

Tracheobronchoscopy

Tracheobronchoscopy is an excellent technique for diagnosis and management of disorders of the respiratory tract. A successful outcome requires knowledge of the instrumentation, airway anatomy, normal appearance of respiratory tract structures, appropriate anaesthetic protocols and monitoring, and acquisition of adequate diagnostic samples during the procedure. The endoscopist should use a standard method of evaluation each time tracheobronchoscopy is performed. This should include standard reporting methods for all findings, standard diagnostic testing and a standard method of navigation through the airways to ensure a complete evaluation. The airway anatomy of the cat and the dog is very similar; however, the airways of the cat are much smaller and therefore visualization of the deeper airways is more difficult. The map of the airways (Figure 7.9) should be kept in mind and referred to during evaluation.

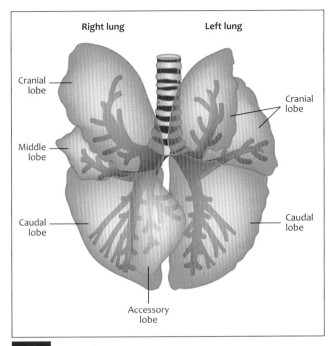

7.9 Lung and airway anatomy.

Larynx

The examination begins with the endoscope being advanced to the larynx; the tongue may need to be pulled forward to aid visualization of the larynx. The soft palate should not extend into the larynx or interfere with respiration. It should sit at the tip of the epiglottis and be level with the tonsils. Care should be taken when evaluating the tongue to avoid pulling on it, as this can alter the normal structures and cause a misleading appearance. The entire oral cavity should be examined. Before assessing the larynx, the epiglottis should be examined to ensure that it is sitting in the correct position. There is a condition called epiglottic retroversion (or epiglottal entrapment), which refers to the displacement of the epiglottis into the lumen of the larynx, resulting in inspiratory airflow limitation and/or distress. This is often part of the brachycephalic syndrome or can be seen alone. This condition often requires surgical correction (Video 7.1; Taylor *et al.*, 2018).

The anatomy, function and motion of the larynx should be assessed. Laryngeal function and motion must be evaluated under a light plane of anaesthesia (see above). The normal laryngeal mucosa is pink and a fine vascular

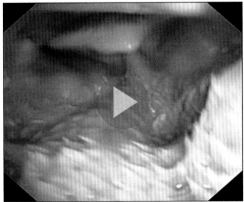

Video 7.1 Epiglottic retroversion – intermittent spontaneous retroflexion of the epiglottis during inspiration causing obstruction of the rima glottidis.

pattern should be visible (Figure 7.10a). There should be no masses, nodules or irregularities of the mucosa. The laryngeal saccules should not be everted and the edges of the vocal folds should be crisp. Salivary secretions should not be excessive. Everted laryngeal saccules, an elongated soft palate and an accumulation of salivary secretions are classic findings in dogs with brachycephalic obstructive airway syndrome (Figure 7.10b). Laryngeal paralysis (Figure 7.10c; Video 7.2) results in thickened arytenoids, blunted vocal fold edges and loss of the mucosal fine vascular pattern; the mucosal surfaces are hyperaemic and

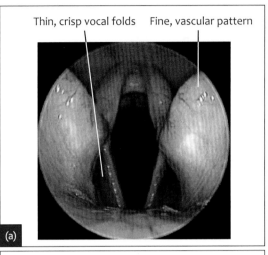

Thin, crisp vocal folds   Fine, vascular pattern

(a)

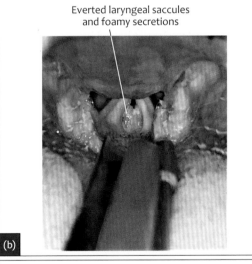

Everted laryngeal saccules and foamy secretions

(b)

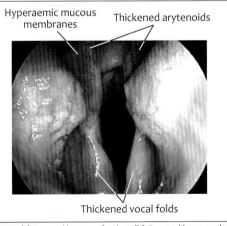

Hyperaemic mucous membranes   Thickened arytenoids

Thickened vocal folds

(c)

7.10 (a) Normal larynx of a dog. (b) Everted laryngeal saccules and an accumulation of foamy saliva are common findings in brachycephalic dogs. (c) Larynx of a dog with laryngeal paralysis.
(a, Courtesy of B McKeirnan; b–c, Courtesy of T McCarthy)

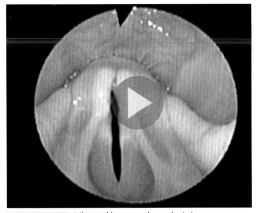

Video 7.2 Bilateral laryngeal paralysis in a cat.
(Courtesy of S Gadson)

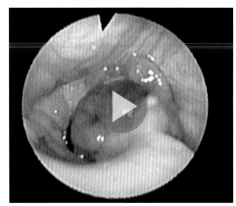

Video 7.3
Laryngeal
carcinoma in a cat.
(Courtesy of S Gadson)

there is often an accumulation of excessive foamy salivary secretions in the larynx. In the normal animal, the arytenoid cartilages should abduct during inspiration and then return to a paramedian position during expiration. In patients with laryngeal paralysis, the arytenoid cartilages (left, right or both) may show decreased motion or may not move at all during inspiration. If the paralysis is complete, motion paradoxical to the phase of respiration (i.e. apparent abduction of the arytenoid cartilages during expiration and a paramedian position during inspiration) can be seen. For more examples of laryngeal abnormalities, see Figure 7.11 and Video 7.3.

Trachea

After examining the larynx, the plane of anaesthesia should be deepened to continue the bronchoscopic evaluation. If the patient is to be intubated, the proximal trachea should be evaluated before intubation. The endoscope is passed through the larynx into the proximal trachea. The tracheal cartilages appear as C-shaped rings that are connected dorsally by the dorsal tracheal membrane. The trachea should have a uniform appearance throughout its length. The dorsal tracheal membrane should be seen as a taut, flat mucosal surface connecting the ends of the C-shaped tracheal rings. This membrane is very helpful to establish proper orientation inside the lumen, as it is centrally located in the most dorsal part of the trachea (Figure 7.12).

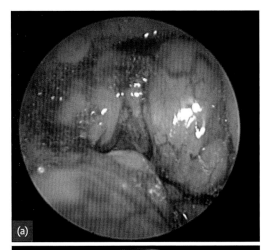

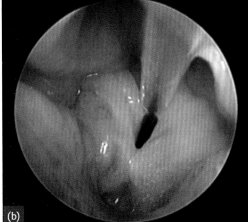

7.11 (a) Laryngeal carcinoma in a cat. (b) Severe laryngeal swelling in a cat. Note the placement of a urinary catheter for airway patency.
(a, Courtesy of L Balmain; b, courtesy of G Brick)

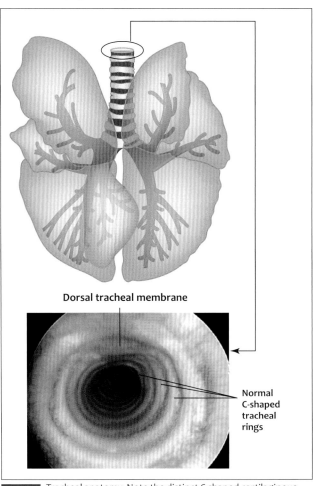

Dorsal tracheal membrane

Normal C-shaped tracheal rings

7.12 Tracheal anatomy. Note the distinct C-shaped cartilaginous rings and the smooth, taut dorsal tracheal membrane.
(Photograph courtesy of T McCarthy)

The patient can be intubated after evaluation of the length of trachea that will be covered by the endotracheal tube. The normal trachea has smooth mucosal surfaces through which small blood vessels can be visualized, and no evidence of masses or excessive secretions. Mucosal oedema or excessive secretions result in poor visualization of the mucosa and vasculature, and indicate inflammation. The tracheal lumen should be relatively round and there should be no excessive dipping of the dorsal tracheal membrane or collapse of the tracheal rings. The endoscope should always be centred in the lumen as it is advanced and care should be taken not to rub or press the endoscope tip against the mucosal surface. The mucosa can be easily scraped by the endoscope, resulting in a distinct line of hyperaemia or occasionally a small superficial mucosal tear. This should be kept in mind when evaluating areas that the endoscope has passed, to help ensure that any such damage is recognized as an artefact. Video 7.4 shows a collapsing trachea in a Chihuahua.

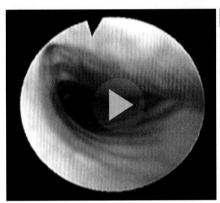

Video 7.4

Grade III collapsing trachea in a Chihuahua.
(Courtesy of T Hoffmann)

Mainstem bronchi

As the endoscope is advanced, the carina or bifurcation of the trachea will come into view. The patient's right side is on the operator's left side; therefore, if the endoscope and camera are correctly positioned, the right mainstem bronchus will be seen on the left side of the image. The bronchial tree should be evaluated as thoroughly and systematically as possible. If orientation is lost, the endoscope should be withdrawn to the level of the carina, which acts as a point of reference, and, if applicable, the video attachment should be checked to ensure that it is in the proper orientation.

If possible, the normal tissues should be examined before the abnormal areas of the lung. All segments of the airways should be round in cross-section and have a shiny, smooth mucosa with a fine vasculature visible, and be free of excessive mucus, oedema or lesions. Occasionally, strands or small clumps of mucus are seen in the normal airways (Figure 7.13). The airways should be examined for the presence of collapse, masses, mucosal irregularities and external compression.

The left and right mainstem or principal bronchi branch off crisply (Figure 7.14a). The principal bronchi branch into lobar bronchi, each of which ventilates a lung lobe. Each lobar bronchus then gives rise to many smaller segmental bronchi. The smaller airways that branch from the segmental bronchi (subsegmental bronchi) can be visualized endoscopically in large dogs. The right mainstem bronchus is in line with the trachea (Figure 7.14b). The first lobar bronchus encountered is that of the right cranial lung lobe (Figure 7.14c). Adjacent is the second lobar bronchus of the right middle lung lobe (Figure 7.14d). The bronchus of

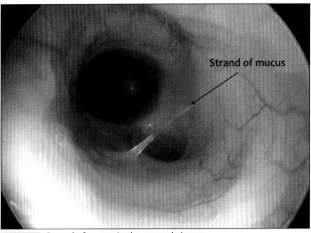

7.13 Strand of mucus in the normal airway.
(Courtesy of T McCarthy)

the accessory lung lobe (Figure 7.14ef) branches off next, and the right main bronchus ends at the caudal lung lobe (Figure 7.14g). Segmental and subsegmental airways should be visualized if possible. After a thorough systematic evaluation of the airways of the right lung, the endoscope should be withdrawn to the carina and the left mainstem bronchus entered.

The left mainstem bronchus branches at an angle (Figure 7.15a). The first lobar bronchus encountered leads to the left cranial lung lobe (Figure 7.15b), where it branches further. Beyond the first lobar bronchus, the left main bronchus becomes the left caudal lobar bronchus (Figure 7.15c), which also branches significantly. Segmental and subsegmental airways (Figure 7.15d) of the left lung should be visualized if possible. Although there are many lobes and branches to evaluate, the entire procedure should take no more than approximately 7–10 minutes, including the time required for diagnostic procedures. The whole procedure should be done with oxygenation and oxygen breaks (by removing the endoscope from the bronchial tree) every 40–50 seconds to ensure that the patient does not develop hypoxaemia.

Once the airways have been visualized, diagnostic procedures such as BAL, brush cytology and biopsy can be performed.

Bronchoalveolar lavage

BAL is a technique used to sample the small airways of patients with lung disease. It can be performed routinely in patients undergoing bronchoscopy. BAL differs from tracheal washes, which collect material only from the larger airways. Therefore, BAL can be a valuable technique for evaluating patients with lung disease involving the small airways, alveoli and interstitial lung tissue. The patient must be under general anaesthesia for BAL, and therefore the technique is not appropriate for patients in respiratory distress. BAL may not be necessary in all patients with small airway disease. For example, a tracheal wash is sufficient for the diagnosis of most cases of pneumonia, and does not require general anaesthesia as it can be performed with the patient under sedation. Although BAL has therapeutic applications in humans, it is used mainly as a diagnostic tool in small animals.

As BAL is typically performed during bronchoscopy, the animal should already be under anaesthesia, positioned and monitored as described above. All supplies and equipment needed (Figure 7.16) should be set up before inducing anaesthesia, to ensure a quick and safe procedure.

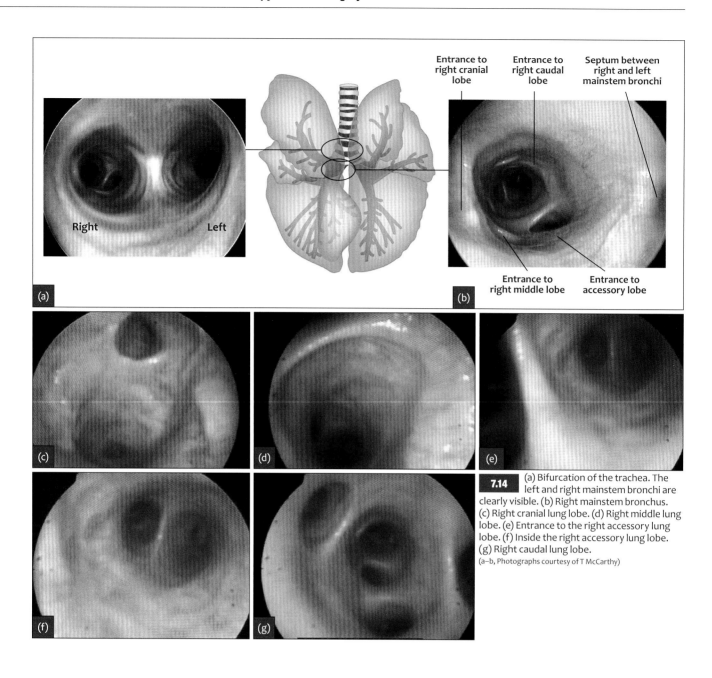

Entrance to right cranial lobe

Entrance to right caudal lobe

Septum between right and left mainstem bronchi

Right   Left

Entrance to right middle lobe

Entrance to accessory lobe

7.14 (a) Bifurcation of the trachea. The left and right mainstem bronchi are clearly visible. (b) Right mainstem bronchus. (c) Right cranial lung lobe. (d) Right middle lung lobe. (e) Entrance to the right accessory lung lobe. (f) Inside the right accessory lung lobe. (g) Right caudal lung lobe.

(a–b, Photographs courtesy of T McCarthy)

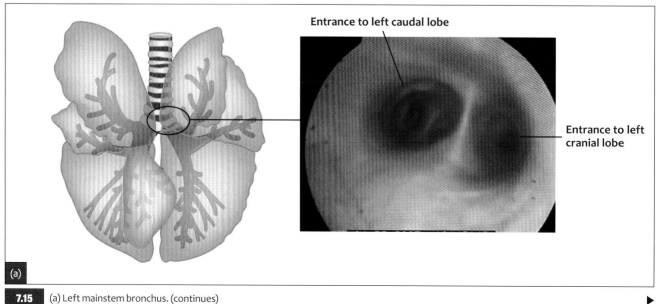

Entrance to left caudal lobe

Entrance to left cranial lobe

7.15 (a) Left mainstem bronchus. (continues)

7.15 (continued) (b) Left cranial lung lobe. (c) Left caudal lung lobe. (d) Deep subsegmental airways.

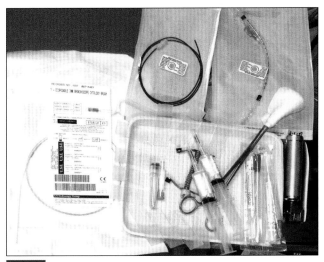

7.16 Equipment required to perform bronchoalveolar lavage.

Technique

Sterile saline (0.9% sodium chloride) should be used to perform BAL. The saline should be non-bacteriostatic to allow bacterial growth during culture of fluid samples. To obtain a diagnostic yield from a BAL requires a seemingly large volume of fluid to be instilled into an airway in order to reach the alveoli. This volume is not standardized, but a total volume of up to 50 ml or sometimes more, divided into two or more boluses, is commonly used in dogs and cats. In dogs with a bodyweight of over 10 kg, two boluses of 25 ml each have been used successfully. In cats and dogs with a bodyweight of less than 10 kg, two to four boluses of 10 ml each typically provide satisfactory results. The first bolus typically collects the most contamination from the larger airways and therefore at least two boluses are recommended.

The preferred technique for BAL requires the use of a flexible endoscope with a sampling channel. The endoscope must be sterile. A bronchoscope with an outer diameter of 4.8 mm is suitable for most patients, but a gastroscope with an 8 mm outer diameter may be used in large dogs. Use of too large an endoscope will make it difficult to reach the deeper, smaller airways and may limit the diagnostic yield. BAL is performed after bronchoscopic examination, so that the visual evaluation of the airways is not affected by the saline infused and so that lung lobes showing gross pathology can be selected for BAL. Brush cytology and/or biopsy should be delayed until after BAL so that they do not alter the fluid retrieved.

Ideally, at least two lung lobes should be evaluated by BAL to increase the chance of retrieving representative samples. Once the lobes to be sampled have been selected based on the findings of either bronchoscopic or radiographic evaluation, the bronchoscope is passed into successively smaller airways until it is seated snugly. Sterile saline that has been pre-drawn into syringes is then instilled via the bronchoscope channel and gently suctioned back through the same channel using a sterile syringe. Alternatively, the procedure can be performed using a lavage catheter (see Figure 7.5) passed through the biopsy channel into the deeper, smaller airways. Negative pressure during aspiration (increased resistance to drawing back on the syringe plunger), would indicate the need to decrease suction to avoid causing airway collapse. If necessary, the endoscope can be repositioned slightly, taking care not to dislodge its tip from the airway in which it is seated. Ideally, 40–90% of the fluid instilled should be retrieved. The fluid is typically slightly turbid with a foamy layer at the top, representative of surfactant.

Fluid obtained by BAL can be evaluated cytologically and microbiologically. In most cases, samples for culture can be pooled from several boluses or lobes. Quantitative aerobic bacterial culture and, in certain cases, culture for fungi, *Mycoplasma* and anaerobes may be warranted. Generally, the first bolus from each lobe should be evaluated separately as it is likely to be more representative of the larger airways (i.e. trachea and bronchi). Cell counts can be made on undiluted BAL fluid, but the interpretation of such counts may be difficult. Cytology results are subjective (i.e. total and differential counts are not determined). Alveolar macrophages are the predominant cell type in BAL samples from healthy dogs and cats, and do not represent granulomatous inflammation; eosinophils are common in samples from healthy cats.

Bronchial and bronchiolar brush cytology

Analysis of bronchial brushings can provide information about airway inflammation in some dogs and cats with chronic cough, and is a more sensitive indicator of airway inflammation than cytological examination of BAL fluid. The brushing procedure is very simple and has a high diagnostic yield. A sterile sheathed brush (see Figure 7.4) is passed through the biopsy channel of the endoscope to the area of interest and the brush is advanced and rubbed lightly on the tissue. The brush is withdrawn into the sheath and then removed from the channel. The brush is then advanced from the sheath and rubbed gently on to a slide for interpretation (Figure 7.17). This procedure is very safe and quick, and identifies cells that do not exfoliate into BAL fluid. It is also an excellent way to evaluate the bronchial epithelium.

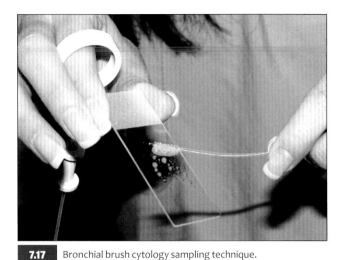

7.17 Bronchial brush cytology sampling technique.

Biopsy

Endoscopic biopsy of the airways may be useful to obtain samples for histopathology when endobronchial lesions are identified during the visual examination. Samples are obtained under direct visualization using forceps passed through the biopsy channel of the bronchoscope. Transbronchial aspiration and biopsy can be performed, with or without fluoroscopic assistance. However, due to the risk of haemorrhage and pneumothorax, transbronchial lung biopsy is not routinely performed. Biopsy within the airway must be performed with caution and consideration of the risks of potentially severe bleeding or development of pneumothorax after the procedure. The benefit and risk must be considered in each circumstance.

Pathological conditions

Tracheobronchitis

Tracheobronchitis is commonly diagnosed in the dog and cat. It is characterized by inflammation, hyperaemia and oedema of the tracheal and bronchial mucosa. The mucosal surfaces are often mottled with excessive secretions, accumulations of mucus or mucopurulent debris; there is epithelial polyp formation and, sometimes, bleeding. The irregular nodular mucosal surfaces and epithelial polyps (Figures 7.18 and 7.19) result from the normal process of tissue repair after chronic damage associated with inflammation, that is, the growth of fibroblasts and production of fibrous tissue. These changes should not be confused with neoplastic or granulomatous lesions. Tracheobronchitis can develop as the result of a number of conditions, such as chronic allergic airway disease or infection; however, in many cases the aetiology is unknown. Bronchial brushing, BAL and biopsy are used to obtain samples for histopathology and culture to enable a complete assessment and determine appropriate treatment.

Asthma, the most common inflammatory lower airway condition in cats, may be associated with a number of findings at bronchoscopy, including airway hyperaemia, stenosis, mucus accumulation, bronchiectasis and irregular epithelial surfaces. However, such findings are not specific for asthma, as they may also be seen in cats with pneumonia or neoplasia.

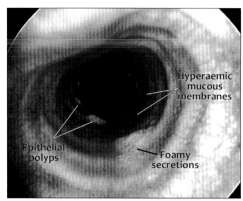

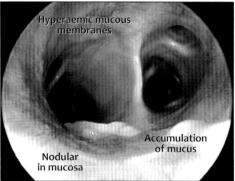

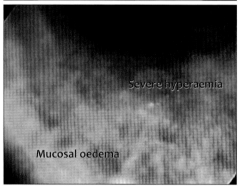

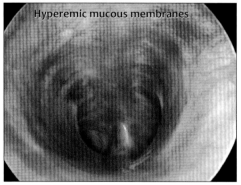

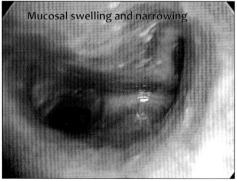

7.18 Changes in the trachea associated with tracheobronchitis. (Courtesy of T McCarthy)

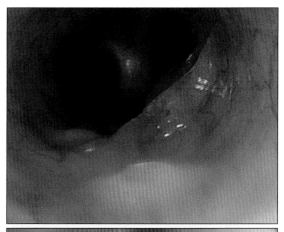

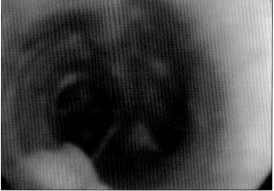

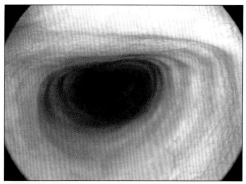

7.20 Mild cervical tracheal collapse.
(Courtesy of T McCarthy)

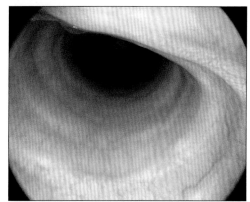

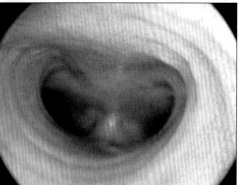

7.21 Moderate intrathoracic tracheal collapse.
(Courtesy of T McCarthy)

7.19 Mucopurulent secretions in the trachea of a cat with tracheobronchitis.
(Courtesy of T McCarthy)

Tracheal collapse

Tracheal collapse is a progressive degenerative disease of the cartilage rings that leads to dynamic tracheal collapse during ventilation. Collapse can occur in the cervical and/or thoracic trachea and may extend into the smaller airways. Cervical tracheal collapse is most evident on inspiration, while collapse of the intrathoracic trachea or mainstem bronchi is more apparent on expiration (Figures 7.20 to 7.24). In dogs with tracheal collapse, the dorsal tracheal membrane becomes pendulous and the tracheal rings become flattened, resulting in airway obstruction and mucosal irritation. The obstruction can range from mild to so severe that it creates a double lumen effect.

Collapse of the cervical trachea can be treated surgically by placement of an extraluminal polypropylene ring (or spiral) prosthesis to open and stabilize the trachea. A newer technique is the placement of an intraluminal stent to prevent tracheal collapse. A number of types of stents have been evaluated in the canine and feline trachea, including balloon-expandable and self-expanding stents. There can be significant complications after stent placement including:

- Irritation of the airway (which can cause cough)
- Laryngeal paralysis
- Stent fracture
- Granulation tissue formation
- Airway and lung infection
- Stent migration (movement of the stent)
- Tracheal rupture
- Collapse of main stem bronchi or non-stented regions of the trachea
- Although rare, animals are at risk of death during or after stent placement.

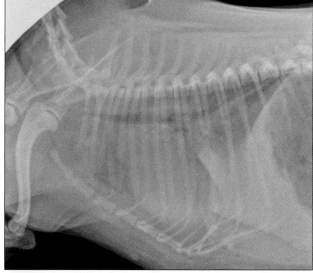

7.22 Lateral view of a dog with severe extrathoracic and intrathoracic tracheal collapse. The dog showed chronic cough and dyspnoea.

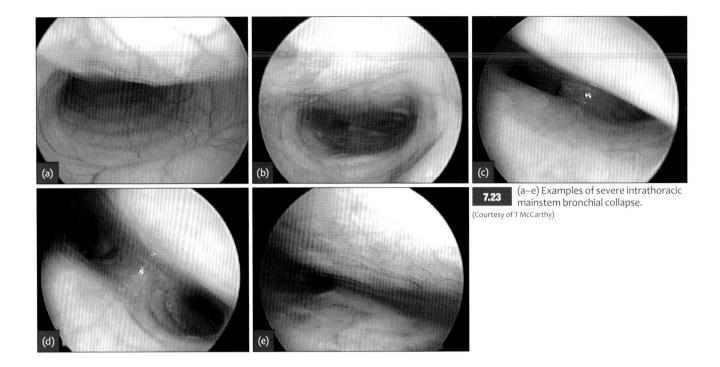

7.23 (a–e) Examples of severe intrathoracic mainstem bronchial collapse.
(Courtesy of T McCarthy)

However, stents can be well tolerated. Stenting is indicated for patients that have extensive cervical and/or intrathoracic collapse that cannot be managed medically (Figure 7.24).

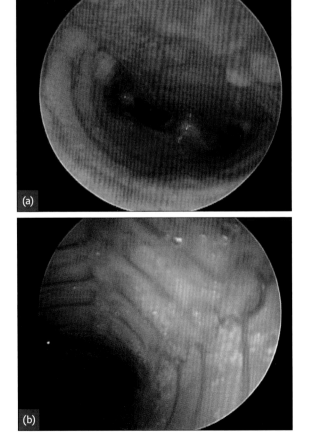

7.24 (a) Severe intrathoracic tracheal collapse in a dog.
(b) Appearance of the trachea following placement of an intraluminal stent.
(Courtesy of T McCarthy)

Brachycephalic obstructive airway syndrome

Brachycephalic obstructive airway syndrome is associated with classic airway changes in brachycephalic dogs as a result of chronic excessive effort upon inspiration. The breeds most commonly affected are English Bulldogs, French Bulldogs, Boston Terriers, Pugs and Pekingese. The syndrome is characterized by the presence of one or all of these features:

- Stenotic nares
- Elongated soft palate extending into the larynx
- Hyperplastic turbinates extending into the nasopharynx
- Everted laryngeal saccules and/or laryngeal collapse (see Figure 7.10b)
- Tracheal hypoplasia
- Excessive foamy airway secretions (Figure 7.25)
- Gastrointestinal signs – regurgitation and/or hiatal hernia.

Tracheal hypoplasia can affect segments of the trachea or its entire length. With hypoplasia, there is overlapping of the ends of the tracheal rings, creating a misshapen and narrowed trachea.

Other conditions

Other abnormalities of the airways include tracheal tears, neoplasia, granulomas and parasitic infections. Infection with the lungworm *Oslerus osleri* or the French heartworm (*Angiostrongylus vasorum*) results in small, irregular polypoid lesions on the tracheal and carinal mucosa (Figure 7.26a). Deformation of the carina can also occur as a result of extramural compression (Figure 7.26b) caused by hilar lymphadenopathy or extraluminal masses such as granulomas, abscesses or neoplasia. Transbronchial needle aspiration or biopsy can be used to obtain a diagnosis in these cases.

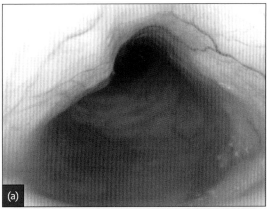

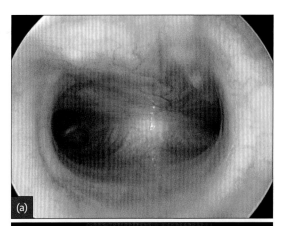

Rounding or blunting of the airway bifurcations can be caused by chronic inflammation, infiltration or oedema of the lung tissue (Figure 7.27). Biopsy of irregularities in the mucosal surface and cytological examination of the tissue samples are essential. Endoscopic examination can also be used to identify sources of bleeding in the airways, lung lobe torsion and causes of airway obstruction. Pulmonary abscessation, granulomatous disease, fungal infection, pneumonia and bronchiectasis can also be identified. Pulmonary oedema can be seen in the airways of animals with heart failure (Figure 7.28).

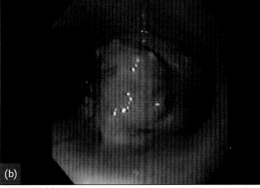

7.25 (a) Deformed tracheal rings and (b) foamy airway secretions in a brachycephalic puppy with tracheal hypoplasia.
(Courtesy of T McCarthy)

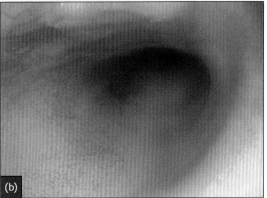

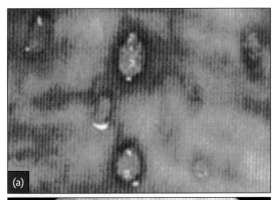

7.27 (a) Blunting at the carina is seen in this chronically irritated airway. (b) Granulomatous inflammation associated with coccidioidomycosis in a young dog.
(Courtesy of K Gulikers)

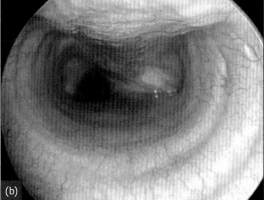

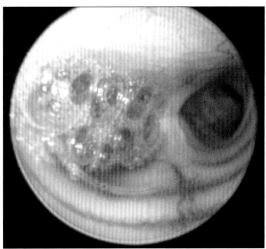

7.26 (a) *Oslerus osleri* nodules on the tracheal mucosal surface. (b) Severe airway collapse at the carina caused by an extraluminal mass.

7.28 Pulmonary oedema seen in the airways of a patient with heart failure.

Foreign body removal

Foreign material in the airways is commonly retrieved under direct bronchoscopic visualization. Removal of foreign bodies from the airways can be very challenging, depending on the shape and location of the object. A range of foreign body retrieval forceps, including basket, rat-toothed, alligator, net and polyp snare-type forceps, may be useful for removal of a variety of foreign objects, such as stones, teeth, plastic, plant material and food (Figure 7.29 and Video 7.5). Adequate ventilation must be provided during the retrieval procedure, because ventilation will be compromised if the bronchoscope blocks the airways for a prolonged period of time. In addition, care should be taken to ensure that the endoscope does not completely fill the lumen of any airway. The veterinary surgeon should be prepared to stop the procedure and refer the patient for surgery if the foreign body cannot be removed swiftly, as the risks of complication will increase with a prolonged procedure. Smooth, round objects are often very difficult to remove with the instrumentation that can fit into the endoscope channel, and may be best removed surgically.

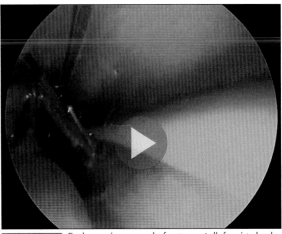

Video 7.5 Endoscopic removal of a grass stalk foreign body from the airway of a dog.

Removal of foreign bodies from the small airways can be very difficult. The procedure must be planned carefully before removal attempts are made. The veterinary surgeon must ensure removal instruments will pass through the endoscope channel, and try to practise grasping a similar object using the selected instruments before attempting the procedure. The most useful devices tend to be rat-toothed forceps, snares, three-pronged graspers and retrieval baskets. During the process, the veterinary surgeon must take care not to disrupt the mucosa surrounding the foreign body, to minimize the risk of bleeding into the lungs and the visual field. The procedure should be as quick as possible and air should be moving through the channel during the procedure to ventilate the area of lung

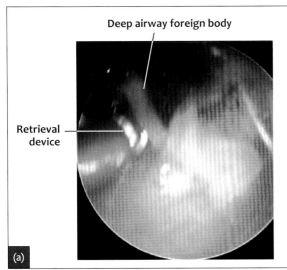

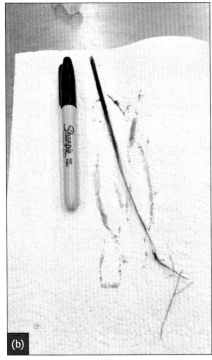

7.29 (a) Removal of a foreign body from a deep airway. (b) The foreign body (a grass stalk) after removal.

Postoperative care

Following bronchoscopy, the patient should remain intubated and should breathe 100% oxygen for 10 minutes, to resolve the hypoxaemia that may occur secondary to procedures performed during bronchoscopy. Pulse oximetry should be used to monitor the patient's oxygenation throughout recovery from anaesthesia and during the postoperative period. Capnography will help to ensure proper ventilation. This is especially important in patients with chronic obstructive pulmonary disease, where airway collapse is common. The patient's body temperature, respiratory rate, respiratory effort and depth should be assessed at regular intervals, and auscultation of the lungs should also be performed at intervals. In patients that have undergone BAL, crackles may be heard on auscultation for up to 24 hours after the procedure.

Complications

When bronchoscopic examination and procedures are performed properly, serious complications are uncommon. Complications that occur may be related to anaesthesia (arrhythmia, hypotension, oesophagitis, tracheitis)

or to the endoscopic procedure itself. Complications of bronchoscopy include hypoxaemia, bleeding in the airways and infection. Hypoxaemia is typically transient, bleeding rarely occurs if the endoscopist is careful to manipulate the endoscope gently, and infection is rare when the equipment is properly sterilized and stored between procedures. It may also be helpful to sterilize equipment immediately before a procedure. Other potential complications include coughing and bronchospasm secondary to irritation of the airways resulting from the procedures performed and manoeuvring of the bronchoscope in the airway. Bronchospasm can be treated with a bronchodilator; in fact, it may be helpful to pre-treat cats (especially those with asthma) with a bronchodilator (terbutaline at 0.01 mg/kg s.c. 30 minutes before the procedure) to decrease the likelihood of bronchospasm. Coughing is typically transient but, in some dogs with airway obstruction exacerbated by coughing, it may be useful to instil 1–2% lidocaine at the carina before completing the bronchoscopic procedure to decrease coughing. Rarely, pneumothorax can occur from trauma caused to diseased airways by the movement of the endoscope or the diagnostic procedures performed.

When performed properly, flexible endoscopy of the respiratory tract is a very low-risk, high-yield diagnostic tool. Careful planning, a thorough and consistent examination technique, and the use of all appropriate diagnostic tools are essential elements of successful flexible endoscopic evaluation of the respiratory tract. Many new diagnostic and treatment possibilities lie ahead for the veterinary patient as veterinary endoscopists embrace the expanding field of interventional endoscopy.

Acknowledgements

The authors would like to thank Robert C. Denovo, S. Dru Forrester, Keven Gulikers, Steve Hill, Timothy C. McCarthy and Brendan McKiernan for their valuable assistance with the preparation of many of the figures for this chapter.

References and further reading

Andreasen CB (2003) Bronchoalveolar lavage. *Veterinary Clinics of North America: Small Animal Practice* 33, 69–88

Ashbaugh EA, McKiernan BC, Miller CJ and Powers B (2011) Nasal hydropulsion: a novel tumor biopsy technique. *Journal of the American Animal Hospital Association* 47, 312–316

Bolliger CT and Mathur PN (2000) Interventional bronchoscopy. In: *Progress in Respiratory Research, Volume 30*, ed. CT Bolliger and PN Mathur, pp. 108–119. Karger, Basel

Coolman BR, Marretta SM, McKiernan BC and Zachary JF (1998) Choanal atresia and secondary nasopharyngeal stenosis in a dog. *Journal of the American Animal Hospital Association* 34, 497–501

Cremer J, Sum SO, Braun C, Figueiredo J and Rodriquez-Guarin C (2013) Assessment of maxillary and infraorbital nerve blockade for rhinoscopy in sevoflurane anesthetized dogs. *Veterinary Anaesthesia and Analgesia* 40, 423–429

Johnson LR (2001) Small animal bronchoscopy. *Veterinary Clinics of North America: Small Animal Practice* 31, 691–705

Johnson LR and Fales WH (2001) Clinical and microbiologic findings in dogs with bronchoscopically diagnosed tracheal collapse: 37 cases (1990–1995). *Journal of the American Veterinary Medical Association* 219, 1247–1250

Johnson LR and Vernau W (2011) Bronchoscopic findings in 48 cats with spontaneous lower respiratory tract disease (2002–2009). *Journal of Veterinary Internal Medicine* 25, 236–243

King LG (2004) *Textbook of Respiratory Disease in Dogs and Cats*. Elsevier, St. Louis

Levitan DM, Matz ME, Findlen CS and Fister RD (1996) Treatment of *Oslerus osleri* infestation in a dog: case report and literature review. *Journal of the American Animal Hospital Association* 32, 435–438

McCarthy TC (2005) *Veterinary Endoscopy for the Small Animal Practitioner*. Elsevier, St. Louis

McKiernan BC (2000) Diagnosis and treatment of canine chronic bronchitis: twenty years of experience. *Veterinary Clinics of North America: Small Animal Practice* 30, 1267–1278

McKiernan BC (2007) Laryngeal function and doxapram HCl (Dopram). *Proceedings: Veterinary Information Network MEDFAQ*. Available from www.vin.com

Mehta AC, Prakash UBS, Garland R *et al.* (2005) American College of Chest Physicians and American Association for Bronchoscopy Consensus Statement: prevention of flexible bronchoscopy-associated infection. *Chest* 128, 1742–1755

Padrid P (2000) Feline asthma: diagnosis and treatment. *Veterinary Clinics of North America: Small Animal Practice* 30, 1279–1294

Payne JD, Mehler SJ and Weisse C (2006) Tracheal collapse. *Compendium on Continuing Education for the Practicing Veterinarian* 28, 373–382

Rha JY and Mahony O (1999) Bronchoscopy in small animal medicine: indications, instrumentation and techniques. *Clinical Techniques in Small Animal Practice* 14, 207–212

Roudebush P (1990) Tracheobronchoscopy. *Veterinary Clinics of North America: Small Animal Practice* 20, 1297–1314

Taylor A, Rozanski E and Gladden J (2018) Epiglottic retroversion: concurrent diseases, management and outcome in 13 cases (2012–2017) (Abstract R06) ACVIM 2018

Willard MD and Radlinsky MA (1999) Endoscopic examination of the choanae in dogs and cats: 118 cases (1988–1998). *Journal of the American Veterinary Medical Association* 215, 1301–1305

 Video extras

- **Video 7.1** Epiglottic retroversion – intermittent spontaneous retroflexion of the epiglottis during inspiration causing obstruction of the rima glottidis
- **Video 7.2** Bilateral laryngeal paralysis in a cat
- **Video 7.3** Laryngeal carcinoma in a cat
- **Video 7.4** Grade III collapsing trachea in a Chihuahua
- **Video 7.5** Endoscopic removal of a grass stalk foreign body from the airway of a dog

Access via QR code or: bsavalibrary.com/endoscopy2e_7

Chapter 8

Principles of rigid endoscopy and endosurgery

Philip Lhermette, Elise Robertson and David Sobel

Introduction

Whereas the use of flexible endoscopes is largely confined to the gastrointestinal and respiratory tracts, where the ability to follow a tortuous lumen is paramount, rigid endoscopes can be introduced into any appropriate body orifice – and if a suitable orifice cannot be found, then the surgeon can create one! Laparoscopy and thoracoscopy have challenged the traditional paradigms in human surgery and have revolutionized the treatment of many common conditions, such as gall bladder disease, reproductive tract disorders, bowel cancer and heart disease.

The advantages of minimally invasive surgery are as valid in veterinary medicine as they have been proved to be in human medicine, but some caution must be exercised. Minimally invasive techniques should be considered only when the procedure can be carried out at least as safely and effectively as the equivalent open surgical procedure. In many cases, minimally invasive techniques are safer and more effective than traditional alternatives, but in order for the veterinary surgeon (veterinarian) to perform them safely and effectively they do require adequate training and practice.

Health and safety considerations

Effective and timely cleaning and sterilization of endoscopes is essential to prevent cross-contamination between patients and possible zoonotic infection of the endoscopist (see Chapter 2). For many endosurgical procedures, particularly laparoscopy and thoracoscopy, the same precautions are taken as for traditional sterile open surgery. The surgeon should be gowned and gloved, and a face mask should be worn as appropriate. Other procedures, such as otoscopy, rhinoscopy, colonoscopy and urethrocystoscopy, have particular requirements for operator and patient safety, not least because these are not sterile procedures and the operator may be exposed to body fluids and exudates, often diluted by copious amounts of saline irrigation fluid. The potential for zoonotic transmission of infection should always be appreciated, and the use of surgical gloves, a face mask and eye protection is advised, together with a surgical gown – preferably worn over a non-absorbent plastic apron.

Anaesthesia is required for nearly all rigid endoscopic procedures, with the possible exception of reproductive vaginoscopy (see Chapter 11) and some otoscopic procedures (see Chapter 10). An anaesthetist is therefore required and should be experienced in monitoring patients undergoing endosurgery, as there are some specific considerations that need to be taken into account (see below). Some laparoscopic and thoracoscopic procedures also require a surgical assistant to act as camera operator, freeing the surgeon to use both hands to manipulate the instruments. It is therefore essential that other members of the team are sufficiently trained in the handling of endoscopic instruments and endoscopes before embarking on these procedures.

Anaesthetic considerations

Any procedure necessitating anaesthesia or sedation requires a thorough knowledge of the condition of the patient and the risks and benefits of the various anaesthetic regimes and protocols available. The reader is referred to the BSAVA Manual of Canine and Feline Anaesthesia and Analgesia for comprehensive coverage of the subject. There are, however, specific considerations that should be taken into account when embarking upon some forms of endoscopic or minimally invasive surgery, in particular relating to endoscopy of the respiratory tract, thoracoscopy and laparoscopy.

Respiratory tract

Anaesthetic technique and airway management will depend entirely on the location of the lesion and the proposed procedure. Adequate monitoring should always include pulse oximetry and capnography.

Tracheobronchoscopy

For rigid tracheobronchoscopy, the usual prerequisites for general anaesthesia apply.

Fasting: Food should be withheld from the patient overnight and water for 3–4 hours. Since certain procedures are undertaken without the reassurance of a protected airway in the form of an endotracheal tube, it should be considered essential that the patient's stomach is empty to prevent regurgitation during anaesthesia and possible aspiration of stomach contents.

Premedication: Premedication with butorphanol/acepromazine helps to provide a smoother induction and recovery while helping to reduce gag reflexes. In cats, due to the sensitive nature of the larynx, topical anaesthesia with 1% lidocaine spray is advisable. Premedication with terbutaline helps to reduce dynamic airway spasms, which can become irreversible, especially when investigating lower airway disease.

Induction and maintenance: In most cases, it is desirable to examine the posterior pharynx and larynx before bronchoscopy, and preferably before intubation. For this reason, it is often preferable to use intravenous alfaxalone or propofol for induction, followed by total intravenous anaesthesia with a continuous infusion or intermittent boluses of alfaxolone/propofol, and/or isoflurane by mask, to maintain anaesthesia.

All patients should receive 100% oxygen by mask or tent/incubator for approximately 10 minutes before starting the procedure, since the presence of the endoscope in the airway will inevitably result in some degree of hypoxia. In routine cases where the procedure is not likely to be prolonged, intubation is unnecessary, but if the procedure is likely to be prolonged, as in the case of foreign body removal, intermittent intubation should be considered.

An alternative method of maintaining adequate oxygenation during bronchoscopy is to pass a canine urinary catheter or small feeding tube into the trachea alongside the bronchoscope and attach this tube to the anaesthetic machine. This does not interfere with visualization of the larynx, and in medium to smaller dogs allows oxygen and anaesthetic gases to be delivered throughout the procedure. This may also be possible in large cats if a very small bronchoscope is used. However, the small diameter of the trachea often precludes the placement of additional instrumentation or catheters alongside the endoscope without risk of blocking the airway. Alternatively, in larger dogs, the endoscope may be passed through the lumen of an endotracheal tube via a T-piece connector. Care should be taken to ensure that there is sufficient space to allow adequate gas flow around the endoscope (between the endoscope and the catheter, or between the endoscope and the endotracheal tube) or an increase in pulmonary pressure could occur, potentially resulting in alveolar rupture. Although these methods are useful for supplying supplementary oxygen, they are unable to maintain the anaesthetic gas concentration in the lungs accurately, since room air is also being breathed in around the endoscope, and so they should not be relied upon exclusively to maintain anaesthesia. Intermittent intubation, mask inhalation or intravenous alfaxolone/propofol may be required to maintain adequate anaesthesia.

Monitoring: The use of pulse oximetry or capnography is strongly advised in all cases. Any drop below 95% oxygen saturation should alert the clinician to stop the procedure and reoxygenate the patient. The patient should be maintained on 100% oxygen for approximately 10 minutes following the procedure.

Rhinoscopy

In addition to the usual prerequisites for general anaesthesia, rhinoscopy requires endotracheal intubation, with close attention to adequate cuff inflation to ensure a good seal and prevent aspiration of fluid and debris from the nose during saline irrigation (see Chapters 7 and 9). A small sterile gauze swab can be used to pack the caudal pharynx and prevent detritus from collecting over the larynx, but it should not inhibit free flow of irrigation fluid around the free edge of the soft palate and out through the mouth. Large throat packs can block fluid drainage and divert it down the oesophagus, especially in cats and small dogs, and this should be avoided.

Thoracoscopy

Thoracoscopy requires the induction of a pneumothorax in order to collapse the lungs and provide a space in which to operate. Thus, the same anaesthetic procedures and precautions will be required as in open chest surgery, with intermittent positive-pressure ventilation (IPPV) and careful monitoring of blood and respiratory gases. Occasionally, it may be necessary to perform selective intubation to ventilate one lung in order to maintain an adequate operative field on the relevant side of the chest (see Chapter 13). Insufflation of the chest has been described but is rarely necessary in the authors' experience. Pressures as low as 3 mmHg significantly reduce cardiac output with very little improvement in visual field.

Laparoscopy

The peritoneum is a *potential* space. In the normal animal, the serosal surfaces are in close approximation and the peritoneal space contains a small amount of fluid. If an endoscope were placed into this space, the end of the instrument would be in contact with various organs and tissues resulting in 'red-out' – a diffuse pale red image over the entire screen. In order to see anything meaningful, it is necessary to fill the peritoneal cavity with an inert gas in order to create a space in which to work – that is, a pneumoperitoneum. Air has been used successfully in the past but is poorly absorbed and therefore carries a higher risk of embolism, and – with the advent of laparoscopic surgery using lasers and electrosurgical techniques – it tends to support combustion rather too well. The most commonly used gas is carbon dioxide (CO_2), as it is cheap, readily available and safe. Any retained CO_2 following the procedure is absorbed by the bloodstream and expelled by the lungs, and CO_2 does not support combustion and is therefore safer when using laser or electrosurgical techniques.

An insufflator is essential for laparoscopy. It is used to create and maintain a pneumoperitoneum and to control the gas pressure during the procedure. It may also be necessary to vent a smoke plume from laser or electrosurgery and replace it with fresh gas.

Gas is supplied from a high-pressure cylinder either directly to the patient, through a pressure-reduction valve in the insufflator, or into a reservoir tank within the insufflator and thence to the patient. A flow-control valve regulates the delivery of gas and monitors intra-abdominal pressure. If the pressure falls below that set by the operator, the valve opens and allows more gas to flow; when the pressure that has been set is reached, the valve closes. Most electronic insufflators allow different flow rates to be set. A low flow rate of 1 litre/minute or less, depending on patient size, is used for initial insufflation to allow the patient to adapt to the increased abdominal pressure slowly. Once insufflation pressure is reached, the flow rate can be increased so that sudden drops in pressure that occur as instruments are inserted and removed are evened out quickly. Insufflators will usually measure the total gas delivered during the procedure, and also monitor the pressure in the CO_2 cylinder itself to warn of low gas supply.

In small dogs (<10 kg), it is recommended to insufflate the abdomen to a maximum pressure of 8 mmHg, and in larger dogs to no higher than 10–12 mmHg. Cats should be insufflated to around 6 mmHg initially for port insertion. These pressures are often used initially when inserting the operating ports, as they give maximum distance between the abdominal wall and underlying viscera, and reduce the ventral deformation of the abdominal wall that inevitably occurs when introducing a cannula. Once the operating cannulae are inserted, intra-abdominal pressure may be lowered to 6 mmHg or below in dogs and to around 2–4 mmHg in cats, as all that is required is a sufficient space to visualize the site of interest.

Technique for abdominal insufflation

Insufflation of the abdomen may be initiated with a Veress needle or via a modified Hasson (paediatric) approach. The Veress needle can also be used to create a pneumothorax before thoracoscopy.

Veress needle approach: The Veress needle (see Chapters 2 and 12) contains a spring-loaded hollow blunt obturator that normally protrudes beyond the sharp point of the needle. As the needle is pressed against the abdominal wall the obturator is pushed back into the body of the needle and the sharp point passes through the muscle and fascia into the peritoneum. As soon as the point of the needle enters the peritoneal space the obturator springs back, exposing the blunt point and reducing the chance of trauma to the internal organs.

1. A small (1 mm) incision is made with a No. 11 scalpel blade in the skin at the chosen site, usually at a prospective port site cranial to the umbilicus in the midline. It is beneficial to introduce a small bleb of local anaesthetic (bupivacaine) at the puncture site and at all the port sites before their introduction, as this will greatly reduce postoperative discomfort.
2. The abdominal wall is grasped with the index finger and thumb of the non-dominant hand and tented upwards. The Veress needle is introduced at an angle to the skin surface by pointing it caudally towards the pelvis and into the pocket created by the tented-up abdominal wall. In this way iatrogenic damage to the spleen is less likely and the fatty falciform ligament is avoided. The bladder should also have been voided either naturally before anaesthesia or by preoperative catheterization to prevent inadvertent puncture.
3. With experience, as the tip of the needle enters the peritoneal space, a slight 'pop' is felt. The tap on the top of the Veress needle is then opened and a syringe of sterile saline is attached to the Luer fitting. Gentle suction is applied to check for fluid or blood. If no blood or fluid is present, 1–2 ml of sterile saline is injected into the abdomen; it should flow freely and easily.
4. The syringe is then removed and, with the tap still open, the abdominal wall is tented up with the distal end of the Veress needle to ensure that the drop of saline sinks into the needle hub via negative pressure (hanging drop method). This should occur if the needle is correctly placed.
5. Once the Veress needle has been correctly placed, sterile tubing is attached to the hub and connected to the insufflator. Abdominal pressure should initially be low (<2 mmHg). If it rises rapidly, this usually indicates that needle placement is incorrect (i.e. subcutaneous) or that the needle is blocked. Initial insufflation should be slow to allow homeostatic mechanisms to compensate for the increased intra-abdominal pressure.

Complications: Problems that may be encountered during insertion of a Veress needle include:

- Placing the needle subcutaneously or subperitoneally (tenting)
- Placing the needle into the omentum or falciform ligament
- Penetrating a solid organ
- Penetrating a viscus.

Subcutaneous placement of the Veress needle can be frustrating but is fairly easily avoided. With practice it is possible to appreciate the feel of the Veress needle penetrating the peritoneum, but inexperienced endoscopists are understandably cautious and may fail to penetrate the abdominal wall completely before starting insufflation. This results in subcutaneous emphysema. Although this is not dangerous, it can impede the technique and make subsequent proper placement of the Veress needle more difficult. The emphysema should resolve over the following 48 hours.

If the Veress needle is inadvertently inserted into the omental bursa, mesentery or falciform ligament, these structures can insufflate and obscure the view when the endoscope is inserted via the primary port. If this occurs and it is not possible to negotiate the tip of the endoscope around the obstruction, it may be necessary to desufflate the abdomen, reposition the Veress needle and try again.

Penetrating a solid organ can be more of a potential problem; if this occurs the initial insufflation pressure will be high, and the operator is alerted via electronic alarm. Penetration of an organ itself is rarely a problem unless a major vessel is damaged, but attempts to insufflate the spleen can readily result in a fatal gas embolism. The abdomen should always be palpated underneath the insertion point and the tip of the Veress needle should be directed away from the spleen. If blood is seen on insertion of the Veress needle, it should be removed and repositioned before insufflation.

Penetration of a hollow viscus may be apparent to the surgeon if blood is seen on insertion of the Veress needle or on applying gentle suction with a syringe, or if a low or zero rate of CO_2 flow is seen (solid organ), or, rarely, if a high rate of CO_2 flow is seen despite a lack of progressive insufflation of the peritoneal space (hollow organ). In this case, the Veress needle should be removed and replaced. The same applies to inadvertent penetration of a viscus with a cannula. The underlying damaged viscus should be examined and, if repair is required, it should be determined whether this can be performed laparoscopically or whether conversion to open surgery is needed.

Modified Hasson (paediatric) approach: An alternative technique for abdominal insufflation is the modified Hasson (or paediatric) technique.

1. A 2 cm incision is made in the skin over the midline at the designated port site and the fascia is dissected from the linea alba.
2. Two stay sutures are placed lateral to the midline and the linea alba is elevated.
3. An incision is made in the linea alba to accommodate the cannula (5 mm incision for a 6 mm cannula) and the cannula is introduced directly into the abdomen with a blunt trocar or without a trocar.
4. The abdomen is then insufflated through the trocar.

This technique requires a larger skin incision than the use of a Veress needle, and is more time-consuming.

However, in cats there may be some advantages with the modified Hasson approach as there is an increased risk of peritoneal tenting when using a Veress needle. This occurs when the Veress needle passes through the abdominal wall but fails to penetrate the peritoneum and pushes it away from the abdominal musculature, which may result in subperitoneal insufflation. Cats also have a very thin abdominal wall, which reduces friction on the cannula and may result in it sliding in and out of the abdominal incision as instruments are introduced and withdrawn. The use of a modified Hasson technique coupled with a disposable balloon cannula circumvents the problem of tenting and slippage: the balloon cannula, which is constructed of lightweight material and has an inflatable flange with a sliding retention disc, helps to keep the cannula in place during the introduction of instrumentation and/or the endoscope (see Chapter 2).

There has been much debate in both the medical and the veterinary literature on the relative benefits of the Veress needle technique *versus* the modified Hasson technique. It is inadvisable to extrapolate from the experience in human medicine, as the anatomy of veterinary patients is considerably different. The abdomen of the dog and cat is more laterally compressed, whereas in humans the abdomen is ventrodorsally compressed. In thin human patients there may be as little as 2 cm between the abdominal wall and the retroperitoneal vascular structures (Krishnakumar and Tambe, 2009); this increases the likelihood of vascular injury to the aorta or vena cava when the Veress needle is used. Such injuries have not been documented in veterinary medicine, probably because of the larger space between the abdominal wall and these structures in veterinary patients. Another relevant anatomical difference is that in humans the spleen is relatively small and located under the rib cage on the left side. In some breeds of dog, such as the German Shepherd Dog, the spleen may be extremely large and extend right across the midline of the central abdomen from left to right, and is therefore more likely to sustain injury from either Veress needle insertion or modified Hasson port placement. Splenic injury will usually necessitate splenectomy in humans, whereas splenic bleeding in the dog is usually relatively easily controlled. Indeed, sometimes the author [PL] takes splenic biopsy samples with biopsy forceps in the same way as liver biopsy specimens are taken. In humans, the modified Hasson technique increases the risk of bowel injury during introduction, as the bowel lies immediately under the site of entry.

In human laparoscopic surgery, meta-analysis of the literature has revealed no evidence that the open entry technique (i.e. Hasson technique) is superior or inferior to the other entry techniques currently available, including the use of a Veress needle (Toro et al., 2012; Ahmad et al., 2019). There is little published research from the veterinary field, although one paper looking at complications occurring during the initial learning process of laparoscopic ovariectomy in the bitch followed four surgeons new to laparoscopic techniques and found that splenic laceration occurred in six of 618 cases (Pope and Knowles, 2014). Four lacerations occurred when placing a cannula by the modified Hasson/paediatric technique and two occurred when introducing a Veress needle. Statistically, there was no significant difference between the two techniques. Ultimately, as in many situations, the technique with which the surgeon is most familiar is often the safest.

Complications: Problems that may be encountered during the modified Hasson (paediatric) approach include:

- Damage to the underlying intestine
- Damage to the spleen
- Poor retention of the cannula in the incision due to reduced retention with the abdominal wall.

Haemorrhage resulting from damage to the spleen is usually immediately obvious and self-limiting. The area under the insertion point should always be inspected for iatrogenic damage following insufflation and insertion of the endoscope.

Anaesthetic considerations with abdominal insufflation

Raised intra-abdominal pressure inevitably has physiological effects, such as aiding capillary venous haemostasis (which can be useful), but care should be taken to ensure that bleeding does not increase once the pressure is reduced at the end of the procedure. In practice, this is rarely a problem. However, pressure on the caudal vena cava can reduce venous return to the heart and thus decrease ejection volume.

Pressure on the diaphragm increases intrathoracic pressure and not only reduces lung capacity, with a corresponding increase in physiological dead space, but also reduces diaphragmatic excursion during breathing and reduces tidal volume. Inspiratory effort is also increased. CO_2 is highly soluble and can form carbonic acid on serosal surfaces during prolonged procedures, resulting in postoperative discomfort. It can also be absorbed into the bloodstream and can potentially cause hypercapnia and respiratory acidosis. However, these effects are relatively minor and rare at the pressures used for laparoscopy, and should not cause problems for the vast majority of patients.

Pressures above 15 mmHg can reduce perfusion of abdominal organs, particularly the kidney, bowel and hepatic portal system. They can also activate the renin–angiotensin system (RAAS), causing renal vasoconstriction. Relatively healthy patients compensate for these changes readily, and an intra-abdominal pressure of <10 mmHg is of minimal consequence, but the surgeon should always be aware of increases in abdominal pressure and use the lowest pressure necessary to perform the procedure. In practice, a pressure of 3–4 mmHg is usually adequate to maintain a working space. Haemodynamic effects are most marked during induction of pneumoperitoneum, and insufflation using low flow rates initially until the maximum inflation pressure is reached should be employed to allow haemostatic mechanisms to slowly adapt to increasing intra-abdominal pressure. Preoperative fluid volume loading can help to limit the haemodynamic effects, especially in dehydrated patients.

Some anaesthetists recommend the use of IPPV for all laparoscopic procedures to help overcome the increase in airway resistance due to insufflation. However, mechanical ventilation introduces additional risks, especially in inexperienced hands, and in the authors' experience IPPV is unnecessary in the vast majority of patients if abdominal insufflation pressures are kept low. An assisted breath, given by gently squeezing the anaesthetic bag once every couple of minutes, coupled with careful monitoring, is usually sufficient.

Since many insufflators do not heat the gas, prolonged procedures can result in hypothermia, and monitoring core body temperature is useful, especially in small patients.

Patient positioning

Detailed information on positioning requirements for rigid endoscopy procedures can be found in the relevant chapters.

Laparoscopy

For laparoscopy, manipulation of tissues and organs can be accomplished to a large extent using grasping forceps or a palpation probe. However, careful patient positioning can facilitate surgery by moving viscera out of the field of view. A rotating cradle or operating table that can be moved in three planes is ideal.

Placing the patient in a head-down Trendelenburg position is useful when operating on the caudal abdomen, as in this position the viscera move towards the diaphragm. It can also be used to move the spleen out of the way when introducing a Veress needle for insufflation. Venous return is increased with this position, but angulation should not be more than about 15 degrees as it increases pressure on the diaphragm, increasing the respiratory effects of pneumoperitoneum. A reverse Trendelenburg position, with the head elevated, facilitates surgery on the cranial abdomen but causes a reduction in venous return.

Rotating the patient to the left or right exposes the kidney and, in bitches, the ovary on the elevated side. The left lateral position is also useful for visualizing the right limb of the pancreas and gives good access to the liver, avoiding the falciform fat. During some laparoscopic procedures, such as ovariohysterectomy, the patient's position is changed intraoperatively to enable access to both sides of the abdomen.

Thoracoscopy

During thoracoscopy from a paraxiphoid transdiaphragmatic approach, rotation of the patient can be useful to move the lungs out of the way, enabling the surgeon to access more of the lateral chest wall and the lateral and dorsal lung surfaces.

Urethrocystoscopy

Urethrocystoscopy may be performed in sternal or dorsal recumbency. Occasionally, manipulation of the bladder through the abdominal wall can be helpful, especially in large patients, where the length of the endoscope can become an issue. A slight reverse Trendelenburg position helps to move the bladder caudally and facilitates entry into the trigone when using a relatively short endoscope such as the 2.7 mm 30-degree cystoscope.

Rhinoscopy

Rhinoscopy is usually performed in sternal recumbency with the nose angled slightly down to facilitate drainage from the pharynx. Otoscopy is usually performed in lateral or sternolateral recumbency with upward traction on the pinna.

Choice of endoscope

The simplest endoscope to use when starting to perform laparoscopy or thoracoscopy is the 0-degree endoscope. This gives a true view along the axis of the endoscope, and instruments introduced through operative ports enter the field of view at the expected angle.

A 30-degree endoscope can be very useful, especially in tight spaces, since it allows the endoscope to be kept somewhat out of the way of the instrumentation and allows the surgeon to look around organs or structures that would otherwise obscure the view. However, the angle of view makes manipulation of instruments a little more complicated. If the endoscope is oriented with the axis of view upwards, instruments introduced from the side will appear on the monitor to be coming in from below and to the side. This takes a little getting used to and requires practice. These endoscopes are commonly used in the nose, joints and bladder, where manipulation of the endoscope is restricted in a small space and the angle of view can be exploited to see around corners and enlarge the field of view by rotating the endoscope around its long axis. In the nose and bladder, the endoscope is invariably used in a sheath, which usually incorporates an instrument channel, so instruments pass directly into the field of view and manipulation does not present a problem.

Special considerations for endosurgery

Endoscopic surgery differs from conventional open surgery in several important ways:

- The surgical field is viewed in two dimensions on a television monitor
- The view is magnified and the angle of view may not be along the long axis of the endoscope
- Instruments are often long and held at a site distant from the point of interest
- There is a fulcrum effect at the port site, such that upward movement of the instrument handle results in downward movement of the tip of the instrument
- There is a lack of direct tactile feedback to the surgeon
- Manipulation of the position of the patient during the operation can be advantageous
- There is limited opportunity to move the positions of the instruments once ports have been placed.

Positioning

Correct positioning of the patient (see above), equipment and monitor in relation to the surgeon is essential. The endoscopy trolley should be positioned such that it is directly in front of the surgeon, with the monitor just below head height. During some procedures it may be necessary for the surgeon to change sides in relation to the patient, and if this is the case the endoscopy trolley should also be moved to afford the optimum view.

Camera orientation

Camera heads are attached to the endoscope by a releasable collar, which allows the endoscope to rotate in relation to the camera. This is useful when using an endoscope with an angled view, such as 30 degrees, since it affords a larger field of view as the endoscope is rotated and enables the surgeon to look around corners. However, it is vital that the camera head itself is kept in the correct orientation. The camera is, in effect, the surgeon's eyes; if it is rotated inadvertently through 90 degrees, this has the same effect as the surgeon turning on their side. If this is not noticed it can be very confusing, as lateral movements of instruments in the field of view are shown as vertical on the monitor. Most camera heads have a flat surface or buttons on the top that help the surgeon to maintain the correct camera orientation.

Use of instruments

One of the first obstacles the novice endoscopist must overcome is learning to operate in a three-dimensional environment with two-dimensional visualization with unfamiliar, long instrumentation. Appreciation of depth and distance can be difficult at first, especially given the high magnification afforded by the endoscope, which exaggerates the smallest movements. Moving the endoscope further away from the site of interest to give a more panoramic view is helpful if an instrument is lost from the field of view or when moving instrumentation towards the site of interest. Moving the endoscope close to the site of interest helps with appreciation of fine movements and depth of field.

Practice is essential and the benefit of endoscopy training sessions in a 'dry laboratory' setting cannot be overemphasized. Handling and manipulation of instruments is key to good operative technique and requires practice. The use of a laparoscopy 'trainer' is extremely useful for the veterinary surgeon in acquiring the skills to manipulate laparoscopic instruments in a two-dimensional video environment. Commercial laparoscopy trainers can be purchased but are expensive. A simple alternative can be manufactured from an opaque plastic box about the size of an average dog's abdomen, with holes cut into the top at locations equivalent to the sites commonly used for port placement (see later for details of port placement). These holes should be covered with thick cloth-covered neoprene through which cannulae can be inserted. An image can be obtained by a suitably placed webcam in the training box and viewed on a laptop placed in front of the box. A desk lamp usually provides sufficient illumination. The only other requirement is some laparoscopic hand instruments, which can be bought cheaply second hand for training purposes.

Simple exercises can then be performed in the training box, such as stacking sugar cubes, placing small objects into a rubber glove or bag, or dissecting holes in pieces of paper following a pre-drawn pattern. A piece of chicken breast, complete with skin, makes a good model for practising biopsy techniques, cutting tissues and suturing. All these exercises help to familiarize the surgeon with camera technique and improve manual dexterity. It is essential that these basic techniques are mastered. Attending wet labs and practising on cadavers should always precede live surgery. Assisting a proficient endoscopic surgeon in live procedures is an extremely useful way for the veterinary surgeon to become acquainted with the necessary techniques in a more realistic environment.

Tactile information

Tactile feedback is used in open surgery to locate solid masses in fat, to differentiate solid from cystic masses, or to detect variations in the texture of a solid organ, such as the liver, that may indicate a pathological change. To some extent tactile information can be gained during laparoscopy with a palpation probe, a blunt-ended probe that can be run over the surface of an organ or used for ballottement of a cystic structure. With practice, a good degree of tactile information can be obtained in this way.

Demisting

Placing a cold endoscope in a warm, humid abdomen or thorax can often lead to misting of the lens. While this can usually be resolved by gently wiping the lens on a serosal surface, it is useful to try to prevent it occurring, as far as possible, by pre-warming the instrument. Placing the endoscope in warm sterile distilled water for a few seconds is ideal, or even just warming the tip of the endoscope in the hand can be effective. Commercial demisting solutions are available and effective but not generally necessary; povidone–iodine is a good substitute.

Port placement

Laparoscopic and thoracoscopic cannulae are often called ports or operative ports. In arthroscopy, they are called portals. The correct placing of ports is vital to a successful surgical outcome. Placement will vary according to the size of the patient and the procedure to be undertaken. Several general principles must be applied:

- Before embarking upon laparoscopy or thoracoscopy, port placement must be carefully planned so that additional ports do not have to be placed during the procedure
- Ports must be placed sufficiently far from the site of interest so as not to overcrowd the area, but not so far that instruments cannot reach easily
- The camera (endoscope) port is placed first and instrumentation or operative ports are placed to the sides, sufficiently far apart that instruments do not interfere with each other, and so that instruments can triangulate down to a focus at the site of interest at a comfortable angle – usually around 45–60 degrees. This is the normal position in which a surgeon would hold hand instruments during an open procedure.
- Where two operating ports are used, they should be equidistant from the camera port (Figure 8.1).

The exact port position on the abdomen or thorax in relation to landmarks such as the umbilicus, pubis or specific ribs will vary according to the size of the patient: in terms of relative position between the umbilicus and pubis, 2 cm caudal to the umbilicus is very different in a cat and a Great Dane. It is important to visualize the operative site in three dimensions and plan the port sites accordingly in each case.

Optimal positioning of ports will considerably improve the ease of manipulation of instruments for dissection and suturing and, ultimately, the speed of surgery. The surgical site is placed at the centre of an imaginary circle, with the ports placed on the periphery; the camera port is usually placed in the centre with operating ports on either side. The angle between the optical axis of the endoscope and an instrument is called the *azimuth angle*. The angle between the two instruments is the *manipulation angle*, and the angle between the instrument and the horizontal is the *elevation angle* (Figure 8.2).

Ideally, the azimuth angles should be the same and the manipulation angle should be approximately 60 degrees. The elevation angle should be the same as the manipulation angle. This positioning will allow the shortest operative time and optimal performance (Supe *et al.*, 2010) as well as allow the surgeon to be in the most ergonomically comfortable position with the elbows at 90 degrees, forearms

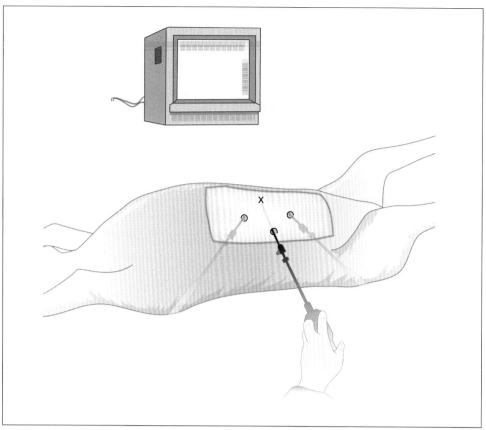

8.1 Port placement for triangulation in laparoscopy. X marks the site of surgical interest.

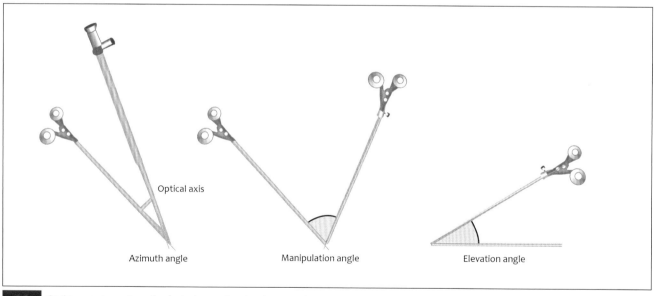

Optical axis

Azimuth angle

Manipulation angle

Elevation angle

8.2 Optimum ergonomic angles for instrument and endoscope placement.

parallel to the floor and the shoulders relaxed. However, patient size and operative site will often dictate different approaches, and if a larger elevation angle is required, a correspondingly larger manipulation angle is required. For complex tasks such as suturing, a relatively small elevation angle is required for manipulation of the needle. Ideally, the operating site should be 15–20 cm from the port site, but this is not always achievable in small patients.

Due to the fulcrum effect of long instruments passing through a fixed port, movements can be exaggerated, especially if more than half the instrument is inside the patient. If more than half the instrument length is outside the body, exaggerated arm movements can lead to fatigue in the surgeon's shoulders and elbows, so in smaller patients it is recommended to use shorter instruments to avoid this problem. Ideally, the length of instrument inside and outside the patient's body should be equal.

When inserting a smooth-sided cannula with a sharp trocar into an insufflated abdomen, there should be a reasonable space between the abdominal wall and the underlying viscera. Care should be taken not to stab the trocar into the abdomen too forcefully. A middle finger extended along the axis of the cannula can ensure safe and controlled abdominal access. Holding the upper end of the cannula in the palm of the hand, gentle pressure is exerted in a twisting motion until the tip of the cannula enters the peritoneal space. Care should be taken not to depress the abdominal wall too far towards the underlying viscera. If undue pressure has to be exerted it may be necessary to slightly enlarge the incision. Once the cannula has entered the peritoneal space, the trocar is removed, and the cannula can be pushed gently a little further into the abdomen if necessary. Only 5 mm or so of the cannula should enter the abdomen, to reduce the blind spot and maximize the operating space. The valve in the cannula closes as soon as the trocar is removed to prevent the escape of gas. An endoscope with a camera head attached to the oculus is then inserted into the cannula and the area immediately underneath the entry point is inspected for iatrogenic damage. The endoscope can then be directed to the site of interest for further inspection.

Ternamian EndoTIP (Karl Storz) cannulae are inserted in a slightly different manner. The blunt tip of the cannula is inserted into the incision in the linea alba and the cannula is gently rotated clockwise until gas is heard escaping from the open tap on the side. Alternatively, an endoscope may be passed down the cannula to 10 mm short of the end, allowing a visual entry into the abdomen. Rubber stops are available to maintain the endoscope in this position. Again, undue pressure should not be exerted, to reduce the risk of inadvertently 'screwing' the cannula into the underlying viscera. If the cannula does not enter the abdomen easily, the tip may not be through the incision in the linea alba, in which case continued rotation will just force the skin and abdominal wall apart. The cannula should be removed and the position of the incision in the linea alba checked with closed haemostats and then the cannula tip should be replaced in the incision and another insertion attempt made.

The gas inlet tubing from the insufflator can be transferred from the Veress needle to the inlet port of the cannula. This allows removal of the Veress needle and means that gas flow is directed away from the endoscope lens, helping to keep it clear. Cold gas contacting the warm peritoneum can, however, sometimes increase fogging of the endoscope lens. If this is a problem, touching the lens to a serosal surface in the abdomen will clear the fogging. Moving the gas inflow to the operative port may also help if the problem persists. Occasionally, it may be necessary to remove the endoscope and wipe the tip with a sterile saline-soaked gauze to remove blood, fat or tissue debris.

Endoscopes should be introduced through the rubber grommet on laparoscopy ports, and the trapdoor seal should be opened manually before inserting the endoscope through the port. Opening the trapdoor simply by pushing the endoscope through it will eventually damage the lens, resulting in the need for costly repair. The same procedure is used for introducing sharp trocars into the port, to prevent blunting. When inserting trocars, care should be taken to ensure that the sharp tip is centrally placed when passing through the rubber grommet, as cuts to the rubber will result in leakage of insufflation gas. Other instruments can generally be passed through directly.

In thoracoscopy, following the insertion of a port and removal of the trocar, the valve mechanism of the cannula is also removed, leaving unsealed access to the thorax. Unlike laparoscopy, where a good gas-tight seal is obligatory, in the thorax a gas-tight seal is not required. On the contrary, air needs to flow in and out of the thorax as the lungs are inflated and deflated by positive-pressure ventilation. Failure to allow this air flow risks creating a tension pneumothorax.

It is usually necessary to create a second port in order to introduce instrumentation (e.g. biopsy forceps). For operative surgery a third port may be required. Additional ports are always inserted under direct visualization through the endoscope and the port site is chosen with respect to the area of interest. The tip of the endoscope is brought up to the proposed site to transilluminate the skin. This allows larger vessels in the skin to be seen so that a relatively avascular area can be selected. Local anaesthetic is injected and a 5 mm skin incision is made. A cannula is introduced through the incision, only this time entry into the abdomen is under direct visualization through the endoscope to avoid trauma to the spleen or other viscera. The trocar is removed and replaced by a blunt palpation probe. If instrumentation or probes are smaller than the port diameter, for instance, where 5 mm instruments are used with an 11 mm cannula, a reducing valve must be used to maintain a gas-tight seal.

Whenever possible, instruments of any kind should be introduced into the abdomen under direct visualization, with the jaws closed, to prevent trauma to the abdominal viscera. The tip of the instrument can then be guided down to the point of interest under visual control. Retracting the endoscope to give a wide-angle survey view is often useful as instruments are introduced. The endoscope can then be advanced along with the instrument to the point of interest to allow a close-up view for fine manipulation.

Rigid endoscopes, particularly those smaller than 4 mm in diameter, are fragile and are easily broken by rough handling or sharp knocks. Endoscopes smaller than 4 mm in diameter should always be used in a protective sheath; failure to do so may result in permanent damage. Torsion or bending of the shaft of the endoscope is a common problem and occurs most often during arthroscopy or rhinoscopy, where the endoscope is manipulated in a small, rigidly enclosed space. The appearance of a dark semilunar shadow at the edge of the image on the video monitor is an indication that excessive torsion is being used and damage to the endoscope is likely to occur.

Dissection and haemostasis

All the tissue manipulations that are undertaken during open surgery can be accomplished endoscopically. Blunt dissection with forceps or sharp dissection with scissors enables lesions to be isolated from surrounding tissues. A wide variety of endoscopic instrumentation is available (see Chapter 2). Many endoscopic instruments are insulated and have terminals for connection to monopolar or bipolar electrosurgery units, enabling bleeding points to be grasped and cauterized. Monopolar dissecting hooks are useful for fine dissection and, in some cases, can obviate the need to change instruments when cauterizing and cutting.

Commercially available Endoloops® (Ethicon) are pre-tied loops of suture material (Vicryl® or PDS) attached to a rigid plastic shaft that acts as a knot pusher to cinch the knot down once the loop has been positioned around the tissue. These can be used for isolating a pedicle of tissue for biopsy or removal of a small mass in the liver or periphery of the lung, or for encircling a bleeding point or organ such as the uterine stump.

Haemostatic gauze such as Gelfoam Plus® (Baxter Healthcare), Traumastem® (Millpledge), Surgicel® (Ethicon) or chitosan-based haemostatic bandages can be placed at biopsy sites to reduce haemorrhage, but this is rarely necessary. Haemorrhage can usually be controlled by simple pressure applied with a palpation probe, or small tonsillar swabs can be introduced down the operative port and used to apply pressure and remove small quantities of blood. It should be remembered that haemorrhage always looks considerably worse under the magnifying lens of the endoscope. In practice it is rarely a problem and is usually easily controlled.

Commercially available dissecting and coagulating instruments, such as the HARMONIC® scalpel (Ethicon) and the LigaSure™ (Medtronic Inc.), enable sealing and sectioning of vessels 5–7 mm in diameter, greatly facilitating dissection using only one instrument. However, these instruments are currently extremely costly and outside the budget of many general practitioners. A more cost-effective alternative is the Lina PowerBlade™ – a 'single-use' disposable instrument that can be attached to a standard electrosurgery unit. This instrument can in fact be reused if it is cleaned with care and gas-sterilized. Autoclavable 5 mm reusable vessel sealer/dividers with replaceable blades are also now available, such as the ROBI plus® (Karl Storz) and VetSEAL (Freelance Surgical), although the latter requires a bespoke generator.

Endoscopic staplers and clip appliers provide a rapid and simple way to ligate vessels and ligate and divide tissues. Most of these are 10 mm instruments, although 5 mm clip appliers are available. A 10 mm linear cutter-type endoscopic stapler can be very useful in resecting lung lobes or anastomosing intestine. These instruments place 4–6 rows of titanium staples either side of a blade that simultaneously cuts and divides the tissue when the stapler is fired. Staple cartridges are quite costly, and although these are generally single-use instruments, they can often be reused after ethylene oxide gas sterilization. Clip appliers usually contain around 20 stainless steel or titanium clips that can be applied individually to ligate vessels.

Electrosurgery

Electrosurgery is probably the main method of haemostasis used in minimally invasive procedures and is commonly used for tissue dissection. There are two types of electrosurgery used in minimally invasive surgery: monopolar and bipolar. Both require a complete circuit in order for current to flow. In all forms of electrosurgery, current passes through the patient's tissue to create the surgical effect; this is in contrast to electrocautery, where an electric current is used to heat a metal probe, which is then applied to the tissue. Monopolar electrosurgery requires the use of a dispersive or return electrode placed remotely on the patient. In bipolar electrosurgery, the two jaws of the bipolar forceps form the active and return electrodes and current passes only through the tissue between the jaws of the instrument.

Monopolar electrosurgery

Many endoscopic instruments are insulated along the shaft and include a monopolar terminal for attachment to a surgical generator. Monopolar electrosurgery is the most commonly used modality in endosurgery and is used for both tissue dissection and haemostasis. An electrosurgical generator provides the voltage to drive the current that is required. The generator is connected to an active electrode or handpiece. The current flows through the patient and natural tissue resistance provides impedance, which generates heat at the tip of the active electrode. A dispersive or return electrode completes the circuit by providing a pathway for the current to flow back to the electrosurgery unit. Since an alternating current is used, current will flow in both directions through the circuit. The large size of the return electrode dissipates heat over a wide area to prevent tissue damage, whereas the active electrode concentrates the heating effect at a small point to provide a controlled surgical effect. The only difference between the active and return electrodes is the area of contact and thus the current density.

The effect of the current on the tissue at the active electrode can be modified by changing the waveform of the alternating current. Most generators can produce several different waveforms, which are generally named after the primary function for which they are used (Figure 8.3).

The 'cut' setting provides a low-voltage constant waveform, which is generally used in open surgery with a very small wire or pointed electrode held just above the tissue.

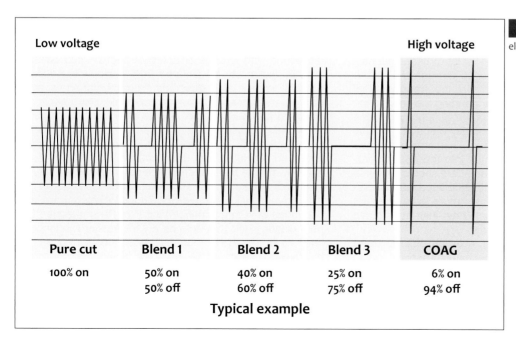

Pure cut	Blend 1	Blend 2	Blend 3	COAG
100% on	50% on 50% off	40% on 60% off	25% on 75% off	6% on 94% off

Typical example

8.3 Voltage and waveforms for common monopolar electrosurgical settings.

This generates a spark to provide intense heat that will vaporize tissue but not penetrate deeply, thus providing a cutting effect. The 'coag' setting provides a high-voltage intermittent waveform, which is usually on for only 6% of the time and off (no current flowing) for 94% of the time. This creates less heat so tissue is not vaporized but instead denatured, to provide a coagulation effect. Most generators also have one or several 'blend' settings or at least a single 'cut and coag' setting. This provides an intermediate waveform with more 'on time' than the 'coag' setting, to provide an increased coagulation effect with some tissue vaporization or cutting effect. Voltage generally increases as 'on time' decreases. However, this description is somewhat simplistic, and in reality the effect on tissues will vary according to a number of factors including:

- Contact or distance from tissue
- Waveform used
- Area of contact (size of electrode)
- Time
- Voltage/power setting
- Tissue type
- Eschar.

These variables affect the rate of heat production, which in turn determines whether the waveform will have more of a cutting or a coagulating effect. For instance, in open surgery a small wire electrode in a handpiece is used with a continuous 'cutting' waveform for skin incision. The tip of the wire electrode is held slightly away from the surface of the skin (or other tissue) and sparks are formed, which cross the gap. Since the current is concentrated at a very small focal point, intense heat is produced, which vaporizes the tissue. This vaporization effect – caused by the cells in the tissue exploding – actually has a cooling effect as the heat is dissipated rapidly, minimizing thermal spread. The tissue is cut with a minimal coagulation effect and minimal collateral damage.

Sparking across a gap can also be used with the 'coag' setting in a process called electrosurgical fulguration. A broader electrode and higher voltage is used but as the current is on for only around 6% of the time less heat is produced. This has the effect of coagulating and charring tissue over a wider area. The longer the generator is activated, the more heat is produced and the deeper the effect on the tissue.

If a continuous 'cutting' waveform is used and the tip of the electrode is bought into contact with tissue, the effect is different again. Because the current is dissipated more rapidly, its density is reduced and consequently less heat is produced. Tissue in contact with the electrode is not vaporized but is desiccated as intracellular water evaporates, and a coagulum forms. Conversely, by using a fine electrode and close proximity, a cutting effect can be achieved using the 'coag' setting to provide improved haemostasis in vascular tissues.

As carbonized tissue (eschar) aggregates on the electrode, its performance can degrade because this material has a high electrical resistance. High-resistance eschar also contributes to arcing as current tries to find the path of least resistance. Eschar can result in increased collateral damage, foreign body reactions and may even ignite. Keeping electrosurgical instruments clean and free from eschar will enable a more consistent effect to be achieved and reduce the likelihood of aberrant current paths causing damage.

Bipolar electrosurgery

In bipolar electrosurgery the current flows from the generator to the bipolar instrument and through the tissue held between the two electrodes (jaws) of the instrument before returning to the generator. The instrument therefore acts as both the active and the return electrode. This is inherently safer than monopolar electrosurgery, as return electrode burns and contact problems are eliminated and current is confined to the tissue grasped by the instrument. Bipolar electrosurgery uses a much lower voltage than monopolar electrosurgery and does not have the option of varying waveforms. Dedicated bipolar instruments, cabling and a bipolar setting on the generator are required.

Use of electrosurgery for minimally invasive procedures

Monopolar and bipolar electrosurgery are used extensively in minimally invasive procedures for both dissection and haemostasis. Monopolar or preferably bipolar forceps can be used for effective haemostasis. Hook electrodes can be used for fine dissection and other instruments, such as scissors or biopsy forceps, can also be connected for monopolar electrosurgical use to maintain a blood-free field and aid dissection. However, there are some hazards inherent to the use of electrosurgery in this context.

Hazards of electrosurgery

Hazards of monopolar electrosurgery: Older electrosurgery units were produced on the assumption that current would flow to ground via the return electrode and thence the generator, which was earthed through the wall socket. Unfortunately, in reality this was not always the case. Current will flow to ground by the easiest route, and this may be through contact points with a metal operating table or other ancillary equipment in contact with the patient, such as towel clips or electrocardiogram leads. The large size of the return electrode dissipates heat over a wide area. If current flows to ground through an alternative route and the point of contact is sufficiently small, burns can occur at this point.

Modern generators are isolated to prevent this problem. The generator recognizes the current from the return electrode and completes the circuit itself, thus removing the ground as a reference for the current. If the circuit from the generator to the patient and back via the return electrode is broken, the generator cuts out, thus preventing burns at alternative sites. However, it is still possible to get burns at the return electrode site if the area of contact is not sufficient; this can be a particular problem in small animals due to poor contact through hair or focal contact over bony prominences. Hair also increases the impedance of the return electrode and thus increases the production of heat. Ideally, the return electrode should have good contact over a large muscle mass near the surgical site. Some generators monitor the impedance of the return electrode at the patient–pad interface and deactivate if the impedance increases unduly. In some high-frequency units, the return electrode acts as a capacitor and does not need such close contact with the patient. In these units, the return electrode is usually a solid plate rather than a flexible pad, and can be placed in close contact with the patient without the use of contact gel or adhesive.

Surgical smoke: Smoke (or plume) is another by-product of electrosurgery that can form a hazard to the surgeon and theatre staff as well as to the patient. Vaporization of tissues produces smoke, which can potentially carry viral DNA, prions, bacteria, carcinogens and other toxic substances. Inhalation of this smoke should be avoided and consideration should be given to using a surgical smoke extraction device.

Direct coupling: Electrical current flows through the path of least resistance. Minimally invasive procedures often involve the use of instruments and cannulae that conduct electricity very well. If the active electrode touches or is placed too near to another instrument or metallic cannula, current may jump to it and then pass to tissue in contact with that cannula or instrument at a remote site, causing injury. If this occurs out of view of the endoscope it may go unnoticed and potentially represents a serious hazard.

Insulation damage: Endoscopic instruments designed for use with monopolar or bipolar electrosurgery are insulated over the entire length of the shaft and handles. However, this insulation can fail though wear and tear or poor handling, allowing current to escape to adjacent tissues where it may cause injury. The use of the 'coag' setting can damage insulation due to the high voltages used, especially if there are weak points in the insulation caused by knocks or abrasions. The relatively low-voltage 'cut' setting is less likely to result in insulation failure and will still provide coagulation when relatively large instruments are used in direct contact with tissue.

Capacitative coupling: A capacitor is a passive electrical component that can store charge in the electric field between two conductors. It consists of two conductive electrodes separated by a non-conductive material that prevents charge from moving between the electrodes. While the plates are connected to an electrical circuit, charge can move through the circuit from one electrode to the other; when the circuit is turned off, charge in the capacitor persists. The separated charges on the electrodes attract each other and an electric field is present between the two electrodes.

From a surgical point of view, a capacitor may be created by surgical instruments. The active electrode being used for electrosurgery is surrounded by non-conductive insulation, which in turn is surrounded by a conductive metal cannula. Current flowing through the active electrode may, through the electrostatic field, induce a current in the metal cannula, which may cause tissue injury at the port site. In practice this is rarely a problem, especially if low-voltage cutting waveforms are being used, as the currents induced are usually dissipated over a reasonably wide area. The problem can be reduced further by using plastic cannulae, but even here the patient's own body tissue is conductive and therefore can induce a capacitor, although the effects are likely to be negligible.

A more serious problem may occur if a hybrid cannula system is used. In this system, a plastic collar anchors the metal cannula at the port site. A capacitor is still formed between the active electrode and the metal cannula, but the plastic collar prevents current from dissipating through the skin and tissue at the port entry site. Instead, current moving to the return electrode escapes from the exposed cannula within the patient to tissues in contact with it. Since the point of contact may be very small, significant damage may be done to internal organs.

Other hazards: High-frequency currents invariably leak from wiring and circuitry, and can induce electrical currents in other metallic objects or instruments. Coiling a cable around a metallic towel clamp, for example, can result in enough current to burn the patient.

Recommendations when using electrosurgery during laparoscopy

- Always check instruments carefully and discard any with damaged insulation. Often just the insulated shaft can be replaced to save costs.
- Use an all-metal or all-plastic cannula system. Avoid hybrid systems.
- Keep instruments well apart and do not activate the generator when instruments are close or touching.
- Always use a 'cutting' waveform when using monopolar electrosurgery to keep the voltage low.
- Use bipolar instruments where appropriate.
- Use the lowest effective power setting. If the desired effect is not achieved, always check the circuit (return electrode) first before increasing the power, as increased power may force the current to seek an alternative pathway.
- Use short bursts rather than prolonged activation of the generator.
- Remove eschar from instruments regularly to avoid sparking and improve efficacy.
- Do not activate the generator when the tip of the active electrode is not in contact with tissue (unless cutting) to avoid sparking to adjacent tissues.
- Avoid metal-to-metal contact of instruments to avoid direct coupling injuries.

Suction and irrigation

Removal of ascitic fluid, blood or thoracic exudates requires suction. Laparoscopic suction/irrigation devices designed to fit the laparoscopic cannulae (5 mm) enable suction and irrigation to be carried out without significant loss of insufflation. The operative site can be irrigated with sterile saline and clots and free blood can be removed by suction to give a clear view of the operative field and ensure that adequate haemostasis has been accomplished.

Specimen retrieval

Concern regarding the seeding of tumour cells at abdominal and thoracic port sites has led to the more common use of specimen retrieval bags. Purpose-made endoscopic retrieval bags can be purchased in a number of sizes. They are rolled into a 5 mm or 10 mm tube for insertion down a standard port; when deployed in the abdomen, the mouth of the bag opens up by means of a plastic spring-loaded mechanism to allow easy insertion of the excised tissue. The mouth of the bag is then closed with a drawstring and the port is removed, allowing the bag to be withdrawn through the abdominal incision, which can be slightly enlarged if necessary. If larger solid organs or tissues are to be removed, a morcellator can be introduced into the retrieval bag while it is still inside the abdomen, and the tissue is morcellated to allow easier removal through a small incision. If commercial retrieval bags are not available, sterile zip-lock bags or the thumb of a surgeon's glove can make a good substitute.

For laparoscopic-assisted procedures where a larger incision is required, a wound retractor such as the Alexis® wound protector/retractor (Applied Medical) may be used to both protect the wound edges and provide radial traction to enlarge the incisional opening. This instrument can be inserted into an extended caudal port site to facilitate exteriorization of intestine/lymph nodes for examination and biopsy. An alternative method could be to use an S-PORT® (Karl Storz) (2–4 cm) mini-laparotomy incision site, or the use of a SILS™ Port (Medtronic Inc.) for the entire procedure as a 'SILS' (single incision laparoscopic surgery) procedure, eliminating the potential need for another port site. These ports allow the passage of three 5 mm instruments through a single larger port site (see Chapter 2).

Knot-tying techniques

Practitioners new to minimally invasive surgery are frequently keen to learn suturing and knot-tying techniques. However, the vast majority of procedures can be carried out with the aid of electrosurgical haemostasis (monopolar or bipolar) or with the use of haemostatic clips or Endoloops®. Knot tying can have specific uses in advanced surgery and may become more useful as procedures are developed. As for most endoscopic skills, a great deal of practice is required to become accomplished at suturing and knot tying using laparoscopic instrumentation. These skills should be practised using an endoscopic 'trainer' (see above) before attempting to operate on a live patient. Some basic knot-tying techniques are included here; more detail can be found in Freeman (1999), Tams and Rawlings (2011) and Fransson and Huhn (2015). Knot tying can be extra-corporeal or intracorporeal.

Extracorporeal knots

The suture material and needle are placed into the abdomen through an abdominal port (usually 10 mm) with the free end remaining outside the body. The suture material is grasped just behind the needle to facilitate passage through the port, and the needle holders are then repositioned to grasp the needle once it is in the abdomen. The needle can then be passed through or around the tissue to be ligated and brought back out through the same cannula, leaving both free ends outside the body.

Extracorporeal knots are formed by pushing individual throws of a surgeon's knot down into the body with a knot pusher, to cinch them down on to the tissue, or by forming a slip knot and introducing it in a similar manner. Alternatively, preformed knotted sutures, such as Endoloops®, may be used; these incorporate a disposable knot pusher and a pre-tied slip knot. Once the knot is positioned correctly, the free ends of the suture material are cut off.

A standard surgeon's knot can be tied extracorporeally and seated down using laparoscopic Babcock forceps (Figure 8.4). A commonly used extracorporeal slip knot is the Roeder knot (Figure 8.5). A modified Roeder knot incorporating an initial double half hitch and two final wraps around just one limb of the suture loop may also be used for added security.

Intracorporeal knots

Intracorporeal knot tying requires a laparoscopic needle holder and receiver forceps. Whereas extracorporeal knot tying requires a long length of suture material, this can be cumbersome when suturing inside the body, and suture length is usually reduced to 10–20 cm or so to facilitate handling. The whole length of the suture material and needle are introduced into the abdomen. Tissue is grasped and sutured in a similar manner as for open surgical techniques.

Standard suture materials can be used with ⅜ circle, ½ circle straight or ½ curved 'ski' needles. Needle size is dictated by the cannula size; it is normally necessary to use a 10 mm cannula with a suitable reducer for endoscopic suturing. Half-circle needles up to CT-1 can be used with 10 mm cannulae. The needle is introduced into the abdomen by grasping the suture material 2–3 cm from the needle with the receiving forceps and passing it down the cannula with the trapdoor held open. The suture material should be grasped outside the abdomen such that the needle lies in the correct plane for suturing when placed inside the abdomen.

In smaller patients, where 5 mm cannulae are used, the needle can be introduced either directly through the skin and abdominal wall, or through a port site by 'backloading'.

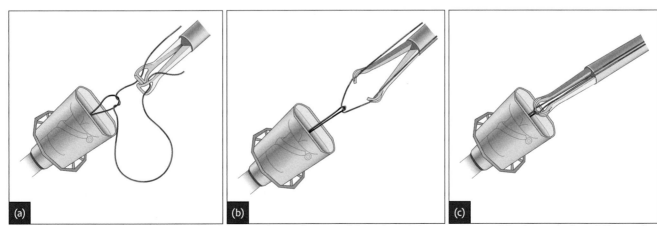

8.4 Extracorporeal knot tied using Babcock forceps. The needle is passed down through the port and around the tissue to be ligated. The needle is then brought out of the port such that both ends of the suture material are outside the body. (a) A single or double half hitch is tied as usual and the free ends of the suture are threaded through the holes in the jaws of the forceps from the inside to the outside. (b) Slight tension is applied to the free ends. (c, d) The knot is slid down into the abdomen with the jaws of the Babcock forceps closed. (continues) ▶

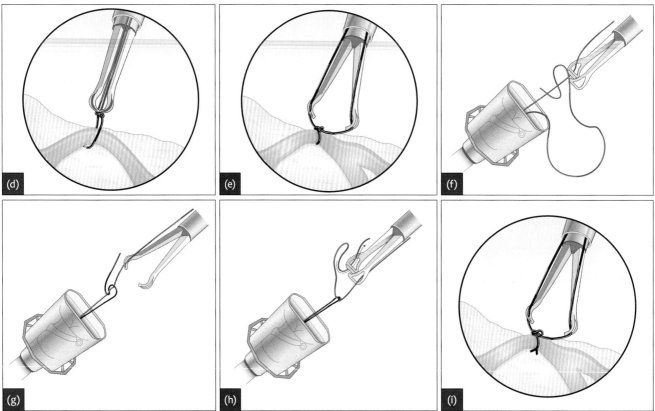

8.4 (continued) Extracorporeal knot tied using Babcock forceps. The needle is passed down through the port and around the tissue to be ligated. The needle is then brought out of the port such that both ends of the suture material are outside the body. (c, d) The knot is slid down into the abdomen with the jaws of the Babcock forceps closed. (e) Once the knot is in place, opening the jaws of the Babcock forceps applies tension to the knot to cinch it down. (f, g) The Babcock forceps are then gently withdrawn and one end of the suture unthreaded from the jaws. (h) A second half hitch is formed, the Babcock forceps are rotated and the free end re-inserted through the jaws as before. (i) The second throw is then pushed down into the abdomen and cinched tight as before.

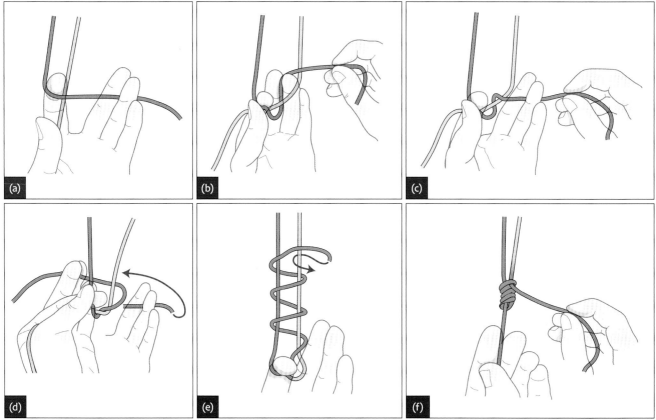

8.5 Roeder knot. (a–d) This is formed by throwing a half hitch which is then held between the index finger and thumb of the left hand. (e) The free end of the suture is then wrapped three times around the two limbs of the loop between the half hitch and the tissue to be ligated. (f) The free end is then wrapped around just one limb of the loop and brought back through the last loop so created.

To do this, the cannula is removed from the abdomen and the needle driver is inserted through the cannula to grasp the end of the suture material (3 mm from the needle) and pull it through the trocar. The needle is introduced into the abdomen through the port incision and the cannula is then slid down the needle driver and back into place in the abdominal wall. In this way, a needle up to CT-1 can be introduced through a 5 mm incision.

Endoscopic needle holders are usually 5 mm in diameter and should have an in-line handle as opposed to a pistol grip, since this facilitates rotation and manipulation of the needle. They should also have a locking ratchet mechanism. A 5 mm reducing valve is required when using a 10 mm cannula. The needle holders are passed through the reducing valve and the suture material is grasped 1–2 cm away from the swaged-on needle. The needle holders are then introduced into the 10 mm operating cannula and the reducing valve is attached to avoid loss of insufflation gas. The valve of the operating cannula should be opened manually to permit passage of the needle and needle holder.

Suturing is easiest with the suture line running from 11 o'clock to 5 o'clock for a right-handed surgeon, or from 1 o'clock to 7 o'clock for a left-handed surgeon (Figure 8.6). The monitor should be placed directly ahead of the surgeon below eye level. Correct ergonomic port placement is essential (see above).

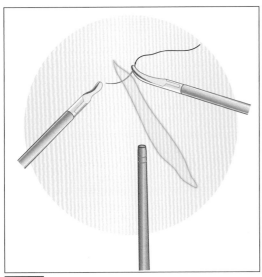

8.6 Intracorporeal knot tying: direction of the suture line.

Once in the abdomen, the needle is manoeuvred into a suitable position and grasped halfway to two-thirds of the way from the tip. The needle should be perpendicular to the long axis of the needle driver and can be manipulated in the jaws of the needle holder by grasping the suture material 2 cm from the needle with the receiving forceps and applying traction in the appropriate direction.

The tissue to be sutured is grasped with the receiving forceps and the needle is passed through by rotating the needle driver around its longitudinal axis in the usual fashion. The open jaws of the receiving forceps can be placed on to the tissue adjacent to the exit point of the needle to stabilize it if required. The needle is then grasped with the receiving forceps and the open jaws of the needle holder can be applied to the tissue adjacent to the needle to apply counter-pressure as required. The needle is then reset in the jaws of the needle holder close to the exit point from the tissue.

If long lengths of suture material are used or space is very limited, it is often easier to wrap the suture material around the closed receiving forceps so they act as a pulley (Figure 8.7). In this way, the needle is pulled away from the wound but the direction of pull on the wound is maintained and tissue trauma is less likely.

Intracorporeal knots are tied in a similar manner to a surgeon's knot or square knot (Figure 8.8) in conventional open surgery.

On some occasions it may be advantageous to create a slip knot to aid in tissue apposition. A square knot can be converted to two half hitches and then slid down on to the tissue to tighten a ligature (Figure 8.9).

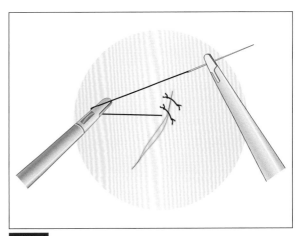

8.7 Applying tension around a pulley.

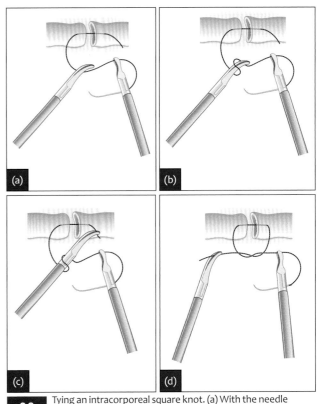

8.8 Tying an intracorporeal square knot. (a) With the needle passed through the tissue from right to left, the needle is brought back over to the right to form a 'C' loop. The receiving forceps are introduced over the suture material and into the loop from the left. (b–d) The suture material is grasped by the needle holders and held parallel to the receiving forceps, which are rotated clockwise around the loop and then used to grasp the free end of the suture to form the first throw as the instruments are drawn apart. (continues) ▶

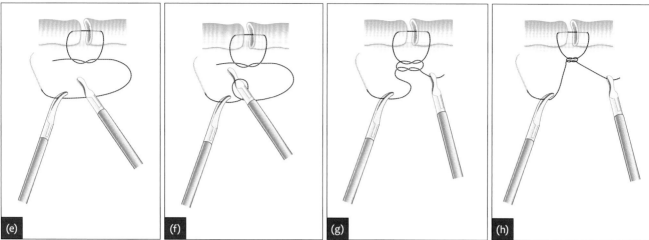

8.8 (continued) Tying an intracorporeal square knot. (e) The needle or long part of the suture material is then grasped again by the needle holders and brought over to the left to create a reverse 'C' loop. (f–h) The suture material is then grasped by the receiving forceps and wrapped around the needle holders, which are rotated clockwise around the loop and then used to grasp the free end of the suture material to complete the second throw. If the suture material is short, the needle can be grasped such that the swaged end is held parallel to the instrument forming the throw; this provides a stable loop with which to work.

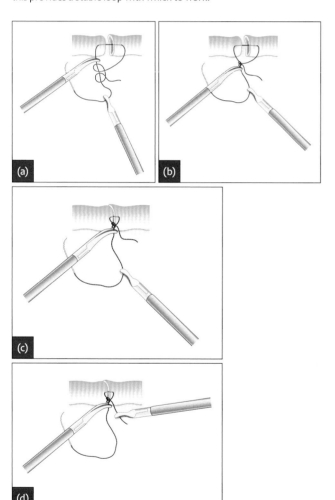

8.9 Converting a square knot to a half hitch. (a) With a loose square knot in place and the long end of the suture grasped in the left hand and the free end to the right, the suture material is grasped between the knot and the tissue on the same side as the long end (i.e. the left), and tension is applied to the knot by moving the receiving forceps and needle holders apart. This converts the knot to two half hitches. (b, c) Maintaining tension with the receiving forceps in the left hand, the needle holders can be placed above the knot and used to slide the knot down on to the tissue. (d) Grasping the free end of the suture material with the needle holders and applying sharp tension to both ends of the suture converts the knot back to a square knot for security. An additional throw can then be formed.

Desufflation

At the end of the procedure, the abdomen is desufflated. This should be done relatively slowly to allow homeostatic mechanisms to compensate for the change in intra-abdominal pressure. Intermittent opening of the trapdoor on one of the cannulae over a minute or so will allow desufflation at a suitable rate.

Human patients sometimes experience shoulder pain postoperatively due to stretching and drying of the phrenic nerve endings in the diaphragm or as a result of a direct irritant effect of CO_2. The leading hypothesis is that residual CO_2 retained in the abdomen postsurgery causes phrenic nerve irritation, which in turn leads to referred pain at the nerve root of C4. In the authors' experience, this does not seem to be a problem in veterinary patients, and lameness postsurgery has not been reported.

It is important to ensure that as much CO_2 as possible is removed at the end of the procedure. This can be achieved by placing the patient in a Trendelenburg position (with angulation of 30 degrees) and performing a pulmonary recruitment manoeuvre consisting of five manual inflations of the lung, with the trapdoor mechanism removed from the cannula to allow gas to flow freely out of the abdomen. If using a Ternamian EndoTIP cannula, this process can be assisted by elevating the abdominal wall with the cannula several times; this produces a bellows effect and flushes the abdomen. The pulmonary recruitment manoeuvre has been shown to reduce shoulder and abdominal pain in humans by more than 50% in the 2 days following laparoscopic surgery (Phelps *et al.*, 2008).

Closure

Most laparoscopic ports require minimal closure. Ternamian EndoTIP cannulae dissect bluntly through tissue planes as they are inserted and allow tissues to re-appose on removal, forming an effective seal. Even traditional 5 mm cannulae do not generally result in large enough wounds to allow herniation, so 5 mm or smaller abdominal ports may be closed with a simple interrupted suture and the skin may be closed with tissue adhesive or an intradermal suture. Ports of 10 mm should be closed in two layers: deeper layers with an absorbable suture material such as polyglactin 910 and the skin with intradermal polyglactin 910, tissue glue or non-absorbable polyamide skin sutures. All ports placed in the linea alba, where the abdominal wall is thinnest and healing delayed, should be closed in two layers to reduce the risk of herniation. If ascites is present, all abdominal incisions should be closed in several layers to prevent seepage of fluid. All thoracic ports should be closed in at least two layers to ensure an airtight seal.

Postoperative care

For the most part, postoperative care is similar to that for conventional open surgical cases, and recovery is usually more rapid. Pain relief should be administered for the first 24 hours postoperatively and then as required depending on the procedure and whether the animal is showing signs of pain.

Following laparoscopy, the abdomen is fully deflated but CO_2 continues to be absorbed during the recovery period and the patient should be monitored until completely recovered. Embolisms are rare but can occur even in recovery. Insufflation results in pressure on the abdominal vascu-lature and an increase in peripheral vascular resistance. As the abdominal pressure drops on desufflation, vascular resistance decreases and there is a resultant hypotension. Most patients compensate readily but this can be potentially dangerous in hypovolaemic patients or patients with pre-existing cardiovascular compromise. The release of intra-abdominal pressure can also rarely lead to increased intra-abdominal bleeding as pressure on the capillaries is reduced.

References and further reading

Ahmad G, Baker J, Finnerty J et al. (2019) Laparoscopic entry techniques. *Cochrane Database of Systematic Reviews* **1**, CD006583

Duke-Novakovski T, de Vries M and Seymour C (2016) *BSAVA Manual of Canine and Feline Anaesthesia and Analgesia, 3rd edn*. BSAVA Publications, Gloucester

Fransson BA and Huhn JC (2015) Minimally invasive suturing techniques. In: *Small Animal Laparoscopy and Thoracoscopy*, ed. BA Fransson and PD Mayhew, pp.12–27. Wiley Blackwell, Philadelphia

Freeman LJ (1999) *Veterinary Endosurgery*. Mosby, St. Louis

Krishnakumar S and Tambe P (2009) Entry complications in laparoscopic surgery. *Journal of Gynecological Endoscopy and Surgery* **1**, 4–11

McCarthy TC (2005) *Veterinary Endoscopy for the Small Animal Practitioner*. Elsevier Saunders, St. Louis

Phelps P, Cakmakkaya OS, Apfel CC and Radke OC (2008) A simple clinical maneuver to reduce laparoscopy-induced shoulder pain: a randomized controlled trial. *Obstetrics & Gynecology* **111**, 1155–1160

Pope JFA and Knowles TG (2014) Retrospective analysis of the learning curve associated with laparoscopic ovariectomy in dogs and associated perioperative complication rates. *Veterinary Surgery* **43**, 668–677

Supe AN, Kulkarni GV and Supe PA (2010) Ergonomics in laparoscopic surgery. *Journal of Minimal Access Surgery* **6**, 31–36

Tams TR and Rawlings CA (2011) *Small Animal Endoscopy, 3rd edn*. Elsevier Mosby, St Louis

Toro A, Mannino M, Cappello G, Di Stefano A and Di Carlo I (2012) Comparison of two entry methods for laparoscopic port entry: technical point of view. *Diagnostic and Therapeutic Endoscopy*, doi: 10.1155/2012/305428

Chapter 9

Rigid endoscopy: rhinoscopy

Philip Lhermette, David Sobel and Elise Robertson

Introduction

Nasal disease is common in the dog and cat, often pre-senting as a nasal discharge with or without sneezing, stertor or stridor. Epistaxis may or may not be a feature, and can be present in the absence of other clinical signs. Access to the nasal cavity is difficult, because it is entirely encased in bone apart from the cranial and caudal nares, and contains numerous turbinate scrolls forming many blind-ending channels in which foreign bodies or pathological changes can be hidden. Excellent coverage of nasal diseases and pathology can be found in the *BSAVA Manual of Canine and Feline Head, Neck and Thoracic Surgery*, and the reader is referred to this Manual for detailed coverage of nasal conditions.

There are only a few direct physical approaches to the nasal cavity: dorsal rhinotomy, ventral rhinotomy and rhinoscopy. Rhinoscopy is minimally invasive, is associ-ated with lower morbidity than the other (surgical) options, and is the best option for visualizing lesions and taking biopsy samples either for initial diagnosis or to confirm a suspected diagnosis. A rhinoscopic approach may also be used to remove foreign bodies and for treatment such as tumour ablation or debulking using a surgical laser (see Chapter 16) or, in cases of nasal aspergillosis, debriding fungal plaques and instilling anti-fungal solutions. Indeed, rhinoscopy is the only method by which a full direct visual examination of the nose can be carried out, and it is therefore the gold standard for diagnosis of intranasal disease.

For the novice endoscopist, rhinoscopy is one of the more accessible and easily learned procedures. Animals with nasal and sinus disease are commonly presented to the first-opinion veterinary surgeon (veterinarian) and these problems are often of significant concern to the owner. Thus, rhinoscopy tends to be among the first – and most useful – procedures to be added to the endoscopic reper-toire of the small animal practitioner.

Anatomical considerations

The diagnosis and management of diseases of the rhinar-ium and associated sinuses is complicated by the anatomy of the region. Many critical structures are in close proxim-ity and the more physiologically important structures are encased in bone, making it difficult to access nasal and sinus pathology readily. In addition, the presenting signs of most nasal diseases are relatively similar, complicating diagnosis. It is therefore essential to have a sound appre-ciation of the anatomy of the nose and sinuses before embarking on any procedure. Although different in terms of external appearance, the nose serves similar physio-logical functions in the dog and the cat, and the anatomy of the two species will therefore be considered together here (Figure 9.1).

The rostral aspect of the nose is formed by the nasal planum, which surrounds the nostrils and leads into the nasal vestibule on each side. The paired nasal bones form the dorsal limits of the nares, while the lateral and ventral limits are formed by the maxillary and palatine bones, respectively. Any or all of these bony structures can be damaged by aggressive nasal disease. Often, gross changes in these bony locales lead to the initial suspicion of disease in the nasal cavities.

The left and right nasal cavities are separated by a midline nasal septum, and each cavity is divided by dorsal, ventral and ethmoidal nasal conchae into the dorsal, middle, ventral and common nasal meatuses. The ventral nasal concha extends rostrally into the lateral part of the vestibule, where it forms the alar cartilage just inside the nasal planum. Located at the most ventral aspect of the alar cartilage is the punctum of the naso-lacrimal duct. In disease, nasolacrimal duct transit is often interrupted, resulting in epiphora. The complex scrolling of the conchal bone and resulting diverticula make full exploration of every part of the nose impos-sible. However, the majority of the dorsal, middle and common meatuses and all of the ventral meatus will be accessible in most patients.

The paranasal sinuses are a series of small, air-filled, mucous membrane-lined bony spaces that communicate to varying degrees with the nasal cavities. The only sinuses that have frequent clinical significance in respir-atory disease are the frontal sinuses, as their natural drainage into the ethmoid concha is often pathologically obstructed in the diseased state. The paired frontal sinuses are divided by a median septum and further subdivided into three chambers on each side – lateral, medial and rostral – which communicate with the nares via separate nasofrontal openings. In the majority of dogs and cats the sinuses cannot be directly accessed with a rigid rhinoscope. The anatomy of the frontal sinuses can vary between breeds and also between individuals in a breed.

The mucous membrane of the nose is well vascular-ized and lined with ciliated columnar epithelium. This,

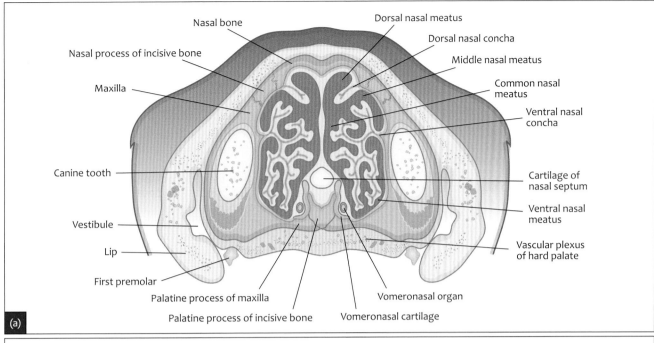

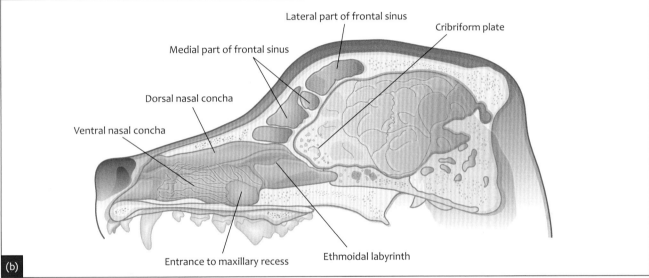

9.1 (a) Transverse section and (b) longitudinal section showing the anatomy of the nose. These illustrations show the typical anatomy of the canine nose; the anatomy of the feline nose is very similar.

coupled with the large surface area of the conchae, results in warming and humidifying of the inspired air and the trapping of airborne particles in a thin layer of nasal mucus, which can then be carried outside the nasal cavity by the action of the cilia. The most posterior aspect of the dorsal nasal meatus forms the cribriform plate of the ethmoid bone, through which the olfactory nerves pass to terminate at the olfactory bulb of the brain.

Indications

Dogs and cats with primary nasal disease may be presented to the veterinary surgeon with a variety of problems, ranging from acute respiratory distress to chronic long-standing disease. The presenting problems that should prompt a diagnostic investigation for nasal disease are listed in Figure 9.2.

Common indications

- Nasal discharge: unilateral/bilateral; mucoid/mucopurulent
- History of a foreign body

Other signs affecting the nares

- Sneezing/reverse sneezing
- Stertor (snoring/snorting)
- Stridor (inspiratory noise/wheezing)
- Epiphora, resulting from blockage of the nasolacrimal ducts
- Facial swelling or deformity
- Epistaxis

Other clinical signs

- Halitosis in the absence of dental disease
- Dental disease
- Exophthalmos
- Dysphagia
- Head shaking
- Pawing at the nose
- Rubbing the face on the ground

9.2 Indications for diagnostic investigation for nasal disease.

Clinical history

It is essential to take a careful history. A history of, for example, sniffing up a foreign body or clinical signs becoming apparent soon after walking through long grass may suggest a possible diagnosis. History taking should include careful questioning of the owner concerning:

- Duration of the clinical signs
- Age of the patient at the onset of clinical signs
- Whether the clinical signs are unilateral or bilateral
- Progression *versus* waxing and waning of the clinical signs
- Use of the animal (e.g. hunting, field work)
- Environmental exposure of the animal to toxins
- Travel history
- Trauma to the nose or surrounding structures
- Other concurrent illnesses.

Figure 9.3 summarizes the diagnostic significance of these factors.

Characteristic	Differential diagnoses and comments
Acute versus chronic onset	
Acute	Foreign body; trauma
Chronic	Neoplasia; fungal rhinitis; lymphoplasmacytic rhinitis (allergic or immune-mediated); trauma; foreign body; coagulopathy; hypertension; hyperadrenocorticism (rare)
Unilateral versus bilateral	
Unilateral	Neoplasia; foreign body; localized infection; tooth root infection; early aspergillosis
Bilateral	Lymphoplasmacytic rhinitis; infection (viral/bacterial); allergy; bronchial infection and coughing leading to secondary nasopharyngeal infection. Early unilateral infections (e.g. aspergillosis) or invasive neoplasia can progress from unilateral to bilateral if the infection/mass breaches the nasal septum. Toxic/irritant inhalation (e.g. smoke)
Age at onset	
Young (0–7 years)	Infection, trauma, allergy or foreign body more likely
Old (>7 years)	Neoplasia increasingly likely
Waxing and waning	Allergic (may be seasonal or geographical); intermittent exposure to toxins (e.g. smoke, dust)
Species/breed	
Cats	Cats are prone to grass foreign bodies sneezed forward over the soft palate. Oriental cats are more prone to sinusitis
Dogs	Dogs tend to sniff up foreign bodies. Dogs are more prone to aspergillosis. Dolichocephalic breeds: increased incidence of neoplasia. German Shepherd Dog: increased incidence of aspergillosis

9.3 Historical factors in cases of nasal disease and their diagnostic significance.

Clinical examination

Before undertaking any form of endoscopic or rhinoscopic examination, it is essential to perform a clinical examination and screening tests. The extent of this evaluation will vary depending on the individual case; however, a full clinical examination should be performed once a comprehensive history has been obtained.

There are a variety of reasons for considering rhinoscopy, including sneezing and reverse sneezing, nasal discharge, epistaxis, abnormal sounds and/or often some degree of airflow obstruction (see Figure 9.2). The physical examination should therefore include an assessment of nasal airflow and palpation of the palate and facial bones for pain, swelling or evidence of bony lysis.

Careful auscultation of the inspiratory and expiratory airflow from the nose may reveal the magnitude of any impairment of airflow and identify whether the pathology is unilateral or bilateral. A neonatal stethoscope is useful for listening to the airflow over the dorsum and lateral aspects of the nose and over the frontal sinuses. Some clinicians use a cold glass slide held close to the nares to demonstrate airflow: misting on the slide from the humid expired air indicates airflow from the nose. Manually closing each nostril in turn with the mouth held shut will elicit a response (sometimes violent) if one nostril is occluded by pathology and the contralateral nostril is occluded. Careful and delicate percussion of the rhinarium and sinuses may help to localize fluid and inspissated mucoid debris or even tissue masses.

A careful aural examination can identify evidence of inflammatory or infectious disease that has extended to, or arisen from, the middle or inner ear. On occasion, nasopharyngeal polyps can be identified on examination of the middle ear without having to embark on a full nasal examination.

Any evidence of epistaxis should lead the clinician to look carefully for evidence of coagulopathies, specifically those resulting from platelet dysfunction. Examination of the oral mucosa, ocular tissues and urogenital tissues for evidence of ecchymoses or petechiation may corroborate suspicions of a coagulopathy.

Dental disease is a common cause of secondary bacterial rhinitis and so a careful examination for periodontal disease is indicated. Dental examination and palpation of the gingival margins may also help to exclude oronasal fistulae associated with periodontal disease as the cause of epistaxis or nasal discharge. However, it should be borne in mind that occult dental disease and/or oronasal fistulae can be missed during the physical examination. If dental disease is suspected, a more comprehensive dental examination and dental radiography under general anaesthesia may be indicated (see later).

If the conscious patient will allow it, examination of the oropharynx can occasionally identify pathology at the level of the posterior nares. Occasionally, mass lesions that arise from the posterior nares can be found hanging over the caudal aspect of the soft palate.

A neurological examination should focus on detecting clinical signs of cerebral dysfunction such as weakness, decreased conscious proprioception and visual deficits, which may be associated with cryptococcosis.

Figure 9.4 summarizes the procedures to be performed as part of the clinical examination and the diagnostic significance of clinical findings.

A first presentation of bilateral nasal disease in a young and otherwise healthy pet is often managed with empirical use of antimicrobials. However, certain findings always suggest the need for further diagnostic investigations. Epistaxis, a consistently unilateral discharge, a unilateral nasal discharge that progresses to bilateral discharge, facial asymmetry, facial pain or a lack of response to previous rational therapy indicate the need for further investigation.

Procedure	Findings and diagnostic indications
Look for discharge	Serous: inflammatory; mucoid: chronic inflammation; mucopurulent: epistaxis
Look for epiphora	Mass or infection affecting nasolacrimal duct
Look for swellings or deformity; compare sides	Trauma; neoplasia; inflammation; invasive fungal rhinitis
Auscultate lungs, trachea and both sides of rhinarium	Lower airway disease; reduced airflow in one/both nares; stertor; stridor
Listen for airflow, particularly for discrepancies between nostrils. Place small twist of cotton wool in front of nares to assess airflow. Place a cold mirror or glass slide in front of nares and look for misting	Neoplasia; foreign body
Palpate eyes	Retrobulbar abscess; neoplasia
Palpate rhinarium for signs of pain/discomfort	Trauma; aspergillosis; neoplasia
Percuss sinuses and rhinarium	Space-occupying lesion: mass/fluid/fungal plaques
Examine the oral cavity, especially the palate and teeth	Dental disease; invasive neoplasia
Examine the ears for polyps or otitis media	Auropharyngeal polyps

9.4 Clinical examination of the animal with nasal disease.

Preoperative diagnostic investigations

Blood pressure measurement

Epistaxis may be a result of hypertension. This is especially the case in cats, where hypertension secondary to hyperthyroidism is not uncommon. Blood pressure measurement should be carried out in a calm and quiet environment and repeated several times to obtain a representative result. The underlying cause of hypertension should be investigated before rhinoscopy unless otherwise warranted. In cats, a serum thyroxine (T4) analysis may be useful to rule out hyperthyroidism as a contributory cause of hypertension.

Clinical pathology

Full haematology and serum biochemistry screens should be carried out before rhinoscopy. If epistaxis is a predominant clinical feature, it is essential to investigate the patient's primary and secondary clotting pathways. This is important not only to rule out clotting disorders as a primary cause of epistaxis, but also to alert the surgeon to the likelihood of certain complications arising during or after the rhinoscopy procedure. The nose is a highly vascular organ and some haemorrhage is to be expected during rhinoscopy, even in a normal patient. Clotting disorders may result in severe uncontrollable haemorrhage, and may need to be addressed before the procedure is performed. The assessment should include at least a platelet count and buccal mucosal bleeding time; if epistaxis is severe, the activated clotting time or prothrombin time and activated partial thromboplastin time

should be determined. In addition, a lungworm SNAP test (Angio Detect, IDEXX) should be considered for dogs in endemic areas that are not currently receiving monthly preventive treatment.

Adrenocortical function testing (adrenocorticotropic hormone stimulation test or dexamethasone suppression test) may be useful in cases where hyperadrenocorticism is suspected.

Microbiology

Bacterial culture of superficial nasal swabs typically yields only normal intranasal bacterial flora, owing to the large number of commensal organisms that reside in the nose. Most infections tend to be secondary and opportunistic; primary bacterial rhinitis is found only very rarely. The results of culture and antimicrobial susceptibility testing are therefore difficult to interpret, and these tests are not generally recommended. However, culture and sensitivity tests may be more useful for guiding therapy if a focal area of infection is found. In such a situation, swabs must be taken before rhinoscopy, as focal areas of infection may be washed away or contaminated during the procedure. Culture of nasal biopsy samples may be more representative in cases of deep mucosal infection, although this has not been definitively proven.

Aspergillus may be cultured from swabs taken from normal dogs, as it is ubiquitous in the environment; conversely, it may not be cultured from swabs from infected dogs, as it is not always shed in large numbers in exudates; false-positives and false-negatives are both common. Serological assays for aspergillosis can be useful, but testing a single sample is of limited value: the assay has 70% cross-reactivity with non-fungal disease (including neoplasia), which may produce a false-positive result, while failure of an infected animal to seroconvert may lead to a false-negative result. However, serology can corroborate other findings of the diagnostic investigation and may therefore be useful. A rising titre in paired serum samples is required to demonstrate *Aspergillus* infection with any certainty.

In cats, pharyngeal swabs for respiratory pathogens such as feline calicivirus (FCV), feline herpesvirus type 1 (FHV-1) and *Chlamydia* may be useful; these agents are common causes of chronic rhinitis. Virus isolation and nucleic acid amplification techniques are often used to identify the presence of FHV-1 and FCV. Polymerase chain reaction (PCR) assays for FHV-1 and reverse transcriptase-PCR assays for FCV are commercially available. However, none of the PCR assays has been shown to distinguish between wild-type virus and vaccine virus, meaning that cats that have been vaccinated against these pathogens may well give false-positive results. In addition, test sensitivity (i.e. limits and rates of detection) varies greatly between tests and between laboratories. Furthermore, these infectious agents can be detected in healthy cats as well as clinically ill cats; thus, the positive predictive value of these tests is low and their diagnostic value is questionable in cats with chronic nasal disease.

If cryptococcosis is suspected on the basis of the clinical findings, especially in cats, then samples of nasal secretions should be obtained for cytology and cryptococcal antigen latex agglutination testing. This is of particular importance in patients residing in geographical locations where *Cryptococcus* is endemic.

Full details of testing methodology can be found in the *BSAVA Manual of Canine and Feline Clinical Pathology*.

Intraoperative diagnostic investigations

Further diagnostic investigations can be performed with the patient under general anaesthesia, before rhinoscopy.

Diagnostic imaging

Diagnostic imaging can reveal: increased density in the nasal cavity or bony lysis that may suggest a neoplastic process; turbinate bone destruction consistent with chronic rhinosinusitis or fungal disease; radiopaque foreign objects (e.g. air gun pellets); and tooth root abscessation. Radiography or advanced imaging techniques should ideally always be carried out before rhinoscopy. Once the nasal cavity has been flushed with saline, and the turbinates have been partially obscured with blood clots from intraoperative haemorrhage (which is almost inevitable during rhinoscopy), effective diagnostic radiography will not be possible for a few days.

Radiography

Radiography is extremely useful for assessing the location, extent and possible cause of disease (Figure 9.5). Several views should be taken as a matter of routine:

- Intraoral dorsoventral occlusal (Figure 9.6)
- Ventrodorsal open mouth to assess the cribriform plate
- Rostrocaudal skyline sinus view of the frontal sinuses and tympanic bullae (Figure 9.7)
- Lateral.

Radiographic finding	Possible causes
Dogs	
Loss of trabecular pattern (ethmoturbinates/maxillary)	Fungal infection; neoplasia; trauma
Increased soft tissue density:	
• Maxilla	Neoplasia; foreign body; blood clot; mucus
• Sinus	Mucus; neoplasia; fungal plaque
Lucency	Fungal rhinitis
Septal deviation	Neoplasia
Tympanic bulla opacity	Polyp; infection
Cats	
Unilateral lucency	Neoplasia
Bilateral lucency	Chronic rhinitis

9.5 Common radiographic findings and their significance.

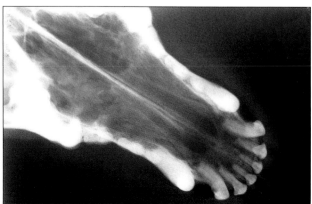

9.6 Intraoral radiograph showing soft tissue opacity in the right caudal nasal cavity of a dog.

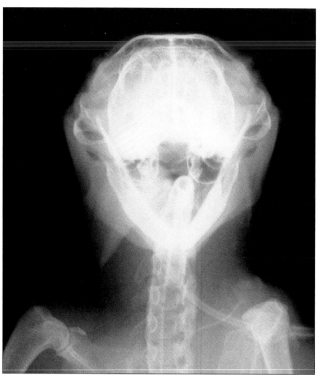

9.7 Radiographic skyline view of the tympanic bullae and frontal sinuses in a cat.

If dental disease is suspected, high-detail dental radiographs or oblique lateral views should also be taken (see Dental examination, below).

Patient positioning for radiography is very important in order to eliminate superimposition of the nasal cavity and frontal sinuses with other structures. Lateral radiographs are frequently unrewarding when assessing animals with unilateral lesions confined to the nasal cavity because superimposition of the normal half of the skull on the abnormal half tends to mask the abnormalities. Lateral radiographs are more useful for the identification of lesions extending through the nasal or frontal bones or the cribriform plate. They are also useful for identifying lesions in the nasopharynx, such as polyps.

It can be difficult to interpret radiographs of the feline nasal cavity. This was highlighted in a study that found that some radiographs of cats with non-nasal disease were erroneously interpreted as showing signs of intranasal disease. This probably occurred because lesions affecting adjacent structures were superimposed on the nasal cavity in one or more of the radiographs evaluated for each cat. Radiography may also be less useful as a means of distinguishing rhinitis from nasal neoplasia in cats than it is in dogs.

Thoracic radiography is used to look for disseminated infectious or neoplastic disease within the pulmonary parenchyma and pleural space (see the *BSAVA Manual of Canine and Feline Thoracic Imaging*).

Advanced imaging

Computed tomography (CT) or magnetic resonance imaging (MRI) are very valuable for examination of the nasal passages (Saunders *et al.*, 2004; Lefebvre *et al.*, 2005). The high level of detail and the ability to localize pathology provided by these modalities can be of tremendous benefit. Limiting factors for both CT and MRI are often their availability and timely access, although veterinary-specific CT and MRI are rapidly becoming more common in both private clinical practice and veterinary teaching hospitals. CT and MRI can be helpful in differentiating neoplasia from infection, and both techniques provide a more precise image of the limits of a mass than radiography, which may help in planning surgical debulking and/or radiotherapy. The ability to take multiple images at regular spacing and in different planes allows a virtual three-dimensional image of the area to be built up, providing further valuable information.

Dental examination

Dental disease is common in dogs and cats and can often be the cause of, be confused with, or contribute to nasal pathology. The deep dorsal recesses of the upper arcade of tooth roots abut the ventral surface of the hard palate and are thus closely associated anatomically with the ventral meatus of the nasal cavity. The intervening bone and mucosa are easily breached by trauma or infection. Periodontal disease, resulting in the resorption of alveolar bone and progressive deepening of periodontal pockets, may lead to communication with the nasal cavity or maxillary sinus. Endodontic disease may lead to lysis of the periapical bone at the tooth root and can be associated with rhinitis.

A full dental examination can be only carried out under general anaesthesia. Visual evidence of fractured maxillary teeth with pulp exposure, exposed dentine, tooth discoloration, shifts in dentition, excessive calculus or periodontal pockets >0.5 mm in depth could suggest periapical root abscessation, an oronasal fistula or neoplasia. The periodontal pockets of each tooth should be explored with a suitable dental probe to assess their depth and to look for evidence of infection, which may have tracked into the nasal cavity. Any haemorrhage should be noted. If probing provokes ipsilateral epistaxis, this confirms the presence of an oronasal fistula although lack of haemorrhage does not rule out a fistula. In cases where dental involvement is suspected to be contributing to the signs of nasal disease, dental radiography should be undertaken using intraoral films and a bisecting angle technique. The apical areas of the tooth roots should be evaluated carefully for evidence of infection, and particular attention should be paid to teeth 104 and 204 (the upper canine teeth). Further details can be found in the *BSAVA Manual of Canine and Feline Dentistry and Oral Surgery*.

Detailed oropharyngeal examination

Examination of the pharynx and larynx may reveal the presence of trauma, neoplasia, nasopharyngeal stenosis or foreign bodies. Enlargement of the tonsils (Figure 9.8) is common in animals with chronic disease. Discharge may be seen passing back from the nose into the oropharynx, whereas it may not be obvious at the nares. Examination and digital palpation of the hard and soft palate may reveal masses either on the surface or palpable through the soft tissues of the soft palate. A spay hook can be used to pull the free edge of the soft palate rostrally (or stay sutures can be placed on the caudal edge of soft palate to assist with rostral retraction), to enable a limited examination of the nasopharynx for foreign bodies or neoplasia.

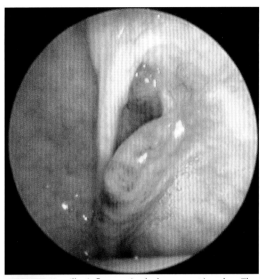

9.8 Tonsillar inflammation/enlargement in a dog. The tonsils can be examined in detail with a rigid endoscope. The tonsillar crypt should be explored with forceps under direct visualization to exclude foreign bodies.

Instrumentation

A full discussion of endoscopic equipment and its care is provided in Chapter 2. Figure 9.9 lists the equipment required for rhinoscopy; specific considerations for different procedures are discussed later, in the relevant sections. An endoscopic video camera is essential for performing any operative or sterile work. Some endoscopists do prefer to look through the eyepiece of the endoscope, but the field is commonly obscured by fluid and blood and is difficult to see without the enlargement the camera affords.

- Camera and monitor
- Xenon, metal halide or LED light source
- 3.5–8 mm flexible endoscope (depending on patient size)
- Fibreoptic light guide cable
- (Dental mirror)
- 2.7 mm, 18 cm HOPKINS® 30-degree endoscope
- 14.5 Fr cystoscopy sheath with 5 Fr instrument channel
- 5 Fr 40 cm biopsy forceps
- 5 Fr 40 cm grasping forceps
- (High-flow arthroscopy sheath for 2.7 mm endoscope)
- 9.5 Fr operating endoscope with 3 Fr instrument channel
- 3 Fr 40 cm biopsy forceps
- 3 Fr 40 cm grasping forceps
- 3 mm cup biopsy forceps
- 'CellSafe' biopsy sample capsules
- Giving set
- Normal saline (1 litre+)

9.9 Equipment required for rhinoscopy. Items in parentheses are not essential but may be useful.

WARNING

Endoscopes sold as 'autoclavable' are designed for the autoclaves used in human hospitals, with a slow heat and cooling cycle. Most veterinary autoclaves heat up and cool down too quickly and will reduce the life of these endoscopes considerably. It is not advisable to autoclave endoscopes in veterinary practice

Premedication and anaesthesia

Rhinoscopy can only be performed with the patient under general anaesthesia. Standard preparation for general anaesthesia should be undertaken, including withholding food for 6–12 hours, depending on the age of the patient, before the procedure. A catheter is placed for administration of intravenous fluids and to provide venous access if needed. The anaesthetic protocols chosen should be those that are standard to the practice given the clinical scenario, although premedication with acepromazine helps to lower the patient's blood pressure and reduce haemorrhage, as well as provide a calm recovery. A combination of 0.02 mg/kg acepromazine and either 0.1 mg/kg butorphanol or 10 μg/kg buprenorphine, administered by intravenous or intramuscular injection, is commonly used. Anticholinergics, such as atropine or glycopyrrolate, may be used as appropriate to counteract bradycardia induced by opioid premedication or the procedure itself.

Rhinoscopic examination

It is good practice to examine the nasopharynx and choanae by using a caudal (posterior) approach before performing rostral (anterior) rhinoscopy. Caudal rhinoscopy is usually performed 'per os' by retroflexing a flexible endoscope over the free edge of the soft palate, in order to look forwards, towards the choanae. This procedure does not require fluid irrigation, and so swabs and samples can be obtained for culture if required, as well as biopsy samples of nasopharyngeal and caudal nasal masses. It may also be pertinent to perform a bronchoscopic examination if tracheal or lower airway disease is suspected (see Chapter 7). Following examination of the nasopharynx (and bronchi), the airway is sealed with a well fitting cuffed endotracheal tube, the seal is tested and anterior rhinoscopy is then performed under saline irrigation to complete the examination.

Caudal rhinoscopy

Caudal (retropharyngeal posterior) rhinoscopy is ideal for direct examination of the retropharynx and posterior nasal cavity. It is particularly useful for obtaining diagnostic tissue samples and for managing and reassessing the progress of problems over time. It is essential to understand the normal anatomy (Figure 9.10) and be able to distinguish normal from abnormal findings.

Caudal rhinoscopy is always performed before anterior (rostral) rhinoscopy because contamination of the nasopharynx with fluid, blood and discharge resulting from the fluid irrigation used during anterior rhinoscopy would otherwise compromise the examination.

Instrumentation

A small flexible endoscope is required to view the nasopharynx and choanae via the caudal approach. The endoscope must be capable of 180 degrees of flexion. A 3.5 mm diameter flexible bronchoscope is ideal for cats and small dogs, although a larger endoscope, such as a gastroscope, may be used in most dogs.

If a flexible endoscope is not available, a dental mirror can be used in conjunction with a light source and a spay hook to pull the soft palate forward and allow a view over the soft palate towards the choanae. This is not really feasible in cats and gives a limited view in large dogs, but is better than nothing. However, it does not allow biopsy sampling or the passing of instruments into the nasopharynx. The soft palate can sometimes be pulled forward sufficiently with a blunt spay hook to reveal a foreign body and allow its removal (see later), but this does not obviate the need to examine the caudal nares properly.

Alternatively, if available, a rigid endoscope with a 270-degree viewing angle can be inserted into the oral cavity beyond the edge of the soft palate to assess the nasopharynx.

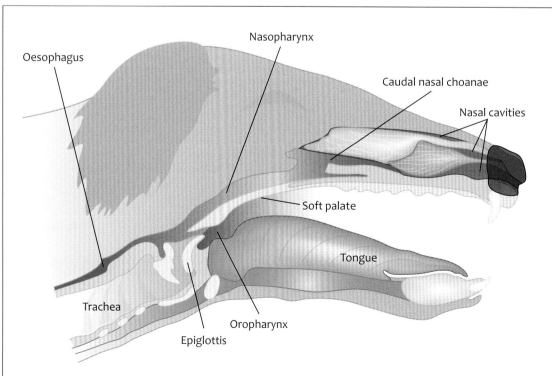

9.10

Anatomy of the retropharynx and posterior nasal cavity.

Oesophagus

Nasopharynx

Caudal nasal choanae

Nasal cavities

Soft palate

Tongue

Trachea

Oropharynx

Epiglottis

Patient preparation and positioning

Caudal rhinoscopy is commonly performed with the patient in sternal recumbency, although some authors advocate positioning in lateral recumbency. The head is propped up slightly with towels to elevate the mouth and nasal planum for easy access. A cuffed endotracheal tube should be placed and checked to ensure an adequate seal to protect the airway from haemorrhage or discharge. The caudal pharynx can be additionally sealed with gauze sponges or cut squares of feminine hygiene products (see later). A mouth gag is essential to keep the mouth open and prevent the patient biting down on to the endoscope in the event of contact with the pharynx stimulating a gag reflex.

The patient's blood pressure should be monitored carefully during rhinoscopy. Caution should be exercised when performing rhinoscopy in patients that are not normotensive or cardiovascularly stable.

Procedure

The flexible endoscope is inserted into the mouth and the oral cavity, laryngeal apparatus and posterior nasopharynx are evaluated. The tip of the insertion tube is advanced towards the larynx so that the free edge of the soft palate is passed, and the endoscope is retroflexed into a 'J' position behind the soft palate to view the nasopharynx (Figure 9.11a). It is also possible to pre-flex the endoscope into the 'J' position before pushing it past the free edge of the soft palate. However, in the author's [PL] experience, passing a non-flexed bronchoscope to the caudal edge of the soft palate and then making a quick downward deflection of the lever (to move the tip upwards) will often eliminate the reflex reverse sneezing that can occur with the flexed manoeuvre. The insertion tube is then gradually withdrawn rostrally, with the tip still flexed, to advance the tip towards the choanae (Figure 9.11b). The tip of the endoscope can easily be viewed by transillumination through the soft palate. Because the endoscope is retroflexed, the view seen on the monitor is upside down and the left and right sides are reversed (Figure 9.12).

There is often a strong gag reflex present during this procedure, which can make manoeuvring frustrating and difficult. This is normal and does not necessarily mean that the patient is not anaesthetized deeply enough. Topical lidocaine sprayed on to the mucosal surfaces may help to

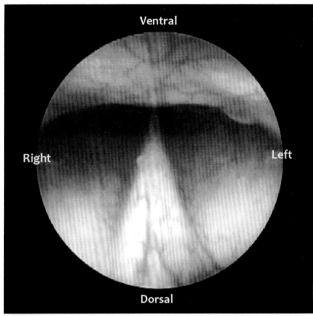

9.12 Normal retroflexed view of the caudal nasal choanae and retropharynx.
(Courtesy of RC Denovo)

blunt this reflex, but should not be expected to abolish it. In addition, bleeding is not uncommon due to the minor trauma caused by the endoscope. If bleeding is expected, for example if biopsy samples are to be taken, it is recommended that gauze be placed in the caudal pharynx to collect the blood.

Normal appearance

During evaluation of the retropharynx, it should be possible to visualize (Figure 9.13):

- The free edge of the soft palate
- The soft palate
- The mucosa of the dorsal nasopharyngeal wall
- The openings of the Eustachian tubes
- The choanae
- The nasal septum
- A number of the turbinates in the posterior nasal cavity.

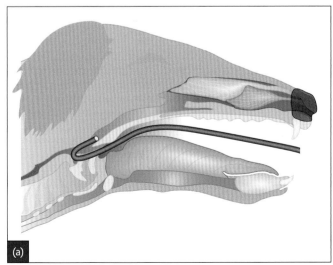
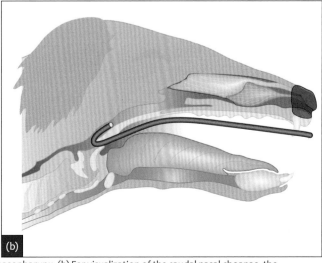

9.11 (a) Use of an endoscope in the retroflexed 'J' position to view the nasopharynx. (b) For visualization of the caudal nasal choanae, the endoscope must be advanced by pulling it towards the endoscopist while keeping it retroflexed.

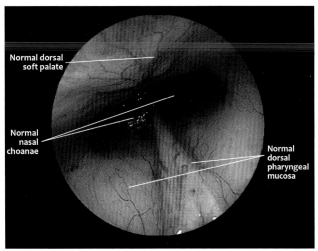

9.13 Normal endoscopic appearance of the dorsal soft palate, the nasal choanae and the dorsal pharyngeal mucosa.
(Courtesy of D Levitan)

Healthy pharyngeal, palatal and retropharyngeal tissue is usually smooth and pink, while diseased tissue is often hyperaemic, irregular or friable or has obvious masses or nodular changes. There should be no obvious discharge from the choanae in the normal animal. A haemorrhagic or mucopurulent posterior nasal discharge can sometimes be seen, even in the absence of discharge from the anterior nares (Figure 9.14), and is always pathological. Raised nodules of benign lymphoid hyperplasia (Figure 9.15) are quite commonly seen if the animal has been sneezing for a prolonged period or if there has been a nidus of chronic inflammation.

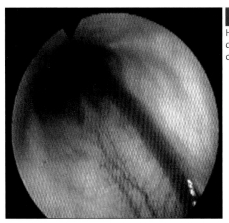

9.14 Haemorrhagic discharge from the choanae.

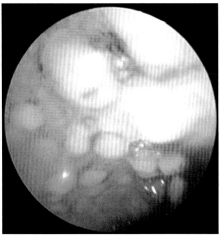

9.15 Nasopharyngeal lymphoid hyperplasia in a Siamese cat. This is commonly found as the result of chronic inflammation.

Biopsy and other sampling

Biopsy samples should be taken from any mass or abnormal tissue. If there are concerns about turbinate bone osteomyelitis, a biopsy sample can be submitted for histopathology following culture and sensitivity testing. Brushings and swabs can also be taken for cytology or culture. Swabs or samples for culture from the nasopharynx, choanae and nares must all be taken before embarking on anterior rhinoscopy, since the fluid irrigation used during that procedure is likely to contaminate the field and wash away debris and infected material.

Biopsy samples can be obtained under direct visualization with the endoscope. It is important to remember that the endoscope should be removed from the patient and the cytology brush or biopsy or grasping forceps introduced via the instrument channel while the tip of the insertion tube is straight. The instrument should be advanced until it is just at the tip of the insertion tube before retroflexing the endoscope tip and taking the sample. Forcing an instrument through an endoscope tip in the 180-degree flexed position, either to insert or withdraw it, may cause expensive and often irreparable damage to the endoscope.

Other methods occasionally used to obtain biopsy samples include aggressive flushing techniques, which may be especially useful for retropharyngeal lesions. An open-ended catheter, Foley catheter or feeding tube is advanced retrograde via the nares to the mass, and sterile saline is flushed manually through the catheter with a syringe under high pressure. Depending on the size of the patient, 10–30 ml of fluid may be instilled per flush. Any tissue dislodged by flushing can be retrieved from the gauze used to pack the pharynx, the nares or the oral cavity.

Foreign body removal

Most foreign bodies can be removed rhinoscopically. Foreign body retrieval from the nasopharynx may be accomplished with a variety of forceps that are designed to fit through the instrument channel of the endoscope. In some cases, nasal or nasopharyngeal foreign material is best removed by flushing as described above for diagnostic sampling, or, in cats, by placing a pharyngeal gauze swab and pushing the foreign material in a rostral to caudal direction, using continuous saline irrigation, directly on to the swab. Blades of grass that have passed rostrally over the soft palate may be difficult to remove via the pharynx due to the directional nature of the barbs on the leaf. In these cases, it is often better to remove the leaf via anterior rhinoscopy to prevent fragments breaking off and being left behind.

Rigid endoscopy via lateral pharyngotomy

In some cases, nasal masses at or near the choanae can be better examined and treated using a rigid endoscope introduced via a pharyngotomy incision. A small incision is made in the lateral pharyngeal pouch in the same manner as is used when introducing a pharyngostomy feeding tube. A 2.7 mm endoscope in a cystoscopy sheath can then be introduced in a rostral direction, giving excellent direct access to the area dorsal to the soft palate.

Anterior (rostral) rhinoscopy

Instrumentation

Small-diameter flexible endoscopes with two-way deflection can be used for anterior rhinoscopy and have the advantage of being relatively easy to manipulate into small crevices. In some medium-sized to large dogs this will allow access to the frontal sinuses. However, the small instrument channel and inability to irrigate effectively makes flexible rhinoscopy ineffective for routine examinations. A rigid 2.7 mm, 30-degree endoscope with a cystoscopy sheath can be used for anterior rhinoscopy in almost all dogs and in most cats. The oval cross-section of the cystoscope allows it to be easily and non-traumatically introduced into the nasal meatuses, and this instrument provides for excellent irrigation and has an integral instrument channel.

For small cats and kittens, a 9.5 Fr operating telescope with a 3 Fr instrument channel may be used. This is essentially a 1.9 mm, 30-degree multi-procedure rigid (MPR) endoscope fused permanently into a cystoscopy sheath. Suitable 3 Fr instrumentation is available for the integrated instrument channel. Another solution is to use a 2.7 mm endoscope with an arthroscopy sheath. This sheath is round in cross-section and smaller than the cystoscopy sheath, and so can be used in smaller cats and dogs. The disadvantage of both the 2.7 mm and 1.9 mm MPR endoscope sheaths is that they have only a very small instrument channel, or none at all; this means that instruments must often be passed alongside the sheath in order to take representative biopsy samples and perform other procedures or remove large foreign bodies.

The disadvantages of flexible endoscopes are their poor light transmission and image quality, coupled with the very small channel diameter, which makes diagnostic sampling or debridement difficult and often non-diagnostic. It is difficult to flush sufficient saline down the instrument channel to clear discharge and haemorrhage, especially when additional diagnostic or therapeutic instrumentation is in place, so visualization is easily compromised. Rigid endoscopes provide a considerably better view and allow the use of larger instrumentation, enabling the surgeon to obtain larger biopsy samples that provide a much better diagnostic yield. The authors recommend the use of rigid endoscopes for nearly all rhinoscopic procedures.

Patient preparation and positioning

It is preferable to place the patient in sternal recumbency as this position reduces the chance of one side of the nose being contaminated by detritus from the other, and the patient is in a more natural position in relation to the image on the monitor (Figure 9.16). The operator must be aware that they will be flushing with a lot of fluid during the procedure and there is likely to be some haemorrhage. If the patient is placed in lateral recumbency, the lower of the two nares will become filled with detritus (i.e. contaminated) from the upper one as it is examined; the lower one

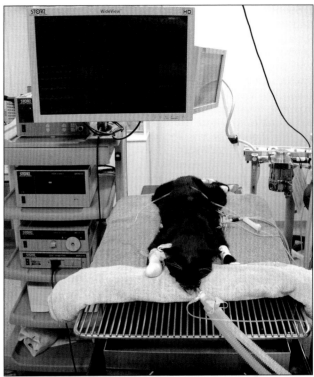

9.16 Theatre set-up for rhinoscopy. The patient is in ventral recumbency on a gridded table with the chin resting on a rolled-up towel. The monitor is positioned at the caudal end of the patient, directly opposite the endoscopist.

should therefore be assessed first to ensure an adequate examination. If there is copious discharge from one nostril, placing that side down will prevent discharge from flowing into the less affected side before the surgeon has had a chance to examine it.

The patient's head is propped up with towels to elevate the nasal planum for easy access. Care should be taken not to elevate the nose too much in an attempt to limit the amount of excess irrigant fluid accumulating around the endotracheal tube cuff.

The procedure is best carried out on a wet table due to the large volumes of irrigant fluid used. A large tray covered with a stainless steel grid will suffice if a wet table is not available, and will also save a lot of mopping up. Towels placed on the floor are also useful to catch additional spillage. Irrigation is usually provided with bags of 0.9% saline fitted with standard giving sets. It is best to avoid performing rhinoscopy in the sterile operating theatre because of the risk of contamination of surfaces with non-sterile irrigant fluid and nasal discharge.

Procedure

Having examined the nasopharynx in detail, as described above, it is important to ensure that the endotracheal tube is well cuffed and forms a good seal with the trachea. This is best done by gently applying pressure to the rebreathing bag as the cuff is inflated and listening for leakage around the endotracheal tube, with the aim of inflating until a good seal is achieved without undue pressure on the tracheal mucosa from the cuff. Large volumes of irrigant fluid will be washed over the soft palate and there will be a continuous flow of fluid through the nostril and out of the mouth, so it is important that the airway is well protected. A gauze swab or a pad may be placed over the larynx to protect the airway from solid debris and clots, being careful not to occlude the pharynx completely. Feminine hygiene products can also be used for this purpose: their high degree of absorbency, small size and low profile are ideal. A single thin mini-pad is cut in half and a slit is made in the centre; this slit is positioned around the endotracheal tube. With larger patients, additional pads can be placed in the caudal pharynx as needed to provide additional absorbency. An assistant should be charged with the task of counting how many pads were placed, to ensure that they are all retrieved before extubation.

The monitor is positioned at about the level of the animal's pelvis with the monitor facing cranially (see Figure 9.16). Using aseptic technique, the endoscope, light guide cable, cannula/sheath and camera are assembled. (See Chapter 2 for details of instrument sterilization procedures.) A bag of sterile saline is hung and connected to one of the stopcocks of the cannula (for a right-handed operator, the right stopcock is used so that it can be operated with the right index finger); 3 litre bags, as used in large animal practice, are preferred to avoid constantly changing bags. The flow of saline is best adjusted with the tap on the ingress port of the rhinoscope, so the normal controls on the giving set can be left open. The shaft of the cannula is coated with sterile water-soluble lubricating jelly, being careful not to get any on the lens of the endoscope.

The endoscope is held in 'pistol' fashion, with the light guide cable and connector facing towards the floor and the camera oriented such that any graphics on the camera head can be read upright. This will ensure that the image produced on the monitor is true.

Rostral rhinoscopy may be carried out directly, viewing the mucosa in air, or under vigorous saline irrigation. Often, the presence of copious discharge or haemorrhage (iatrogenic or otherwise) obscures the view and is difficult to remove with suction. In the majority of cases the procedure is carried out under saline irrigation, as this washes away any debris or haemorrhage and allows a clear view of the mucosa. However, when viewing a relatively large cavity, such as in the presence of extensive turbinate damage in animals with aspergillosis, or when entering the nasopharynx, turbulence in the saline flow can obscure the view. In these situations, turning off the saline flow and reverting to direct viewing through air may greatly improve visualization. It should be noted that the use of saline irrigation, especially if the saline is cold, tends to blanch the mucosa somewhat, so the normal appearance in air will be different from that under irrigation. The nasal cavity is richly supplied with blood vessels and is an ideal heat-exchange mechanism. Persistent flushing of the nasal cavity with cold saline can significantly reduce the core body temperature of smaller patients (e.g. cats) under general anaesthesia, and so core temperature should be monitored if the procedure is at all prolonged.

Beginning with the normal or less affected side (as determined by preoperative radiographs and clinical signs), the nasal planum is deflected dorsally and the endoscope is introduced into the nostril. Fluid flow is started. The dorsal meatus is examined first and is clearly seen as a simple vaulted channel that narrows as the endoscope is advanced towards the ethmoidal area. It is not possible to pass the endoscope as far back as the cribriform plate, although this area can be visualized. The endoscope is withdrawn slightly into the common meatus and the middle meatus will be seen laterally. The endoscope is moved up and laterally into the middle meatus, which can be examined caudally to the area of the opening of the frontal sinuses, which is usually obscured by scrolls of turbinates. The ventral meatus is examined last (Figure 9.17). The tip of the endoscope is withdrawn nearly to the nasal planum and redirected

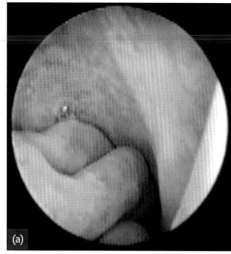
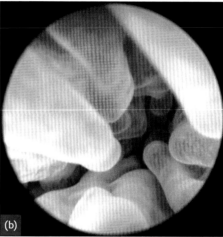

9.17 Normal ventral meatus. (a) Cat. (b) Dog: note the smooth pink turbinates, which appear to almost interdigitate.

(a)

(b)

ventrally into the ventral meatus. When using a 30-degree viewing endoscope, care should be taken to ensure the lumen remains at the bottom of the image on the monitor (see below) to prevent trauma to the floor of the ventral meatus, resulting in haemorrhage. It should be possible to pass the endoscope to the level of the posterior nares and nasopharynx. On entering the nasopharynx, just caudal to the posterior nares, the opening of the Eustachian tube can be seen on the lateral wall (Figure 9.18). Rotating the light guide post from side to side will enable the operator to see both Eustachian tube openings.

The mucous membrane should be uniform and pink/red in colour with no obvious nasal discharge. If thick mucus is present (Figure 9.19) and hampers the view, it may be preferable to remove the endoscope and forcefully flush the nose several times with saline from a 60 ml catheter-tipped syringe before reintroducing the endoscope. Alternatively, attaching a 20 ml or 60 ml syringe of saline to the free port on the rhinoscope sheath will allow a forced jet of saline to be directed more accurately. It is important to close the other ports first or the saline will be directed back up into the bag or, worse, through the instrument port into the endoscopist's face!

Haemorrhage occurring with little or no trauma from the endoscope may be an indication of inflammation. In cases where inflammation is a feature, the meatuses are narrowed due to mucosal congestion. Destructive rhinitis due to bacterial or fungal infection leads to open, enlarged airways and may allow visualization of the duct into the frontal sinuses. Ulcerative lesions (Figure 9.20) should be noted as the endoscope is advanced for the first time, to avoid confusion with any iatrogenic damage.

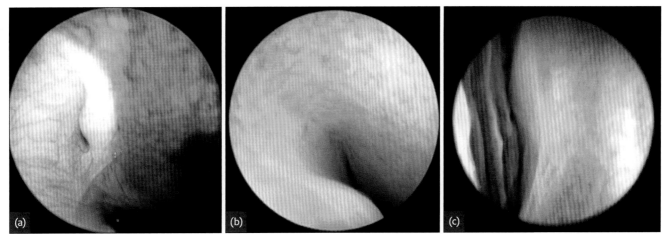

9.18 (a) Normal Eustachian tube opening in a dog. (b) Normal dorsal meatus in a dog. Note the smooth vaulted appearance. (c) Normal ethmoid turbinates in a dog. Note the corrugated appearance of the turbinates on the left compared with the nasal septum on the right.

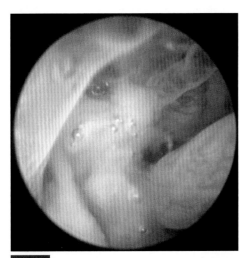

9.19 Mucus in the anterior nares is always abnormal.

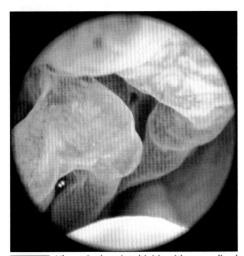

9.20 Ulcerative/erosive rhinitis with generalized swelling and erythema of the turbinates. Multiple small erosions are evident and bleed easily on contact.

The endoscope should be handled carefully to avoid causing trauma to the patient. The nasal mucosa and turbinate bones are very delicate, and careful control of the endoscope tip is essential. For a right-handed endoscopist, the left hand is placed flat on the bridge of the nose, with the shaft of the endoscope held between the forefinger and thumb at the nostril. The camera is held in the right hand and controls the angle of insertion, while the left hand stabilizes the tip of the endoscope and prevents exaggerated movements. In this way, a controlled examination can be performed with minimal trauma. It must be remembered that the 30-degree angle of view of the endoscope is directed away from the light guide post. When passing the endoscope down the narrow meatuses with the light guide post hanging down, the lumen of the meatus should be at the bottom of the image on the video monitor. If the lumen is kept central in the image, then the endoscope will be directed into the ventral surface of the meatus, causing unnecessary trauma and haemorrhage.

A thorough examination must be completed before biopsy samples are taken. Once the biopsy procedures are initiated, haemorrhage will be much more profuse and will greatly obscure the view and increase observational artefact. Many authors and practitioners have suggested techniques to reduce these problems associated with bleeding, but they have all been of limited value. These techniques include using very cold (refrigerated) saline for irrigation and adding a dilute solution of adrenaline (epinephrine) to the irrigant, all in an effort to produce vasoconstriction.

Recently, an attempt has been made to develop techniques for performing 'dry' rhinoscopy. With these techniques, fluid irrigation is used in a very limited fashion. An endoscopic air pump is connected to one port on the endoscope sheath and puffs of air under low pressure are used to blow haemorrhage, fluid and other nasal detritus from the visual field. While dry rhinoscopy requires some delicacy and experience to perfect the technique, it has the advantage of reduced postoperative epistaxis, which in turn minimizes the risk of aspiration of the irrigation fluid and nasal material. In addition, air insufflation appears to provide a more 'true' appearance of the nasal structures than that provided by endoscopy under irrigation. At the time of writing, further evaluation of this technique is in progress.

WARNING

Care should be exercised if using cold irrigant solutions, especially in small patients. The high surface area and excellent vascular supply of the nose act like a heat sink, and hypothermia can result if the procedure is prolonged. Careful monitoring of the patient's core body temperature is advisable

Biopsy

Once a full initial exploration has been made, areas of pathology are returned to and biopsy samples are taken. It is important to take samples from multiple sites, as diagnosis is frequently based on histopathology and there is little correlation between the visual appearance of the mucosa and specific disease entities (Johnson *et al.*, 2004). Inflamed mucosae have a similar appearance with a wide range of underlying pathology. Even normal nasal mucosa will bleed profusely, and the appearance of the haemorrhage will be greatly magnified by the camera. Aggressive irrigation during biopsy is imperative and, while all nasal mucosa is delicate and tends towards haemorrhage, note should be taken of any tissue that seems to bleed particularly easily.

Biopsy samples can be taken from apparently normal and altered nasal mucosa and any polyps or masses at this time. The operator can use either flexible cup biopsy forceps that are introduced via the instrument channel or larger rigid biopsy forceps with a 3 mm cup passed alongside the shaft of the endoscope. Because of the highly reactive nature of nasal mucosa, it is advisable to take repeated samples and to be somewhat aggressive in sample taking in order to obtain deeper tissue samples. It is not unusual for histopathological evaluation of superficial tissues to reveal only inflammation, while deeper samples reveal more problematic pathology. It is often helpful to take several samples at the same spot, sampling progressively deeper tissues, to try to ensure that a diagnostic sample has been achieved.

Biopsy forceps designed to pass through the instrument channel of the endoscope may be too small to get a representative sample from deeper tissues. In these cases, 3 mm clamshell biopsy forceps with a small-diameter shaft can be used alongside the endoscope. The biopsy forceps are first held alongside the endoscope sheath to align the hinge of the forceps with a prominent point on the sheath when the tips of the biopsy forceps are level with the tip of the endoscope. In this way, it is possible to estimate when the biopsy forceps should be coming into view, to avoid pushing them too deep. The endoscope is then inserted to the point of interest and the forceps are 'walked' along the top of the endoscope until they come into view. It is important to pass the biopsy forceps along the top edge of the rhinoscope and in contact with it. Since a 30-degree endoscope looks upwards, if the forceps are passed along the side or bottom of the endoscope they will be easily missed and may be inadvertently passed far beyond the tip of the endoscope, increasing the likelihood of causing iatrogenic damage. It is relatively easy to pass the forceps along the other side of a turbinate from the endoscope and fail to visualize it. If this is the case, the forceps can be removed and the procedure tried again.

In smaller patients where it is not possible to pass the forceps alongside the endoscope sheath, it is useful to measure the position of the lesion by assessing the direction and depth of the tip of the endoscope, and then take samples 'blind'. Markings on the endoscope sheath allow a measurement of depth to be made, and the tip of the endoscope can often be seen by transillumination through the rhinarium if the lighting in the room is kept low. A pair of 3–5 mm biopsy forceps (depending on patient size) can then be placed to the same pre-measured depth and direction, to obtain a large sample. When using this technique, it is very important to ensure that the tips of the biopsy forceps do not pass beyond the level of the medial canthus of the eyes. Measuring this distance on the outside of the rhinarium and marking it with a piece of sticky tape on the forceps themselves will prevent inadvertent penetration of the cribriform plate and potential subsequent trauma to the frontal lobes of the brain.

Tissue specimens that contain spicules of turbinate bone are demonstrative of an aggressive biopsy technique, which is necessary if sufficiently deep diagnostic samples are to be obtained. Samples should be carefully placed in foam-lined tissue cassettes and sent for evaluation by veterinary pathologists experienced in the processing and evaluation of endoscopic samples. Biopsy samples obtained through the channel of the endoscope are necessarily small, and can get lost in a large pot of preserving fluid or be overlooked by the histopathologist. 'CellSafe'-type biopsy capsules (Figure 9.21), available from laboratories, are ideal for biopsy samples collected endoscopically. The specimens are placed in the capsules, which are then clipped shut before being placed in preservative fluid for transport to the laboratory. The capsules consist of two interlocking plastic frames, which can be clipped together in two different ways, one giving a larger space than the other, in order to cater for samples of different sizes. The samples are fixed and prepared in the capsules at the laboratory, so there is little danger of any specimens going astray. Larger samples should be left free-floating and not placed in these capsules as they may be crushed, creating compression artefacts. If the sample recovery process has been relatively atraumatic and sterile, a sample of mucosa can be sent in sterile fashion for bacterial culture and sensitivity testing. However, interpretation must be made cautiously, as even the best technique rarely maintains complete sterility in this anatomical locale.

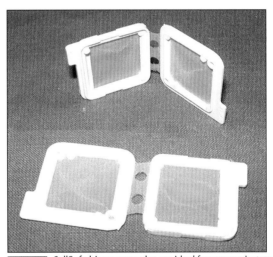

9.21 CellSafe biopsy capsules are ideal for preserving small biopsy samples collected endoscopically.

Frontal sinus exploration

If the diagnostic investigations before rhinoscopy – in particular, CT, MRI or radiography (frontal sinus skyline view) – indicate that the frontal sinus is diseased, it is prudent to examine it endoscopically. A 3 cm x 3 cm square area at the level of the top of the orbit, just medial to the bony prominence, is clipped and aseptically prepared. An incision just large enough to accommodate the rhinoscope (approximately 10–12 mm) is made. A 6–8 mm hole is then drilled halfway between the midline and the zygomatic process of the frontal bone, using a Steinmann pin and

Jacobs chuck, a Hall-type air drill or a Michel trephine (Figure 9.22). Care must be taken to avoid going too far into the sinus; the sinus cavity can be deceptively small and the wall on the far side of the sinus separates the sinus from the calvarium. If too much pressure is applied to the Steinmann pin or drill, it is possible to end up in the brain case.

The endoscope is introduced into the sinus and the walls of the sinus are explored. Between 5 and 7 o'clock to the point of entry into the sinus is the aperture of the sinus into the middle meatus. The use of an appropriately sterilized flexible endoscope can facilitate the examination of this small opening. In the diseased state, where there has been turbinate destruction, it is often possible to pass a rigid endoscope from the nose directly into the frontal sinus without recourse to sinusotomy.

It is the authors' experience that, because of the relative paucity of the membranes of the sinus compared with the nose, the diagnostic yield from biopsy samples taken in the frontal sinus may be greater than for samples taken from the nose when there is radiographic evidence of disease in both locations.

Therapeutic irrigation is performed to flush the sinus adequately. At the end of the procedure, no attempt is made to replace the resected core of bone; the skin incision is closed with a simple interrupted suture.

Pathological conditions

Pathological conditions of the nose are covered in some depth in the *BSAVA Manual of Canine and Feline Head, Neck and Thoracic Surgery*, and the reader is referred to that Manual for additional information. Common conditions found in dogs and cats are summarized in Figure 9.23.

Nasopharyngeal conditions

Foreign bodies

Foreign bodies are not infrequently found lodged in the nasopharynx, having been coughed up over the free edge of the soft palate (Figure 9.24). Smaller or narrow foreign bodies, such as grass awns, may travel rostrally down the nares and can be extracted via anterior rhinoscopy.

Lymphoid hyperplasia

In chronic rhinitis it is not unusual to see lymphoid hyperplasia throughout the pharynx, presenting as multiple small raised nodules in the mucosa (see Figure 9.15). This is purely reactive and should not be mistaken for underlying pathology.

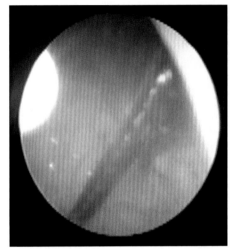

9.24 A blade of grass lodged in the nasopharynx of a cat dorsal to the soft palate.

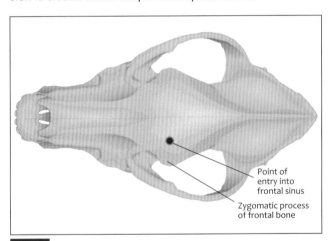

Point of entry into frontal sinus

Zygomatic process of frontal bone

9.22 Position of entry into the frontal sinus.

Disease	Species	Causes	Characteristics	Treatment
Lymphoplasmacytic rhinitis	Dogs, cats	Allergy; viral/bacterial; secondary to obstructive nasal disease or foreign body	Common. Chronic discharge, sneezing	Steroids; antibiotics based on results of culture and sensitivity testing; nasal drops are often more effective
Dental disease	Dogs, cats	Periodontal disease; fistulas; apical granuloma	Common	Appropriate dental treatment, e.g. extraction
Foreign bodies	Dogs, cats	Grass blades; grass awns; sticks	Common	Removal by traction; flushing if necessary to remove fragments
Traumatic disease	Dogs, cats		Uncommon	As appropriate
Nasopharyngeal stenosis	Dogs, cats		Uncommon (more common in cats)	Surgical: balloon dilation (with or without laser surgery); stent placement
Coagulation disorders	Dogs, cats	Genetic; drug-induced; hyperadrenocorticism	Uncommon	Medical
Parasitic rhinitis	Dogs, cats	*Capillaria aerophila*	Rare	Ivermectin
	Dogs	*Pneumonyssoides caninum*	Rare	Ivermectin
Allergic rhinitis	Dogs		Rare	Corticosteroids (systemic ± nasal drops)
Ciliary dyskinesia	Dogs, cats		Rare	Palliative: mucolytic agents (bromhexine hydrochloride 2 mg/kg q12h in dogs; 1 mg/kg q12h in cats)

9.23 Common nasopharyngeal conditions of dogs and cats.

Fungal infection

Fungal plaques of *Aspergillus* can sometimes be seen at the choanae, but the most common finding at this site is neoplasia (Billen *et al.*, 2006). In some cases, fungal infection may be mistaken for neoplasia or *vice versa* (Figure 9.25), so diagnosis must be based on impression smears or biopsy. See below for a discussion of therapy for fungal rhinitis.

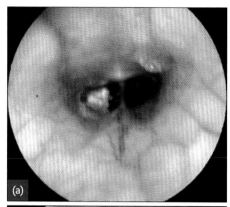

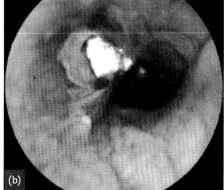

9.25 (a) *Aspergillus* colonies at the choanae, viewed by posterior rhinoscopy. The endoscope is retroflexed through 180 degrees, giving an inverted image, so this colony is in the right nostril. (b) Posterior rhinoscopic view of nasal lymphosarcoma in a dog (same dog as in Figure 9.31). Note the similarity in appearance to (a).

Nasopharyngeal polyps

Nasopharyngeal polyps are fairly common, especially in cats. They can often be visualized without the use of an endoscope, by using a blunt spay hook to pull the free edge of the soft palate rostrally to expose them (Figure 9.26). However, when they are small, an endoscope is useful (Figure 9.27).

These inflammatory tissues can originate in the Eustachian tubes, the middle ear or the ventral nasal meatus. They can be associated with chronic inflammatory conditions (chronic otitis, chronic rhinitis) but are often idiopathic. When found, nasopharyngeal polyps are almost always attached to the underlying tissues by a thin fibrous stalk. This means that they can almost always be removed by grabbing them with forceps (e.g. tonsil forceps) and applying gentle continuous traction. In some cats, this can be achieved by the retropharyngeal approach described above, but in other cases it can be accomplished more easily via anterior rhinoscopy. When they originate within the nasal cavity, polyps can be sessile and may become quite large. Laser or electrocautery resection can be attempted in these cases. Removal is often curative, but new polyps can occur, especially if there is underlying chronic inflammation.

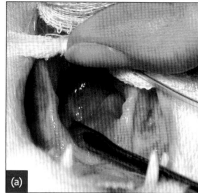
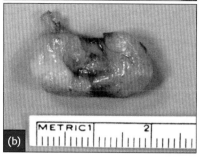

9.26 (a) A nasopharyngeal polyp seen during examination above the soft palate. A spay hook is being used to pull the soft palate forward so that the nasopharynx can be viewed. (b) The polyp after removal. (Courtesy of RC Denovo)

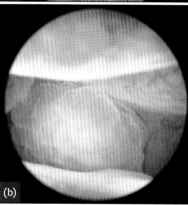
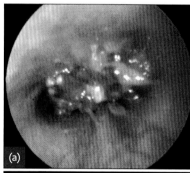
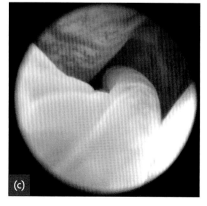

9.27 Benign nasal polyps in the dog. (a) At the choanae the appearance may be vascular and erosive, especially in the presence of secondary infection. With anterior rhinoscopy, polyps may be (b) single and confined to a small area or (c) present throughout most of the nasal passage.

Nasopharyngeal stenosis

Nasopharyngeal stenosis may be an underdiagnosed condition, especially in cats, and should be considered whenever there are signs of chronic respiratory disease. These cases are often misdiagnosed as chronic sinusitis but can easily be differentiated from other causes of upper respiratory disease by retropharyngeal flexible endoscopy.

Stenosis may occur as a congenital anomaly, similar to choanal atresia, or secondary to an inflammatory condition (e.g. foreign body, chronic rhinitis from regurgitation), pharyngeal or palatine surgery or a space-occupying lesion. The size of the pharyngeal aperture may be dramatically reduced to as little as 2 mm or so, causing mucus and discharge to accumulate rostral to the stenosis, with secondary infection and rhinitis resulting. As cats are obligate nasal breathers, this condition causes considerable distress.

Treatment can be attempted by balloon dilation and the placement of a suitable stent. However, if the stenosis is fairly caudal and the stent approaches the free edge of the soft palate, complications can result from hair becoming trapped around the stent during grooming. Balloon dilation alone is usually sufficient (Berent *et al.*, 2006) but may need to be repeated after 1–3 weeks if the stenosis reforms. A rigid endoscope is passed through one nostril to the choana to visualize the stenosis, and a balloon catheter is passed through the contralateral nostril and inflated with saline under direct visualization. Laser resection of the lateral edges of the opening followed by careful balloon dilation allows a more controlled dilation of the stenosis with less haemorrhage and conservation of some of the mucosal margin to facilitate healing (see also Chapter 16). If a laser is used, it is usually passed through the instrument channel of the endoscope. Some degree of re-stenosis is to be expected as healing occurs and scar tissue shrinks. Intralesional injection of a long-acting steroid, such as methyl-prednisolone, following dilation may help to reduce the likelihood of further stricture formation (see also Chapter 15).

Allergic rhinitis

Histopathologically, this disease may present in several forms. Any combination of lymphocytic, plasmacytic, lymphoplasmacytic or eosinophilic rhinitis is suggestive of primary immunological disease. It is critical to be confident that there is no other concurrent primary disease process to make this diagnosis. Idiopathic lymphoplasmacytic rhinitis is also considered to be a relatively common cause of chronic nasal discharge in the dog and is often a bilateral disease, even where nasal discharge is unilateral (Windsor *et al.*, 2004).

Corticosteroids have been the mainstay of treatment for many years. Treatment is usually started with 2 mg/kg prednisolone q12h. Experience has shown that this early aggressive immunosuppressive therapy makes relapses later in the taper period less likely. The dose is tapered after 3 weeks to once-daily treatment. Often, when steroids are the sole therapy, the induction phase of treatment can take up to 6 months. In the authors' experience, topical treatment using corticosteroid drops marketed for ophthalmic use can be more effective in some cases than oral treatment, but this does require a cooperative patient: nasal drops are often resented by the patient and difficult for owners to administer in the longer term. Nebulizers are available for both dogs and cats and can be used with steroid inhalers, which makes them a more attractive option for some patients.

For patients that are poorly tolerant of steroid therapy, a lower dose of prednisolone can be used in conjunction with chlorambucil at a dose of 2 mg/m^2 every other day. Complete blood counts should be performed every 2 weeks to check for leucopenia.

With the standardization of serum allergy testing, it has become increasingly possible to identify some environmental allergens that may play a role in the pathogenesis of this allergic rhinitis. If substantial positive results are obtained to allergens that are likely to be in the patient's environment, then hyposensitization therapy may be instituted. This requires substantial client compliance but, when successful, this safe and well tolerated therapy may provide an opportunity to use minimal immunomodulatory drug therapy.

Bacterial rhinitis/sinusitis

Primary bacterial rhinitis is rare in dogs and cats. When a primarily suppurative response is noted on histopathology, and no other infectious or neoplastic disease is apparent, then a diagnosis of primary bacterial disease can be made. The clinician should always be circumspect in making a diagnosis of primary bacterial rhinitis. It is critical to obtain good-quality samples for bacterial culture. Samples of both exudate and tissue, from multiple locations in the nose, should be submitted for analysis to confirm the presence of a single or multiple infectious agent(s). Careful interpretation of these results, to be sure that the findings are not consistent with contamination, is necessary. When antimicrobial sensitivity testing identifies a drug with appropriate activity against the offending organism(s), long-term antibiotic therapy is often indicated.

Unfortunately, bacterial rhinitis is one of the more frustrating bacterial diseases to treat, and clinicians often have to resort to more extreme measures to rid the patient of the disease. Turbinectomy is an aggressive therapeutic option for refractory rhinitis in dogs. Traditionally, turbinectomy has been performed via an open rhinotomy. The turbinates are removed using rongeurs or a similar instrument. The rostrum can then be left open for a period of time to allow daily irrigation with antimicrobial solutions before primary closure at a later date. A similar procedure using endoscopic techniques may be performed. Using an arthroscopic shaver system (a mechanized rotating shaving device, with a small diameter, designed for curetting bone and cartilage during arthroscopy; see Chapters 2 and 14), a turbinectomy can be performed without the need for a rhinotomy. The debrided material is removed by using the suction function of the shaver. Different blades for the shaver are available to ensure adequate curettage. As a more refined and complete turbinectomy can be performed with this technique, less bleeding and postoperative pain is likely to be encountered. Alternatively, laser turbinectomy may be performed using a diode laser. This may result in less pain and haemorrhage as nerves and vessels are sealed by the laser energy, but the procedure can take longer for a complete turbinectomy and requires experience to prevent collateral damage to adjacent tissues. Laser resection of nasopharyngeal turbinates has been successfully carried out in brachycephalic dogs as part of brachycephalic obstructive airway syndrome (BOAS) surgery (Oechtering *et al.*, 2016).

Foreign body rhinitis

Nasal foreign bodies are common in dogs (Figure 9.28) and cats. The presentation tends to be variable, but chronic mucopurulent nasal discharge is a common

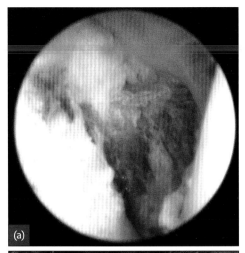

(a)

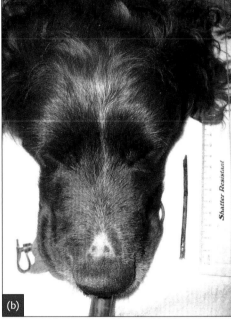

(b)

9.28 (a) A piece of stick embedded in the nose of a spaniel (middle of the image). (b) The piece of stick following removal from the dog's nose.

feature. Radiographically, the soft tissue densities noted may mimic mass effects.

When rhinoscopy is performed, if the foreign body is not seen, it may be embedded under the mucosa and often the only obvious findings are thickened oedematous proliferative mucous membranes, with substantial mucopurulent exudates. If biopsy is performed on these tissues, the results of histopathological examination are likely to be reported as lymphoplasmacytic rhinitis, often with an eosinophilic or a secondary neutrophilic component. These results can be misleading, and foreign material must be suspected in cases of rhinitis that do not resolve with treatment that would be appropriate for the histopathological findings. Often, multiple rhinoscopic examinations or open nasal exploratory surgeries are needed to identify the foreign material. It is worth noting that by the time rhinoscopy is performed the offending foreign material has often been sneezed out, and the resultant foreign body reaction is the only lesion seen by the endoscopist.

Cats tend to present with nasopharyngeal foreign bodies, such as blades of grass, which have been inadvertently coughed up over the soft palate into the caudal nares, from where sneezing may cause passage to a variable degree along the nasal cavity. Dogs may acquire nasal foreign bodies in this manner, but are also prone to sniffing up foreign bodies such as grass seeds, or running on to pieces of sticks.

Plant material may become very friable after a few days incubating in a warm and moist nose and, particularly if it is barbed or rough in texture, may be difficult to remove intact. Barbed material will often move in only one direction and should be removed accordingly. If the foreign body breaks up and is impossible to remove completely, the nose should be flushed vigorously with 60 ml of sterile saline on each side. The packing material in the throat should be removed to allow fluid to drain freely over the soft palate and into the mouth (a small swab may be left over the larynx if there is room) and the nose lowered to allow drainage. The endotracheal tube cuff should be checked to ensure it is fitting snugly. The tip of a 60 ml syringe filled with sterile saline is introduced into the nostril. The nostril is pinched tight around the syringe and the saline is instilled as rapidly as possible to flush the nasal cavity. Debris collected via the mouth can be examined for further foreign material. The nose can also be flushed in a rostral direction by placing a Foley catheter through the oral cavity and up over the soft palate, inflating the bulb to seal the caudal nares and packing the pharynx with gauze swabs. The procedure may be repeated on the contralateral nostril if necessary.

Neoplasia

It is beyond the scope of this Manual to give a detailed account of the oncological management of nasal neoplasia, and the reader is referred to the *BSAVA Manual of Canine and Feline Oncology*. However, a brief overview of the common nasal cancers (Figure 9.29) is in order.

Many nasal tumours are locally invasive and slow to metastasize. However, the gross appearance is often misleading, and histology is always required to differentiate between benign polyps and malignancies. Tumours may be staged to help predict the likely prognosis (Figure 9.30).

Lymphoma

Nasal lymphoma (Figure 9.31) is occasionally encountered. When it does occur, the nasal presentation is almost always the only manifestation; it is rarely multicentric. Nasal lymphoma can be treated with a standardized L-COPA protocol with moderate success (see the *BSAVA Manual of Canine and Feline Oncology* for more information on protocols). The authors' anecdotal observation is that nasal lymphomas are more frequently of a large lymphoblastic type, and are more locally aggressive, although not as aggressively metastatic as lymphomas found elsewhere in the body.

Adenocarcinoma

Nasal adenocarcinoma (Figures 9.32 to 9.35) is an aggressive tumour of the glandular epithelium of the nasal passages. Some surgeons have suggested surgical debulking of these tumours before adjunctive therapy, but the results do not bear out the utility of this approach. Surgery should not be routinely considered unless vital structures of the head are likely to be compromised by local invasion. However, tumour debulking may be of significant benefit to a patient that is experiencing

Site	Disease	Age affected	Characteristics	Treatment
Neoplasia of the nasal planum	Most commonly squamous cell carcinoma	Middle to old age dogs and cats	Locally invasive, slow to metastasize	Surgical resection ± radiation therapy
Nasal cavity – dogs	Adenocarcinoma	Middle to old age	Locally invasive, slow to metastasize	Surgical resection ± radiation therapy ± chemotherapy
	Chondroscarcoma	Middle to old age	Locally invasive, slow to metastasize	Surgical resection ± radiation therapy
	Osteosarcoma	Middle to old age	Locally invasive, slow to metastasize	Surgical resection ± radiation therapy ± chemotherapy
	Squamous cell carcinoma	Middle to old age	Locally invasive, slow to metastasize	Surgical resection ± radiation therapy
	Melanoma	Middle to old age	Locally invasive, slow to metastasize	Surgical resection ± radiation therapy
	Lymphosarcoma	Young to middle age	May be generalized	Chemotherapy ± local debulking
	Nasopharyngeal polyp	Middle to old age	Benign, recurrent	Traction, surgical removal
	Chondroma	Middle to old age	Benign, recurrent	Surgical resection
	Osteoma	Middle to old age	Benign, recurrent	Surgical resection
Nasal cavity – cats	Lymphosarcoma	Middle to older age	May be generalized	Check other sites and FeLV/FIV status
	Adenocarcinoma	Middle to old age	Locally invasive, slow to metastasize	Surgical resection ± radiation therapy
	Nasopharyngeal polyp	Young to middle age	Benign, recurrent	Traction, surgical removal

9.29 Common nasal tumours of dogs and cats. FeLV = Feline leukaemia virus; FIV = Feline immunodeficiency virus.

Stage	Presentation	Prognosis
I	Unilateral	Reasonable medium term with surgery/radiation
II	Bilateral	Guarded medium term with surgery/radiation
III	Associated external mass	Guarded short term with surgery/radiation
IV	Brain involvement	Poor

9.30 Staging of nasal tumours.

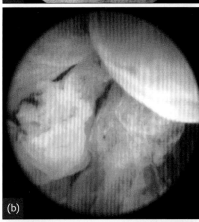

9.32 Adenocarcinomas in the dog. (a) Appearance of an adenocarcinoma at the choanae viewed in air. (b) Opaque irregular pale adenocarcinoma with swelling and erythema of the surrounding turbinates. (c) Appearance of an adenocarcinoma under irrigation (same dog as in (a)). The adenocarcinoma is pale and relatively smooth and translucent (compare with (b)), giving the appearance of a polyp.

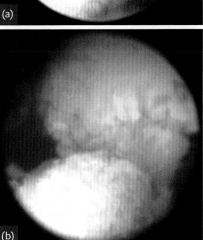

9.31 Nasal lymphosarcoma in a Rottweiler. (a) Initial appearance of the lesion. (b) Cut surface of the lesion following biopsy. Note the 'cotton wool' appearance.

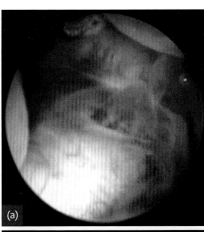

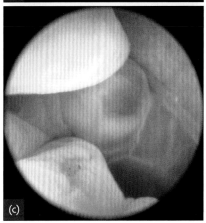

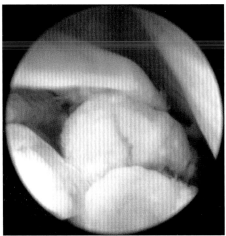

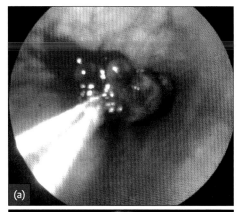

9.33 Adenocarcinoma in a cat showing a pale lobulated appearance and vascularity.

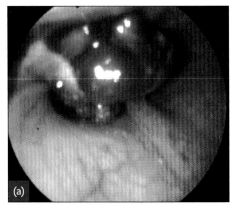

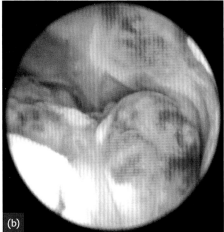

9.34 Nasal adenocarcinoma at the choanae viewed by (a) posterior rhinoscopy and (b) anterior rhinoscopy. Note the difference in appearance when viewed under saline irrigation.

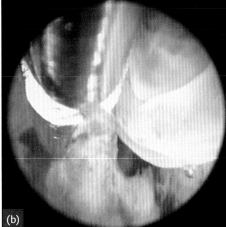

9.35 (a) Biopsy of an adenocarcinoma at the choanae, using posterior rhinoscopy. The biopsy forceps should be preplaced at the tip of the endoscope before retroflexing the endoscope around the free edge of the soft palate to prevent damage to the biopsy channel. (b) Biopsy of a nasal adenocarcinoma using anterior rhinoscopy.

substantial facial/nasal pain and difficulty breathing. The authors have used endoscopic diode laser surgery to effectively debulk this type of tumour for many years. The procedure is well tolerated and, while it is by no means curative, many patients achieve a substantial clinical improvement. The tumour is radiation sensitive, although cobalt linear accelerators are likely to be more effective than orthovoltage radiotherapy. More and more success is being reported using chemotherapy as monotherapy. Carboplatin is used at a dose of 30 mg/m² every 3 weeks for three cycles. The drug is very well tolerated, not aggressively nephrotoxic and easy to administer; however, its cost is a limiting factor. There is an increasing body of evidence that photodynamic therapy may be of value in treating these tumours, but this therapy is not routinely clinically available.

Melanoma

Nasal melanoma is an unusual extension of melanomas of the skin of the rostrum and/or the mucocutaneous junction. This type of tumour is radiosensitive.

Chondrosarcoma

This is a common nasal tumour (Figure 9.36). Its major clinical manifestation is based upon its space-occupying nature. Although chondrosarcoma is not highly metastatic, it is locally aggressive, and can cause tremendous damage to facial symmetry and the normal functional anatomy of the nose and head. Laser debulking (Figure 9.37) is potentially of some benefit. However, since these are relatively avascular tumours, the response to laser debulking alone is often disappointing, with palliation resulting from removal of overlying inflammatory tissue. A combination of laser debulking and aggressive curettage will remove more tumour tissue. Aggressive surgery could theoretically be considered curative, but it is very difficult to achieve clean surgical margins in this anatomical region. This type of tumour is moderately radiosensitive.

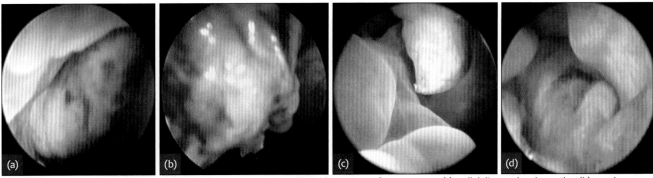

9.36 Nasal chondrosarcomas in the dog. Nasal masses can present with a variety of appearances: (a) well delineated and vascular; (b) poorly delineated and invasive; (c) ulcerative; and (d) pale, almost translucent and relatively avascular. Histopathology is always required for diagnosis as the morphology is so varied.

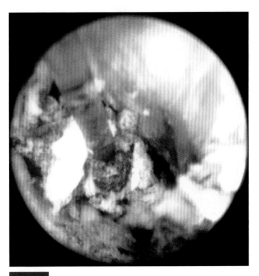

9.37 Laser debulking of a nasal chondrosarcoma in a dog.

Osteosarcoma

Osteosarcoma in the nose (Figures 9.38 and 9.39) behaves similarly to osteosarcomas of the flat bones elsewhere in the body. It is less aggressive and less metastatic than those in the long bones, but it causes considerable local damage. Palliative surgical debulking can be undertaken to improve the patient's breathing through the nose. Fair to good success has also been reported with carboplatin (30 mg/m^2 every 3 weeks for four cycles) either as monotherapy or in conjunction with doxorubicin (300 mg/m^2) given approximately 4 days before the carboplatin. The use of doxorubicin increases the potential toxicity of the treatment (it is associated with increased myelosuppression and cardiotoxicity) and its potential efficacy is controversial. The author [DS] does try to use this protocol, however, as the two drugs appear to have a synergistic beneficial effect on the cell cycle. Whether this is borne out statistically remains to be seen.

Benign tumours

Of the benign processes, both chondromas and osteomas are occasionally seen. If they are identified early and surgical removal can be achieved, along with appropriate reconstructive techniques, the prognosis can be good.

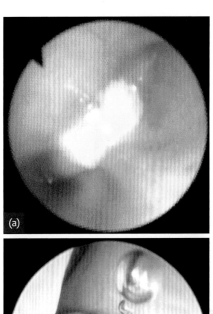

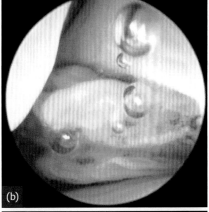

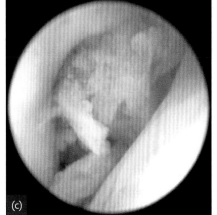

9.38 Osteosarcomas in the cat: (a) at the choana; (b) well circumscribed vascular nasal mass; and (c) pale, friable, relatively avascular appearance of a nasal mass.

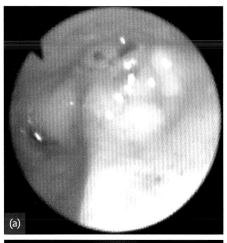

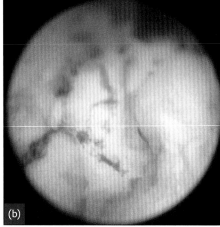

9.39 Osteosarcomas in the dog: (a) at the choana; and (b) nasal.

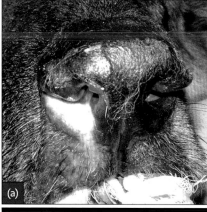

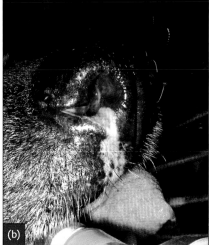

9.41 (a) Swelling and depigmentation of the nasal planum, characteristic of *Aspergillus* infection, in a German Shepherd Dog. (b) Resolution of swelling and depigmentation 1 month after initial treatment.

Fungal rhinitis

Dogs

Aspergillus is the most common nasal fungal pathogen in the dog and cat (Figure 9.40) and should be suspected any time there is chronic non-resolving rhinitis, especially with radiographic evidence of bony destruction mimicking neoplasia. Fungal serology is usually included as part of the preoperative diagnostic investigations but is not always diagnostic (see above). Swelling and depigmentation of the nasal planum (Figure 9.41) coupled with a mucopurulent nasal discharge, epistaxis and pain over the rhinarium are common presenting clinical signs.

The rhinoscopic appearance of fungal rhinitis is quite characteristic (Figure 9.42). Diagnosis is easily confirmed in the laboratory from impression smears and/or culture.

Treatment with oral fungicides, such as itraconazole at 5 mg/kg q12h, is both expensive and potentially hepatotoxic. Serial blood chemistry measurements must be performed in order to be vigilant with regard to liver disease, and therapy must be continued for 2–3 months. Success rates of up to 60–70% have been reported for oral treatment alone, but these rates can be greatly improved if oral fungicides are used in conjunction with non-invasive topical treatment (Smith *et al.*, 1998). This treatment protocol compares favourably with surgical trephination of the

Fungal pathogens	Species affected	Age affected	Characteristics	Treatment
Aspergillus spp: *A. fumigatus* (less commonly *A. niger,* *A. nidulans,* *A. flavus,* *A. terreus*)	Dogs and cats	Any	Chronic unilateral, then bilateral mucopurulent nasal discharge ± epistaxis; facial pain	Debridement + clotrimazole or enilconazole infusion (Oral itraconazole) Cats: oral posaconazole
Cryptococcus spp.	Cats (and rarely dogs)	Any	Chronic unilateral, then bilateral mucopurulent nasal discharge ± epistaxis; facial pain	Debridement + clotrimazole or enilconazole infusion (Oral itraconazole)
A. felis	Cats (and rarely dogs)	Any	Chronic unilateral, then bilateral mucopurulent nasal discharge ± epistaxis; facial pain	Debridement + clotrimazole or enilconazole infusion (Oral itraconazole) Often very refractory to treatment

9.40 Fungal infections of the nasal tract in dogs and cats.

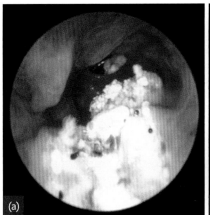
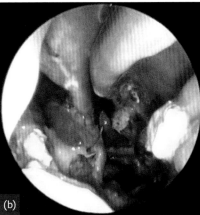
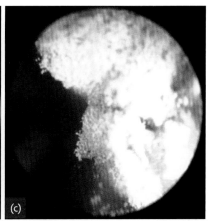

9.42 Nasal aspergillosis in dogs. (a) Classic white plaques. (b) Plaques showing a greenish tinge due to secondary infection. Note the extensive turbinate damage, leading to an abnormally large airspace. In (a), turbinate destruction has exposed the frontal sinus and *Aspergillus* plaques can be seen within the sinus cavity (rear of the image). (c) Close-up view of an *Aspergillus* colony showing the 'cotton wool' appearance of the fungal hyphae.

sinuses to place indwelling cannulae in the frontal sinuses for the application of antifungal solutions (Mathews *et al.*, 1998). Treatment will normally require general anaesthesia, and can be carried out following rhinoscopic examination and diagnosis.

It is imperative to carefully debride as much of the fungal plaque as possible under direct observation, before administering the antifungal treatment (Figure 9.43). This will allow good exposure of the remaining fungal material to the antifungal solution. Failure to remove fungal plaques is the most common reason for poor response to treatment. Following good debridement, 85–90% of cases should resolve with a single treatment.

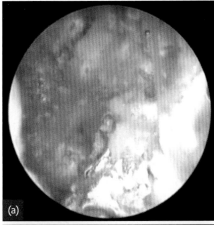

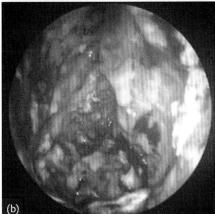

9.43 Nasal *Aspergillus* plaque (a) before and (b) after debridement.

Following debridement of the fungal plaques, the throat pack is removed and a suitably sized Foley catheter is introduced through the mouth and retroflexed over the soft palate. The bulb of the catheter is inflated with saline to seal off the caudal nares from the pharynx, and a fresh gauze pack is placed in the pharynx to ensure a good seal. Tampons may also be used to pack the throat to good effect. A canine urinary catheter or red rubber feeding tube is introduced into each nostril, and a small Foley catheter is then introduced alongside it such that the bulb is just inside the nostril. The bulbs are then inflated with saline to seal off the rostral nares and the Foley catheters are all clamped shut. The nares may require further sealing with cotton wool, cotton buds or (in larger patients) tampons to ensure a good seal.

Enilconazole has been used as a nasal infusion, and has been demonstrated to be 80–90% effective. It is freely available in the UK, where it is marketed as an antifungal wash for horses and dogs (Imaverol™, Elanco). However, in the USA it is available only as the chemical-grade solution, which is difficult to obtain and is very caustic to healthy tissues. Enilconazole is more active in vapour form than clotrimazole and gives good results. Care must be taken to carefully pack off the oral and pharyngeal cavities to minimize contact of the antifungal agent with healthy tissues. Clotrimazole has been used extensively in the USA to good effect. It is readily available in a pre-made solution containing polyethylene glycol (Macrogol 400) (marketed for the treatment of athlete's foot fungus in humans) or as a gel, and is available without prescription.

> **WARNING**
>
> Formulations of clotrimazole containing isopropyl alcohol and propylene glycol (Canesten® Solution) should be avoided as they may result in pharyngeal irritation and oedema. Polyethylene glycol is a relatively non-irritant vehicle

Two 60 ml syringes are filled with 1–5% enilconazole (or 1% clotrimazole) and attached to the urinary catheters placed in the nostrils; antifungal solution is then infused into each nostril until it is filled and starts to leak out (up to 50 ml depending on the size of the patient) and left for 15 minutes. The dog is then rotated through 90 degrees (e.g. into left lateral recumbency) and the process is repeated, again allowing 15 minutes after the infusion. The dog is then rotated again into dorsal recumbency and finally into right lateral recumbency, instilling more of the solution per nostril as required, and allowing 15 minutes each time. In this way, almost all of the nasal mucosa and sinuses should be bathed in the antifungal solution (Figure 9.44).

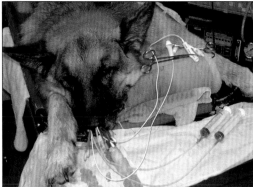

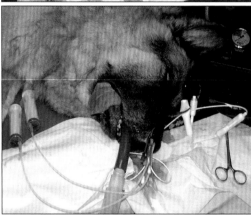

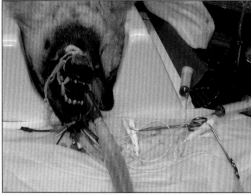

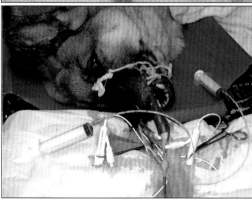

9.44 Treatment of nasal aspergillosis using an intranasal infusion of enilconazole. After each infusion, the patient is left for 15 minutes and then rotated by 90 degrees for the next infusion, to ensure that as much of the nasal mucosa and sinuses as possible comes into contact with the antifungal solution.

After the treatment, as much of the remaining solution as possible is drained through the anterior nares. Enilconazole and clotrimazole can irritate the trachea, larynx and oesophagus, so care should be taken to avoid drainage back into the pharynx as much as possible.

In 85–90% of cases one treatment will be successful, but some dogs may require two or three treatments for a cure. It is always advisable to repeat rhinoscopy after 1 month (Figure 9.45) to assess the effectiveness of treatment and repeat it if necessary.

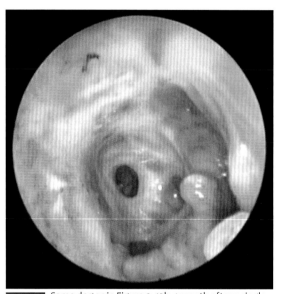

9.45 Same dog as in Figure 9.42b, 1 month after a single enilconazole treatment. No fungal plaques are visible.

In some cases, fungal infection may extend into the sinuses or may even be restricted to the sinuses with no fungal plaques seen on anterior rhinoscopy. If there is evidence of disease in the frontal sinus(es), and access to the frontal sinuses from the middle meatus is obstructed, small holes are trephined to enable fungal plaques to be removed as before. A Michel trephine, Steinmann pin and Jacobs chuck or Hall-type air drill can be used for this purpose. Red rubber feeding tubes are inserted and the skin is closed around the tubes to reduce leakage. The antifungal solution is then infused into the frontal sinuses and nasal passages, initially with a dose of 30 ml in each side, under pressure, and the treatment is continued as described above. This topical therapy is generally quite well tolerated, with only mild cutaneous reactions reported at the sites of infusion.

Cats

Aspergillosis in the cat was historically considered rare, but may be becoming more common (Goodall *et al.*, 1984; Smith and Hoffman, 2010). Two forms of aspergillosis affect the upper respiratory tract of cats: sinonasal aspergillosis (SNA) and sino-orbital aspergillosis (SOA). SOA is reported to be the more common form in cats, comprising 65% of reported cases, and is invasive; this contrasts with the situation in dogs, in which SNA accounts for virtually all cases and is considered to be non-invasive.

The clinical signs of SNA in cats are similar to those reported for chronic rhinosinusitis, including sneezing, nasal discharge and epistaxis. There appears to be a predilection for aspergillosis among purebred brachycephalic cats, but no sex predilection has been reported and animals of all ages have been affected (Tamborini *et al.*, 2016).

The treatment of SNA in cats is similar to that in dogs: it includes debridement of fungal lesions along with systemic antifungal therapy (e.g. itraconazole, posaconazole) and/or intranasal infusion of a topical antifungal agent (clotrimazole). As in dogs, adequate debridement of fungal plaques is the key to successful resolution of SNA in cats. The topical antifungal treatment protocol for cats is also similar to that used in dogs, although a much smaller volume of 1% clotrimazole solution is used (approximately 1 ml per nasal cavity per 15-minute rotation). Solutions containing isopropyl alcohol or propylene glycol should be avoided due to its extremely irritant effects on the soft tissues and larynx, which can be life-threatening.

Postoperative care

Having completed the examination of the nasal cavities (and the sinuses, if necessary) and taken any samples, the endoscope is removed. If there is heavy bleeding, it may be pertinent to maintain the patient under anaesthesia for a few minutes until it has subsided. Recovery from anaesthesia should be slow to avoid exacerbating nasal bleeding. A postoperative dose of acepromazine can also be given to keep the blood pressure low and prevent excitement, thereby reducing postoperative haemorrhage. The nose is then lowered to prevent the accumulation of blood and fluid in the pharynx, the throat packing is removed and the nasopharynx is swabbed or suctioned before extubation. Extubation is left until the last minute to ensure the patient's gag and cough reflexes will protect the airway, and the endotracheal tube is removed with the cuff partially inflated. Recovery with the patient in sternal recumbency and the head tilted slightly down will help to prevent any exudate collecting in the pharynx and obstructing the airway.

Some practitioners advocate the use of cold irrigant fluids, an infusion of dilute adrenaline or pseudoephedrine, or packing the nose to limit haemorrhage. In any event, bleeding tends to be ongoing for several hours after rhinoscopy. The addition of irrigant fluid to the mucus and blood tends to make the haemorrhage look worse than it really is, but the sneezing that inevitably occurs after rhinoscopy can produce what looks like an alarming amount of blood. In patients without a coagulopathy, ongoing haemorrhage is rarely of concern. If the veterinary surgeon is concerned about potential blood loss, serial measurements of packed cell volume can be made. It is prudent to recommend overnight hospitalization or at the very least to advise the owner about the messy nature of the first day or so after rhinoscopy. Bleeding generally abates within 72 hours. There is inevitably some postoperative mucosal swelling, and the owner should be warned that the patient's breathing may be worse for a day or two postoperatively.

Postoperative discomfort in dogs and cats is managed with buprenorphine (10–20 μg/kg i.m. q2h) or morphine (0.2–0.5 mg/kg i.m. q2–4h). Ongoing pain relief is provided with non-steroidal anti-inflammatory drugs (NSAIDs) such as meloxicam (0.1 mg/kg orally q24h) or carprofen (2 mg/kg orally q24h). In selected cases, a single dose of dexamethasone (0.2 mg/kg i.v. or i.m.) can be given to reduce mucosal swelling, but should not be given in conjunction with NSAIDs.

Complications

Haemorrhage is the most common complication of rhinoscopy but is rarely long-lasting or significant. Overnight hospitalization after the procedure allows a chance for haemorrhage to resolve adequately before the excitement of returning to the owners raises the patient's blood pressure and potentially dislodges a clot. Postoperative acepromazine can also help to reduce postoperative haemorrhage.

Aspiration of fluid and detritus during the procedure can be prevented by ensuring adequate inflation of the cuff on the endotracheal tube and packing the pharynx with gauze sponges or other suitable absorbent material, leaving enough space for the free flow of fluid over the free edge of the soft palate and out through the mouth. Taking the steps described above to prevent the accumulation of blood and fluids in the airway during recovery will also help to prevent aspiration.

References and further reading

Barrs VR, van Doorn TM, Houbraken J et al. (2013) Aspergillus felis sp. nov., an emerging agent of invasive aspergillosis in humans, cats, and dogs. PLOS ONE 8, e64871

Berent AC, Kinns J and Weisse C (2006) Balloon dilatation of nasopharyngeal stenosis in a dog. Journal of the American Veterinary Medical Association 229, 385–388

Billen F, Day MJ and Clercx C (2006) Diagnosis of pharyngeal disorders in dogs: a retrospective study of 67 cases. Journal of Small Animal Practice 47, 122–129

Brockman D, Holt D and ter Haar G (2018) BSAVA Manual of Canine and Feline Head, Neck and Thoracic Surgery, 2nd edn. BSAVA Publications, Gloucester

Dobson JM and Lascelles DX (2011) BSAVA Manual of Canine and Feline Oncology, 3rd edn. BSAVA Publications, Gloucester

Freeman LJ (1999) Veterinary Endosurgery. Mosby, St. Louis

Goodall SA, Lane JG and Warnock DW (1984) The diagnosis and treatment of a case of nasal aspergillosis in a cat. Journal of Small Animal Practice 25, 627–633

Johnson LR, Clarke HE, Bannasch MJ and De Cock HEV (2004) Correlation of rhinoscopic signs of inflammation with histologic findings in nasal biopsy specimens of cats with or without upper respiratory tract disease. Journal of the American Veterinary Medical Association 225, 395–400

Johnson LR, Drazenovich TL, Herrera MA and Wisner ER (2006) Results of rhinoscopy alone or in conjunction with sinuscopy in dogs with aspergillosis: 46 cases (2001–2004). Journal of the American Veterinary Medical Association 228, 738–742

Lefebvre J, Kuehn NF and Wortinger A (2005) Computed tomography as an aid in the diagnosis of chronic nasal disease in dogs. Journal of Small Animal Practice 46, 280–285

Mathews KG, Davidson AP, Koblik PD et al. (1998) Comparison of topical administration of clotrimazole through surgically placed versus nonsurgically placed catheters for treatment of nasal aspergillosis in dogs: 60 cases (1990–1996). Journal of the American Veterinary Medical Association 213, 501–506

McCarthy TC (2005) Veterinary Endoscopy for the Small Animal Practitioner. Elsevier Saunders, St. Louis

Oechtering GU, Pohl S, Schlueter C and Schuenemann R (2016) Novel approach to brachycephalic syndrome. 2. Laser-assisted turbinectomy (LATE). Veterinary Surgery 45, 173–181

Reiter AM and Gracis M (2018) BSAVA Manual of Canine and Feline Dentistry and Oral Surgery, 4th edn. BSAVA Publications, Gloucester

Saunders JH, Clercx C, Snaps FR et al. (2004) Radiographic, magnetic resonance imaging, computed tomographic, and rhinoscopic features of nasal aspergillosis in dogs. Journal of the American Veterinary Medical Association 225, 1703–1712

Schwarz T and Johnson V (2008) BSAVA Manual of Canine and Feline Thoracic Imaging. BSAVA Publications, Gloucester

Smith LN and Hoffman SB (2010) A case series of unilateral orbital aspergillosis in three cats and treatment with voriconazole. Veterinary Ophthalmology 13, 190–203

Smith SA, Andrews G and Biller DS (1998) Management of nasal aspergillosis in a dog with a single, noninvasive intranasal infusion of clotrimazole. Journal of the American Animal Hospital Association 34, 487–492

Tamborini A, Robertson E, Talbot JJ and Barrs VR (2016) Sinonasal aspergillosis in a British Shorthair cat in the UK. Journal of Feline Medicine and Surgery Open Reports 2, doi: 10.1177/2055116916653775

Tams TR (1998) Small Animal Endoscopy, 2nd edn. Mosby, St. Louis

Tomsa K, Glaus TM, Zimmer C and Greene CE (2003) Fungal rhinitis and sinusitis in three cats. Journal of the American Veterinary Medical Association 222, 1380–1384

Villiers E and Ristić J (2016) BSAVA Manual of Canine and Feline Clinical Pathology, 3rd edn. BSAVA Publications, Gloucester

Windsor RC, Johnson LR, Herrgesell EJ and De Cock HEV (2004) Idiopathic lymphoplasmacytic rhinitis in dogs: 37 cases (1997–2002). Journal of the American Veterinary Medical Association 224, 1952–1957

Zonderland JL, Störk CK, Saunders JH et al. (2002) Intranasal infusion of enilconazole for treatment of sinonasal aspergillosis in dogs. Journal of the American Veterinary Medical Association 221, 1421–1425

Chapter 10

Rigid endoscopy: otoendoscopy

Michela De Lucia, Laura Ordeix and Fabia Scarampella

Introduction

Ear diseases are among the most common health problems seen in dogs, and are also commonly (although less frequently) observed in cats (O'Neill *et al.*, 2014; O'Neill *et al.*, 2019). Most acute cases of otitis can be managed with topical polyvalent medications, but the condition can be refractory to treatment and progress to chronic disease, which represents a diagnostic and therapeutic challenge for the veterinary surgeon (veterinarian). Failure to identify, remove or control the primary cause of otitis (e.g. atopic dermatitis or ear masses), spreading of the inflammatory process from the ear canal to the middle ear and infection with multiresistant strains of *Pseudomonas aeruginosa* and *Staphylococcus pseudintermedius* are frequently responsible for treatment failure and the development of chronic otitis in dogs. In cats, chronic otitis is most commonly associated with diseases arising in the middle ear (e.g. inflammatory polyps) or neoplasia of the external ear canal (adenoma or adenocarcinoma of the ceruminous glands).

Otoscopic examination of the ear canal can increase the chances of successful management of otitis because it facilitates the identification of treatable primary causes (e.g. foreign bodies, ear mites, inflammatory polyps) and evaluation of the severity and extent of the pathological process (e.g. by assessment of the integrity of the tympanic membrane). In cases of mild disease, a hand-held otoscope can be appropriate for examining the ear canal, but it is not suitable when intense inflammation or abundant discharge is present, as occurs in severe acute otitis and chronic otitis. In these cases, video-otoscopy in the anaesthetized patient is more appropriate. Video-otoscopy systems use components of endoscopic technology to acquire, project and record video images of the ear canal and tympanic membrane, as well as pathological changes of the tympanic cavity. They provide a high degree of magnification so that, after appropriate cleaning of the ear canal, these structures can be examined in detail. Video-otoscopes also have a working channel specific for small instruments, such as catheters or forceps, which can be used to remove and collect exudate and tissue samples under direct visualization. Moreover, video-otoscopes designed for use in the dog and cat are equipped with specific flushing and suction systems that allow thorough cleaning and drying of the ear, which is highly recommended as part of therapeutic management in cases of treatment failure or chronic otitis.

The recording capability of the video-otoscopy system means that images can be stored for comparison at subsequent re-evaluations of the patient. These images/videos can also be used to improve communication with the client and compliance with the treatment plan, to share patient information with veterinary colleagues and for educational purposes.

Instrumentation

A video-otoscopy imaging chain comprises a video camera, camera control unit, light source, light guide cable, monitor and endoscope together with an otoscope to examine the external and middle ear (Figure 10.1). Different rigid telescopes with various diameters can be used, ranging from larger otoendoscopes (5 mm) to multipurpose rigid telescopes with a diameter of 2.7 mm and, for very small animals, a mini rigid telescope with an outer diameter of only 9.5 Fr (3.17 mm) Specific instruments including flushing catheters, ear curettes and brushes, biopsy forceps, grasping forceps, polypectomy snares and myringotomy needles can be passed through the working channel of the otoscope or the sheath of the telescope to perform diagnostic and therapeutic procedures in the anaesthetized patient. For ear cleaning and drying, a suction/irrigation machine (Figure 10.2) with a 5 Fr red

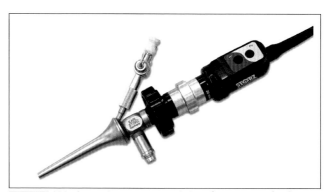

10.1 Veterinary otoscope set consisting of an otoscope for dogs and cats and a stopcock attachment with an integrated working channel. This otoscope is a straightforward telescope with a length of 8.5 cm, a tip diameter of 5 mm and a 5 Fr (1.65 mm) working channel. The configuration of the lens at the otoscope tip provides a 110-degree field of view and the long focal length of the instrument allows deep examination of the ear canal.
(Courtesy of Karl Storz SE & Co. KG)

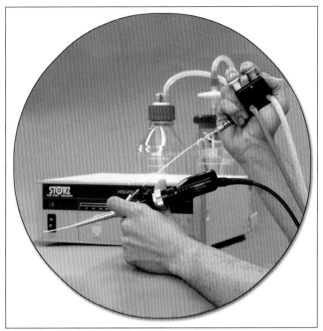

10.2 VETPUMP® 2 flushing and suction apparatus.
(Courtesy of Karl Storz SE & Co. KG)

rubber urinary catheter or a 'Y'-shaped stopcock attachment with an integrated operating channel can be connected to the infusion channel.

To obtain good-quality images during video-otoscopy, frequent cleaning with alcohol-soaked swabs or the application of commercial anti-fogging agents to the tip surface of the lens are recommended.

Indications

Video-otoscopy is indicated whenever a thorough examination of the ear canal and the tympanic membrane is needed. More generally, any clinical sign suggestive of ear disease, such as head shaking or aural pruritus, pain, erythema, swelling or discharge, is a valid indication for video-otoscopy. Depending on the severity of the disease and the animal's temperament, the procedure can be performed in the conscious patient or under general anaesthesia. However, in the conscious patient only a cursory examination can be performed, and this is suitable only for the evaluation of an apparently healthy ear or for initial identification of problems requiring a more detailed examination. It is recommended that the patient be under general anaesthesia for diagnostic and therapeutic otoscopy in cases of:

- Otitis externa in which a foreign body or an ear mass is suspected
- Chronic or recurrent otitis externa
- Neurological signs compatible with middle or inner ear disease.

It should be noted that a proper evaluation of the middle and inner ear requires a combination of otoscopy and an advanced diagnostic imaging technique, that is, computed tomography (CT) or magnetic resonance imaging (MRI). The contraindications to video-otoscopy are limited to those cases in which anaesthesia would pose a risk to the life of the patient.

Patient preparation

Before performing otoscopy, a short course of systemic glucocorticoids may be needed to reduce ear canal stenosis associated with severe or chronic inflammation, particularly in the dog. Prednisone or prednisolone administered orally at a dose of 1–2 mg/kg once a day for 4–7 days will reduce swelling and inflammation, allowing a more complete examination of the ear canal. Steroid administration should be postponed until the results of the preoperative diagnostic work-up (see below) have been obtained.

In cases where samples of ear exudate are to be collected during otoscopy and submitted for bacterial culture and sensitivity testing, it may be appropriate to discontinue any topical antibacterial products a few days before the procedure. Unfortunately, specific recommendations regarding withdrawal times are lacking.

Preoperative diagnostic investigation

Imaging studies should be performed before the otoscopic examination, as ear cleaning and flushing during otoscopy may unintentionally rupture the tympanic membrane and deposit fluid within the bullae, which may be misinterpreted as middle ear pathology.

CT and MRI are essential for thorough investigation of the inner ear and the bony and soft tissue structures surrounding the ear. They are also recommended to evaluate the middle ear in cases of chronic otitis or space-occupying lesions (Figures 10.3 and 10.4). In fact, cross-sectional imaging (i.e. CT or MRI) has a higher diagnostic value for middle ear diseases than video-otoscopy. In particular, the observation of an intact and flat tympanic membrane during otoscopic examination does not exclude the presence of middle ear disease (Figure 10.5). Caution should be exercised when interpreting CT and MRI findings of the middle ear in brachycephalic dogs: recent studies have shown that French Bulldogs, English Bulldogs and Pugs without clinical signs of ear disease have a significantly thicker tympanic bulla wall, a smaller bulla lumen size and a higher prevalence of subclinical middle ear effusion than non-brachycephalic dogs (Mielke *et al.*, 2017).

MRI may be more useful than CT in patients with neurological signs relating to disease of the middle or inner ear because of its potential to detect extension of the pathological process to the nerves, the cochlea, the semicircular canals and the meninges (Figure 10.6)

Radiographic and ultrasonographic examination of the middle ear can also be considered and are much more widely available and cheaper than CT and MRI. Radiographic assessment of the tympanic bulla can be helpful in identifying changes attributable to otitis media, such as a thickened, irregular bulla and soft tissue opacities within the middle ear cavity. However, radiography is not very sensitive for the diagnosis of otitis media, with false-negative results reported in 25% of cases (Remedios *et al.*, 2004). Positive-contrast ear canalography has been described as a more sensitive method than either otoscopy or radiography for determining the status of the tympanic membrane in dogs with chronic otitis externa and secondary otitis media. Owing to its low sensitivity, ultrasound imaging of the tympanic bulla should not be used as a substitute for cross-sectional imaging for the diagnosis of otitis media (Bischoff *et al.*, 2004).

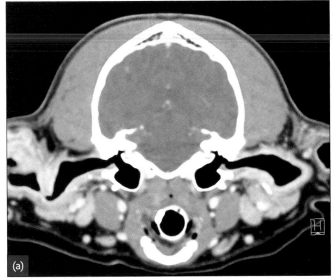

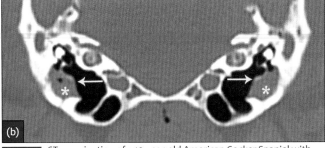

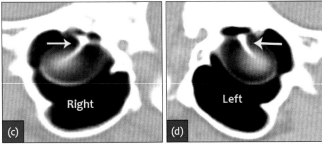

10.3 CT examination of a 10-year-old American Cocker Spaniel with external bilateral chronic otitis. (a) Transverse post-contrast image of the head. (b) Transverse image of the tympanic bullae (bone algorithm). Both tympanic cavities are normally aerated and sections of the tympanic membrane are visible (arrowed). Note the dense material in the pre-tympanic segment of the external meatus (asterisks). (c, d) Multioblique multiplanar images from CT volume data show that the left and right tympanic membranes are intact (arrowed).
(Courtesy of Dr Bertolini, Diagnostic and Interventional Division, San Marco Veterinary Clinic, Padova, Italy)

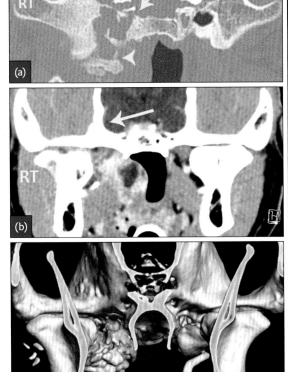

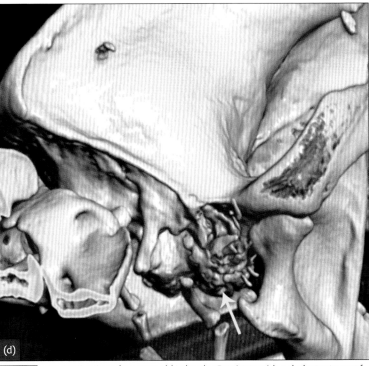

10.4 CT examination of a 9-year-old Labrador Retriever with a cholesteatoma of the right middle ear. (a) Transverse pre-contrast image (bone algorithm). The tympanic cavity is filled with material of soft tissue density and the ventral wall of the bulla (arrowhead) and the petrosal portion of the temporal bone (arrowed) show bone lysis and destruction accompanied by extensive surrounding sclerosis. (b) Post-contrast image (soft tissue algorithm) showing the involvement of peripharyngeal soft tissue leading to pharyngeal eccentric stenosis (arrowed). (c, d) Three-dimensional volume rendering segmentation (frontal view) showing bony proliferative changes of the right bulla (arrowed).
(Courtesy of Dr Bertolini, Diagnostic and Interventional Division, San Marco Veterinary Clinic, Padova, Italy)

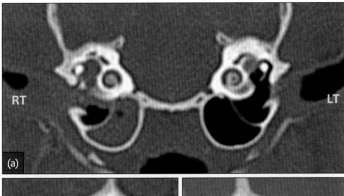

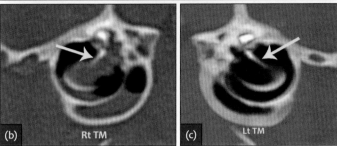

10.5 CT examination of a 4-year-old Domestic Shorthaired cat with right external and middle ear otitis but an intact tympanic membrane. (a) Transverse image through the tympanic bulla. There is increased opacity of the pre-tympanic segment of the right external acoustic meatus. The tympanic membrane is barely visible in this section. (b) Multioblique multiplanar reformatted (MPR) image of the right tympanic cavity, showing a normal tympanic membrane profile. There is increased opacity and thickening of the membrane, and some fluid in the tympanic and epitympanic cavities. (c) Multioblique MPR, thin maximum intensity projection image of the left middle ear, showing a normal appearance of the tympanic membrane and middle ear cavities. Arrows indicate the manubrium of the malleus.
(Courtesy of Dr Bertolini, Diagnostic and Interventional Division, San Marco Veterinary Clinic, Padova, Italy)

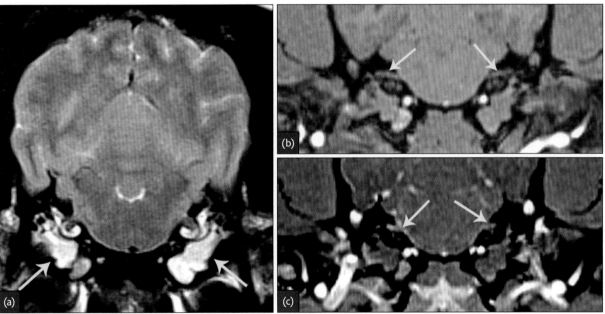

10.6 MRI examination of a 6-year-old Cavalier King Charles Spaniel with right-sided facial nerve paralysis. (a) T2-weighted transverse image showing both tympanic cavities filled with hyperintense fluid material (arrowed). (b) Pre-contrast and (c) post-contrast T1-weighted images showing contrast enhancement of the facial nerves (arrowed) and meninges, suggesting their possible involvement in the inflammatory process.
(Courtesy of Dr Bertolini, Diagnostic and Interventional Division, San Marco Veterinary Clinic, Padova, Italy)

Premedication, anaesthesia and patient positioning

Whenever irrigation and suction of the ear canal is to be performed, the patient must be under general anaesthesia, and should have a properly placed and inflated endotracheal tube to avoid aspiration of exudate and flushing fluids draining through the Eustachian tubes into the nasopharynx, as this might result in aspiration pneumonia (Figure 10.7a).

The anaesthetized patient is placed in lateral or sternal recumbency. A towel can be used to slightly raise the caudal head and the neck in relation to the muzzle; this will allow fluid exiting the tympanic bulla through the auditory tube to flow rostrally and out through the nares when the ear is flushed. The patient's eyes should always be covered with gauze to protect them from flushing solutions containing cleaning agents and pathogens during the procedure (Figure 10.7b). It is also recommended to standardize the orientation of the video-otoscope relative to the position of the animal.

Appropriate pain management is essential when performing video-otoscopy in dogs and cats. This includes anticipatory analgesia, monitoring the patient according to the current pain management guidelines for the species and early intervention if the animal demonstrates signs of pain.

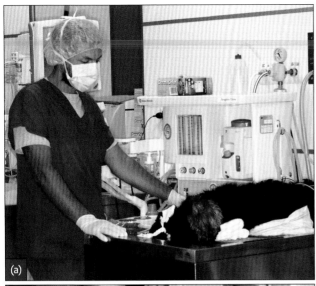

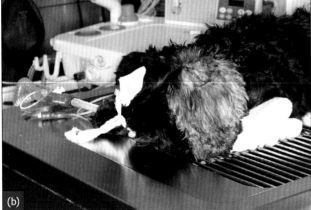

10.7   (a) Patient positioning for an otoscopic examination. The patient under general anaesthesia is positioned in lateral recumbency and properly intubated. (b) Pads have been placed under the neck to slightly raise the caudal portion of the neck, and gauze has been applied over the eye as protection against exudate and washing fluid. (Courtesy of San Marco Veterinary Clinic, Padova, Italy)

Procedure for otoscopy of the external and middle ear

The video-otoscope is inserted into the ear at the inter-tragic incisure. To visualize the entire length of the ear canal up to the level of the tympanic membrane, the ear canal should be straightened to minimize occlusion of the lumen by the cartilage fold at the junction between the vertical and horizontal canals. This is done by pulling the pinna up and outward while inserting the video-otoscope. The otoscope and the pinna must be held straight throughout the examination to maintain complete visualization of the ear canal up to the tympanic region.

Normal findings

On video-otoscopic examination, the normal ear canal of dogs and cats appears pale pink and smooth, with fine blood vessels on its surface (Figure 10.8). Fine hairs are frequently present at the entrance to the external ear canal and may also be present in the vertical and horizontal canals. In

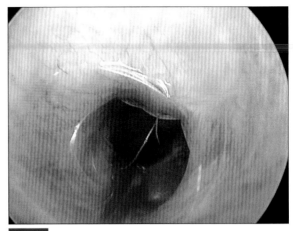

10.8   Normal canine ear canal.

some dogs a tuft of hair is present in front of the tympanic membrane. The diameter of the ear canal and the density of hairs varies between species and between breeds.

A minimal amount of cerumen is present in normal ears and the tympanic membrane is easily identified. In dogs, visualization of the entire tympanic membrane is normally difficult because it forms a 45-degree angle with the horizontal canal. In cats, the tympanic membrane can normally be visualized completely because it is oriented at a 90-degree angle with the ear canal. Using the video-otoscope, both the pars flaccida and the pars tensa of the tympanic membrane are visible (Figure 10.9). The pars flaccida is a small pink region forming the upper quadrant of the tympanic membrane. It contains a fine network of small blood vessels and may appear dilated and prominent in some dogs. It has been suggested that this bulging region may be a product of increased air pressure within the middle ear, most commonly seen in dogs with hypersensitivity disorders. The significance of this observation is not clear. Inexperienced examination of an engorged pars flaccida may result in the mistaken identification of a mass. Alternating inflation and deflation of the pars flaccida can occasionally be observed during video-otoscopy of a normal ear.

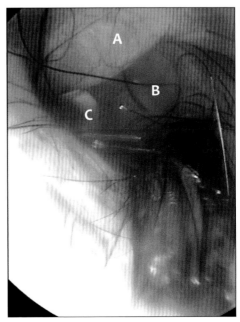

10.9

Normal canine tympanic membrane. A = pars flaccida; B = pars tensa; C = stria mallearis.

The pars tensa is the thin, translucent, tense portion of the tympanic membrane; it constitutes the majority of what is seen of the tympanic membrane when it is examined with the video-otoscope. In a normal ear, the outline of the manubrium of the malleus (the stria mallearis) is visible through the pars tensa. In the dog, the manubrium has a hook that points rostrally. Given this anatomical characteristic, images from the right or left canine ear can be easily distinguished. Blood vessels in the pars tensa may be seen associated with the manubrium, and striations are often visible radiating away from this structure (Figure 10.10). The region of the tympanic membrane overlying the manubrium is reported to be the location of the germinal epithelium in dogs and cats, which is responsible for the healing of a damaged tympanic membrane.

Other structures of the middle ear can occasionally be visualized through a normal tympanic membrane. These structures are the bony ridge that separates the tympanic bulla from the tympanic cavity proper, which appears as a whitish discoloration through the lower to mid-section of the tympanic membrane, and the opening of the tympanic bulla, which can sometimes be seen as a dark area above the bony ridge. For the purposes of this chapter, a brief description of the middle ear anatomy is provided in Figure 10.11.

It is essential that the clinician becomes confident with the normal structures of the ear and their otoscopic appearance before attempting to interpret abnormal findings. 'Practice makes perfect': only with repetition and experience can the practitioner easily recognize and evaluate the different structures of the ear.

Abnormal findings

During the otoscopic examination, the condition of the ear canal should be evaluated. Any foreign bodies or masses should be noted, as should the presence and character of the discharge, and the presence and appearance of the tympanic membrane should be evaluated.

Ear canal

Otitis externa and discharge

During the otoscopic examination, it is very important to evaluate the ear discharge. The amount, consistency and colour of the exudate should be recorded. Although the character of the exudate may suggest an aetiological agent, the practitioner should always confirm their suspicion with appropriate diagnostic tests, such as microscopic and cytological examination of samples of exudate.

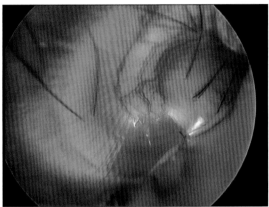

10.10 Blood vessels in the pars tensa associated with the manubrium.

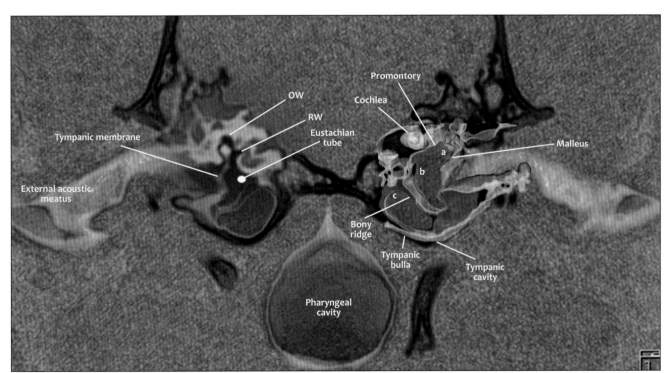

10.11 Middle ear anatomy. Overlay of two-dimensional and three-dimensional CT images of the ear of a dog to emphasize the most relevant structures. The middle ear consists of three parts: the small dorsal epitympanic recess (a), which is occupied almost entirely by the head of the malleus and the incus; the tympanic cavity proper (b), adjacent to the tympanic membrane; and a large ventral cavity within the tympanic bulla (c). On the medial wall of the tympanic cavity proper there is a bony prominence, the promontory, which houses the cochlea. The cochlear (round) window (RW) and the vestibular (oval) window (OW) are located on the caudolateral and dorsolateral surfaces of the promontory, respectively. The Eustachian tube, a short canal that extends from the nasopharynx to the middle ear, opens in the rostral portion of the tympanic cavity proper.
(Courtesy of Dr Bertolini, Diagnostic and Interventional Division, San Marco Veterinary Clinic, Padova, Italy)

After removing the exudate (see Cleaning/flushing procedures, below), the skin surface of the ear canal can be examined. In cases of acute otitis externa, signs of inflammation such as oedema and erythema are evident along the skin surface of the ear canal. Clinically, the swelling caused by the oedema appears as narrowing of the ear canal. Ulceration is commonly observed in cases of bacterial infection, particularly those that are due to rod-shaped bacteria such as *P. aeruginosa*. Progressive histopathological changes occur in chronic otitis externa, which results in stenosis of the ear canal (Figure 10.12). The sebaceous and ceruminous glands may become elongated, producing a multifocal to diffuse nodular dermatosis (Figure 10.13). The subcutaneous tissues thicken as a result of fibrosis and, over time, the auditory cartilages may become calcified. Calcification manifests as a loss of flexibility of the ear canal, which causes difficulty in passing the video-otoscope. There are breed-related differences in the prevalence of histopathological changes in canine chronic otitis externa. In one study, more than 70% of Cocker Spaniels showed a glandular pattern of changes rather than a fibrotic pattern, whereas a glandular pattern was present in only 28% of dogs of the other breeds evaluated (Angus *et al.*, 2002).

Foreign bodies

Foreign bodies may be observed in the ear canal or in the middle ear. Some of the more common foreign bodies include plant awns and impacted wax. Plant awns can be removed using grasping forceps passed through the working channel of the video-otoscope (Video 10.1). Concretions of impacted wax (ceruminoliths) occurring in the absence of inflammation are more common in dogs that have previously been affected by otitis externa. This is possibly because of a decrease in the physiological migration of the epithelium on the lateral surface of the tympanic membrane, leading to the accumulation of cerumen, hairs and cellular detritus (Figure 10.14). Soft and hard wax concretions should be dissolved with a ceruminolytic agent and then gently flushed out of the ear canal (see Cleaning/flushing procedures, below). In some instances, ceruminoliths need to be removed under direct visualization using grasping forceps or an ear brush introduced through the working channel of the video-otoscope. Because these aggregates are frequently attached to the lateral wall of the tympanic membrane, removal may be associated with iatrogenic perforation of the tympanic membrane. It can be helpful to soften the ceruminoliths by applying a ceruminolytic agent for several days before attempting physical removal.

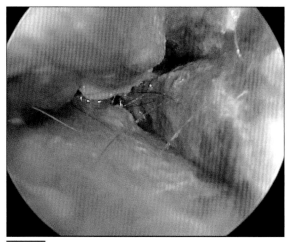

10.12 Stenosis of the ear canal of a dog with chronic otitis externa.

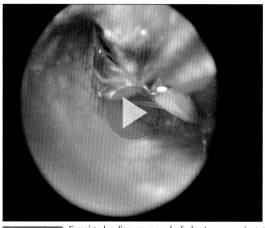

Video 10.1 Foreign bodies: removal of plant awns using grasping forceps passed through the working channel of the video-otoscope.

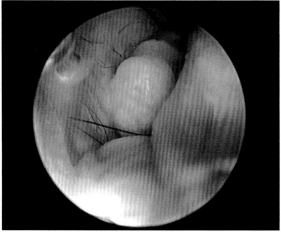

10.13 Glandular proliferation of the horizontal ear canal of a dog with a history of chronic otitis externa.

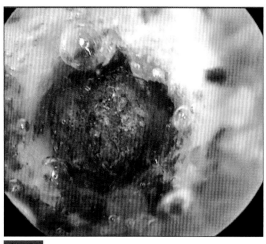

10.14 A hard concretion of wax at the eardrum of a dog.

Masses

Occasionally, during video-otoscopic examination (after proper cleaning of the ear canal) a mass may be observed (Figure 10.15). Any mass in the ear canal should be sampled for histopathological examination using specific instruments passed through the working channel of the video-otoscope. An incisional biopsy can be performed using biopsy forceps in cases where the mass cannot be entirely removed; where it is possible to remove the whole mass, as is often the case for inflammatory polyps in cats, an excisional biopsy can be performed.

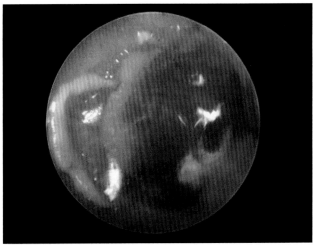

10.16 Inflammatory polyp in a cat. Note the smooth pink to red surface.

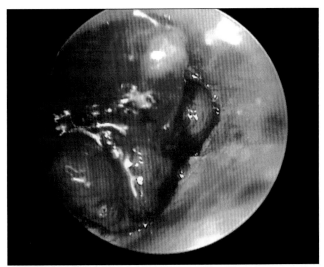

10.15 Mass of neoplastic origin discovered by video-otoscopy in the ear canal of a cat.

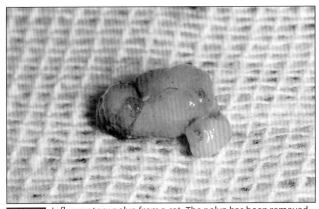

10.17 Inflammatory polyp from a cat. The polyp has been removed using the grasping and traction technique. The presence of a small peduncle at one end of the mass suggests that it has been correctly removed.

Masses in the ear canal can be neoplastic or inflammatory (e.g. inflammatory polyps) in origin. They can arise in the tissues of the ear canal or the middle ear, and may originate in one part of the ear and then progress (from the ear canal to the tympanic cavity, or *vice versa*). More importantly, any proliferative lesion observed in the external or middle ear might also involve the surrounding tissues, including the bony and/or central nervous tissues. Therefore, in addition to diagnostic histopathological examination of biopsy samples, imaging studies to investigate possible middle ear and nasopharyngeal involvement is recommended to establish an appropriate therapeutic approach. This is particularly important in cases where malignant neoplasia is diagnosed histopathologically.

Inflammatory polyps are common in cats. They originate from the middle ear mucosa and can extend into the horizontal canal. They appear as pink to red nodular pedunculated lesions with a smooth surface (Figure 10.16). This presentation is usually characteristic, although inflammatory polyps may sometimes have an irregular and multinodular appearance. Histopathological differentiation from a neoplastic lesion arising from the tympanic bulla is essential. In dogs, true inflammatory polyps arising from the middle ear are uncommon. One of the authors [MDL] has seen several cases of fibroepithelial polyps originating from the external ear in dogs.

Removal of a polyp by traction and avulsion can be attempted during the video-otoscopic examination. The patient is positioned in lateral recumbency and, after thorough cleaning of the ear canal, the polyp is grasped with grasping forceps and removed by firm traction with rotation until it detaches at the stalk (Figure 10.17 and Video 10.2). Alternatively, a polypectomy snare can be

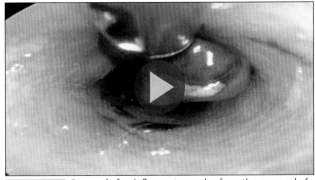

Video 10.2 Removal of an inflammatory polyp from the ear canal of a cat.

used to capture the polyp and cut it as close as possible to the stalk. Where available, laser ablation is another effective technique for the removal of ear polyps (see Chapter 16).

It can be difficult to remove multilobulated polyps because they tend to rupture and bleed. Repeated grasping and traction may be necessary to debulk the mass. In such cases, a portion of the stalk may remain, and this increases the risk of polyp recurrence.

Tympanic membrane

On video-otoscopic examination, the tympanic membrane may appear normal, intact but abnormal, ruptured or completely absent. It may appear opaque, white or grey as the consequence of a persistent inflammation (myringitis) associated with chronic otitis (Figure 10.18). It is not uncommon for the tympanic membrane to be intact in dogs and cats with middle ear otitis. Otoscopic examination of 41 ears with chronic external ear otitis and middle ear otitis showed an intact tympanic membrane in 15% of the cases, while in the remaining cases the tympanic membrane was ruptured (39%) or not visible (34%) (Lorek *et al.*, 2020). This presentation can be the consequence of an external otitis with rupture of the tympanic membrane that healed, trapping microorganisms and exudates in the middle ear, or it can be due to a primary infection of the middle ear caused by the entry of pathogens via the Eustachian tube. This might be the case for feline middle ear otitis associated with *Mycoplasma* spp. colonization or infection (Achermann *et al.*, 2017). In these cases, the tympanic membrane may appear intact but altered in colour, opacity or outline. The tympanic membrane can sometimes have a bulging appearance caused by the presence of fluid in the tympanic cavity (e.g. in cases of infectious otitis media or primary secretory otitis media) (Figure 10.19).

In some cases, where middle ear otitis is present, the tympanic membrane is ruptured (Figure 10.20). It can be difficult to assess the integrity of the tympanic membrane visually, even with the high resolution and magnification provided by the video-otoscope, and so holes or partial tears may not be readily recognized. An easy technique for evaluating the integrity of a visualized but diseased tympanic membrane is to fill the ear canal with sterile saline solution while the patient is placed in lateral recumbency with the suspected ruptured membrane uppermost. The tip of the video-otoscope is then positioned under the fluid, near the membrane. If small perforations are present, air from the tympanic cavity will escape from the middle ear and air bubbles will be seen by the examiner when the animal breathes.

To confirm the absence of the tympanic membrane, the inexperienced examiner should compare the appearance of the diseased ear with the depth and position of the healthy contralateral tympanic membrane. However, if the tympanic membrane is not visualized when the tip of the video-otoscope is advanced as far as possible, it is likely that the membrane is absent. Sometimes, a small ring of granulation tissue may be seen at the annulus fibrosus, where the tympanic membrane attaches to the ear canal (Figure 10.21). When the tympanic membrane is

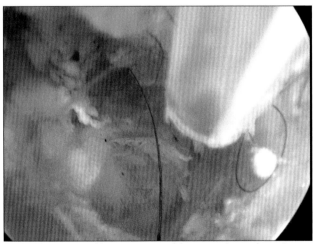

| 10.18 | Opaque, white appearance of the tympanic membrane in a dog with chronic otitis externa. |

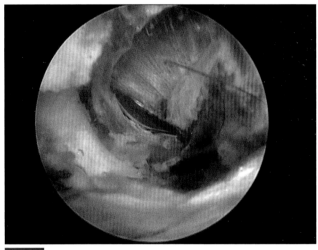

| 10.20 | Rupture of the tympanic membrane in a dog. |

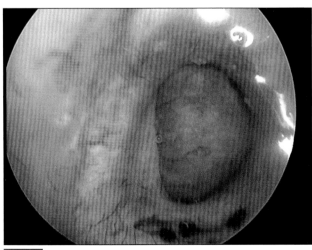

| 10.19 | Bulging appearance of the tympanic membrane in a dog. |

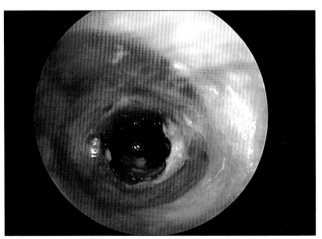

| 10.21 | Otitis media in a dog. Note the absence of the tympanic membrane and the small ring of granulation tissue at the annulus fibrosus. |

absent, the medial wall of the tympanic cavity appears as a dark space at the end of the canal. The mucoperiosteum lining the clean tympanic cavity may occasionally reflect enough light to appear shiny and white; this may be erroneously interpreted as a diseased but intact tympanic membrane. To determine the nature of the structure, a small-diameter soft feeding tube can be gently advanced and directed ventrally towards the observed structure until it stops. If the tympanic membrane is intact, it resists gentle pressure and may distort slightly. If the tympanic membrane is absent, the tip of the tube disappears ventrally into the tympanic bulla. The absence of the tympanic membrane can also be inferred if the fluid used for flushing exits through the nostrils when the ears are flushed.

The practitioner must be aware of a condition described in dogs called 'false middle ear'. In some instances, the examiner may have the impression that the tympanic membrane is absent, when in fact it has been displaced medially into the middle ear cavity. This alteration may develop as a result of two changes that occur simultaneously. The first of these is increased pressure on the tympanic membrane due to obstruction along the horizontal ear canal from inflammation, neoplasia, impacted wax or hypertrophic or cystic glands, which stretches the tympanic membrane so that it bulges into the middle ear cavity. Second, negative pressure inside the tympanic bulla as a result of poor air movement through the Eustachian tube pulls the tympanic membrane even further into the middle ear cavity. This condition is easily recognized on CT imaging, which reveals a 'finger' lesion protruding into the bulla. These patients can also be retrospectively diagnosed at a 2-week recheck after cleaning of the ear canal, when the previously unseen tympanic membrane returns to a normal location. The normal tympanic membrane has been shown experimentally to heal in 21–35 days. Therefore, if the tympanic membrane were truly absent, re-examination 2 weeks later should show the membrane to be still incomplete.

It may be difficult to visualize the tympanic membrane otoscopically in some dogs with chronic otitis externa where the ear canals are stenotic or occluded. The tympanic membrane was visible by routine otoscopic examination in 28%, 40% and 66% of dogs with chronic otitis externa in three different published studies. Other techniques, such as positive-contrast ear canalography and tympanometry, have been used to determine the integrity of the tympanic membrane when it cannot be visualized. Tympanometry uses a sensor that measures the compliance of the tympanic membrane in response to sound waves. It is used frequently in the evaluation of otitis media in human patients, but it has poor sensitivity and specificity in evaluating canine otitis media.

Middle ear

If the tympanic membrane is ruptured or completely absent, an accumulation of whitish or yellow exudate may be observed in the tympanic cavity (Figure 10.22). In the case of cholesteatoma, abundant keratin debris, produced by the stratified squamous epithelium of the lateral wall of the tympanic membrane that migrates into the tympanic cavities, is evident. There may be abnormal tissue in the tympanic cavity, indicating the presence of an inflammatory or neoplastic condition.

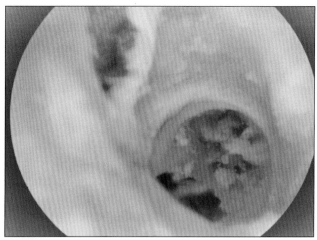

10.22 Tympanic cavity filled with whitish debris in a dog with otitis media.

Cleaning/flushing procedures

After the patient is anaesthetized and imaging studies have been performed (see above), the practitioner may begin the video-otoscopic examination. In many, if not all cases, an ear flush will be necessary before examination is possible. In addition to allowing visualization of the structures within the ear, the ear flush removes exudates and biofilms that cause irritation and promote the persistence of chronic infections; allows sampling from the horizontal canal; and allows sampling and cleaning of the tympanic cavity, either through a ruptured tympanic membrane or after a myringotomy.

All the clinicians involved in ear flushing procedures should wear gloves, a face mask and, ideally, eye protectors to avoid contact with contaminated fluid and aerosols.

Sampling

Samples of exudate from the ear canal for cytological examination should be collected before the cleaning process. Culture and susceptibility testing of the exudate in cases of otitis externa may not be necessary and, if carried out, the results should be interpreted with caution. Different bacterial organisms and different antimicrobial susceptibility patterns have been observed in up to 20% of samples taken from the same site within the external ear canal; in the same study, the findings of cytological examination agreed with culture results in only 68% of case (Graham-Mize *et al.*, 2013). Moreover, the value of bacterial culture results in directing the selection of the most appropriate topical antibiotic treatment has been questioned. A study evaluating the effectiveness of empirical antibiotic treatment of otitis externa associated with *Pseudomonas* infection reported a treatment success rate of 91% despite the reported *in vitro* resistance of the pathogen; these results were considered to be due to the high local concentrations of antibiotics that can usually be achieved with topical therapy (Pye *et al.*, 2013).

With cases of otitis media, bacterial culture and susceptibility testing of samples from the horizontal ear canal and the middle ear should be performed. Different microbial isolates and antimicrobial susceptibility patterns have been reported from the middle ear and the external ear canal of dogs with otitis affecting the external and middle ear.

Preliminary ear cleaning

After samples of exudate have been collected, the ear canal should be filled with a ceruminolytic agent to soften and loosen ear wax, making it easier to remove. A combination of a ceruminolytic and an anti-biofilm agent may be useful when the presence of a biofilm is suspected. Due to the possible ototoxicity of ceruminolytic agents in patients with ruptured tympanic membranes, these products should be completely removed from the ear canal and middle ear by thorough flushing with an inert fluid, such as sterile saline, at the end of the procedure. The use of ceruminolytic agents in cats is not recommended, as cats are very sensitive to ototoxic effects and may show neurological side effects. There are many ear-cleaning preparations on the market and the clinician should choose the most appropriate product based on the characteristics of the exudate. For ears with mild waxy exudates or deposits, products containing propylene glycol are suitable. Hard waxy secretions are broken down better with an oily squalene-based preparation (Figure 10.23); this organic oil is relatively safe and unlikely to cause ototoxicity. When a purulent exudate is present in the ear, a ceruminolytic surfactant such as dioctyl sodium sulphosuccinate is probably the best option (Figure 10.24).

Products containing foaming agents such as urea and carbamide peroxides are quite potent, and should be reserved for tenacious secretions and when biofilm is suspected.

After the ceruminolytic agent has been instilled and enough time allowed for it to act, a flushing solution is used to remove it, and the loosened waxy secretions, from the ear. An ear bulb syringe (or alternatively a Spruells needle and syringe) filled with sterile isotonic (0.9%) saline or warm water can be used to dislodge large amounts of debris, gently flushing the ear until the solution that runs out is relatively clean. The bulb syringe should never completely occlude the ear canal; a gap should be left between the nozzle and the wall of the canal because complete occlusion may cause excessive fluid pressure and iatrogenic rupture of a weakened tympanic membrane. Once most of the exudate has been removed, ear cleaning may continue using a three-way tap connected to a syringe, a saline supply and a urinary catheter, tomcat catheter or feeding tube of an appropriate length and diameter. The authors prefer to use a feeding tube because it is softer and will cause less trauma if it comes into contact with a damaged tympanic membrane. The catheter/tube tip is placed at the level of the tympanic membrane under otoscopic visualization and the ear canal is flushed and suctioned until completely clean. The ear should be examined with the video-otoscope at this point, and further flushing can be performed if needed.

Flushing

A relatively simple technique of suctioning and flushing with the video-otoscopy system involves the use of a three-way tap connected to a long polypropylene catheter and two 20 ml syringes, one for flushing and the other for suctioning. The operator advances the catheter through the working channel of the video-otoscope until the tip is visible in the video field and directs it towards the remaining exudates. Flushing can be performed by an assistant, who fills one syringe with saline, attaches it to the three-way tap and empties the syringe in short pulses through the catheter. The operator can move the tip of the catheter within the ear canal to target tenacious debris. The fluid is then suctioned out using the second syringe. Several cycles of flushing and suctioning are generally needed to remove all debris from the ear canal (Videos 10.3 and 10.4). If available, a VETPUMP® 2 (see Figure 10.2) automatic suction/irrigation system allows a more accurate and controlled cleaning procedure.

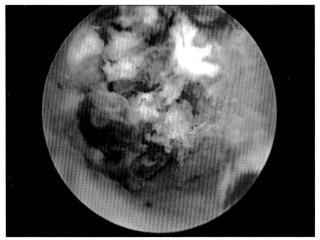

10.23 Hard waxy secretions in the ear of a dog with ceruminous otitis externa.

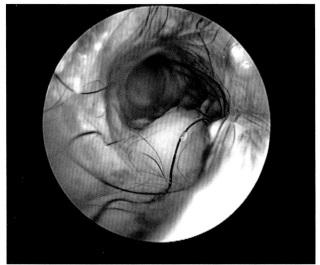

10.24 Purulent exudates in the ear of a dog with *Pseudomonas aeruginosa* infection.

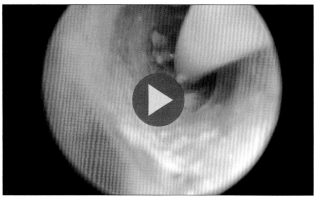

Video 10.3 Flushing technique: flushing and suctioning cycles in the external ear canal of a dog with otitis externa.

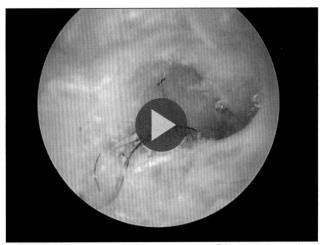

Video 10.4 Flushing technique: appearance of the intact tympanic membrane after the flushing procedure.

Hairs or other debris that is not dislodged by flushing may be removed with instruments such as brushes, grasping forceps or ear curettes specifically designed for use with the video-otoscope. Although the tip of the video-otoscope can be advanced only as far as the level of the tympanic membrane, the catheter can be advanced further, into the bulla, if the tympanic membrane is absent. Samples of material from the middle ear for diagnostic investigations should be obtained before middle ear flushing. When the tympanic membrane is absent or spontaneously ruptured, samples from the middle ear can be obtained with the tube technique. This technique utilizes an open-ended sterile urinary catheter, a 3.5 Fr tomcat catheter or a polypropylene catheter attached to a syringe and passed through the working channel of the video-otoscope. Under visualization, the operator passes the tip ventrally into the tympanic bulla while applying gentle suction with the syringe. If necessary, 1 ml of sterile saline can be flushed into the middle ear cavity and then aspirated, to help collect samples where there is very little exudate, or where there is thick material in the cavity. The tube is then removed from the working channel and disconnected from the syringe. In some cases, only a small amount of material, entrapped in the tip of the tube, is collected. In these cases, the syringe is filled with air and re-attached to the tube, and the material is expressed.

Part of the material collected should be cultured and part processed for cytological examination. The role of anaerobic bacteria in recurrent otitis externa and otitis media is unknown. However, there are some reports of the isolation of anaerobic bacteria from the horizontal ear canal and tympanic cavity of dogs with otitis media undergoing total ear canal ablation or lateral bulla osteotomy (Hettlich *et al.*, 2005). Therefore, both aerobic and anaerobic cultures are recommended in cases of infectious otitis media.

If the tympanic membrane is intact but the index of suspicion for otitis media is high (because of compatible clinical signs, an abnormal tympanic membrane or compatible results of imaging studies) a myringotomy should be performed for diagnostic and therapeutic purposes.

Myringotomy

Myringotomy, a deliberate focal rupture of the tympanic membrane to allow collection of material from the middle ear and, in some cases, to administer treatment, can be performed using either a hand-held otoscope or a video-otoscope. However, the video-otoscopy system is better, as it allows continuous visualization and accurate positioning for the procedure. It is very important to identify the correct site for performing the myringotomy incision. The incision must be made in the caudoventral portion of the pars tensa (at 6–7 o'clock or 5–6 o'clock depending on which ear is being subjected to the procedure) to avoid damaging the tympanic germinal epithelium and the structures of the middle ear, such as the ossicles or the cochlear promontory (Figure 10.25), as well as iatrogenic damage to nerves arborising across the pars tensa in cats. Turning the otoscope upside down so the light guide cable is dorsal, with the camera maintained in the same position, will ensure that the opening of the instrument channel is ventral in the horizontal canal, and this will help with correct positioning for the incision.

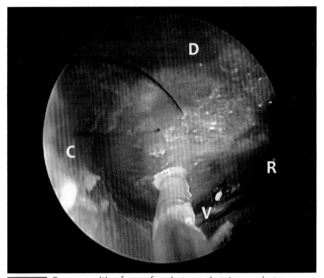

10.25 Proper position for performing a myringotomy using an open-ended tomcat catheter. The incision is made in the caudoventral portion of the pars tensa (at 6–7 o'clock). C = caudal; D = dorsal; R = rostral; V = ventral.

After thorough cleaning and drying of the ear canal, a flexible myringotomy needle provided with an outer tube, or a 3.5 Fr tomcat catheter or a polypropylene catheter selected according to the length of the ear canal, is placed through the working channel of the video-otoscope. When using a myringotomy needle, the needle is used to make an incision and then the outer tube is pushed into the middle ear. The needle is then removed, and material from the middle ear is collected by connecting a syringe to the tube. When using a catheter, the tip is cut at an angle to make it sharper, and the tip is then used to make the incision (Video 10.5). After the tip of the catheter has passed through the tympanic membrane into the middle ear, material can be collected using a syringe as described above.

To facilitate the sampling procedure, 1 ml of sterile saline solution can be infused into the bulla and then aspirated. The fluid obtained is then used to make cytological preparations and for culture and sensitivity testing. When a biofilm-associated infection is suspected, cytology can be used to look for bacterial aggregates and to select the most representative sample for bacterial culture and sensitivity testing. After sample collection, the tympanic cavity should be gently flushed using sterile saline instilled by a catheter introduced through the myringotomy incision and directed ventrally, until the fluid that is aspirated is clear.

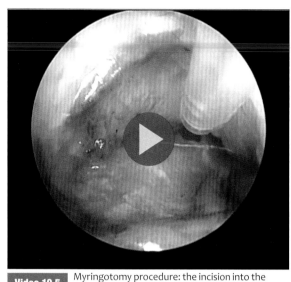

Video 10.5 Myringotomy procedure: the incision into the caudoventral quadrant of the pars tensa is made with a 3.5 Fr tomcat catheter.

Myringotomy is recommended in cases of primary secretory otitis media where manual removal of the mucoid effusion from the tympanic cavity and the administration of topical glucocorticoids is required and secondary secretory otitis seen in cats associated with ascending infection from the nasopharynx via the eustachian tubes. The insertion of tympanostomy tubes to provide continual ventilation and drainage of the tympanic cavity has been proposed in Cavalier King Charles Spaniels with primary secretory otitis media, but as yet there is insufficient evidence to recommend this procedure as an alternative to repeated myringotomy for the treatment of this condition.

Myringotomy can also be successfully performed using diode lasers. As discussed elsewhere in this text, diode lasers using a fiberoptic delivery system can be employed for a variety of surgical procedures. Lasers of both 980 nm and 810 nm have successfully been employed in performing therapeutic myringotomy in both dogs and cats.

Under otoendoscopic guidance, the laser fibre is used to incise the bulging tympanum in a cruciate pattern, from the cranio-dorsal aspect to the caudo-ventral aspect, and then in the reverse manner. This provides excellent drainage of the middle ear. As one of the great frustrations in aural surgery is early closure of the incised tympanum, the use of thermal energy associated with the diode laser provides some degree of delayed healing, which, in this case, is advantageous in allowing a longer period of patency and, as such, a longer period of therapeutic drainage (Sobel, 2017) .

Biofilm-related infections

The critical role of bacteria in the pathogenesis of external and middle ear otitis has long been acknowledged. The mechanisms through which bacteria promote recurrence or persistence of the disease have not yet been completely unravelled. However, recently the possible role of biofilms in chronic ear infections has been highlighted.

What is a biofilm?

The term 'biofilm' refers to a community of bacteria that lives in an extracellular polymer matrix composed of poly-saccharides, DNA and proteins. This matrix allows them to survive even in the presence of high concentrations of antibiotics. The common mechanisms of antibiotic resistance, such as efflux pumps, modifying enzymes and target mutations, do not seem to be responsible for the protective effect of a biofilm; even bacteria that do not carry any of the known genes for antibiotic resistance can have a profoundly reduced susceptibility to antibiotics when they form a biofilm. Biofilms generally inhibit or delay the penetration of antimicrobials, resulting in a considerable decrease in the antimicrobial concentration to which the bacteria in the biofilm will be exposed. This in turn leads to the survival of the more resistant strains within the community, and these strains will be responsible for treatment failure and recrudescence of the infection.

Although this mechanism clearly plays an important role in the inability of antibiotics to fully eradicate biofilm-forming bacteria, there must be other mechanisms involved. For example, experimental studies have shown that fluoroquinolones are unable to eradicate biofilms, even though these antibiotics can easily diffuse throughout the biofilm matrix (Pye *et al.*, 2013). In this case, the presence of a subpopulation of tolerant bacteria, termed 'persister cells', has been suggested as the reason for the biofilm's resistance to antibiotics. Once antibiotic treatment is withdrawn, persister cells 'hiding' in the matrix can resume growth and repopulate the biofilm, causing recurrence of the infection. Strains of *P. aeruginosa* and *S. pseudintermedius* isolated from cases of otitis in dogs have been shown to be capable of producing biofilms. Data from *in vitro* studies indicate that the minimum inhibitory concentrations (MICs) for biofilm-embedded bacteria are significantly higher than those for their planktonic (free-living) counterparts (Lebeaux *et al.*, 2014).

Diagnosis of the presence of biofilm in otitis

It can be difficult to identify biofilms in clinical samples owing to their small size (4–200 μm in tissues). In human medicine, direct microscopic examination with fluorescence *in situ* hybridization (FISH) and immunostaining are used to identify biofilms in mucosal specimens from the middle ear. More recently, optical coherence tomography, a high-resolution, real-time biomedical imaging technology, has been proposed as a non-invasive method to detect the presence of biofilm *in vivo* in human patients with chronic otitis media. These techniques are not yet routinely available in veterinary medicine. Thus, when the presence of biofilm is suspected on the basis of previous antibiotic treatment failures and recurrence of the infection, cytology should be used to look for the presence of bacterial aggregates. These aggregates have been suggested as a valid indicator of the possible presence of biofilm, especially with *P. aeruginosa* infections (where aggregates are 8–40 μm in size) (Figure 10.26) (Griffin *et al.*, 2017). Interestingly, some microorganisms in bio-films may be viable but cannot be cultured in routine culture media, which may explain discrepancies between the results of cytology and culture. Culture-independent methods (e.g. polymerase chain reaction) should be used in such circumstances. Since neither culture nor culture-independent techniques can distinguish between biofilm-located and planktonic microorganisms, the clinician must rely on microscopic detection of microbial aggregates located in a matrix for the identification of biofilms.

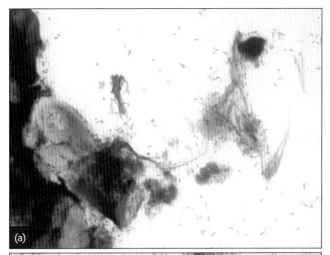

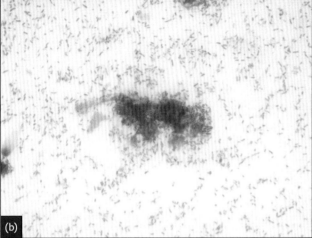

10.26 Ear cytology of a dog with *Pseudomonas* otitis. (a) Numerous planktonic bacteria (rods) are present in the smear. (b) Probable biofilm formation. Note the aggregate of bacteria.

Management of biofilm-related infection in the ear

Biofilms in the ear canal can be physically broken up and partially removed by extensive flushing and aspiration. Several products have been shown to be useful in the management of biofilms, particularly Tris-EDTA (tromethamine), colloidal silver and topical and systemic *N*-acetylcysteine (NAC). The results of a recent *in vitro* study have shown that Tris-EDTA may be a useful adjunctive treatment for chronic *Pseudomonas* otitis where biofilms may have developed if topical gentamicin or neomycin has been used (Pye *et al.*, 2014).

NAC has important mucolytic and antibacterial properties, and has been shown to inhibit the formation of *P. aeruginosa* biofilms. Clinical trials in humans and a recent systematic literature review (Dinicola *et al.*, 2014) have suggested that NAC might be useful as an adjuvant treatment to remove bacterial biofilms, with an excellent safety and efficacy profile. NAC has also been shown in an *in vitro* study to have inhibitory activity against clinically relevant and drug-resistant bacteria associated with canine otitis externa.

In dogs, systemic administration of NAC is well tolerated and can help to dissolve biofilm in the middle ear when otitis media is present. The initial dose of NAC is 140 mg/kg as a 5% solution, injected intravenously or administered orally (diluted in 5% dextrose or sterile water)

(Viviano *et al.*, 2013). Giving NAC by intravenous injection avoids the risk of losing the medication due to vomiting or gastrointestinal upset, which is a common side effect when the drug is given orally. The initial dose is followed by maintenance doses of 70 mg/kg administered orally four times a day for seven or more treatments. NAC can also be administered topically after the ear canal has been cleaned in cases where a biofilm is suspected. A 1–2% solution of NAC is instilled in the ear canal and left for 2 minutes, then rinsed out with Tris-EDTA, before instilling a topical antibiotic.

Postoperative care

Oral glucocorticoid therapy started before the video-otoscopic examination is normally continued after the procedure to reduce inflammation and pain. The duration of glucocorticoid therapy depends on the type of ear disease and its severity. For acute disease in which the primary cause of the inflammation has been removed (e.g. foreign body) or medically controlled (e.g. ear mites), a few days on a once-daily dose of glucocorticoids is sufficient before discontinuation. On the other hand, systemic glucocorticoids may be used for a few weeks in cases of otitis externa with secondary otitis media. As well as controlling the inflammation and pain associated with ear disease, glucocorticoids may reduce the amount of mucus produced in the bulla and its viscosity; changing the quality of the mucus in this way aids in its removal. Glucocorticoids may also reduce swelling of the auditory tube wall, increasing the drainage of mucus from the middle ear into the nasopharynx. Prednisone or prednisolone is often administered orally at a dose of 1–2 mg/kg once a day for 2 weeks, then decreased to 0.5 mg/kg every other day until discontinuation.

Successful medical management of infectious otitis media may require long-term (6–8 weeks) antibiotic treatment. Systemic antibiotics should be selected based on the results of culture and sensitivity tests, and used in combination with topical antimicrobial therapy. However, empirical antibiotic treatment should be started soon after the video-otoscopic procedure, based on the results of cytology, while waiting for the culture and sensitivity test results. The systemic treatment can be modified accordingly once the results of the tests are known. Selection of an antimicrobial agent based on the results of susceptibility tests that measure the MIC or the use of maximal doses of oral antibiotics may increase the therapeutic success rate. However, the efficacy of systemic antimicrobials to treat otitis media may be lower than would be expected on the basis of the test results, due to the low concentrations of antibiotics that reach the middle ear via the bloodstream. Direct application of antibiotics into the middle ear can overcome this problem as they achieve a higher concentration at the site of infection. Therefore, topical antibiotic treatment alone following thorough lavage of the tympanic bulla has been suggested as a suitable treatment. However, some experts still consider the combination of systemic and topical therapy to be the best option in cases of middle ear otitis.

There are several techniques for supplying topical antibiotics into the bulla. Gotthelf (2004) described the application of 1 ml of an aqueous solution containing non-toxic antibiotics directly on to the infected muco-periosteum through a small catheter placed into the bulla. Most of the topical antibiotic solution will remain within the bulla for several days after infusion; however, the entire procedure of flushing, suctioning and bulla infusion should be repeated weekly during the course of therapy. Other clinicians have recommended performing lavage of the tympanic bulla under video-otoscopic guidance once, followed by application into the ear canal of 1–2 ml of an aqueous solution of the antibiotic every 12 hours plus application of a relatively large volume (2–4 ml) of an antiseptic solution at least every 48 hours; this treatment can be administered at home by the owner. Application of this volume of aqueous solution should cause continuous flushing of the tympanic bulla as long as the tympanic membrane is perforated. However, neither clinical evidence nor an expert consensus has been published regarding the utility of such frequent lavage or the most appropriate protocol to use. Two of the authors [LO and FS] prefer to use an antimicrobial solution such as Tris-EDTA to dilute antibiotics and to flush the ear canal and tympanic bulla; some people use depot silver ointments/solutions for *Pseudomonas* infections as a post-procedure option. For further discussion of therapeutic options, the reader is referred to articles on infectious otitis media listed in the References and further reading.

In cases of infectious otitis media, therapy can be discontinued only when weekly examination reveals no signs of inflammation in the ear canal and the results of cytological examination are negative for the presence of micro-organisms and inflammatory cells. At this point, regular monthly rechecks are recommended. Complete healing of the tympanic membrane should not be regarded as a criterion indicating a cure, because in some cases the tympanic membrane may not regenerate (e.g. if the germinal epithelium is damaged or the vascular supply supplied by the pars flaccida is impaired).

Complications

Complications of video-otoscopy are mainly those caused by ear flushing and myringotomy. These problems are infrequent in dogs but common in cats. Pain and head shaking after the procedure may be seen as a result of aggressive flushing and inadequate analgesia. Neurological signs may be a consequence of mechanical trauma from instruments used to clean the middle ear, or high fluid pressure on the nerves in or in close proximity to the middle ear. These signs may include enophthalmos, ptosis, miosis and protrusion of the nictitating membrane (Horner's syndrome), or a drooped lip and ear, inability to close the eyelid and a decreased palpebral reflex (facial nerve injury). Severe neurological signs such as head tilt, loss of balance and circling (vestibular syndrome) and deafness may be seen after overly aggressive irrigation of the tympanic cavities or the use of ototoxic agents that are not removed appropriately from the ear.

Fortunately, most complications are transient, but owners should be made aware that complications may occur and that some of them may be permanent. For these reasons, ear flushing should never be done in a patient that is under anaesthesia for another purpose without the owner's written consent. The owner should also be informed of the need for myringotomy to evaluate and treat middle ear disease in many cases. On the other hand, the owner should be made aware that complications similar to those associated with video-otoscopic procedures may also arise from untreated ear disease.

References and further reading

Ackermann AL, Lenz, JA, May ER and Frank LA (2017) Mycoplasma infection of the middle ear in three cats. *Veterinary Dermatology* **28**, 417–e102

Angus JC, Lichtensteiger C, Campbell KL and Schaeffer DJ (2002) Breed variations in histopathologic features of chronic severe otitis externa in dogs: 80 cases (1995–2001). *Journal of the American Veterinary Medical Association* **221**, 1000–1006

Bischoff MG and Kneller SK (2004) Diagnostic imaging of the canine and feline ear. *The Veterinary Clinics of North America. Small Animal Practice* **34**, 437–458

Bjarnsholt T, Alhede M, Alhede M et al. (2013) The in vivo biofilm. *Trends in Microbiology* **21**, 466–474

Classen J, Bruehschwein A, Meyer-Lindenberg A and Mueller RS (2016) Comparison of ultrasound imaging and video otoscopy with cross-sectional imaging for the diagnosis of canine otitis media. *The Veterinary Journal* **217**, 68–67

Cole LK (2004) Otoscopic evaluation of the ear canal. *Veterinary Clinics of North America: Small Animal Practice* **34**, 397–410

Cole LK, Kwochka KW, Hillier A, Kowalski JJ and Smeak DD (2005) Comparison of bacterial organisms and their susceptibility patterns from otic exudate and ear tissue from the vertical ear canal of dogs undergoing a total ear canal ablation. *Veterinary Therapeutics* **6**, 252–259

Cole LK, Kwochka KW, Kowalski JJ and Hillier A (1998) Microbial flora and antimicrobial susceptibility patterns of isolated pathogens from the horizontal ear canal and middle ear in dogs with otitis media. *Journal of the American Veterinary Medical Association* **212**, 534–538

Cole LK, Samii VF, Wagner SO and Rajala-Schultz PJ (2015) Diagnosis of primary secretory otitis media in the Cavalier King Charles Spaniel. *Veterinary Dermatology* **26**, 459–466

Corfield GS, Burrows AK, Imani P and Bryden SL (2008) The method of application and short term results of tympanostomy tubes for the treatment of primary secretory otitis media in three Cavalier King Charles Spaniel dogs. *Australian Veterinary Journal* **86**, 88–94

Dinicola S, De Grazia S, Carlomagno G and Pintucci JP (2014) N-acetylcysteine as powerful molecule to destroy bacterial biofilms. A systematic review. *European Review for Medical Pharmacological Sciences* **18**, 2942–2948

Doust R, King A, Hammond G et al. (2007) Assessment of middle ear disease in the dog: a comparison of diagnostic imaging modalities. *Journal of Small Animal Practice* **48**, 188–192

Epstein ME, Rodan I, Griffenhagen G et al. (2015) 2015 AAHA/AAFP Pain Management Guidelines for Dogs and Cats. *Journal of Feline Medicine and Surgery* **17**, 251–272

Garosi LS, Dennis R and Schwarz T (2003) Review of diagnostic imaging of ear diseases in the dog and cat. *Veterinary Radiology & Ultrasound* **44**, 137–146

Gortel K (2004) Otic flushing. *Veterinary Clinics of North America: Small Animal Practice* **34**, 557–565

Gotthelf LN (2004) Diagnosis and treatment of otitis media in dogs and cats. *Veterinary Clinics of North America: Small Animal Practice* **34**, 469–487

Graham-Mize CA and Rosser EJ Jr (2004) Comparison of microbial isolates and susceptibility patterns from the external ear canal of dogs with otitis externa. *Journal of the American Animal Hospital Association* **40**, 102–108

Griffin CE (2006) Otitis techniques to improve practice. *Clinical Techniques in Small Animal Practice* **21**, 96–105

Griffin C and Aniya J (2017) Otitis controversies. In: *Advances in Veterinary Dermatology, Volume 8*, eds. S Torres and P Roudebush, Wiley Blackwell

Hall-Stoodley L, Hu FZ, Gieseke A et al. (2006) Direct detection of bacterial biofilms on the middle-ear mucosa of children with chronic otitis media. *Journal of the American Medical Association* **296**, 202–211

Hettlich BE, Boothe HW, Simpson RB et al. (2005) Effect of tympanic cavity evacuation and flushing on microbial isolates during total ear canal ablation with lateral bulla osteotomy in dogs. *Journal of the American Veterinary Medical Association* **227**, 748–755

Jones WS (2006) Video otoscopy: bringing otoscopy out of the 'black box'. *International Journal of Pediatric Otorhinolaryngology* **70**, 1875–1883

Lebeaux D, Ghigo JM and Beloin C (2014) Biofilm-related infections: bridging the gap between clinical management and fundamental aspects of recalcitrance toward antibiotics. *Microbiology and Molecular Biology Reviews* **78**, 510–543

Lewis K (2008) Multidrug tolerance of biofilms and persister cells. *Current Topics in Microbiology and Immunology* **322**, 107–131

Little CJ, Lane JG, Gibbs C and Pearson GR (1991) Inflammatory middle ear disease of the dog: the clinical and pathological features of cholesteatoma, a complication of otitis media. *Veterinary Record* **128**, 319–322

Lorek A, Dennis R, van Dijk J et al. (2020) Occult otitis media in dogs with chronic otitis externa – magnetic resonance imaging and association with otoscopic and cytological findings. *Veterinary Dermatology* **31**, 146–e28.

May ER, Conklin KA and Bemis DA (2016) Antibacterial effect of N-acetylcysteine on common canine otitis externa isolates. *Veterinary Dermatology* **27**, 188–e47

Mielke B, Lam R and ter Haar G (2017) Computed tomographic morphometry of tympanic bulla shape and position in brachycephalic and mesaticephalic dog breeds. *Veterinary Radiology and Ultrasound* **58**, 552–558

Morris DO (2004) Medical therapy of otitis externa and otitis media. *Veterinary Clinics of North America: Small Animal Practice* **34**, 541–555

Nguyen CT, Jung W, Kim J et al. (2012) Noninvasive in vivo optical detection of biofilm in the human middle ear. *Proceedings of the National Academy of Sciences of the United States of America* **109**, 9529–9534

Nuttall T and Cole LK (2004) Ear cleaning: the UK and US perspective. *Veterinary Dermatology* **15**, 127–136

O'Neill DG, Church DB, McGreevy PD *et al.* (2014) Prevalence of disorders recorded in dogs attending primary-care veterinary practices in England. *PLoS ONE* **9**, e90501

O'Neill DG, Romans C, Brodbelt DC *et al.* (2019) Persian cats under first opinion veterinary care in the UK: demography, mortality and disorders. *Scientific Reports* **9**, 12952

Palmeiro BS, Morris DO, Wiemelt SP and Shofer FS (2004) Evaluation of outcome of otitis media after lavage of the tympanic bulla and long-term antimicrobial drug treatment in dogs: 44 cases (1998–2002). *Journal of the American Veterinary Medical Association* **225**, 548–553

Pye CC, Singh A and Weese JS (2014) Evaluation of the impact of tromethamine edetate disodium dihydrate on antimicrobial susceptibility of Pseudomonas aeruginosa in biofilm in vitro. *Veterinary Dermatology* **25**, 120–e34

Pye CC, Yu AA and Weese JS (2013) Evaluation of biofilm production by *Pseudomonas aeruginosa* from canine ears and the impact of biofilm on antimicrobial susceptibility in vitro. *Veterinary Dermatology* **24**, 446–449

Remedios AM, Fowler GD and Pharr JW (1991) A comparison of radiographic *versus* surgical diagnosis of otitis media. *Journal of the American Animal Hospital Association* **27**, 183–188

Rohleder JJ, Jones JC, Duncan RB *et al.* (2006) Comparative performance of radiography and computed tomography in the diagnosis of middle ear disease in 31 dogs. *Veterinary Radiology & Ultrasound* **47**, 45–52

Salgüero R, Herrtage M, Holmes M *et al.* (2016) Comparison between computed tomographic characteristics of the middle ear in nonbrachycephalic and brachycephalic dogs with obstructive airway syndrome. *Veterinary Radiology & Ultrasound* **57**, 137–143

Sobel D (2017) Otoscopy, ear flushing and myringotomy. In: *Textbook of Veterinary Internal Medicine, 8th edn*, ed. SJ Ettinger *et al.* pp. 339–347, Elsevier, Philadelphia

Spoering AL and Lewis K (2001) Biofilms and planktonic cells of *Pseudomonas aeruginosa* have similar resistance to killing by antimicrobials. *Journal of Bacteriology* **183**, 6746–6751

Stern-Bertholtz W, Sjöström L and Håkanson NW (2003) Primary secretory otitis media in the Cavalier King Charles Spaniel: a review of 61 cases. *Journal of Small Animal Practice* **44**, 253–256

Trower ND, Gregory SP, Renfrew H and Lamb CR (1998) Evaluation of the canine tympanic membrane by positive contrast ear canalography. *Veterinary Record* **142**, 78–81

Viviano KR and VanderWielen B (2013) Effect of *N*-acetylcysteine supplementation on intracellular glutathione, urine isoprostanes, clinical score, and survival in hospitalized ill dogs. *Journal of Veterinary Internal Medicine* **27**, 250–258

Zhao T and Liu Y (2010) *N*-acetylcysteine inhibit biofilms produced by *Pseudomonas aeruginosa*. *BMC Microbiology* **10**, 140

Video extras

- **Video 10.1** Foreign bodies: removal of plant awns using grasping forceps passed through the working channel of the video-otoscope
- **Video 10.2** Removal of an inflammatory polyp from the ear canal of a cat
- **Video 10.3** Flushing technique: flushing and suctioning cycles in the external ear canal of a dog with otitis externa
- **Video 10.4** Flushing technique: appearance of the intact tympanic membrane after the flushing procedure
- **Video 10.5** Myringotomy procedure: the incision into the caudoventral quadrant of the pars tensa is made with a 3.5 Fr tomcat catheter

Access via QR code or: bsavalibrary.com/endoscopy2e_10

Chapter 11

Rigid endoscopy: urethrocystoscopy and vaginoscopy

Julie K. Byron and Gary C.W. England

Introduction

Endoscopic examination of the lower urinary tract and reproductive tract can be an important part of the diagnostic evaluation and treatment of a number of disorders in dogs and cats. The female urinary tract of both species is usually examined using rigid endoscopy, which allows direct visualization of the vestibule, urethra, bladder and vagina. Because of its long and tortuous anatomy, the urinary tract of the male dog is examined with flexible endoscopy, although some procedures are performed using a surgical perineal approach and percutaneous cystoscopy of the bladder is performed through a transabdominal approach. Endoscopic evaluation of the lower urinary tract of the male cat is particularly challenging, due to the very narrow urethra, and is rarely performed except via a percutaneous transabdominal approach. Over the past 15 years, a range of interventional procedures has been developed to address a variety of conditions of the lower urinary tract, including ectopic ureter, urethral sphincter mechanism incompetence, urolithiasis and neoplasia (see Chapter 16).

Instrumentation

Rigid and flexible endoscopes may be used to perform urethrocystoscopy and vaginoscopy. Rigid cystoscopes consist of three parts: a telescope, a sheath and a bridge. These may be separate components or integrated by the manufacturer. The glass fibre telescope provides an angled view of 0, 12, 30 or 70 degrees from the tip of the scope. The authors prefer to use a 30-degree telescope, as it allows all areas of the bladder to be visualized with less manipulation, as well as good visualization of the working field when using instruments (Figure 11.1). The sheath contains the irrigation and operating channels, and the bridge has the light source and camera connections as well as the instrument port (Figure 11.2). Some smaller endoscopes have the bridge and sheath integrated into one piece. Rigid endoscope systems are available in a variety of diameters and lengths. For urethrocystoscopy of small animals, three telescope sizes are generally recommended: 4.0 mm x 30 cm for medium to large bitches, 2.7 mm x 18 cm for small and medium bitches, and 1.9 mm x 18 cm for very small bitches and queens, and for male cats with a perineal urethrostomy.

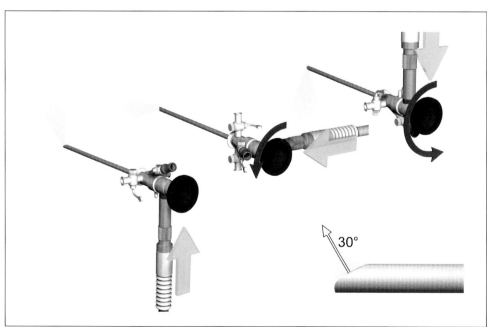

11.1 Artist's rendition of the view through a telescope with a 30-degree viewing angle by rotating the endoscope along its longitudinal access, keeping the camera head fixed and rotating, using the light guide cable.
(Drawing by Tim Vojt. Reproduced with the permission of The Ohio State University)

30°

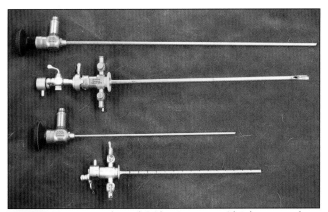

11.2 Two commonly used rigid cystoscopes with telescope and accompanying sheath. The upper scope is a 4.0 mm diameter x 30 cm telescope with a separate sheath and bridge (shown assembled), and the lower one is a 2.7 mm x 18 cm telescope with an integrated sheath and bridge.
(Reproduced with the permission of The Ohio State University)

A flexible or semi-flexible 5 Fr endoscope may be used to examine the urethra of male cats; however, these instruments have only a fluid infusion port and are not equipped with an instrument channel. Male dogs with urethras that will accommodate an 8–10 Fr catheter can be examined using a flexible 7.5–9.5 Fr x 45 cm human ureteroscope or a flexible endoscope of similar size.

A large variety of accessories and instruments are available for use with rigid endoscopes. At least one high-quality biopsy forceps that fits through the operating channel is required for obtaining tissue samples. In addition, stone retrieval baskets, grasping forceps to retrieve stone fragments and foreign bodies, and cautery tips are available (Figure 11.3).

The care of uroendoscopic equipment is similar to that of any other endoscope. Rigid endoscopes are relatively durable; however, the small size of many of the instruments makes them especially fragile and the glass fibres within them can be broken if they are subjected to fulcrum forces. Caution must be exercised to prevent over-flexion of the flexible instruments, and the use of excessive force when deploying and retracting them must be avoided. This is most likely to occur when levering the telescope against the pubis to improve visualization of the ventral aspect of the bladder. It is safer to have an assistant gently place external pressure on the ventral aspect of the bladder to bring it into the visual field rather than to angle the telescope excessively. The very small flexible and semi-flexible endoscopes are also extremely fragile and need additional protection during cleaning and sterilization.

Rigid endoscope systems require a light source, a camera head, camera control unit, a video monitor and preferably an image capture system that allows data to be stored on a hard drive or DVD. There are several manufacturers of these systems, and they are often purchased as part of a package with the endoscopes. Some incompatibilities exist between different systems, so it is best to use components from the same manufacturer or verify their compatibility before purchase.

The best light sources for video-uroendoscopy are xenon with automatic or manual intensity adjustment. Although many rigid and flexible endoscopes have eye-pieces, a camera and video system are essential for proper detailed viewing and documentation of uroendoscopic studies. Cameras are generally available in one- or three-chip models, and now high definition (HD). Three-chip models have better image quality because they have three-colour capture and processing, and produce better images in low-light conditions; however, one-chip models are adequate for most applications. Ideally, the camera should have a focusing system and image capture controls mounted on the operating head, although some cameras have foot-pedal operation. A wide range of image capture systems are available, from state-of-the-art HD video to those that record still images only. Since dynamic imaging is desirable in uroendoscopy, a system that can capture and record both still images and video clips is preferable.

Clinical history

Urethrocystoscopy in the dog and cat may be performed for a variety of reasons (Figure 11.4). The procedure allows the clinician to visually assess the urethra, ureteric openings and bladder in all patients, as well as the prostatic urethra in the male dog and the vestibule and vagina in the bitch and queen.

Dysuria is a common indication for urethrocystoscopy in small animals. This can range from stranguria and signs of voiding obstruction to pollakiuria and painful urination. Urinary incontinence is also a frequent indication for endoscopic investigation of the lower urinary tract, particularly in animals with juvenile incontinence. A thorough history of the clinical signs, including their onset and frequency, will often narrow the clinical suspicion to a particular part of the lower urinary tract.

The character of the clinical signs is a key part of the evaluation of a patient for urethrocystoscopy. Patients with stranguria tend to have either urethral obstruction or significant inflammation involving the urethra and possibly the bladder. Neoplasia must be considered in such cases, especially in older dogs and cats.

11.3 An assembled 4.0 mm x 30 cm cystoscope with compatible grasping and biopsy forceps.
(Reproduced with the permission of The Ohio State University)

- Haematuria of unknown origin
- Stranguria
- Pollakiuria
- Painful urination
- Dysuria
- Urolithiasis
- Recurrent urinary tract infection
- Urethral obstruction of unknown origin
- Urethral mass
- Urinary bladder mass
- Unresponsive urinary incontinence
- Vulvar discharge
- Penile discharge

11.4 Indications for urethrocystoscopy in the dog and cat.

In patients with haematuria, the timing of the appearance of blood in the urine stream can be of diagnostic significance. If the urine is grossly haemorrhagic at the start of urination and then clears, it is likely to be originating from the urethra, the prostate in males, or the vagina or vestibule in females. Urine that is clear at the start and contains blood at the end of the stream may indicate a lesion in the bladder or the upper urinary tract, since blood is generally denser than urine and may settle to the dependent portion of the bladder and be evacuated at the end of the stream. Patients with haematuria throughout the urine stream may have a lesion anywhere along the urinary tract. Patients with haematuria without dysuria may have a lesion in the upper urinary tract, such as renal neoplasia or idiopathic renal haematuria.

It is important to question the client about whether the patient has ever had normal micturition or has always exhibited the clinical sign. This is particularly important for patients with urinary incontinence, as lack of continence in the juvenile animal, and particularly before neutering, may indicate ectopic ureter or congenital abnormalities of the urethra. Some breeds of dog appear to be predisposed to ectopic ureters, although they have been found in many breeds (Figure 11.5). Many cats with juvenile incontinence have more severe anatomical abnormalities of the urogenital tract, such as fusion of the bladder and uterus, and ectopic ureters are very rare in the cat.

Patients presenting with recurrent urinary tract infections despite appropriate antimicrobial therapy may have a lesion within the urogenital tract that is providing a nidus for the bacteria, such as prostatic disease, polypoid cystitis/urethritis or urolithiasis (Figure 11.6). Endoscopic evaluation of these cases may reveal a urachal diverticulum that may serve as a source of infection due to incomplete emptying of the bladder.

- Siberian Husky
- Labrador Retriever
- Golden Retriever
- Newfoundland
- Miniature Poodle
- Toy Poodle
- English Bulldog
- West Highland White Terrier
- Fox Terrier
- Skye Terrier
- Soft Coated Wheaten Terrier

11.5 Breeds of dog with a higher risk of ectopic ureter.

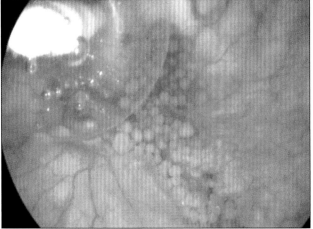

11.6 Laparoscopic-assisted cytoscopic view of uroliths. The round structure at the top left of the image is the inflated bulb of a Foley catheter.
(Courtesy of P Lhermette)

Since many clinical signs of urogenital disease can be treated without urethrocystoscopy, it is important to try medical non-invasive options first, and to move on to this procedure only after these options have failed. In some cases, such as patients with urolithiasis, there are also more invasive surgical options. A desire to limit the number of open surgical procedures in a patient that chronically forms non-dissolvable stones, such as those composed of calcium oxalate, may lead to the use of laser lithotripsy and voiding urohydropulsion to remove them. Finally, an assessment of the previous treatments and their success may indicate the nature of the underlying problem and assist the clinician in determining whether there is a need for urethrocystoscopy.

Clinical examination

The evaluation of a patient before urethrocystoscopy must include observation of the patient urinating or attempting to urinate. There are subtle changes in the posture of the patient and the strength and width of the urine stream, as well as signs of discomfort, which may not be apparent to the client; however, these signs may indicate to the veterinary surgeon (veterinarian) the nature of the disorder.

A thorough general physical examination should be performed, with careful attention being paid to the urogenital system. The prepuce, penis, vulva and anal area must be examined to assess and identify any conformational abnormalities. Careful abdominal palpation should also assist in determining the size of the bladder, especially if it is abnormally large or palpable after a urination attempt. Lumbosacral or coxofemoral pain may lead to difficulty passing urine and urine retention. A rectal examination is one of the most important parts of the examination of a patient with lower urinary tract disease. Palpation of the urethra through the rectal mucosa may indicate a mass, urethrolith or other abnormality. An assessment of the prostate in male animals and of anal tone in animals of both sexes can also be made. It is difficult to perform a rectal examination in the conscious feline patient; however, it is of value to perform this examination while the cat is under general anaesthesia. The prepuce of male dogs and cats should be gently retracted to assess for abnormalities such as a persistent frenulum, and the penile and perineal urethra should be externally palpated. Digital palpation of the vestibule and vaginal opening of bitches may be performed with the patient conscious in some cases; however, many will require heavy sedation, and some patients may be too small for digital examination to be performed safely and comfortably without general anaesthesia. It is important to remember that palpation must be performed gently, with adequate sedation and lubrication, and care taken to prevent iatrogenic lesions.

Preoperative diagnostic investigations

Depending on the presenting clinical complaint, a variety of diagnostic evaluations may be performed before diagnostic or therapeutic urethrocystoscopy. Urinalysis and urine culture are frequently performed, as well as survey and contrast radiography and ultrasonography of the urinary tract.

A complete blood count and serum chemistry may be done to assess the patient's kidney function and overall health before anaesthesia. Thoracic radiography should be performed to exclude metastases in cases where neoplasia is suspected. The preoperative diagnostic plan will vary with each patient and depends on the clinical problem being assessed.

Intraoperative diagnostic imaging

Once the animal is under general anaesthesia, further diagnostic imaging can be performed.

Radiography

Radiography can be an important component of the evaluation of these cases. The position of the bladder is better assessed by radiography than by ultrasonography. Plain three-view survey abdominal radiographs are the easiest way to evaluate the urethra for stones and may also reveal nephroliths, ureteroliths and cystoliths. Cystography, particularly double-contrast cystography, will provide useful structural information that assists in the planning of further procedures. In cases of urolithiasis, cystography may be used preoperatively to quantify the number of stones present before their removal, and then postoperatively to check they have all been retrieved. In cases of lower urinary tract disease, retrograde urethrography (in males) and vaginourethrography (in females) are useful to demonstrate urethral abnormalities and obstructive lesions, and also to identify congenital anatomical defects. In cases of urinary incontinence, excretory urography, particularly if evaluated with computed tomography (CT), provides additional information about renal and ureteral changes.

Ultrasonography

Ultrasonography is a critically important adjunct to both radiographic and endoscopic evaluation of the lower urinary tract. It provides information about the structure of solid organs, in particular the prostate and kidneys, as well as information about the wall of fluid-filled organs, such as the bladder, that may not be detectable by other imaging modalities. Ultrasonography is also valuable for investigating organs that are not accessible endoscopically, such as the prostate and the uterus when the cervix is closed. Aspirates or needle biopsy specimens can be obtained from these organs under ultrasound guidance, although care must be taken when infection or neoplasia is suspected to prevent seeding along the needle track.

Computed tomography

CT has become widely used in the imaging of anatomical abnormalities of the lower urinary tract over the past two decades. It can be performed under heavy sedation or general anaesthesia. Many CT systems have software that provide three-dimensional image reconstruction. If intravenous contrast medium is administered, a CT excretory urogram can be performed. This is considered more accurate than contrast radiography or ultrasonography in determining the course of ectopic ureters and whether they are intramural or extramural (Figure 11.7).

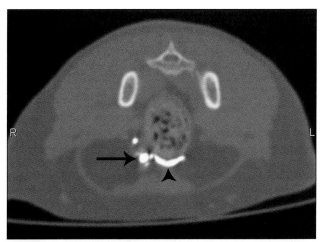

11.7 Extramural ectopic ureter. Computed tomographic excretory urogram of a 10-month-old male neutered Domestic Shorthaired cat with a chronic history of urinary incontinence. The transverse image shows the bladder and the entry of the left ureter (arrowhead) laterally into the urethra (arrowed) distal to the neck of the bladder.
(Reproduced with the permission of The Ohio State University)

Fluoroscopy

Fluoroscopy with a C-Arm imaging system is sometimes performed during interventional procedures, such as ureteral stent placement, sclerotherapy for idiopathic renal haematuria and ectopic ureter ablation. This imaging procedure provides a 'bird's eye' view of the anatomy that complements the direct visualization of endoscopy and can provide greater detail to guide the clinician (see Chapter 15).

Conditions of the lower urinary and reproductive tracts

Vestibule

Lymphoid follicles

A common finding in the bitch is the presence of lymphoid follicles on the vestibular or vaginal wall (see Figure 11.8). These lesions are usually multiple, small (1–3 mm in diameter) and pale or white in appearance. Some bitches have a concurrent urinary tract infection (UTI). The follicles appear to be a normal response to vaginal bacteria and do not require treatment. These lesions need to be differentiated from herpesvirus vesicles, which may initially be vesicular in nature (2–3 mm in diameter) and if ruptured may develop into smaller focal red raised lesions. Herpesvirus lesions are most commonly observed in previously infected bitches that are in pro-oestrus or oestrus, as viral recrudescence can occur at these stages of the oestrous cycle.

Remnant hymen/persistent hymen/paramesonephric septum

Some bitches that show signs of pain during coitus may have remnant tissue immediately cranial to the external urethral orifice, which may be detected using vaginoscopy. The normal hymen is a thin membrane separating the vagina from the vestibule and failure of this membrane to break down completely may result in thin 'strings' of tissue obstructing the vaginal cavity. A complete (imperforate) hymen with bulging of the membrane because of trapped fluid in the vagina is occasionally seen.

In some bitches, where there has been abnormal development of the paramesonephric duct system, a ventrodorsal band of tissue or a partial vaginal septum may be present (Figure 11.8). In some cases, the band of tissue divides the vagina over a significant part of its length; this is termed a bifid vagina.

Vaginoscopy may be used to place ligatures around small band-like hymenal remnants to allow them to be sectioned. Alternatively, the remnant can be sectioned with a diode laser or even with scissors under endoscopic control. Rarely, an episiotomy may be required.

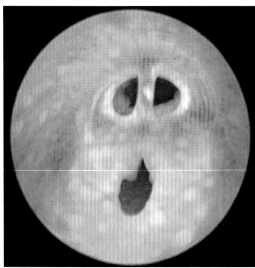

11.8 Endoscopic appearance of a paramesonephric remnant. Note the presence of multiple nodules due to lymphoid hyperplasia. (Courtesy of P Lhermette)

Vestibulovaginal stenosis

In some cases, there may be an appreciable narrowing of the vestibulovaginal junction; this is often better appreciated by digital palpation or contrast radiography than vaginoscopy. It is normal for this area to be approximately half the diameter of the vagina. In cases of vestibulovaginal stenosis, there may be evidence of fluid pooling cranial to the stenosis and signs of vaginitis. The clinical importance of this condition is often minimal; although it has been reported to be associated with urinary incontinence, the epidemiological evidence for this is poor.

Vagina
Vaginal hyperplasia

Thickening of the vaginal wall during oestrus is normal; however, in a small number of bitches there is excessive proliferation of tissue. Often this originates immediately cranial to the external urethral orifice, and a tongue-shaped mass of hyperplastic vaginal tissue may be identified. The tissue is present only during oestrus and regresses in the luteal phase. These bitches are normally presented because they show signs of pain at attempted coitus. It is often difficult to advance the endoscope into the vagina in these cases because it persistently abuts the ventral margin of the hyperplastic tissue. In some bitches, vaginal hyperplasia may first be recognized when the tissue becomes so large that it protrudes from the vulval lips.

Vaginal polyps

Vaginal polyps are relatively common, particularly in older intact bitches. They most commonly do not cause clinical signs, although they may be associated with vaginitis. Polyps usually have a thin stalk-like attachment to the vaginal wall, and the polyp itself is usually rounded, smooth and pink/white in colour.

Vaginal neoplasia

Vaginal tumours are not uncommon. The most frequently seen are leiomyomas. In the USA and some countries in Europe and Africa, a transmissible venereal tumour may be identified. Tumours may be intraluminal or extraluminal. Intraluminal leiomyomas usually have a wide-based attachment, while extraluminal tumours often press on and distort the normal outline of the vagina. Both types have a thick fibrous white capsule, although there may be prominent vessels visible. Transmissible venereal tumours are often irregular, red and have ulcerated areas.

Abnormalities of the cervix

Observation of the cervix may identify abnormalities that interfere with the establishment of normal pregnancy. Non-patency of the cervix or severe adhesions or fibrosis may cause such problems. Examination of the cervix may also be useful in the investigation of bitches with a vulvar discharge. During pregnancy, this discharge may be associated with resorption or abortion, or bleeding from the marginal haematoma of the placenta. Identification of the site and the nature of the discharge may influence the management of these cases. In non-pregnant bitches the nature of the discharge can be assessed and it may be possible to collect material for cytological and bacteriological screening.

Endometrial disease

For an accurate assessment of endometrial disease, it is necessary to catheterize the cervix, either to allow direct endoscopic visualization of the endometrial surface or to enable the collection of material for cytological and bacteriological investigations.

Prostate

Prostatic disease is common in older male dogs, particularly entire animals, but may not be readily diagnosed on urethroscopy. However, prostatic carcinoma is often advanced at the time of examination and may be recognized by the presence of proliferative tissue protruding into the lumen of the prostatic urethra. In most cases, diagnosis of prostatic disease is more readily achieved by a combination of retrograde urethrography, ultrasonography and biopsy.

Urethra

Disorders of the urethra are generally classified as functional or structural. The important functional disorders result in urinary incontinence or dysuria. Urinary incontinence can also be due to structural disorders but often is a result of overall loss of the sphincter mechanism of the urethra.

Urethral sphincter mechanism incompetence

Urethral sphincter mechanism incompetence (USMI) is a multifactorial disorder that is more commonly encountered in bitches than in male dogs or in cats of either sex. It is typically seen as an acquired disease of adult neutered bitches but also occurs less commonly in young animals, where it may be considered congenital, and in entire adults. Although USMI is often associated with a short urethra and intrapelvic bladder neck, this is not invariably the case, and in some cases there is no detectable anatomical abnormality. In these animals, urethrocystoscopy will be unremarkable and, although a measurement of urethral length can be made endoscopically, a comparable judgement of both urethral length and bladder neck position can be obtained with retrograde contrast vaginourethrography. Since USMI is often a disease of neutered bitches and is thought to be related to the absence of endogenous oestrogens, endoscopy may reveal a relative lack of folding of the urethral mucosa, although this finding is not invariably present and can be difficult to appreciate. Other animals with USMI may have structural abnormalities of the urethra, such as cystic urethral dilatation, which is encountered more commonly in males than females. USMI may be exacerbated by UTI and by obesity. In general, however, most animals with USMI show no abnormalities on physical or endoscopic examination.

Urethral dyssynergia

Inappropriate contraction of the urethra (urethrospasm) during micturition is a possible cause of dysuria and overflow incontinence in males and, rarely, females. Generally classified as urethral dyssynergia, this is a poorly characterized disorder that may involve the reticulospinal tracts of the central nervous system. It may involve the smooth and/or skeletal muscle portions of the urethra and results in focal dilatation of the urethra just proximal to the affected area. The resulting difficulty in passing urine, urine retention and overflow incontinence in the absence of structural or mechanical obstruction is usually indicative of the diagnosis. Endoscopic examination of the urethra is rarely necessary in these cases, unless contrast urethrography is inconclusive. In these cases, the prognosis is guarded because of the tendency for the disease to recur, even though each episode is usually self-limiting. Urethral spasm also occurs in animals with other urethral conditions (e.g. irritation after the use of an indwelling catheter) and in males with prostatic disease.

Urethral obstruction

Physical obstruction of the urethra is more common than dyssynergia. The most frequent cause in males is the presence of calculi (in dogs) or plugs of mineral debris and mucus (in cats). The urethra of the male cat is not amenable to endoscopy (except with very specialized endoscopes of very small diameter) but in dogs it may be possible to identify the calculi by urethroscopy. In most instances, radiographic evaluation may be more appropriate for diagnosis, since the bladder and urethra are examined concurrently. Retrograde urethrography and double-contrast cystography are recommended in cases of radiolucent calculi and obstructions of soft tissue opacity. These contrast procedures are also helpful in identifying extramural urethral compression caused by a mass or other lesion.

In the bitch, urethral obstruction is more commonly associated with mucosal lesions of the urethra, in particular neoplasia and proliferative urethritis. Endoscopic or radiographic examination will reveal proliferative mucosal lesions obscuring the urethral lumen, usually circumferentially and along variable lengths of the urethra. In most cases, biopsy is required for a definitive diagnosis.

Urethral stricture may be identified in dogs and cats of both sexes. Recent catheterization, surgical manipulation or trauma should increase suspicion of stricture in an animal with difficulty emptying its bladder (Figure 11.9). Contrast urethrography may also reveal this abnormality.

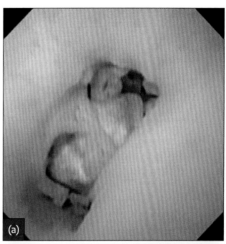
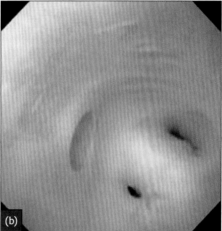

11.9 (a) Urethral stricture in a 5.5-year-old male entire English Bulldog with a 3-day history of straining to urinate. Note the urethroliths trapped proximal to the stricture. (b) Partially imperforate perineal urethra in a 1-year-old male entire English Springer Spaniel with a history of difficulty urinating since weaning.
(Reproduced with the permission of The Ohio State University)

Ureters
Ureteral ectopia

Ureteral ectopia is the second most common cause of urinary incontinence in dogs, especially in bitches. It is most frequently diagnosed in juvenile animals, most often with a history of urinary incontinence preceding neutering. In normal animals, the ureters enter the bladder at the trigone. With an ectopic ureter, the ureteral opening is distal to this, typically in the urethra. In most male dogs, the ureteral opening is in the prostatic urethra; in bitches its position varies and may be anywhere from the bladder neck to the vestibule (Figure 11.10). Entrance into the vagina or the uterus has been reported but appears to be rare. The situation in the cat is similar, although the condition is much rarer in this species. In dogs, the course of the ectopic ureter is usually intramural, whereas in cats it is typically extramural. Intramural ureters enter the serosal surface of the bladder at the trigone, in the normal position, but do not perforate the bladder wall fully; rather, they run within

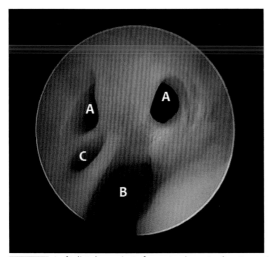

11.10 Left distal opening of an ectopic ureter in a 5-month-old female entire Golden Retriever. The dog had a history of urinary incontinence noticed soon after birth. A = The vaginal os partially occluded by a paramesonephric septal remnant. B = The urethra. C = The ectopic ureter.
(Reproduced with the permission of The Ohio State University)

the bladder and urethral wall. Extramural ectopic ureters do not enter the bladder at all but run within the retroperitoneal space and pelvic canal to enter the urethra directly. Fluoroscopy or CT excretory urethrography are necessary to differentiate intramural from extramural ureters, and this is an important diagnostic step because the two conditions may be corrected differently. It is not uncommon for the ectopic ureter to have several openings (or fenestrae) into the urethral lumen, and urethroscopy is the best method to assess this. Urethroscopy is a very sensitive tool in the diagnosis of ureteral ectopia, since the ectopic openings can be readily identified and the trigone can be examined to confirm the absence of the normal ureteral orifice.

Ectopic ureters may be abnormal in ways other than the location of their distal orifice. In male animals, ectopic ureters that open in the high-pressure zone of the prostatic urethra may become dilated, and if the pressure is transferred to the renal pelvis this can result in severe hydronephrosis. In females, some ureteral openings are very large and will develop into ureterocoeles, and the dilatation may extend to the proximal ureter. Imaging before urethroscopy will assist in planning for corrective action and prognosis.

Ureterocoeles

Ureterocoeles are cystic dilatations of the terminal ureter, usually occurring concurrently with ureteral ectopia. They have also been reported to accompany blind-ending ureters and possibly normal ureters with terminal strictures. The significance of ureterocoeles is not always clear but they have been associated with both incontinence and dysuria. Urethroscopy can assist in the diagnosis and correction of some types of ureterocoeles, although, as noted above, preoperative imaging is crucial.

Bladder and urethra
Urinary tract infection

Cystoscopy of animals presenting with acute UTI is unlikely to be helpful, but in chronic cases significant abnormalities may be encountered in both the urethra and the bladder that contribute to the persistence of the infection. Small

'fried egg' lesions are often seen lining the bladder mucosa in cases of chronic UTI. These have a pale central area ringed by hyperaemic inflamed tissue; examination of biopsy samples often reveals them to be lymphoid (Figure 11.11). In established cases it is important to rule out the possibility of complicating factors, including polypoid cystitis (Figure 11.12), neoplasia of the bladder or urethra and urolithiasis. Polypoid cystitis and most cases of bladder neoplasia produce proliferative lesions of the bladder epithelium that can be detected on cystoscopy. The site of predilection for each condition varies, although significant overlap exists: polypoid cystitis often affects the ventral pole of the bladder but transitional cell carcinoma (the most frequent neoplasm) is typically centred on the trigone. Both neoplasia and polypoid cystitis can prevent complete clearance of a UTI or predispose to recurrence. Careful evaluation of the bladder apex may reveal a urachal diverticulum, another potential cause of recurrent UTI.

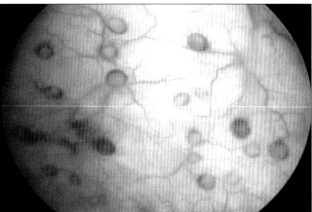

11.11 Inflammatory 'fried egg' lesions in the bladder of a 5-year-old female entire Golden Retriever with urinary incontinence and recurrent urinary tract infections.
(Reproduced with the permission of The Ohio State University)

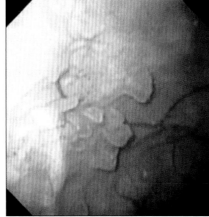

11.12 Polypoid cystitis in a 1-year-old male entire English Springer Spaniel (same dog as in Figure 11.9b). This dog had urolithiasis and a partially imperforate urethra.
(Reproduced with the permission of The Ohio State University)

Urolithiasis

Urolithiasis (Figure 11.13) is encountered in cats and dogs of both sexes, although males tend to present with urethral obstruction and females with signs of cystitis or haematuria. Several types of stone are reported (see the *BSAVA Manual of Canine and Feline Nephrology and Urology*) but the most common are struvite and calcium oxalate. The diagnosis of urolithiasis can be established by various imaging modalities, but cystoscopy has the advantage of offering the possibility of both diagnosis and treatment by retrieval of the stones in selected cases.

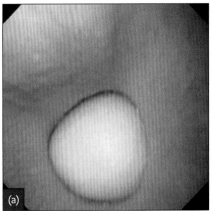

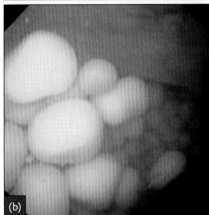

11.13 (a) Urethrolith in the penile urethra of a 2.5-year-old male entire Rottweiler with a history of urethral obstruction. The urolith is lodged at the base of the os penis. (b) Further uroliths in the bladder of the same dog. These were determined by analysis to be cysteine uroliths. (Reproduced with the permission of The Ohio State University)

Neoplasia

Transitional cell carcinoma is the most common neoplasia found in the bladder and urethra of both the dog and cat, although bladder neoplasia is rare in the cat. It is usually present in the trigone area and may invade the ureters and the urethra (Figure 11.14). It is very difficult to distinguish this proliferative neoplasia from an inflammatory process without examination of biopsy samples. Frequently, cytological examination of the urine sediment will reveal cellular atypia consistent with neoplasia. Obtaining a sample via cystoscopy or catheterization is safer than needle aspiration, as this latter method carries the risk of seeding the tumour along a needle track.

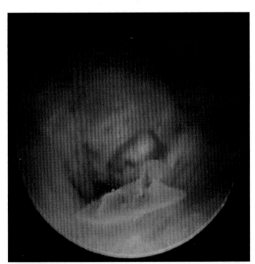

11.14 Transitional cell carcinoma extending into the vaginal vestibule from the urethra in a 10-year-old female neutered Dachshund with a 4-month history of straining to urinate. (Reproduced with the permission of The Ohio State University)

Proliferative urethritis

Proliferative urethritis may be of infectious or immune-mediated origin. The lesions may be granulomatous, lymphoplasmacytic or suppurative in nature. The urethra may be partially occluded by the abnormal tissue and lesions may extend into the vestibule (Figure 11.15). The bladder is not usually involved; however, secondary infection and other consequences of urine retention may be evident. Diagnosis must be made by examination of biopsy samples or by cytology to differentiate the condition from neoplasia. Cystoscopic re-evaluation may be needed to document resolution of the condition.

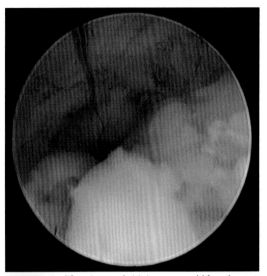

11.15 Proliferative urethritis in a 7-year-old female neutered mixed-breed dog with a 2-week history of straining to urinate. A biopsy taken at the time of cystoscopy confirmed that the lesion was inflammatory and not neoplastic. (Reproduced with the permission of The Ohio State University)

Urethrocystoscopy and vaginoscopy of the female animal

Urethrocystoscopy of the bitch or queen can be performed with the patient in ventral, dorsal or lateral recumbency. The endoscopist stands or sits at the caudal end of the animal and the tail is secured out of the operating region. The external genitalia of the anaesthetized patient are shaved and surgically prepared. It is important to use sterile technique to minimize iatrogenic contamination of the urinary tract. The endoscope is either gas or steam sterilized, and the caudal half of the patient is draped in sterile fashion. The endoscopist should wear a sterile surgical gown and sterile gloves during the procedure, and some practitioners also prefer to wear a surgical hat and mask. The endoscopist assembles the endoscope and its components, and attaches the light and camera cables. The irrigation and efflux lines are attached and the endoscope is liberally coated with sterile water-based lubricant. The authors prefer to use passive drainage on the efflux lines, but some practitioners use low-pressure suction to assist the evacuation of fluid. The endoscope is passed into the vaginal vestibule and sterile 0.9% saline is passed through the irrigation channel to distend the anatomy and improve visualization; the vulvar folds are gently grasped around the endoscope to enable fluid distension of the chamber.

Vaginoscopy of bitches that are in pro-oestrus or oestrus can normally be performed without sedation and with the patient standing on a table. For cervical catheterization (see later), it may be helpful to have the table tilted so that the hindlegs are higher, which tends to move the abdominal viscera out of the pelvis and appears to facilitate manipulation.

The mucosa of the vestibule is light pink and smooth in texture (Video 11.1). The vaginal opening, which is surrounded by a ridge of tissue, the cingulum, is seen at the craniodorsal aspect of the vestibule. Ventral to this is the smaller urethral opening. There may be a thin band of tissue crossing the opening of the vagina dorsoventrally, which has been termed a hymenal membrane (Figure 11.16). A thicker band, referred to as the mesonephric remnant, is often associated with abnormalities of development of the urethra and ureter. Most patients with ureteral ectopia have this thicker band of tissue (Cannizzo et al., 2003). In the entire bitch, the urethral opening is often covered by a dorsal fold of tissue, which is often exaggerated in size during oestrus and should not be interpreted as a mass lesion. Lateral to the urethral opening are the fossae, which may contain crypt-like areas.

The endoscope is directed into the urethra and slowly passed cranially into the bladder. The urethra has a dorsal fold, which is particularly pronounced in the queen, and generally has smooth, light pink mucosa. The length of the urethra may vary between normal dogs. Once the vesicourethral junction is reached, the bladder is drained of urine and debris and re-distended with saline to provide a clear view. Urine is generally heavier than saline and pools in the dependent aspect of the bladder, obscuring structures in this area. Distension of the bladder is essential to obtain an adequate evaluation of the ureters and bladder wall; however, over-distension may lead to tearing of the urothelium and result in iatrogenic haemorrhage. To prevent this, the bladder should be manually palpated through the abdomen by an assistant while saline is being introduced, and distension should be ceased when the bladder is slightly firm. If bleeding occurs, the bladder should be drained of fluid and chilled saline infused to induce vasoconstriction and reduce the impact of haemorrhage on visibility.

With the bladder almost fully distended, the trigone is examined. The ureters are located dorsolateral to the midline as two crescent-shaped slits in the bladder wall. These two C-shaped structures should be facing each other as mirror images (Figure 11.17). An inverted V- or Y-shaped ridge may extend cranially from the openings and join at the midline. Verification of the patency of the ureters should be made by observing the pulsatile flow of urine from each ureter.

The endoscope is then passed cranially to the apex of the bladder and the entire bladder wall is examined. The bladder mucosa is light pink with a fine vascular pattern. Occasionally the bladder wall will be semi-transparent and abdominal organs may be faintly visualized from the lumen. In patients without this transparency, there may be fibrosis of the bladder wall. It is important to examine all areas of the interior of the bladder to ensure that small lesions or calculi, which may fall to its dependent aspect, are not missed. Manual palpation and manipulation of the bladder through the abdomen by an assistant can help with a full evaluation. After completion of the examination, the efflux channel of the endoscope is opened and the fluid is drained from the bladder.

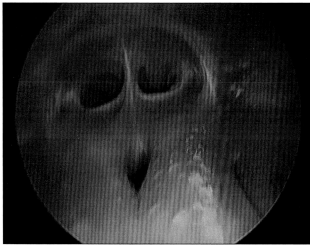

Video 11.1 Normal urethrocystoscopy of the neutered bitch.
(Reproduced with the permission of The Ohio State University)

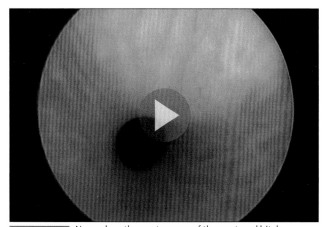

11.16 Mesonephric remnant in a 5-month-old female entire English Bulldog with a history of urinary incontinence. This dog was diagnosed with bilateral ectopic ureters. Note the lymphoid follicles in the vestibule.
(Reproduced with the permission of The Ohio State University)

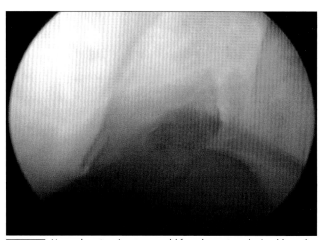

11.17 Normal ureters in a 3-year-old female neutered mixed-breed dog. Note the pulsatile flow of urine from the right ureter.
(Reproduced with the permission of The Ohio State University)

Uroendoscopy of the male animal

Uroendoscopy of the male dog is generally performed with a flexible endoscope, although some procedures have been developed that use a rigid endoscope passed through a surgical incision into the perineal approach. When performing flexible endoscopy, an assistant may be required to exteriorize the penis from the prepuce, and atraumatic haemostats or stay sutures may be necessary to maintain this retraction, particularly in the male cat. The endoscope is prepared and lubricated as described above and is introduced directly into the external urethral orifice. Infusion of saline facilitates distension of the urethra ahead of the endoscope. It is important not to use the endoscope tip itself to dilate the urethra as this can cause injury to the delicate urothelium, which may be interpreted as lesions. As the endoscope is passed from the perineal urethra into the prostatic urethra of the dog, tiny prostatic duct openings may be noted in the mucosa. These indentations are generally not seen in the male cat.

Examination of the trigone, ureters and bladder lumen proceed as described above for female animals, but may be difficult due to the small size of the endoscope in relation to the size of the bladder lumen. Care must be taken to keep the tip of the endoscope close to the bladder wall to avoid missing lesions. Identification of the ureteral openings and complete examination of the bladder lumen may be facilitated by having an assistant move the bladder via external palpation while the endoscopist keeps the endoscope stationary (Video 11.2).

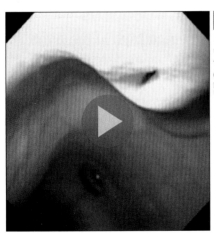

Video 11.2

Normal urethrocystoscopy of the neutered male dog.
(Reproduced with the permission of The Ohio State University)

Operative techniques

All operative procedures are performed after the endoscopist has completed a thorough examination and documented it with video and still images. Most interventions will lead to haemorrhage, which can easily obscure the view through the endoscope and may be difficult to clear adequately to achieve a good-quality image.

Biopsy

A variety of biopsy instruments that fit the instrument channels of rigid endoscopy sets are available. Clamshell cup biopsy forceps are the most commonly used. It is important to keep in mind that the samples obtained will be much smaller than those taken during gastrointestinal biopsy procedures, and care must be taken to handle them carefully and not crush them during preparation for transport to the laboratory. The author [JB] recommends placing the samples in a hinged biopsy cassette (e.g. CellSafe) for transport in formalin, to minimize the risk of damage or loss.

When the endoscopist has identified an area for biopsy, an assistant passes the biopsy instrument through the instrument channel, being careful not to place too much pressure on the endoscope and resulting in excessive movement. Once visualized, the tip of the biopsy instrument is guided to the appropriate area and the jaws are opened and then closed around the tissue. Twisting the instrument slightly while pulling it away from the wall will facilitate the removal of the sample. The biopsy instrument is withdrawn through the instrument channel and the sample is carefully removed using a needle and a stream of saline from a syringe.

Laser lithotripsy

A holmium:YAG laser can be used to break down large calculi so they can be flushed using voiding urohydropulsion or removed using a stone basket accessory. All types of calculi commonly found in the dog and cat, including calcium oxalate, struvite and urate, can be shattered with this type of laser; however, some, such as cysteine and calcium phosphate calculi, are particularly challenging to break apart. The decision to perform cystoscopy-assisted laser lithotripsy on these types of calculi must be made with consideration of the number and size of stones and the associated longer anaesthesia time that will be needed. Care must be taken to break the stones down to a size that will easily pass through the urethra, to minimize trauma and inflammation.

The laser fibre is sheathed in a sterile 5 Fr ureteral catheter before being passed through the endoscope instrument channel. This stabilizes the laser fibre, which provides more precise control during the procedure. The tip of the fibre is placed against the calculus, in a crevice on its surface if possible, and the laser is fired. Rapid vaporization of the fluid at the end of the fibre leads to an explosive force that breaks the mineral down (Figure 11.18). This is more easily done when the calculus is lodged in the urethra, since the force generated by the laser can push the stone away from the tip of the fibre when loose in the bladder. Directing the fibre in such a way as to gently push the calculus against others or the bladder wall may stabilize it and result in more effective fragmentation. Care must be taken not to damage the bladder mucosa with the laser, since it has the ability to cut tissue.

Once the calculi are sufficiently broken down, the bladder is distended with saline and the fragments are flushed using voiding urohydropulsion or removed with a stone basket passed through the instrument channel. It is not advised to use the basket for multiple retrievals, since the repeated passing of the endoscope through the urethra to remove each fragment may cause additional trauma unnecessarily (see also Chapter 16).

Ectopic ureter ablation

The holmium:YAG laser and both 980 nm and 810 nm diode lasers can be used to manage intramural ectopic ureters. A 5 Fr ureteral catheter is passed into the ectopic ureteral orifice and threaded proximally until resistance is met. This catheter shields the lateral wall of the ureter and prevents damage to it and the urethral wall. A guidewire should not

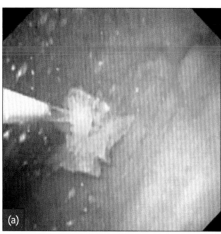

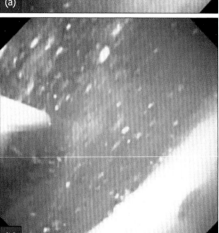

11.18 Laser lithotripsy of calcium oxalate cystoliths in a 7-year-old female neutered Shih Tzu. (a) The tip of the laser fibre is positioned in a crevice in the urolith. (b) As the laser is fired, the fluid at the tip of the fibre is superheated and vaporizes, producing a shockwave that shatters the urolith. (Reproduced with the permission of The Ohio State University)

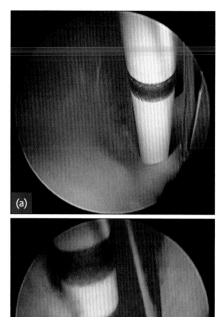

11.19 Laser ablation of an ectopic ureter in a 7-month-old female neutered Soft Coated Wheaten Terrier. (a) The ureteral catheter is shown in place and the tip of the laser fibre is positioned at the leading edge of the medial ureteral wall. (b) As the laser is fired, it cuts along the medial ureteral wall, moving the terminal ureteral opening proximally. (Reproduced with the permission of The Ohio State University)

be used for this purpose because of the risk of thermal injury to the ureter and the potential for subsequent stricture. The tip of the laser fibre is placed against the leading medial edge of the ureteral wall. The laser is fired and the medial wall of the ureter is opened to the level at which the ureter begins to deviate laterally (Figure 11.19). Ideally, this occurs at the level of the natural trigone; however, this may not be the case, and the endoscopist should be prepared for the possibility of malformation of the bladder neck making it challenging to identify the best level at which to leave the final opening. This decision can be assisted by the use of C-Arm fluoroscopy during the procedure to elucidate the path of the ureter and the level at which it enters the bladder wall. Extramural ureters cannot be managed with laser ablation because they enter the lower urinary tract very close to their external orifice, leaving little or no tissue to ablate.

Cystoscopy-assisted placement of a ureteral guidewire

Urethrocystoscopy can be used to assist in the placement of a ureteral guidewire for the passing of stents and other devices (see Chapter 15). A 0.4572–0.889 mm (0.018–0.035 inch) hydrophilic semi-flexible wire is passed through the instrument channel of the endoscope and directed through the ureteral opening. Additional guidance can be provided by using C-Arm fluoroscopy to monitor the passage of the wire through the ureter. The endoscope is withdrawn off the wire, leaving the wire in place for further procedures such as renal pelvic sclerotherapy or the placement of a ureteral stent.

Reproductive procedures
Assessment of breeding time in the bitch

The most common cause of apparent infertility in the bitch is that the bitch is normal but is simply being mated at an inappropriate time. Bitches ovulate approximately 12 days after the onset of pro-oestrus, but some normal bitches may ovulate as early as day 5 while others ovulate as late as day 30. Many dog breeders try to impose standard mating regimes, for example, on days 10 and 12. For many bitches this is not appropriate and, even though both the male and female are normal, pregnancy does not result from mating on the designated days. Careful monitoring of oestrus is important to establish the time of ovulation and therefore the most appropriate time for mating (Figure 11.20). Observation of the behaviour of the bitch has limited value and, while the gold standard for evaluation is measurement of plasma progesterone, the use of vaginoscopy to assess physical features of the reproductive tract provides a rapid, simple and cost-effective method of assessing the underlying hormonal changes. Examination is normally performed with the bitch standing. In most cases it can take as little as 2 minutes to make an evaluation of the stage of the oestrous cycle. One specific advantage of vaginoscopy is the ability to detect the end of the fertile period – something that is difficult to achieve by measurement of plasma hormone concentrations.

Vaginoscopic evaluation is based upon assessment of the appearance of the vaginal wall (the mucosal fold contours and profiles, the colour of the mucosa and the appearance of any fluid present) and changes in the appearance of these features at specific times of the oestrous cycle. A specific scoring system was devised by Lindsay et al. (1988) and has been modified by the author [GE] as follows (Figure 11.21):

Period	Days from LH surge	Days from ovulation
Period of potential fertility – the 'fertile period'	–3 to +7 (or later)	–5 to +5 (or later)
Period of potential fertilization of mature oocytes – the 'fertilization period'	+4 to +6 (or later)	+2 to +4 (or later)
Time of oocyte maturation (estimated)	+4 to +5	+2 to +3
Period of peak fertility in bitches of high fertility at natural mating	0 to +6	–2 to +4
Preferred time for managed breeding of natural service or fresh semen insemination	+2 to +6	0 to +4
Time for critical managed breeding or frozen semen artificial insemination	+4 to +6	+2 to +4
Period of reduced fertility with matings or inseminations late in oestrus	+7 to +9	+5 to +7

11.20 The timing of peak fertility in relation to the day of the luteinizing hormone (LH) surge and the day of ovulation.

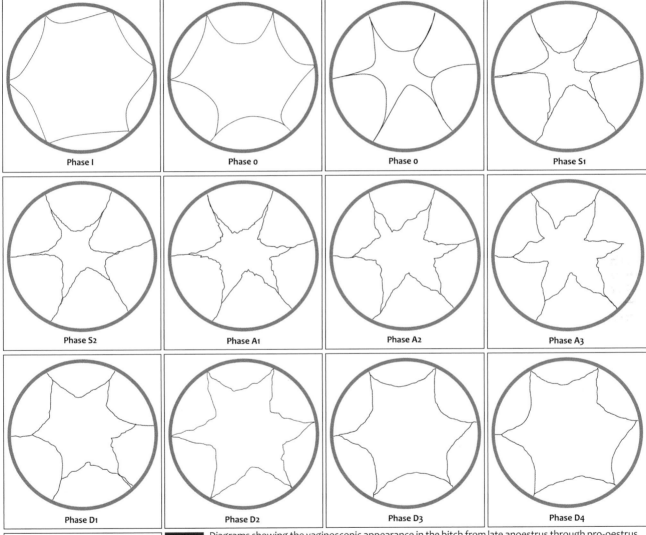

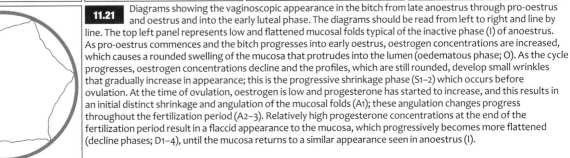

11.21 Diagrams showing the vaginoscopic appearance in the bitch from late anoestrus through pro-oestrus and oestrus and into the early luteal phase. The diagrams should be read from left to right and line by line. The top left panel represents low and flattened mucosal folds typical of the inactive phase (I) of anoestrus. As pro-oestrus commences and the bitch progresses into early oestrus, oestrogen concentrations are increased, which causes a rounded swelling of the mucosa that protrudes into the lumen (oedematous phase; O). As the cycle progresses, oestrogen concentrations decline and the profiles, which are still rounded, develop small wrinkles that gradually increase in appearance; this is the progressive shrinkage phase (S1–2) which occurs before ovulation. At the time of ovulation, oestrogen is low and progesterone has started to increase, and this results in an initial distinct shrinkage and angulation of the mucosal folds (A1); these angulation changes progress throughout the fertilization period (A2–3). Relatively high progesterone concentrations at the end of the fertilization period result in a flaccid appearance to the mucosa, which progressively becomes more flattened (decline phases; D1–4), until the mucosa returns to a similar appearance seen in anoestrus (I).

- Inactive phase: characterized by a thin, red and dry mucosa with low and flattened mucosal folds. This appearance is designated I
- Oedematous phase: characterized by a thickened and oedematous mucosa that appears turgidly swollen, rounded and grey/white in colour. Mucosal folds with this appearance are designated O
- Shrinkage phase: characterized by a thickened mucosa that is normally white but with reduced turgidity, with progressive furrowing, wrinkling and indentations. The mucosal fold profile is still rounded rather than angular. The progressive nature of this phase means that the early changes are designated S1 and the later changes S2
- Angulated phase: characterized by a thickened mucosa that is normally white but with significant reduced turgidity; in profile, the mucosal folds have progressive shrinkage and angulation, such that the peaks are sharp-tipped and irregular in appearance. The mucosa is wrinkled and shrunken in appearance. The progressive nature of this phase means that the early changes are designated A1 and the later changes A2 and A3
- Declining phase: characterized by a progressive decline in the size of the mucosal fold profile. Early in the phase (designated D1) there is a flaccid appearance to the mucosal fold profile. Subsequently, the folds become more rounded (D2) and there is sloughing of the cornified layers of the epithelium (D2 and D3), resulting in a thin mucosa that is variegated in colour, with flattened folds and a rosette appearance to the mucosa (D4)
- Inactive phase: the declining phase is followed by a return to a phase characterized by a thin, red and dry mucosa with low and flattened mucosal folds. This appearance is also designated I. There may be more debris present at this stage than is observed in phase I before the onset of pro-oestrus.

Studies that have related the appearance of the vaginal wall to the underlying endocrinology have demonstrated a progression as described above in all bitches. The specific timing of some events is variable, but good correlations have been demonstrated between the onset of ovulation and phase A1, and between the fertilization period and phases A1–A3 (Figure 11.22). Generally, the onset of the fertile period can be detected by observing the onset of mucosal shrinkage without profound angulations, while gross shrinkage of entire mucosal folds with obvious angulation (phases A2 and A3) is characteristic of the fertilization period.

Mating is best planned approximately 4 days after the first detected mucosal shrinkage, or at the onset of the period of obvious angulation of the mucosal folds. The end of the fertilization period can be detected by observing sloughing of the vaginal epithelium and the development of a variegated appearance to the colour of the mucosal surface.

Cervical catheterization

It is difficult to place a catheter through the cervix of a bitch because the vagina is long and narrow, and the cervical opening is small and at an angle to the vagina. The procedure is not possible in queens.

For cervical catheterization in the bitch it is normal to use a semi-flexible urinary catheter with terminal rather than side holes. A guidewire will help with introducing the catheter through the cervix. In most cases a 2.5 mm diameter catheter is suitable, although in small breeds or bitches that have not been pregnant a 2 mm diameter catheter may be necessary.

Using a rigid endoscope, the cervix can be visualized; the endoscope is then manipulated under the cervix until the cervical os can be identified. The os is usually located in the centre of a rosette of wrinkles/furrows but sometimes its location can be identified only by the presence of fluid originating from it. A fine catheter may then be placed through the endoscope towards the cervical os. In many cases it is necessary to place a guidewire inside the catheter to increase its rigidity. Once the catheter tip is placed into the os, the guidewire may be withdrawn slightly and the catheter is pushed forward, using a rotating action. The catheter can normally be introduced into the full length of the uterine body. This technique requires training and practice before catheterization can be achieved reliably.

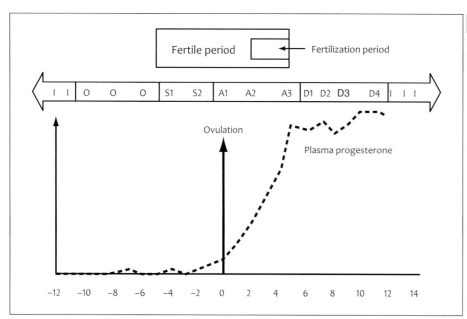

11.22 Relationship between vaginoscopic score, time of ovulation, fertile and fertilization periods, and plasma progesterone concentrations in bitches.

Catheterization is simplest in medium-sized dogs and most difficult in giant breeds (with a very long vagina) and toy breeds (where the diameter of the catheter may be too large). Some bitches need to be sedated to prevent movement during the procedure, which makes placement of the catheter very difficult. The cervix is simplest to catheterize during oestrus; however, the cervix is also relaxed during anoestrus and pro-oestrus. Catheterization during the luteal phase can be difficult in some bitches. Catheterization during oestrus is most commonly performed for the purpose of artificial insemination. However, it may also be performed to collect material for microbiological and cytological investigation from the endometrial surface by aspiration or by the use of small brushes passed through the catheter. In the postpartum bitch the endoscope may be passed directly through the cervical os to enable visualization of the endometrial surface.

Postoperative care

Postoperative care varies between institutions and between individual patients, but generally consists of analgesia and, potentially, anti-inflammatory medication. Postoperative analgesia may not be immediately necessary in patients that have received epidural analgesia for the procedure, but is important in all other cases and should be provided for at least 2–3 days. Signs of discomfort while urinating and over-grooming of the penis or vulva may indicate the need for additional pain management. Anti-inflammatory medication (such as non-steroidal anti-inflammatory drugs) is often used postoperatively, particularly after manipulation procedures such as extraction of uroliths. The use of antibiotics is controversial and is discussed in more detail below. There are no specific guidelines for peri-procedure antibiotic administration in the absence of active infection. Some practitioners administer a single dose or every-90-minute dose of ampicillin or a first-generation cephalosporin; however, careful thought should be given to the necessity of antibiotic treatment in the individual patient.

Complications

Complications may arise during uroendoscopy. Lodging of the endoscope in the urethra can be avoided by selecting an endoscope of suitable size for the patient and lubricating the endoscope properly before insertion. The endoscope, whether flexible or rigid, should never be forced proximally through the urethra. Forcing the endoscope can lead to urethral damage or, for a flexible endoscope, 'hairpinning' and lodging in the urethra. Gentle pressure and, especially in male patients, proper use of saline to dilate the urethra ahead of the endoscope should be sufficient to allow its passage; if this is not successful, a smaller diameter endoscope should be used.

The endoscopist must be attentive to the degree of fluid distention of the bladder and release any over-filling through the efflux channel of the endoscope. Over-filling may cause haemorrhage of the bladder wall even in a normal bladder. An over-distended bladder will show signs of petechial haemorrhage and splitting of the glycosaminoglycan layer and the mucosal layer. Bleeding can make visualization very challenging, even with repeated drainage of the bladder and refilling with fresh saline. The use of chilled saline may reduce active bleeding by causing vasoconstriction of the superficial vessels.

Iatrogenic damage to the mucosa is common, and small iatrogenic lesions should be recognized as such and not mistaken for pathology. The endoscopist must carefully observe the appearance of the urethral, vaginal and bladder mucosa as the endoscope is passed into each of these areas, to assist in making an assessment before such injuries may occur. The linear nature of these lesions and their appearance in areas of otherwise normal tissue are indicators of their nature. In general, lesions that involve only the superficial layers will not need specific treatment post procedure; however, the use of careful controlled movements throughout the procedure, an appropriately sized endoscope, and adequate lubrication and fluid distension will reduce their occurrence in general.

Perforation of the lower urinary tract is also a potential complication of uroendoscopy. This is particularly a risk in patients with a severely diseased urethral or bladder wall. A rupture of the urethra with a rigid endoscope may not be as obvious as a tear in the wall, but may be recognized by the sudden appearance of multi-layered tissue structures rather than a smooth mucosal surface (Figure 11.23). Depending on the size of the damage, surgical repair may be necessary to correct a bladder tear. Rupture of the urethra can also occur but may not require surgical intervention. Placing a urinary catheter for several days after the procedure may be sufficient to allow the defect to heal. Careful selection of an appropriately sized endoscope and the use of gentle technique will minimize these risks.

As with any minimally invasive procedure, there is some risk of development of infection after the procedure. No studies have evaluated the risk of cystitis or pyelonephritis after urethrocystoscopy in dogs or cats thus far. Data from human patients indicate an incidence of 1–10%, with higher risk if the patient had recently been hospitalized, had been treated with antibiotics in the previous 6 months or was immunosuppressed. There also appears to be increased risk if manipulations such as stent removal are performed during the procedure (Gregg *et al.*, 2018). While there is no agreed standard of care, most veterinary surgeons who perform urethrocystoscopy will treat the patient with a single injection of antibiotics administered at the time of the procedure. In cases where the patient already has evidence of a UTI, or there is substantial risk of pyelonephritis, such as with laser ablation of ectopic ureters, it is prudent to treat based on the results of culture and susceptibility tests, and/or treat for a longer period, such as 7–14 days.

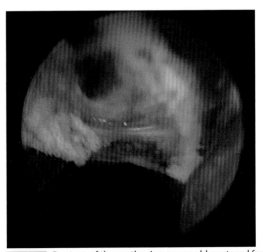

11.23 Rupture of the urethra in a 2-year-old neutered female Welsh Corgi during laser ablation of ectopic ureters. Note the fibrous bands as the tissue separates. The dog was managed with a urinary catheter for 2 days and recovered uneventfully.

References and further reading

Cannizzo KL, McLoughlin A, Mattoon JS *et al.* (2003). Evaluation of transurethral cystoscopy and excretory urography for diagnosis of ectopic ureters in female dogs: 25 cases (1992–2000). *Journal of the American Veterinary Medical Association* **223**, 475–481

Elliott J, Grauer GF and Westropp JL (2017) *BSAVA Manual of Canine and Feline Nephrology and Urology, 3rd edn*. BSAVA Publications, Gloucester

Gregg JR, Bhalla RG, Cook JP *et al.* (2018). An evidence-based protocol for antibiotic use prior to cystoscopy decreases antibiotic use without impacting post-procedural symptomatic urinary tract infection rates. *Journal of Urology* **199**, 1004–1010

Lindsay FEF, Jeffcoate IA and Concannon PW (1988) Vaginoscopy and the fertile period in the bitch. *Proceedings of the 11th International Conference on Animal Reproduction and Artificial Insemination*. Dublin, June 26–30, 1998. Abstract 565

Moxon R, Batty H, Irons G and England GCW (2012) Periovulatory changes in the endoscopic appearance of the reproductive tract and teasing behavior in the bitch. *Theriogenology* **78**, 1907–1916

Video extras

- Video 11.1 Normal urethrocystoscopy of the neutered bitch
- Video 11.2 Normal urethrocystoscopy of the neutered male dog

Access via QR code or: bsavalibrary.com/endoscopy2e_11

Chapter 12

Rigid endoscopy: laparoscopy

Philip Lhermette, Eric Monnet and Philipp D. Mayhew

Introduction

Exploratory laparotomy is a major invasive procedure, often carried out on a sick or debilitated patient. Clinicians may hesitate to subject a patient to such a procedure for purely diagnostic purposes, and may therefore rely on incomplete information from indirect observations such as blood tests and imaging studies to form a diagnosis. Owners may also be reluctant to subject their pet to major surgery 'just to get a sample'.

Laparoscopy is a minimally invasive surgical technique that is becoming increasingly widely used in veterinary practice for diagnostic procedures and surgical treatment of a wide variety of conditions. It is a very safe technique if the basic rules are followed. It minimizes soft tissue trauma, allows very good visualization of abdominal organs and enables good tissue samples to be obtained by biopsy (Johnson and Twedt, 1977; Wildt and Lawler, 1985; Richter, 2001; Cole *et al.*, 2002; Rothuizen and Twedt, 2009). These factors in turn allow more accurate diagnosis, treatment of abdominal disease and staging of tumours.

Biopsy samples obtained via laparoscopy are larger and more diagnostically valuable than percutaneous Tru-Cut biopsy specimens and haemorrhage can be controlled directly (Cole *et al.*, 2012). Patients recover more quickly than following conventional surgery, and the smaller incisions required for laparoscopy result in a lower incidence of wound interference and infection. In addition, postoperative pain is significantly reduced (Davidson *et al.*, 2004; Hancock *et al.*, 2004; Devitt *et al.*, 2005; Culp *et al.*, 2009; Gauthier *et al.*, 2015), partly as a result of the smaller incisions but also due to the more delicate tissue handling during laparoscopic procedures.

Laparoscopy requires a basic set of specialized equipment (see below). This equipment can also be used for other rigid endoscopic applications, such as thoracoscopy, urethrocystoscopy, rhinoscopy and video-otoscopy. Laparoscopy also requires the induction of a pneumoperitoneum to allow distension of the abdominal cavity with an inert gas to obtain a working space sufficient to perform diagnostic and surgical procedures.

After the veterinary surgeon (veterinarian) has mastered the basic technique of diagnostic laparoscopy and learned the appropriate indications, these procedures become an easy and rewarding addition to any small animal veterinary practice. With more experience, advanced surgical procedures can be performed via laparoscopy in dogs and cats. Laparoscopic-assisted surgery is also possible and helps minimize the impact of surgery on patients.

Indications

Many abdominal surgical procedures carried out via conventional laparotomy can be performed either entirely laparoscopically or be laparoscopically assisted. These are listed in Figure 12.1.

- Exploratory laparoscopy
- Liver biopsy
- Kidney biopsy
- Pancreatic biopsy
- Lymph node biopsy
- Intestinal biopsy
- Ovariectomy/ovariohysterectomy
- Cryptorchidectomy
- Gastropexy
- Laparoscopic-assisted cystoscopy
- Intestinal/gastric foreign body removal
- Examination of the gall bladder and biliary tree
- Cholecystectomy or cholecystocentesis
- Vasopexy and colposuspension
- Inguinal hernia repair
- Staging and/or removal of intra-abdominal neoplasia
- Splenic biopsy/splenectomy
- Investigation of intra-abdominal trauma
- Adrenalectomy
- Extrahepatic shunt attenuation
- Nephrectomy

12.1 Examples of laparoscopic and laparoscopic-assisted abdominal surgical procedures that can be performed in dogs and cats.

Instrumentation

The basic equipment required for diagnostic laparoscopy is listed in Figure 12.2. Much of this equipment is also used for other minimally invasive procedures, such as video-otoscopy, rhinoscopy, urethrocystoscopy and thoracoscopy.

Telescopes

Telescopes are classified according to their diameter and angle of view. The angle of view can be fixed or variable. Fixed-angle telescopes are available with an angle of view from 0 degrees (these are also known as forward-viewing telescopes) to 120 degrees. The angle of view of variable-angle telescopes can also vary from 0 degrees to 120 degrees. Angled telescopes enable the operator to look around fixed structures or masses in the abdominal cavity and are useful in tight spaces where there is a restricted view.

Essential equipment

- Endoscopic camera and monitor
- Xenon (or metal halide/LED) light source
- Light guide cable
- Electrosurgery unit (monopolar/bipolar)
- 5 mm bipolar cutting device (e.g. LigaSure™, ENSEAL®, Robi® plus)
- Carbon dioxide insufflator
- Veress needle
- Sterile insufflation tubing
- 2.7 mm, 18 cm HOPKINS® 30-degree endoscope
  - (14.5 Fr cystoscopy sheath with 5 Fr instrument channel)
  - (7 Fr, 40 cm biopsy forceps)
  - (7 Fr, 40 cm grasping forceps)
- 3 mm examination sheath
- 3.9 mm Ternamian ENDOTIP cannula or 3 mm operating cannula and sharp trocar
- 5.0 mm, 29 cm HOPKINS® 0-degree endoscope
  - (5.0 mm, 29 cm HOPKINS® 30-degree endoscope)
- 6 mm laparoscopic cannula with sharp trocar (x3) or 6 mm Ternamian ENDOTIP cannula (x3)
- 11 mm laparoscopic cannula with sharp trocar
- 11/6 mm reducing valve
- 5 mm endoscopic biopsy forceps (cup and/or punch type)
- 5 mm endoscopic grasping/dissecting forceps (Marylands)
- 5 mm endoscopic Babcock forceps
- 5 mm endoscopic scissors
- 5 mm palpation probe with centimetre markings
- Normal saline or sterile deionized water (≥1 litre)
- Standard laparotomy surgical kit

Useful additions

- Image capture device (still and video)
- 5 mm suction/irrigation cannula
- Monopolar hook dissector
- 5 mm intestinal handling forceps
- 5 mm endoscopic clip appliers
- 12 mm Endo GIA™ stapler
- 5 mm needle holders

12.2 Equipment required for laparoscopy.

The telescope most commonly used by the author [PL] for laparoscopy is a 5 mm, 0-degree forward-viewing telescope; however, a 5 mm, 30-degree endoscope can be advantageous for some complex procedures, as it allows the operative site to be viewed from different angles and is especially useful where space is limited. Practice is required to use this type of endoscope effectively, and it is recommended to use a 0-degree telescope while learning laparoscopic procedures to reduce the risk of unnecessary complications.

A 5 mm, 0-degree forward-viewing telescope can be used in dogs of all sizes and even cats, although a 2.7 mm, 30-degree telescope is often used in cats and small dogs (<6 kg) as it is less cumbersome and requires a smaller incision. The 2.7 mm, 30-degree telescope is too short and provides too little illumination in dogs larger than 6–8 kg. If the telescope is to be used through a 3.9 mm cannula, it is essential to place it in an examination sheath first, as any leverage on the unsheathed insertion tube is very likely to damage the telescope irreparably. The 5 mm telescopes are more robust and do not require a protective sheath, so they can be used directly through the operating cannula.

Operating telescopes with an integrated working channel through which instruments can be passed into the abdominal cavity are available, but are not generally recommended for surgical interventions as tissue handling becomes a limiting factor. These instruments are usually 11 mm in diameter and therefore not really suited for use in smaller dogs and cats. They also do not provide practice in instrument handling and triangulation, which are skills that can be useful for the more advanced procedures that

are performed less frequently. Laparoscopes as large as 10 mm in diameter can be used for examining large- and giant-breed dogs, but are generally unnecessary. As a rule, the larger the diameter of the telescope, the bigger the resultant image is on the display screen and the more light is conducted into the abdominal cavity to illuminate the field of view.

Light source

A high-intensity xenon light source is considered to give the brightest, whitest light and truest representation of the colours of the abdominal viscera, and is highly recommended (Magne and Tams, 1999; Brandão and Chamness, 2015). Newer LED lighting systems offer an excellent alternative at a more affordable price and the bulbs are very long lasting. However, if a metal halide light source is already available for flexible endoscopy, then this can be used instead. Older halogen light sources are not suitable for laparoscopy.

Camera and video monitor

The use of a camera and video monitor allows excellent visualization of the abdominal cavity by the operator and the assistant, and is essential for the maintenance of a sterile field.

Equipment for insufflation

The most common method of inducing initial insufflation of the abdominal cavity requires a Veress needle (see Chapters 2 and 8). This instrument contains a spring-loaded hollow blunt obturator that normally protrudes past the sharp point of the needle. As the needle is pressed against the abdominal wall, the obturator is pushed up into the body of the needle and the sharp point passes through the muscle and fascia into the peritoneum. As soon as the point of the needle enters the peritoneal space, the obturator springs back to its original position, revealing its blunt point and reducing the chance of iatrogenic trauma to the internal organs.

Automatic insufflators are designed to deliver gas at a predetermined pressure and flow rate (see Chapter 2). The insufflation tubing may be either single use or sterilized and reused. The tubing usually incorporates a single-use filter that prevents fluid from refluxing up the tube and damaging the electronics of the insufflator, and also prevents particulate matter entering the abdominal cavity of the patient.

Carbon dioxide (CO_2) is the gas of choice for insufflation for safety reasons: it has a lower risk of air emboli and of spark ignition when using electrocautery or surgical lasers (Magne and Tams, 1999; Brandão and Chamness, 2015).

Trocars and cannulae

Access to the peritoneal cavity can be accomplished with a multi-port or a single-port access system (see Chapter 2). The terms 'port' and 'cannula' are used interchangeably to refer to the access point into the abdomen.

- The multi-port access system requires trocar–cannula units to be placed independently directly through the abdominal wall.
- Single-port access systems (e.g. the SILS™ system (Medtronic); see Chapter 2) are placed through a single

incision. Several cannulae can then be placed through the single-port access system. This system is used where a larger incision is required (e.g. for laparoscopic-assisted intestinal surgery where organs or masses are to be exteriorized for surgical intervention).

A wide variety of trocar–cannula units are available. Trocars can be sharp, blunt or optical. The type of trocar–cannula unit used depends on the selected entry technique. Blunt trocars are mostly used for open entry with a modified Hasson (or paediatric) technique (see below and also Chapter 8). Sharp and optical trocars are mainly used for closed entry following insufflation with a Veress needle. Ternamian tipped cannulae (Karl Storz) are used without a trocar and enable blunt entry into the abdomen with or without visual guidance.

Trocar–cannula units can also come with a sleeve. The sleeve is initially placed over the Veress needle. Following placement of the Veress needle with the sleeve and insufflation of the abdominal cavity, the needle is removed and the sleeve is kept in place across the abdominal wall. A blunt trocar is then advanced into the lumen of the sleeve and radial forces are applied to stretch the muscle fibres of the abdominal wall without cutting them.

Trocar–cannula units allow the telescope and operating instruments to be introduced into the abdomen. In addition, the CO_2 insufflation tubing can be connected to the cannula to maintain insufflation of the abdominal cavity during the procedure. The tubing is often connected to an instrument port to reduce the flow of cold gas over the telescope, which could result in fogging. Diagnostic procedures usually require two cannulae, while surgical procedures may require two, three or more cannulae, depending on the specific procedure to be performed.

Accessory instruments

A number of accessory instruments are essential during laparoscopy. A palpation probe is required to move, palpate and ballotte the abdominal organs. Almost all palpation probes are marked with centimetre graduations so that the size of organs or lesions can be estimated. Biopsy forceps are used for biopsy of the liver, spleen, abdominal masses, lymph nodes and pancreas. For surgical interventions, commonly used instruments include grasping forceps, dissection forceps, scissors, aspiration/irrigation tubes, monopolar 'J' or 'L' hooks, bipolar vessel sealers/cutters and clip applicators. Many biopsy and surgical instruments also have the capability for monopolar electrosurgery at the distal tip. Ultrasonic dissectors and radiofrequency units are now available to establish safe and reliable haemostasis during laparoscopy.

Patient preparation

Before laparoscopy, the patient should be prepared for general anaesthesia by having food withheld for 12 hours. This will allow emptying of the stomach, which reduces the chances of it being punctured during placement of the trocar–cannula units or Veress needle, and also reduces the risk of regurgitation. If the patient has not passed urine in the hours before surgery, then the bladder should be emptied following the induction of anaesthesia to prevent iatrogenic trauma. In small patients, a full bladder can also take up an appreciable amount of the working space. The surgical field should be clipped, prepared and draped as for routine surgery.

Anaesthetic considerations

Laparoscopy is usually performed under general inhalation anaesthesia. Most patients tolerate general anaesthesia well during laparoscopy, but it is to be expected that the pneumoperitoneum from CO_2 insufflation will increase intra-abdominal pressure and may interfere with ventilation (Duke *et al.*, 1996; Bufalari *et al.*, 1997; Mayhew *et al.*, 2013b). The increase in intra-abdominal pressure associated with laparoscopy can also cause compression of the caudal vena cava and liver, decreasing venous return to the heart and reducing cardiac output. It also reduces diaphragmatic movement, increasing respiratory effort and reducing tidal volume. In healthy animals, at the intra-abdominal pressures recommended, these effects are minimal. However, the patient's haemodynamic status should always be carefully evaluated before laparoscopy. When operating in the cranial abdomen, a 15-degree reverse Trendelenburg position (with the patient's head elevated) will help to relieve some of the pressure on the diaphragm, as well as move the viscera out of the surgical field. However, these advantages must be balanced with the effect of gravity, which will further reduce blood flow to the heart when the head is elevated.

CO_2 is absorbed by the peritoneal lining, contributing to hypercapnia, so end-tidal CO_2 (ETCO$_2$) should be monitored with a capnograph during laparoscopy. ETCO$_2$ will often be increased by 5–20% (from a normal level of approximately 35–45 mmHg). When ETCO$_2$ is elevated to about 50 mmHg, or in cases in which ventilation becomes compromised, it will become necessary to ventilate the patient. Either a mechanical ventilator or manual ventilation achieved by applying intermittent pressure to the rebreathing bag can be used. If a mechanical ventilator is used, care must be taken not to over-ventilate in order to mitigate the possibility of pulmonary damage. For most routine elective laparoscopic procedures, providing an assisted breath once every 1–2 minutes by compressing the rebreathing bag is all that is required. However, for longer procedures, and especially if there is pre-existing cardiorespiratory compromise, a mechanical ventilator is recommended.

Initially, insufflation should be at a low flow rate to allow the patient's homeostatic mechanisms to compensate for the increased intra-abdominal pressure. The flow rate will depend of the size of the patient and may be as low as 0.2 litres/minute in cats and small dogs, or as high as 2 litres/minute in giant-breed dogs. Once insufflation is complete, the flow rate can be increased to 1–4 litres/minute (depending on the size of the animal) to allow rapid replacement of gas and to maintain a near-uniform pressure in the event of gas leakage during the insertion of instruments. Intra-abdominal pressure should always be maintained below 10 mmHg in dogs and 6–8 mmHg in cats. Usually a pressure of 4–6 mmHg is sufficient for excellent visualization. It may be necessary to use a higher pressure (10 mmHg in dogs, 6 mmHg in cats) during initial placement of the cannulae to reduce indentation of the abdominal wall during their insertion and thereby reduce the risk of iatrogenic damage to the abdominal organs by the sharp trocar. Once the cannulae are in place, the intra-abdominal pressure can be reduced. A local anaesthetic block with bupivacaine or lidocaine is recommended at each cannula site at the beginning of the procedure to aid in analgesia and balanced anaesthesia. Bupivacaine has a slower onset (30 min) and a longer duration of action (3–8 h) and is therefore a better option for postoperative pain. Lidocaine acts faster (10–20 min), although it has a shorter duration of action (1–2 h). However, this is usually sufficient for small wounds with minimal trauma.

Procedure

Insufflation

A working space has to be created by introducing CO_2 into the peritoneal cavity. Initial entry into the peritoneal cavity is associated with the risk of puncture of an abdominal organ or a large blood vessel. Both closed and open entry techniques have been described and are associated with a low risk of puncture of the abdominal organs and major vasculature in human patients (Garry, 1999; Alkatout, 2017). Most of the time, the choice of technique is dictated by the surgeon's preference.

- Veress needle technique – this is the most common method of inducing initial insufflation of the abdominal cavity.
- Hasson or modified Hasson (paediatric) technique – this approach avoids the blind insertion of a sharp Veress needle into the peritoneal space. The cannulae used for the Hasson technique have a blunt trocar. This technique should theoretically minimize the risk of trauma to the abdominal organs that can occur with a Veress needle or sharp trocar.

Veress needle technique

If a Veress needle is used, it is usually placed in the site to be used by the first (telescope) port or an instrument port. It is beneficial to introduce a small bleb of local anaesthetic (bupivacaine or lidocaine) at the puncture site (and indeed at all port sites) before the introduction of the Veress needle, as this greatly reduces any postoperative discomfort.

1. A small (1 mm) stab incision using a No. 11 scalpel blade is made in the skin at the chosen site, either in the ventral midline or in the paralumbar fossa of the side corresponding to the site of the surgical approach.
2. The external fascia can also be incised with a No. 11 scalpel blade to facilitate placement of the needle.
3. The abdominal cavity should be palpated to localize the spleen before placing the Veress needle. The spleen can sometimes be manipulated out of the surgical field by moving it to the left side, but in any case it must be avoided.
4. The skin and abdominal wall are grasped with the thumb and forefinger of the non-dominant hand and tented upwards.
5. The Veress needle is grasped by the barrel, allowing the central blunt obturator to move freely. It is then introduced into the incision at an angle to the skin surface by pointing it caudally towards the pelvis and into the pocket created by the elevated abdominal wall (Figure 12.3). In this way, iatrogenic damage to the spleen is less likely and the fatty falciform ligament is avoided.
6. Alternatively, stay sutures can be placed through the external fascia of the abdominal wall to provide counter-traction while the Veress needle is inserted, or towel clamps can be used to elevate the abdominal wall adjacent to the point of insertion.

The Veress needle consists of a spring-loaded obturator surrounded by a sheath with a sharp cutting tip. The obturator retracts into the needle shaft as it traverses the abdominal wall, exposing the sharp cutting tip. Once the needle has penetrated the wall and entered the abdominal cavity, the obturator advances beyond the tip and is intended to reduce the risk of iatrogenic injury to the internal abdominal organs.

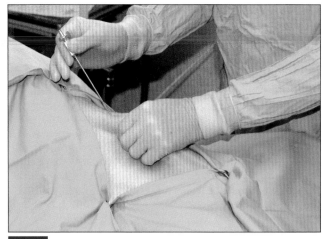

12.3 Introducing the Veress needle.

- The Veress needle is introduced with a quick controlled stabbing movement rather than a continuous push, which often results in deeper penetration. It may be helpful to allow the heel of the hand to rest gently on the abdominal wall to permit a more controlled entry into the abdomen.
- With experience, the tip of the needle can felt entering the peritoneal space with a slight 'pop' as the blunt obturator springs back into place. Several tests can be performed to confirm appropriate placement of the needle in the peritoneal cavity (Vilos, 2006; Vilos et al., 2007; Kroft et al., 2009).
  - The lever on the top of the Veress needle is opened and a syringe of saline is attached to the Luer fitting.
  - Gentle suction is applied; if fluid or blood is apparent, the needle is withdrawn 1 cm or so and repositioned, as it may indicate entry into the spleen or a large blood vessel. Intestinal content may be aspirated if a loop of intestine has been penetrated, although this is extremely rare. If intestinal content is aspirated, a laparotomy may be required to close the puncture site in the intestine.
  - If all is well, 1–2 ml of sterile saline is injected into the abdomen. It should flow freely and easily. The syringe is then removed and, with the tap still open, the abdominal wall is tented up with the distal end of the Veress needle to ensure that the drop of saline sinks in the needle hub as a result of the negative pressure created (hanging drop method). This should occur if the needle is correctly placed.
- Once the Veress needle has been placed correctly, sterile tubing is attached to the hub and connected to the insufflator. The insufflator should register a reasonably high gas flow (around or just below the flow rate set on the insufflator) and abdominal pressure should initially be low (<2 mmHg). If the abdominal pressure rises rapidly or gas flow is low/zero, this usually indicates that the needle is incorrectly placed (i.e. subcutaneously, retroperitoneally or in the falciform ligament) or blocked (Vilos, 2006; Vilos et al., 2007; Kroft et al., 2009). Gentle manipulation of the tip of the needle or replacement may be required in such instances.
- The abdomen is slowly insufflated to a pressure of about 8–10 mmHg in dogs or 6–8 mmHg in cats. Once the initial ports have been placed, it is often possible to reduce the intra-abdominal pressure to 4–6 mmHg in dogs or 2–4 mmHg in cats to maintain a sufficient operating space.

Optical Veress needles are available that can be used to monitor the placement of the needle into the abdominal cavity. A small endoscope is placed within the lumen of the Veress needle to visualize its introduction into the peritoneal cavity. A closed approach can also be performed with an optical trocar, without placement of a Veress needle and insufflation of the abdominal cavity. The abdominal wall is lifted with two stay sutures placed in the linea alba, close to the site of introduction of the optical trocar, to provide counter-traction. A small incision is made in the linea alba and the optical trocar is advanced through the body wall under direct visualization via an endoscope placed with the tip just inside the distal end of the trocar. A Veress needle is not required if an open approach is used (see below).

Complications: Penetration of the spleen will result in haemorrhage, which can obscure visualization and interfere with surgery. It is rarely dangerous and will usually cease unaided or with gentle pressure from the tip of a palpation probe. Insufflation of gas into a mass, organ or vessel can result in a fatal gas embolism, so it is essential to ensure that the Veress needle is correctly placed before commencing insufflation.

Problems that may be encountered with Veress needle placement include:

- Placing the needle subcutaneously or peritoneal tenting (especially in cats)
- Placing the needle into the omentum or falciform ligament
- Penetrating a viscus.

Subcutaneous placement of the Veress needle can be very frustrating but is fairly easily avoided. With practice, it is possible to appreciate the feel of the Veress needle penetrating the peritoneum, but inexperienced endoscopists are understandably cautious and may fail to penetrate the abdominal wall completely before starting insufflation. This may result in subcutaneous emphysema. Although this is not dangerous, it can impede technique and make subsequent proper placement of the Veress needle more difficult. The emphysema will resolve over approximately 48 hours.

In the cat, the peritoneum is relatively loosely attached to the overlying musculature and it is not uncommon for peritoneal tenting to occur, especially if the Veress needle is not inserted with a controlled quick stabbing motion. The Veress needle passes through the musculature but fails to penetrate the peritoneum and instead pushes it away, creating a space between the peritoneum and the abdominal musculature.

If the Veress needle is inadvertently inserted into the omental bursa, mesentery or falciform ligament, these structures can be insufflated and obscure the view when the endoscope is inserted via the primary port. If this occurs, and it is not possible to negotiate the tip of the endoscope around the obstruction (which happens occasionally), it may be necessary to desufflate the abdomen, reposition the Veress needle and try again.

Hasson (paediatric) technique

The Hasson (or paediatric) technique is an open approach that requires a mini-laparotomy to be performed (Hasson, 1984; Kassir *et al.*, 2014). A midline incision of 2 cm is made at the port site, and the skin over the midline and the fascia is dissected from the linea alba. Two stay sutures are placed lateral to the midline and the linea alba is elevated. An incision is made in the linea alba to accommodate the cannula (5 mm for a 6 mm cannula) and the cannula is introduced with or without a blunt trocar. The abdomen is then insufflated through the cannula.

The disadvantages of this technique are that it creates a much larger incision than is needed for the placement of the first cannula, it is more time-consuming than the Veress needle technique and it increases the risk of the cannula moving in and out of the abdomen as instruments are passed through it, since friction with the abdominal wall is reduced. Care must be taken as iatrogenic damage to abdominal organs may still occur during insertion of the cannula. Hasson cannulae are commercially available; traditionally these had flanges to allow the cannula to be sutured in place to prevent movement, although newer modifications are now available with an inflatable cuff at the tip and a moveable plastic buffer to slide down the shaft and secure the abdominal wall against the cuff. Alternatively some have cone-shaped anchoring devices that slide down into the incision. Standard laparoscopic cannulae can also be used with this approach.

Cats have a very distensible abdomen, which makes them good candidates for laparoscopy as there is more working space in a 4 kg cat than a dog of comparable size. However, the abdominal wall is thin and incision sites tend to stretch with insufflation, allowing cannulae to slip in and out as instruments are inserted and removed. A balloon cannula (e.g. Kii® Fios, First Entry Advanced Fixation Disc, Applied Medical (5 mm x 75 mm)) is extremely useful in cats, as the balloon/retention disc keeps the cannula in place even during insufflation and instrument use.

Comparison of the Veress needle and Hasson techniques

There has been much debate in both the medical and the veterinary literature about the relative benefits of the Veress needle technique *versus* the Hasson (paediatric) technique. Extrapolation of data from human medicine should be avoided, as the anatomy of veterinary patients is considerably different. The abdomen of dogs and cats is more laterally compressed, whereas the human abdomen is compressed anteroposteriorly. In thin human patients, there may be as little as 2 cm between the abdominal wall and the retroperitoneal vascular structures; this increases the likelihood of vascular injuries to the aorta or vena cava when the Veress needle technique is used. Such injuries have not been documented in veterinary medicine, probably because of the larger space between the abdominal wall and these vascular structures in veterinary patients.

Another relevant anatomical difference is that in humans the spleen is relatively small and located under the rib cage on the left side. In some breeds of dog, such as the German Shepherd Dog, the spleen may be extremely large and extend across the midline of the central abdomen, and is therefore more likely to suffer iatrogenic injury from both Veress needle and port placement. In humans, splenic injury will usually necessitate splenectomy, whereas splenic bleeding in the dog is quite easily controlled. Indeed, splenic biopsy samples are sometimes taken with biopsy forceps in the same way as liver samples. In addition, in humans, the Hasson/paediatric technique has been shown to increase the risk of intestinal injury during introduction, as the loops of intestine lie immediately under the site of entry.

In short, certainly in human laparoscopic surgery, meta-analysis of the literature has revealed no evidence that the open entry (i.e. Hasson) technique is superior or inferior to other entry techniques currently available (Ahmad *et al.*, 2019; Toro *et al.*, 2012). There is little published research from veterinary medicine, although one paper looking at complications occurring during the initial learning process of laparoscopic ovariectomy in the bitch followed four surgeons new to laparoscopic techniques and found that splenic laceration occurred in six of 618 cases (Pope and Knowles, 2014). Four lacerations occurred during placement of a cannula by the Hasson/paediatric technique, and two during the introduction of a Veress needle. Ultimately, the safest technique is the one with which the surgeon is most familiar.

Surgical approaches

The two most common approaches are the right lateral and the ventral midline approach. Wherever possible, the author [PL] uses a ventral midline approach through the linea alba to reduce postoperative discomfort and give access to both sides of the abdomen. When placing a midline port cranial to the umbilicus, it is helpful to angle the port at 45 degrees to the vertical so that it enters the abdomen lateral to the falciform fat to prevent instruments getting entangled in the fat.

Lateral approach

The lateral approach is usually performed with the patient in an oblique position to use gravity for retraction of the abdominal organs. The patient is placed at a 30-degree angle with the dorsal spinous processes elevated to increase exposure of the kidney, adrenal gland and pancreas. The right lateral approach is recommended for diagnostic evaluation of the liver, gall bladder, right lobe of the pancreas, duodenum, right kidney and right adrenal gland. The left lateral approach is used for exposure of the left kidney, left adrenal gland and oesophageal hiatus. It should be noted that because the spleen lies directly under the normal entry sites for this approach, there is the potential for trocar/cannula insertion to cause splenic trauma.

Ventral approach

A ventral approach is often used for surgical procedures and offers good visualization of the whole of the liver, gall bladder, pancreas, kidneys, adrenal glands, stomach, intestines, reproductive system, urinary bladder and spleen. With the ventral approach, the primary (telescope) port is placed on the midline caudal to the umbilicus. A disadvantage of the ventral approach is that the falciform ligament may impair visualization of the cranial abdomen, especially in obese animals. Placement of the telescope port caudal to the umbilicus will usually allow the surgeon to withdraw the telescope sufficiently to manoeuvre around the caudal boundary of the falciform ligament and visualize both sides of the cranial abdomen. With a ventral approach, it is not unusual to tilt the patient laterally to a 30-degree or 45-degree angle, to allow gravity to move the abdominal organs from the surgical field of view and improve visualization (e.g. of the ovaries during an ovariectomy).

Port positions

In all cases, careful preoperative planning of port positions is essential. Port positioning varies according to the size of the patient and the procedure to be undertaken. It is essential to imagine the operative site in three dimensions and plan the procedure such that the ports are at a sufficient distance from the site of interest so that instruments are not crowded together and can be introduced at a comfortable angle for the surgeon (usually at 45–75 degrees to each other) (Manasnayakorn *et al.*, 2008). Ideally, the target organ should be 15–20 cm from the trocar used for placing the telescope (the optical trocar) and the same distance from the operating trocars, which are placed either side of the optical trocar on an arc with the target organ at the centre; however, these distances may be constrained by the size of the patient. For maximum ergonomic efficiency, the angle of elevation between the instruments and the target organ should be the same as the angle between the instruments, and the azimuth angles between the instruments and the optical port should be equal (see Chapter 8).

Cannula placement

The first trocar–cannula unit (or Ternamian ENDOTIP cannula; see below) placed via either an open or a closed technique is usually the cannula that receives the telescope (Garry, 1999). It is very important to avoid the spleen when placing the first cannula, especially if using a sharp trocar. Abdominal palpation to locate the spleen before insufflation, together with careful insertion technique, will help prevent iatrogenic damage. Selection of the site for the telescope port is determined by the relative importance of being able to visualize the different abdominal structures. The entry site is determined and, following local analgesia by infiltration of a local anaesthetic agent (e.g. bupivacaine, or lidocaine – see above), a single stab incision is made with a No. 11 blade through the skin and linea alba. Due to the pointed shape of the blade, the incision in the linea alba will be slightly smaller than the skin incision.

The skin incision should be just large enough to accommodate the diameter of the cannula. It is important to ensure that the initial incision is the correct size. If a smooth cannula is used, an over-large incision will allow the cannula to move in and out of the incision as instruments are inserted and withdrawn due to repeated instrument exchange via port. A practical way to assess the correct incision size is to make an impression of the open cannula end on the skin (with the trocar removed). If the cannula end is cut at an angle the impression will be oval. The incision should be made just smaller than the narrowest diameter of the impression to ensure a tight fit.

Once the skin incision has been made, the trocar–cannula unit is passed through the abdominal wall in a controlled manner. Holding the upper end of the trocar in the palm of the hand, pressure is exerted with a twisting motion until the tip of the cannula enters the peritoneal space. The depth of penetration of the cannula is limited by a finger placed along the shaft (Figure 12.4). Immediately after entry into the abdomen, the sharp trocar is removed from the cannula to prevent organ trauma and the cannula is pushed gently into the abdominal cavity a little further. Ideally, the tip of the cannula should be just inside the peritoneal space to provide the largest working area and limit the blind spot behind the tip of the endoscope. The valve in the cannula closes as soon as the trocar is removed to prevent the escape of gas.

If a Ternamian ENDOTIP cannula (which has no sharp trocar) is used, the technique is slightly different. This type of cannula is introduced with a clockwise screwing motion to allow it to bluntly dissect through the abdominal wall with the telescope in place, permitting visual entry into the

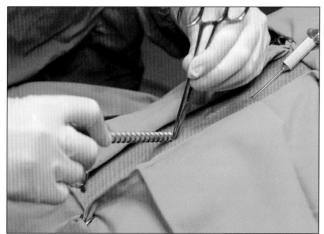

12.4 Location of the incision in the linea alba with blunt haemostats before placement of a Ternamian tipped cannula.

peritoneal cavity. The initial incision should be the same size as the diameter of the body of the cannula but smaller than the diameter of the thread, as an incision smaller than the diameter of the body of the cannula will result in skin being caught up in the thread and rotated as the cannula is screwed in. The incision must penetrate any fascial sheath below the skin incision to facilitate blunt dissection through the deeper tissue planes. The blunt tip of the cannula must be placed into the incision in the linea alba or the cannula will just push the abdominal wall away from the skin as it is inserted. It can be surprisingly difficult to locate the incision in the linea alba, especially in overweight dogs; localization can be greatly facilitated by inserting closed blunt haemostats into the incision (Figure 12.4). This technique is also useful to locate the abdominal wall incision when placing sutures. The threaded barrel of the ENDOTIP cannula helps prevent displacement during surgery.

The insufflation tubing can now be transferred from the Veress needle to the inlet port of the cannula, and the Veress needle can then be removed. This allows gas flow to be directed away from the telescope lens, helping to keep it clear. However, cold gas can sometimes cause fogging of the lens. If this is a problem, moving the gas inflow to an instrument port may help. The telescope is then connected to the light source and the camera and advanced through the rubber seal of the cannula and into the abdomen. The trapdoor valve in the cannula is opened manually to reduce the risk of trauma to the lens of the telescope. Upon entry into the abdominal cavity, the image may be blurred due to fogging of the telescope lens. To prevent fogging it is recommended to use a commercially available antifogging solution or alternatively a povidone–iodine solution. It is also helpful to immerse the telescope in warm saline or sterile water for a minute or two before it is introduced into the abdomen, to reduce fogging. In addition, if fogging becomes a problem during a procedure, gently touching the lens of the telescope on a serosal surface will usually clear the lens.

Examination technique

Once the telescope is in the abdominal cavity, careful examination of the viscera is performed. First, the region directly below the cannula site and the Veress needle site is evaluated for any evidence of haemorrhage or other iatrogenic damage (Figure 12.5). Then a quick examination of the whole ventral abdomen is carried out to look for additional pathology. The site of entry for the second

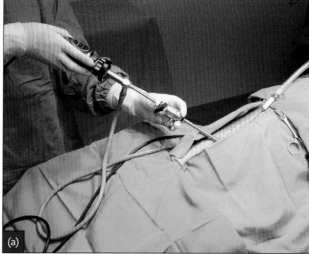

(a)

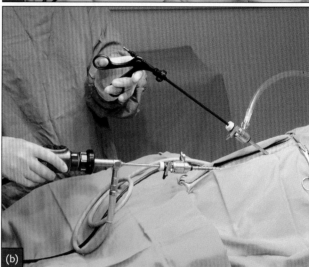

(b)

12.5 (a) Following insertion of the telescope, the area immediately underlying the primary port and Veress needle is examined for iatrogenic damage. (b) A secondary port has been inserted for the introduction of biopsy forceps.

(instrument) port is then selected under direct visualization and percutaneous palpation of the body wall. This location depends upon the procedures that are to be performed. Transillumination of the abdominal wall using the telescope light source will enable any large blood vessels to be avoided when making the incision for the second port. The second cannula is then placed through the abdominal wall in the manner described above, and is observed directly through the telescope as it enters the abdomen to avoid damage to the underlying viscera.

Exploration of the abdominal cavity is assisted by using a palpation probe to 'feel' and move the organs as needed. The use of other instruments, such as grasping forceps, should be avoided when exploring the abdomen and moving organs and tissues, as they are likely to cause iatrogenic damage to the delicate tissues. Instruments should never be passed blindly into the abdomen, but rather viewed via the endoscope and camera as they pass through the cannula, and directed to the area of interest. Using this technique will help prevent serious tissue trauma by the probe or other accessory instruments. If an instrument is lost from the field of view, it is important not to try to manipulate it back into view, but rather to withdraw the endoscope to give a more panoramic view until the instrument is visualized, and then follow it back down to the operative site. It may sometimes be helpful to tilt the patient from side to side or by 10–20 degrees in a Trendelenburg/reverse Trendelenburg position to allow gravity to move the viscera out of the field of view and facilitate the examination. The endoscope and instruments should always be retracted from the abdomen before rolling the patient to prevent iatrogenic damage.

Ending the procedure

At the conclusion of the laparoscopic procedure, the instruments and telescope are removed. The pneumoperitoneum is relieved by discontinuing CO_2 insufflation and opening the two-way stopcocks on the cannulae. The abdomen is desufflated slowly to allow homeostatic mechanisms to adapt to the reduced abdominal pressure. The trapdoor valves on the cannulae are then removed. Gentle pressure on the abdominal wall will help to remove any gas that is not removed by the natural elasticity of the body wall as it reverts to its normal position. Care should taken that the tip of the cannula does not traumatize abdominal viscera as the abdomen desufflates.

Human patients can experience shoulder pain following laparoscopy. The leading hypothesis is that residual CO_2 retained in the abdomen after surgery results in phrenic nerve irritation, which causes referred pain to the nerve root at C4. This does not appear to be a problem in veterinary patients, and the authors have never seen a patient showing lameness as a sign of pain after laparoscopy. However, it is generally recommended never to exceed a maximum intra-abdominal pressure of 15 mmHg (10 mmHg routinely in dogs and 8 mmHg in cats) and to ensure that as much CO_2 as possible is removed at the end of the procedure. Removal of residual CO_2 can be facilitated by placing the patient in a Trendelenburg position (with the head lowered at an angle of 30 degrees) and performing a pulmonary recruitment manoeuvre (PRM) consisting of five manual inflations of the lungs with the trapdoor mechanism removed from the cannulae to allow free flow of gas out of the abdomen. If using a Ternamian ENDOTIP cannula, this can be assisted by elevating the abdominal wall using the cannula several times, which produces a bellows effect and flushes the abdomen. The PRM has been shown to reduce shoulder and abdominal pain in human patients by more than 50% in the 3 days after laparoscopic surgery (Toro *et al.*, 2012). After removal of the cannulae, the incision sites are sutured in two layers in a routine manner.

Additional considerations

If appreciable ascites is present, it is best partially drained before laparoscopy. Gas-filled loops of intestine floating on top of ascitic fluid are more prone to damage by the Veress needle or the introduction of cannulae, and will make visualization difficult during surgery. Drainage by syringe and three-way tap with a large-bore intravenous catheter placed in the midline will usually suffice. If ascites is present, all abdominal incisions should be closed in at least two layers to prevent seepage of fluid postoperatively.

With any laparoscopic procedure, the surgeon should always be prepared to convert to conventional open surgery should it be required. For instance, persistent haemorrhage, unforeseen complications or removal of a large mass may all require conversion to open laparotomy. A full laparotomy kit should be available in the operating theatre at all times.

Biopsy techniques
Liver biopsy

Liver biopsy is one of the most common indications for diagnostic laparoscopy and with practice can be completed very rapidly and with minimal trauma to the patient. Most diseases of the liver will be managed medically, but often a definitive diagnosis can only be obtained histologically. Laparoscopy enables tissue samples to be taken under direct visualization from lesions in the liver, and images of the entire organ or specific lesions to be captured and then sent to the laboratory along with the samples to aid the pathologists with their diagnosis. Any haemorrhage can be seen and dealt with directly. Laparoscopic and wedge-style biopsy samples have been shown to provide superior histopathological results than specimens obtained using a Tru-Cut-style needle (Cole *et al.*, 2002; Kimbrell *et al.*, 2018). The quality of biopsy samples collected laparoscopically is considered superior to any other type because the biopsy specimen is taken from the region of interest under direct visualization, and a significant amount of tissue is obtained for histopathological analysis (Cole *et al.*, 2002; Harmoinen *et al.*, 2002; Twedt and Monnet, 2005; Case, 2015). Furthermore, there is less risk of iatrogenic damage than with percutaneous needle biopsy, any haemorrhage can be controlled and, as an added bonus, the entire abdomen can be examined in detail during the same procedure.

Before undertaking a liver biopsy, a coagulation profile should be obtained. This should include the prothrombin time, partial thromboplastin time and an accurate platelet count. Determination of the buccal mucosal bleeding time is also advised. Although coagulopathies are a relative contraindication to liver biopsy, the coagulation status does not necessarily predict whether the animal will bleed from a liver biopsy (Ewe, 1981; McGill, 1981).

Liver biopsy is most commonly performed via a ventral midline approach with the patient in dorsal recumbency. The camera port is placed just caudal to the umbilicus to allow manipulation of the endoscope to both sides of the falciform fat. The instrument port is placed a few centimetres cranial to this position. This approach enables access to both sides of the liver.

Alternatively, a right lateral approach with the patient in left lateral recumbency can be used; this approach avoids the falciform fat but gives access to only the right side of the liver. For a lateral approach, the first cannula for the telescope is placed in the caudodorsal abdominal wall in the region of the paralumbar fossa. A second cannula is then placed at the same level as the first, but more towards the midline (Figure 12.6), on a line between the iliac crest and the xiphoid. (A left-handed surgeon may do the opposite so as to have the biopsy instrument in the dominant hand.) As much as 85% of the liver, the extrahepatic biliary system and the right lobe of the pancreas can be visualized with this approach.

The telescope and palpation probe are moved cranially, with the tip of the probe in view. The diaphragm and the diaphragmatic surface of the liver can then be examined. The telescope is then withdrawn slightly and the gall bladder can be seen between the right lateral and right medial lobes of the liver, which are elevated to expose the visceral surface and the proximal biliary tree. The gall bladder can be palpated with the probe and the patency of the biliary tree assessed. The cystic duct can be traced down to the common bile duct where it enters the duodenum. The other lobes of the liver are then elevated in turn to visualize the visceral surfaces (Figure 12.7) and

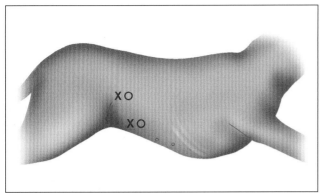

12.6 Port positions for liver biopsy (O) and pancreatic biopsy (X) in left lateral recumbency.

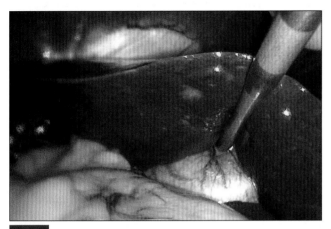

12.7 Inspecting the liver with a palpation probe.

hilium. The normal liver should be of a uniform deep red colour and should not be friable or bleed easily on palpation. The gall bladder should be thin walled and easily compressible. Any swellings or areas of discoloration or obvious pathology should be noted and the gall bladder should be palpated.

The use of 5 mm cup biopsy forceps is recommended. The biopsy forceps are directed to the area of the liver to be sampled; either an edge or the surface of the liver can be sampled with forceps (Figure 12.8). It is always important to take samples from three or four areas, including some that appear grossly normal. If the liver pathology is diffuse and generalized, biopsy samples are taken from the edge of the liver lobes.

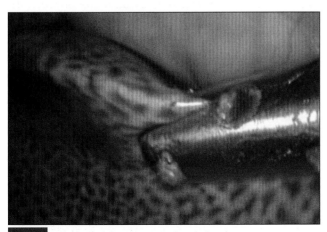

12.8 Biopsy of the liver using cup biopsy forceps.

The biopsy forceps are advanced to a position just below the border of the lobe to be biopsied. The cups of the forceps are opened and the forceps are slowly withdrawn with slight upward pressure, such that the edge of the liver lobe naturally falls within the cups as the forceps come to the edge of the lobe. The cups are then closed. The author [PL] generally holds the cups tightly closed for approximately 15–30 seconds before pulling the sample away from the liver. The normal liver capsule is quite tough and a reasonably firm tug is often needed to detach the sample. This does not cause damage to the liver or sample and there is rarely much haemorrhage.

The biopsy area is then closely monitored for excessive bleeding. Generally, most biopsy sites bleed very little (Figure 12.9), although the magnified image observed on the monitor can often make a slight seepage of blood seem like a lot; usually it is only a maximum of approximately 5 ml and bleeding stops within 2–3 minutes. If bleeding is considered to be excessive, pressure can be applied with the palpation probe, or a small piece of saline-soaked Gelfoam® can be placed into the biopsy site. These options are usually sufficient to control excessive bleeding. On occasion, the judicious use of electrocautery is of benefit. Cautery can be applied with the biopsy forceps if they are attached to a monopolar energy source, but the biopsy sample should be removed first to prevent thermal damage to it.

Endoscopic needles or long spinal needles can be used to drain and flush cysts and abscesses or to take samples from cysts under direct visual guidance.

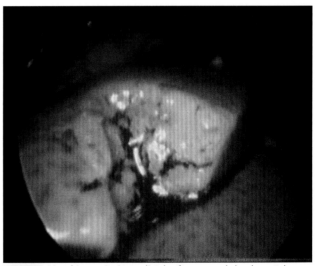

12.9 Liver biopsy site immediately after a sample has been taken, showing minimal haemorrhage.

Cholecystocentesis

Cholecystocentesis is often performed at the same time as liver biopsy. A percutaneous cholecystocentesis can be performed under laparoscopic guidance via a right lateral or ventral midline approach (Figure 12.10). Two 5 mm cannulae are needed, especially if liver biopsy samples are to be taken at the same time, which is usually the case. The site of puncture is determined under direct visualization within the abdominal cavity, while pressure is applied outside on the abdominal wall, as the shortest distance from the abdominal wall to the gall bladder. It is also important to identify the line of attachment of the diaphragm; the needle should not penetrate through the diaphragm to

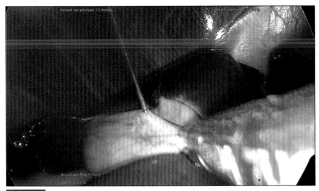

12.10 Aspiration of the gall bladder under laparoscopic control.

avoid a pneumothorax. It is often helpful to partially desufflate the abdomen to a pressure of 3–4 mmHg to reduce the distance between the abdominal wall and the gall bladder, especially in medium-sized to large dogs. A 20 G, 3 inch (80 mm) spinal needle is used to aspirate the gall bladder. After penetration through the abdominal wall, the needle is directed to the gall bladder under direct visualization with the endoscope. It is possible to first penetrate through the liver parenchyma before entering the lumen of the gall bladder to limit leakage of bile, although this is not strictly necessary. Grasping forceps may be needed to stabilize and expose the gall bladder within the abdominal cavity. The gall bladder should be emptied as much as possible to reduce the internal pressure and limit the risk of leakage. A cholecystostomy tube can also be placed laparoscopically (Murphy *et al.*, 2007).

Pancreatic biopsy

The right lobe of the pancreas lies adjacent to the duodenum, between two layers of the mesoduodenum. The body of the pancreas, adjacent to the pylorus, unites the left and right lobes, and the left lobe is in the deep leaf of the greater omentum.

Pancreatic biopsy is performed via a right lateral or ventral midline approach. The right lateral approach gives an excellent view of the duodenum and the right lobe of the pancreas, as well as the extrahepatic biliary system and the liver (Twedt, 1999; Harmoinen *et al.*, 2002). A midline approach with the patient rolled 45 degrees to the left gives excellent access to the right lobe and body of the pancreas. A ventral midline approach enables examination of the whole pancreas but requires considerably more dissection to access the left lobe, and is rarely necessary. Access to the left lobe in the omental bursa is gained by blunt dissection through the avascular part of the greater omentum just caudal to the gastroepiploic vessels. The greater curvature of the stomach may need to be elevated a little first and cranial traction applied to the omentum in order to see the left lobe of the pancreas. If the patient is rolled 45 degrees to the right, the left lobe of the pancreas can be accessed by moving the spleen medially with a palpation probe.

As for liver biopsy (see above), two cannulae are required for this procedure. They are placed in the caudal part of the abdomen in sites similar to those for liver biopsy, but it is often beneficial to place each cannula 3–5 cm caudal to the sites used for liver biopsy (see Figure 12.6). The endoscope is introduced to the level of the pylorus, and the mesentery is moved cranially and to the left with a gentle raking movement of a blunt probe. The duodenum is identified and elevated, revealing the right lobe of the pancreas for inspection.

The normal pancreas is pale pink and uniformly nodular in texture. Swelling and oedema may indicate acute pancreatitis, whereas extensive nodularity or calcification may indicate chronic pancreatitis. Masses may also be seen, although islet tumours are often too small to be seen macroscopically. Punch-type laparoscopic biopsy forceps are preferred for sample collection (Figure 12.11), as they cut through the mesenteric covering of the pancreas better, although cup biopsy forceps can also be used. The biopsy site selected should be at the edge of the pancreas, away from the location of the pancreatic ducts that traverse the centre of the gland and subsequently enter the duodenum with the common bile duct.

As with all pancreatic surgery, minimal manipulation will minimize the risk of iatrogenic mechanically induced pancreatitis. In practice, this is rarely a problem. Haemorrhage from biopsy sites is minimal and can be controlled as for liver biopsies (Figure 12.12).

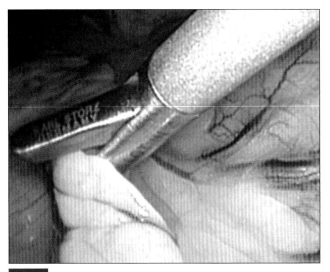

12.11 Biopsy of a normal pancreas using punch-type biopsy forceps.

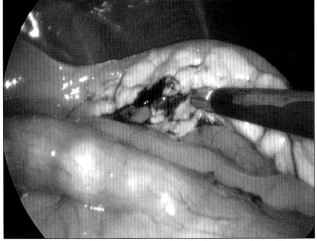

12.12 Pancreatic biopsy site immediately after a sample has been taken, showing minimal haemorrhage.

Renal biopsy

Laparoscopy is well suited for evaluation and biopsy of the kidney (Grauer *et al.*, 1983; Rawlings *et al.*, 2003a). An automatic core-type biopsy needle is recommended for sample collection. Direct visualization of the kidney allows the operator to navigate the biopsy needle to the desired site to be sampled and also to monitor and control excessive postoperative bleeding.

Before performing renal biopsy, adequate evaluation of the kidneys is necessary, including techniques such as contrast excretory urography and ultrasonography. This is vital to determine whether specific pathology is present in one or both kidneys and to determine the functional integrity of the kidney(s) in question. Unless there is a specific indication to sample the left kidney, the right kidney is preferred because it is less mobile. A left kidney biopsy performed through a left lateral approach is more difficult because the spleen is located beneath the usual cannula entry site.

The ventral abdomen and right abdominal wall to just below the lateral processes of the lumbar vertebrae are clipped and prepared for surgery. The patient is positioned in partial or complete left lateral recumbency. Using a right lateral mid-abdominal telescope placement, the right kidney is easily visualized (Figures 12.13 and 12.14). Alternatively, a midline approach with the patient rolled 45 degrees to the left gives excellent access to the right kidney and enables the cannulae to be placed in the linea alba, reducing perioperative discomfort. The author [PL] always places a second cannula so that a palpation probe is available to provide tamponade at the biopsy site. The palpation probe is placed in the abdomen above the kidney. The entry site for the biopsy needle is determined by percutaneous palpation of the abdominal wall while viewing with the telescope internally. When kidney biopsy samples are taken,

the needle entry site through the abdominal wall should be caudal to the diaphragm. If the needle penetrates the diaphragm, a pneumothorax may result from leakage of the pneumoperitoneum into the thorax.

A 1 mm stab incision is made in the skin at the desired entry site and the needle is directed into the abdominal cavity and to the kidney. The usual location for sample collection is the cranial or caudal pole of the kidney; it is important to obtain predominantly cortex with little medulla. The needle should be introduced at a tangential angle and should not penetrate deep into the kidney because the arcuate arteries are located in the corticomedullary junction. The biopsy needle is seated through the renal capsule and the needle is 'fired'. Use of a 14 G Tru-Cut biopsy needle is recommended to collect good samples for pathological evaluation. The surgeon must be aware of the 'throw distance' of the needle when fired, to avoid perforating right through the kidney and causing iatrogenic damage to the structures beyond (adrenal gland, vena cava, liver). The needle is then removed from the abdominal cavity. Generally, several millilitres of blood will flow from the biopsy site; this haemorrhage can appear alarming due to the magnification provided by the display screen, and is usually greater than that seen with liver or pancreatic biopsy samples taken with biopsy forceps. The palpation probe should be quickly moved over the bleeding area and pressure applied for several minutes (Figure 12.15). Although this procedure can be done single-handedly, it may be useful to consider having an assistant to pre-place the palpation probe at the intended biopsy site to then quickly apply pressure upon removal of the needle to reduce subcapsular haemorrage. Additional samples can be taken if the first is not considered suitable. Once the haemorrhage has been controlled, the palpation probe is removed and the abdomen is desufflated. Finally, the camera and primary port are removed and the cannulae are withdrawn. Port closure is routine.

Intestinal biopsy

Full-thickness small intestinal biopsy samples can be obtained at laparoscopy using the technique of grasping and then exteriorizing a portion of intestine through the abdominal wall. The intestinal biopsy sample is then

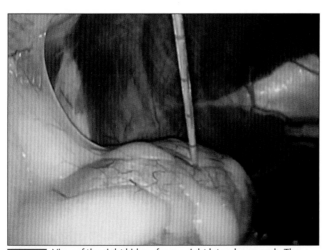

12.13 View of the right kidney from a right lateral approach. The Tru-Cut needle is placed in the cranial pole of the kidney.

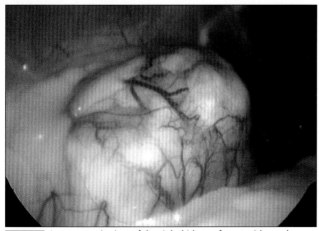

12.14 Laparoscopic view of the right kidney of a cat with renal lymphosarcoma.

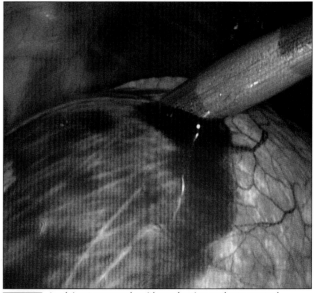

12.15 Applying tamponade with a palpation probe to control haemorrhage following renal biopsy.

obtained from the exteriorized intestine, as would be done for a standard full-thickness surgical biopsy (Case, 2015).

Intestinal biopsy requires three cannulae. One is used for the telescope and the other two are used to introduce two pairs of grasping forceps to examine the intestine. Generally, this procedure is performed in dorsal recumbency from a standard ventral midline approach. The camera port is placed just cranial to the umbilicus along the ventral midline and the two operative ports are placed either caudal to the umbilicus on the midline, or lateral to the midline, depending on the site to be examined and operator preference (Figure 12.16). It is helpful to place an 11 mm port at the site selected for exteriorization as this will require less enlargement and may even be of a sufficient size in cats and small dogs.

The technique involves using 5 mm atraumatic grasping forceps with multiple teeth to grasp the intestine. It is better to grasp the intestine along the antimesenteric border to avoid iatrogenic trauma to the jejunal arcades. It is important to inspect the entire length of the intestine to decide where to take the biopsy samples. This is done in much the same way as when performing intestinal biopsy via an open laparotomy. An assistant manipulates the telescope and camera, while the surgeon uses atraumatic grasping forceps in the other two ports to 'run the bowel' until a suitable area is found for biopsy. Most of the intestine, with the exception of the duodenocolic curvature, can be visualized with laparoscopy. The author [EM] prefers to start the inspection of the intestine with the caecum. The caecum is located medial to the duodenum. Pulling the omentum away from the right side of the abdominal cavity should uncover the caecum. The ileum and then the jejunum are visualized. The duodenum can also be visualized. If a biopsy of the duodenum is required, an extra cannula may need to be placed in the right cranial quadrant of the abdomen to be able to exteriorize the duodenum.

After identifying the loop of intestine to be biopsied, it is grasped by the antimesenteric border and pulled against the 11 mm cannula. The cannula incision is carefully enlarged with a scalpel blade or cautery enough to exteriorize the loop of intestine. This should be performed under direct visualization from within the abdomen to make sure that the scalpel blade does not puncture the loop of intestine. A Gelpi retractor is placed to keep the abdominal wall open. A 4–5 cm length of the loop of intestine is exteriorized, and stay sutures are used in the intestine to prevent it falling back into the abdominal cavity (Figure 12.17). It is important not to exteriorize too much intestine as this can make replacement into the abdomen difficult through a small incision. A small full-thickness biopsy sample is then obtained in the same manner as during open abdominal surgical biopsy (Case, 2015).

The small intestine is generally closed in the standard manner in two or three layers. If there is any question of contamination of the peritoneal space with intestinal contents during the procedure, lavage with warm saline can be performed using a laparoscopic suction cannula with ports for inflow and egress. The intestine is then returned to the abdominal cavity. This technique results in loss of the pneumoperitoneum and it is therefore difficult to take multiple intestinal biopsy samples. However, if multiple biopsy samples are required it is possible to re-insert the 11 mm cannula and place a temporary purse-string suture in the abdominal wall around it to form a seal. The abdomen can then be re-insufflated and the procedure repeated to obtain further samples. Alternatively, if several samples need to be taken from different areas of the small bowel, consideration should be given to placement of an Alexis wound retractor at one of the port sites to facilitate handling and examination of the bowel and 'run the bowel' as required.

Following collection of the final sample, the abdomen is re-insufflated and all operative sites are inspected for haemorrhage. The abdomen is then desufflated and the telescope and ports are removed. Closure of the abdominal wall is performed in the standard manner.

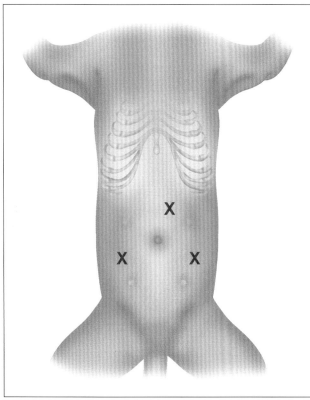

12.16 Port positions for full-thickness intestinal biopsy. Alternatively, all ports maybe placed in the midline.

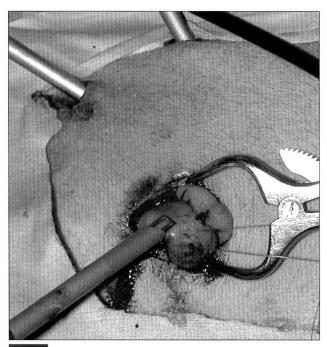

12.17 Biopsy of an exteriorized loop of small intestine.

Feeding tube placement

Duodenal/jejunal feeding tube placement has been described as a modification of percutaneous endoscopic gastrostomy (PEG) tube placement techniques. Following routine PEG tube placement, a duodenal feeding tube is inserted through the PEG tube into the gastric lumen and grasped by a pair of forceps placed through the flexible endoscope. The end of the feeding tube can then be guided through the pylorus and into the duodenum/jejunum as required (see also Chapter 5).

An alternative method of laparoscopic duodenostomy or jejunostomy tube placement does not require the use of a flexible endoscope or PEG tube. The patient is positioned in dorsal recumbency and the abdomen is shaved, prepared and draped for surgery.

The abdomen is insufflated with a Veress needle placed at the site of the proposed feeding tube placement, just caudal and lateral to the umbilicus on the right side. A primary telescope port is then introduced cranial to the umbilicus in the midline a comfortable distance away (as for intestinal biopsy; see above). The insufflation tubing is transferred to the telescope port and the Veress needle is removed from the abdomen. A secondary port, preferably 11 mm with a 5 mm reducer to accommodate the instruments, is introduced under direct visualization on the right side at the position of insertion of the Veress needle. A third port may be required to 'inspect' the intestine and select a suitable site for the duodenostomy/jejunostomy tube. This also facilitates identification of the direction of the intestine, to allow the duodenostomy/jejunostomy tube to be placed correctly in an aboral direction. This tertiary port is placed at the same level as the secondary port on the other (i.e. left) side of the midline.

Once the desired site for placement of the tube has been identified, the respective piece of intestine is exteriorized through the abdominal wall to allow the tube to be inserted externally (Rawlings et al., 2002; Hewitt et al., 2004; Case, 2015). The technique for exteriorization is similar to that described above for intestinal biopsy. However, instead of placing three cannulae on the midline as for intestinal biopsy, one of the cannulae where the feeding tube will be placed is outside the midline. After exteriorizing the desired loop of proximal jejunum or duodenum, four pexy sutures are placed between the edge of the incision into the abdominal wall and the loop of intestine. A purse-string suture is placed on the antimesenteric border, and an 8 Fr infant feeding tube is advanced through the centre of this suture and 10–15 cm aborally in the jejunum or duodenum. The purse-string suture is then tightened, along with the four pexy sutures. The skin is closed around the feeding tube in the usual fashion. The tube itself is sutured to the skin with a Chinese finger-trap pattern of suture material placed around the tube. The duodenostomy/jejunostomy site is visualized through the endoscope before desufflating the abdomen and removing the endoscope and cannula. Port closure is routine.

A gastrostomy feeding tube can also be placed using laparoscopy by exteriorizing the body of the stomach through the left abdominal wall and then inserting the tube externally following a gastropexy (see below). A Foley catheter is used as the gastrostomy tube. A purse-string suture is placed in the stomach wall and the abdominal wall to prevent dislodgement of the Foley catheter. The author [EM] has experienced some instances of dislodgement of the tube because of weakness of the abdominal wall at the level of the gastrostomy tube.

Gastropexy

Laparoscopic-assisted gastropexy

A prophylactic gastropexy is recommended for animals at high risk of developing gastric dilatation–volvulus and can be performed alone or at the same time as laparoscopic ovariectomy. Laparoscopic-assisted gastropexy is performed by exteriorizing the pyloric antrum through the right abdominal wall (Rawlings, 2002). The animal is placed in dorsal recumbency and the abdomen is shaved, prepared and draped for surgery. The abdomen is insufflated with a Veress needle placed on the midline just caudal to the umbilicus, and a primary telescope port is then introduced at this site. The instrument port is placed 2 cm behind the last rib on the right side, at the junction of the distal and proximal third of the last rib. It may be helpful to use an 11 mm port with a 6 mm reducer at this site. Fine-toothed grasping forceps or Babcock forceps are used to grasp the pyloric antrum between the greater and smaller curvatures, 5–6 cm from the pylorus. The abdominal cavity is then desufflated to minimize tension on the wall of the stomach. The port for the grasping forceps is enlarged parallel to the last rib. A 5–6 cm incision is adequate. A portion of the pyloric antrum is exteriorized and stay sutures are placed in the gastric wall. A 3 cm incision is made into the muscularis of the gastric wall to develop a seromuscularis flap, without penetrating the gastric lumen. The edges of this incision are then sutured to the transverse abdominal muscle with a simple continuous pattern of 3 metric (2/0 USP) monofilament absorbable suture material (Figure 12.18). The internal and external oblique muscles are then closed. Subcutaneous tissue and skin are closed in a routine fashion. The abdomen is reinsufflated to 2 mmHg and the pexy site examined. If all is well, the abdomen is dessuflated, cannulae removed and port closure is routine.

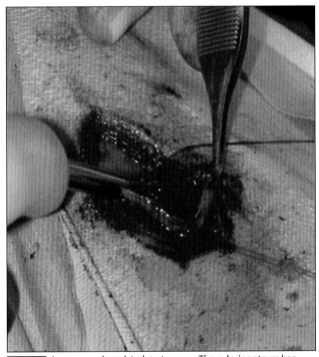

12.18 Laparoscopic-assisted gastropexy. The pyloric antrum has been exposed through a 3 cm incision caudal to the last rib on the right side. Two flaps are being created in the seromuscularis layers of the pyloric antrum.

Laparoscopic gastropexy

Laparoscopic gastropexy is performed with intracorporeal suturing (Mayhew and Brown, 2009; Spah *et al.*, 2013; Imhoff *et al.*, 2015; Coleman *et al.*, 2016; Takacs *et al.*, 2017). The availability of unidirectional barbed sutures has greatly facilitated the development of laparoscopic gastropexy. The animal is placed in dorsal recumbency and the telescope port is established on the midline 2 cm caudal to the umbilicus. Another port is placed 2 cm cranial to the umbilicus. A third cannula is placed in the caudal right abdomen at the level of the umbilicus.

After identifying the pyloric antrum, a stay suture on a straight needle is partially introduced into the abdominal cavity at the level of the gastropexy on the right side of the abdomen caudal to the last rib. The straight needle is grasped in the abdominal cavity with a needle holder. The needle is advanced through the pyloric antrum close to the lesser curvature. The needle is then advanced through the abdominal wall at the entry point and the suture is tensioned to bring the pyloric antrum against the abdominal wall.

Scissors are then introduced into the abdominal cavity through the port in the caudal right abdomen and used to make a 3 cm incision in the transverse abdominal muscle in the caudocranial direction. The incision should end at the stay suture. A 3 cm seromuscularis incision is made in the pyloric antrum from the greater curvature towards the stay suture and two seromuscularis flaps are undermined.

Two 3 metric (2/0 USP) monofilament unidirectional barbed sutures are used to suture the seromuscularis flaps to the edges of the incision in the transverse abdominal muscle. A continuous suture pattern is used (Figure 12.19). Two needle holders are required to complete the suturing. The more lateral suture is completed first, followed by the more medial suture (Figure 12.20). As an alternative to using needle holders, an endoscopic suturing device can be used to complete the two simple continuous sutures (Mayhew and Brown, 2009; Coleman and Monnet, 2017).

After completion of the gastropexy the cannulae are removed and each cannula site is closed in a routine fashion.

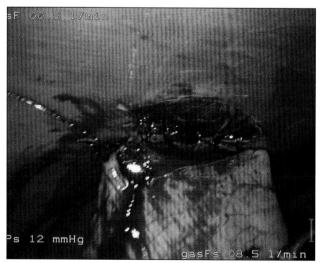

12.19 Laparoscopic gastropexy. An incision has been made in the transverse abdominal muscle and two seromuscularis flaps have been created in the pyloric antrum. Unidirectional barbed suture has been used to complete the more lateral continuous pattern between the edge of the transverse abdominal muscle and one of the seromuscularis flaps of the pyloric antrum.

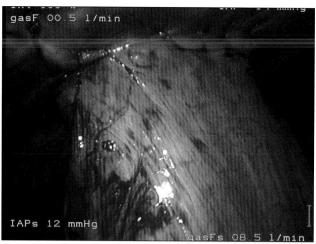

12.20 The laparoscopic gastropexy has been completed with the second suture between the edge of the transverse abdominal muscle and the more medial seromuscularis flap of the pyloric antrum.

Intestinal foreign body removal

A single non-linear foreign body in the intestinal tract can be removed laparoscopically if the animal has no signs of peritonitis. It is inadvisable to remove linear foreign bodies laparoscopically because the duodenocolic curvature cannot be evaluated appropriately with laparoscopy.

Three cannulae are placed on the midline close to each other. The small intestine should be evaluated along its entire length (except for the duodenocolic curvature). The author [EM] prefers to start from the caecum and inspect the intestine in the oral direction to evaluate its integrity and localize the foreign body. The loop of intestine containing the foreign body is exteriorized after extending a cannula incision or connecting two cannula incisions together. A Gelpi retractor is helpful to keep the abdominal wall open. An enterotomy or enterectomy is then performed as with a laparotomy. After flushing the loop of intestine with sterile saline, it is returned into the abdominal cavity. The abdominal cavity is lavaged with warm saline and the midline is closed in a routine fashion.

A modification of this laparoscopic-assisted approach can be used for gastric foreign body removal, if this cannot be achieved with a flexible endoscope (see Chapter 5). Following insufflation of the abdomen, a 6 mm port is placed 2–3 cm cranial to the umbilicus in the midline, and a 6 mm or 11 mm secondary port is placed 2–3 cm cranial to the primary port on the midline. The mid-body of the stomach is grasped with Babcock forceps introduced though the secondary port. The cannulae are removed and the two incisions are joined to make a 5 cm incision; this may need to be extended depending on the size of the foreign body to be removed. The stomach wall is exteriorized and held in place with stay sutures. The stomach wall is incised and the endoscope, cannula and forceps are introduced to retrieve the foreign body. The gastric wall is then sutured with a continuous suture of polyglactin (Vicryl) or polydioxanone (PDS) in the normal fashion, and the stomach returned to the abdomen. The abdominal incision is closed routinely. In very overweight dogs, the falciform ligament can interfere with a midline approach somewhat, but this can be partially obviated by introducing the operating ports at an angle to the right of the midline to try to penetrate through the side of the falciform ligament at its attachment to the body wall.

Ovariohysterectomy

The peritoneum is very sensitive to painful stimuli, and tearing the ovarian ligament from its peritoneal insertion during a routine open ovariohysterectomy results in considerable postoperative discomfort. This is completely eliminated by using a laparoscopic technique and postoperative pain is therefore greatly reduced, partly due to less intraoperative trauma and partly due to the smaller wound size. Laparoscopic studies following routine open ovariohysterectomy in bitches have shown a high incidence of adhesions between the kidney and the abdominal wall due to the trauma of ovarian ligament rupture during surgery, which does not occur following laparoscopic ovariectomy or ovariohysterectomy.

Ovariohysterectomy is performed where there is evidence of uterine pathology, such as cystic endometritis or early pyometritis, and may also be used for routine neutering of bitches and queens, although the authors recommend ovariectomy (see below) for this purpose. Ovariohysterectomy can be performed laparoscopically in all sizes of dogs and cats. Limitations of laparoscopic-assisted ovariohysterectomy relate to the size of the patient and the surgeon's experience, as the 'lack of space' in the abdominal cavity of very small animals can make the procedure technically more difficult. The advantages of laparoscopic ovariohysterectomy are the ability to examine the whole abdomen, little or no tension on the tissues, reduced postoperative pain and rapid recovery of the patient following the procedure (Hancock *et al.*, 2004; Devitt *et al.*, 2005; Culp *et al.*, 2009).

Ovariohysterectomy is performed with the animal in dorsal recumbency, with ventral midline placement of the cannulae. A 15-degree Trendelenburg position can be helpful to move the abdominal viscera to the cranial part of the abdomen, especially during insertion of the caudal cannula. It is also necessary to tilt the patient to the right side to work on the left ovary and then tilt the patient to the left side to work on the right ovary. This can be facilitated by the use of positioning aids. In most cases, the patient is placed with the shoulders in a positioning trough or supported by sandbags and is then rotated on the table by simply grasping the torso through the drapes. In large and giant breeds of dog this can be difficult, and the use of a bespoke laparoscopy positioner is helpful. This is a commercially available V-shaped trough that attaches to the operating table and allows the patient to be rotated to 45 or 90 degrees to either side by means of a lever and ratchet mechanism operated by the theatre staff.

The procedure requires three cannulae (Figure 12.21). The author's [PL] preference is to place the cannulae along the midline. The abdomen is insufflated using a Veress needle placed 3–4 cm cranial to the umbilicus in the midline. A primary telescope port is then established in the midline 1–2 cm caudal to the umbilicus, behind the falciform fat. The area under the point of insertion is examined for any iatrogenic damage and the insufflation tubing is transferred to the telescope port. The Veress needle is removed. A second 6 mm port is established under direct visualization at the site of the Veress needle. Entry here may be through the falciform ligament, and it is helpful to introduce the cannula at a slight angle towards the right side so that it enters the abdomen to the side of the falciform ligament. The final port is established in the midline 2–3 cm cranial to the pubis, under direct visualization and being careful not to damage the bladder, which lies just underneath the point of entry. In medium to large bitches, an 11 mm port with a reducer is used here to facilitate removal of the ovaries and uterus.

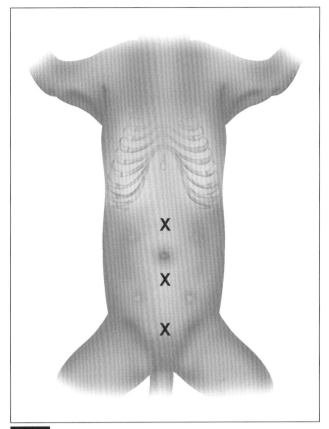

12.21 Port positions for laparoscopic ovariohysterectomy.

The surgeon (and assistant if required) stands to one side of the patient, and the patient is rotated towards them by approximately 45 degrees. The uterine horn on the contralateral side is visualized (Figure 12.22) and traced forward to the ovary. The ovary is grasped with Babcock forceps passed through the caudal port. Gentle caudal traction and elevation are applied, and the ovarian suspensory ligament and associated ovarian blood vessels are identified. If preferred, the handle of the Babcock forceps can be laid down, maintaining the position of the ovary unaided and allowing the surgeon to operate the camera and instrumentation through the other ports. This enables a surgeon to carry out the procedure without a surgical assistant. A bipolar vessel sealer or a bipolar

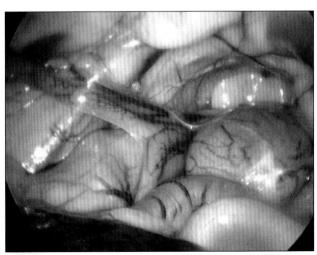

12.22 Laparoscopic view of the caudal abdomen of a bitch, showing the uterine body and horns emerging from beneath the urinary bladder.

vessel sealer/cutting device is passed through the cranial port, and the ovarian artery and vein are sealed and sectioned close to the ovary. The ovarian ligament is also sectioned, freeing the ovary from the abdominal wall.

If a simple bipolar vessel sealer is used, it will be necessary to intermittently change instruments and insert scissors to dissect the tissues following vessel sealing. A bipolar cutting device (such as the Robi® plus, LiNA PowerBlade™, ENSEAL® or LigaSure™) (Figure 12.23) can be used if available; this makes surgery a lot simpler as it removes the need to change instruments to dissect the ovary free. In addition, a variety of 'single-use' vessel sealer/cutting devices are available. However, these instruments are expensive and require gas sterilization to enable them to be reused up to 30–40 times. Autoclavable instruments are also available with replaceable blades, such as the Robi® plus and VetSEAL, although the latter requires its own generator.

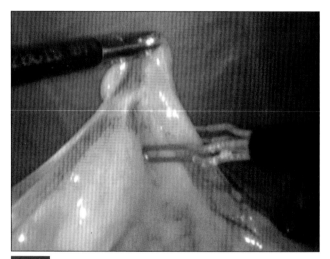

12.23 Transecting the ovarian pedicle with a bipolar cutting device.

Once the ovary is free, the area is checked for bleeding and any small bleeding vessels are grasped with bipolar forceps and cauterized. Gentle cranial traction is applied to the ovary to keep the uterine horn straight and under slight tension to allow the round ligament, broad ligament and associated mesentery to be dissected from their uterine attachments, applying cautery as necessary, right down to the uterine body. The Babcock forceps are then withdrawn until the ovary lies just under the point of entry of the caudal port, where it can be released.

The patient is then rotated to 45 degrees on to the other side, the surgeon changes sides and the process is repeated for the other ovary and uterine horn. This time, however, the ovary is not released. The patient is rotated back into dorsal recumbency and, maintaining a firm hold on the ovary, the forceps, cannula and ovary are all withdrawn from the abdomen together. If the ovary is very large or surrounded by a lot of fat, it may be necessary to enlarge the port slightly before the ovary can be withdrawn from the abdomen. This is performed under direct visualization by passing a No. 11 scalpel blade cranial to and alongside the cannula in the midline with the sharp edge facing away from the cannula. Entry of the blade into the abdomen can be monitored through the telescope. In this way, the caudal port is enlarged just enough to exteriorize the ovary.

The ovary can be grasped with a pair of Allis tissue forceps or haemostats at this point to enable removal of the cannula, ensure a firm grip and facilitate traction. Once

the ovary and one uterine horn are exteriorized, gentle traction is applied to exteriorize the uterine body and cervix. The uterine body is then clamped and ligated using a transfixing suture before transection and removal in the usual fashion. The uterine stump is replaced into the abdomen, and the remaining uterine horn and ovary are exteriorized to complete the procedure. Alternatively, if the ovaries and uterus are small, both uterine horns can be exteriorized before transection of the cervix (Figure 12.24). The caudal port is held closed manually in order to insufflate the abdomen sufficiently for a final inspection for haemorrhage and to ensure that the uterine stump has been fully returned to the abdomen. When the surgeon is satisfied that all is well, the abdomen is desufflated and the ports are removed. All the incisions are closed using 2 metric (3/0 USP) or 3 metric (2/0 USP) absorbable suture material; usually only one suture is necessary for 6 mm ports, and two for 11 mm ports. The skin is closed using tissue adhesive (Figure 12.25).

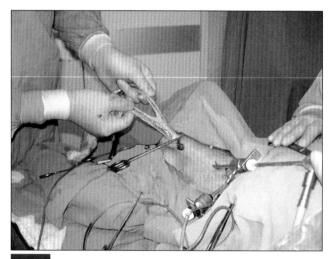

12.24 Exteriorizing the uterus through the caudal port position.

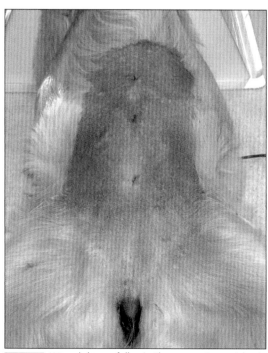

12.25 Wound closure following laparoscopic ovariohysterectomy in a 2-year-old Retriever.

An alternative technique is to dissect the ovaries as described above and then place a pre-tied loop of suture material (Endoloop® Ligature) in the abdominal cavity through one cannula. Both ovaries and uterine horns are passed through the loop (Figure 12.26), which is then tightened down at the level of the cervix. The uterus is transected and the uterus and ovaries are removed through one of the ports, which is enlarged if necessary.

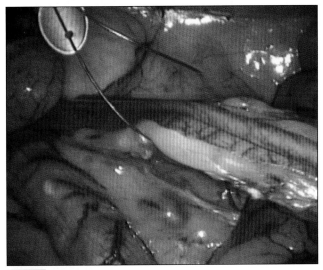

Parameter	Single port	Two ports	Three ports
Surgery time (minutes)	24–36	14–22	16–22
Postoperative pain scores (mean (range); low = 0; high = 18)	2 (0–6)	1 (0–5)	3 (0–8)
Owner-reported comfort scores (worst pain = 1; normal comfort = 10)	8.5	10	8

12.27 Comparison of one-, two- and three-port laparoscopic ovariectomy techniques in the dog.
(Data from Case *et al.*, 2011)

12.26 Both uterine horns have been passed through an Endoloop®.

Ovariectomy

Ovariectomy can also be performed via laparoscopy. This is a simpler and faster procedure than ovariohysterectomy and is recommended for routine neutering of bitches and queens. Ovariectomy has been standard practice in many European countries since 1981 and is becoming more common in the UK, USA and elsewhere. A literature review by Goethem *et al.* (2006) concluded that:

> '[Ovariohysterectomy] is technically more complicated, time consuming, and is probably associated with greater morbidity (larger incision, more intraoperative trauma, increased discomfort) compared with [ovariectomy]... making [ovariectomy] the preferred method of gonadectomy in the healthy bitch.'

It has been shown that pyometra and cystic endometritis do not occur in the absence of ovarian tissue and, therefore, there is no need to remove a healthy uterus. In addition, there are no published data to show any benefit from removal of the uterus.

Single-port, two-port and three-port techniques for laparoscopic ovariectomy have been described. Each technique has its advantages and disadvantages. A recent comparison of single-, two- and three-port techniques in a double-blinded study showed that a two-port technique was quicker and associated with less pain than either a single- or three-port technique in dogs (Case *et al.*, 2011; Figure 12.27).

Single-port ovariectomy

There has been a recent resurgence in the popularity of single-port laparoscopy for biopsy and ovariectomy. Single-port laparoscopic surgery requires the use of an operating laparoscope: this is a 10 mm device that incorporates an instrument channel and an endoscope into a single unit. The oculus is offset, allowing the passage of 5 mm instrumentation into the abdomen directly along the same axis as the endoscope, as is the case with flexible gastroscopes.

The single-port approach has both advantages and disadvantages for the surgeon. The procedure is considered by some to be safer for the inexperienced laparoscopist as all instrumentation is introduced under direct visualization, thereby reducing the risk of iatrogenic damage, which can occur if instruments are introduced through remote ports without directly viewing their entry into the abdomen. A single abdominal incision is required, rather than two or more. This is a benefit in large and giant breeds where the operating port is required to be 11 mm because of the size of the ovary, but it is a disadvantage in cats and the majority of dogs, in which a 3 mm or 6 mm port would suffice. In the author's [PL] experience, two 6 mm ports cause less pain than one 11 mm port.

If the surgeon wishes to perform only ovariectomies and biopsies in medium to large breeds, then an operating laparoscope may suffice. However, this instrument is limited in its application, and if other procedures or more advanced surgery that requires more than one hand instrument are contemplated, then a separate 5 mm endoscope and cannulae must be purchased, which considerably increases the overall cost of equipment. Separate ports are much more versatile. Many surgeons also prefer to have instrumentation approaching the surgical site from the side rather than in the same axis as the line of sight, which will partially obstruct the view of the surgical site and make manipulation of instruments and tissues somewhat awkward and time-consuming. Use of a single-port operating laparoscope does not provide practice in triangulation and instrument handling. This is a major disadvantage of the single-port technique, since routine laparoscopic procedures performed using a multi-port approach provide excellent training and transferable skills that can be invaluable when performing less common procedures.

An alternative is to use a single-port multiple-access device (SILS™) (Manassero *et al.*, 2012). This is a relatively large device designed to provide access to the abdomen via the human umbilicus, which uses a single 2 cm incision to provide three or more entry ports for instrumentation and an endoscope. Although articulated instruments are available for this device, conventional straight instruments can be used, but their proximity to each other makes manipulation more difficult. Since three ports are available, a suspensory needle or hook is not required to fix the ovary for dissection, but access, manipulation and dissection are more challenging. There is little advantage to using this device for ovariectomy, but it can be of use in cases where a larger incision will be needed to remove an abdominal organ or mass in a laparoscopic-assisted procedure.

Two-port ovariectomy

The two-port ovariectomy is the author's [PL] preferred procedure for routine ovariectomy in the bitch and queen. The instrumentation required for ovariectomy is essentially the same as for ovariohysterectomy, with the addition of an ovariectomy hook. This is a sharp curved needle attached to a heavy handle. It is passed percutaneously and used to fix the ovary in place against the body wall to facilitate dissection. Alternatively, a large curved suture needle with suture material attached can be used for the same purpose, but is a little more challenging to do single-handedly.

A wider than normal surgical clip is required to give access to the body wall in the mid-lateral abdomen. The clip follows the line of the costal arch up to a point in the mid-upper abdomen over the ovary and then back to the midline near the pubis. Four drapes are placed accordingly with the corners of the aperture in both flanks and on the midline. When clipped in this way, the wide clip is less noticeable in the standing dog. Alternatively, if an EndoGrab™ device is to be used (see below), such a wide surgical clip is not required as the instrument is introduced through the cranial port (Figure 12.28). The ventral abdomen should always be clipped sufficiently to allow the insertion of a third port near the pubis should conversion to an ovariohysterectomy become necessary in the event of uterine pathology being discovered.

The procedure and port placements are similar to those for a laparoscopic ovariohysterectomy, but the caudal port is not required. Generally, a 5 mm, 0-degree endoscope and two 6 mm cannulae are used, but in small bitches (<6 kg) a 3.9 mm cannula may be used caudal to the umbilicus with a 2.7 mm, 30-degree endoscope. In larger bitches (>30 kg), especially if they are obese, an 11 mm port may be required as the cranial port, placed midway between the umbilicus and the xiphoid, to allow removal of the ovaries and bursa. The author [PL] prefers to use a Ternamian ENDOTIP cannula for initial entry into the abdomen caudal to the umbilicus and a straight-sided 6 mm cannula cranial to the umbilicus for the instrument port, as this is easier to remove and replace when the ovary is extracted from the abdomen.

Following insufflation of the abdomen and placement of the cannulae, the patient is rotated 45 degrees to the left, towards the surgeon. The right ovary is visualized just caudal and lateral to the kidney and grasped with Babcock

forceps introduced through the cranial port. It is usually possible to place one jaw of the forceps within the ovarian bursa, which affords a good grip on the fibrous tissue directly over the ovary and allows the ovary to hang free. The opening of the bursa can be seen as a pink slit on the medial side of the bursa. If the opening is not visible, the bursal fat should be grasped and reflected laterally towards the abdominal wall.

The ovary is held against the abdominal wall and the handle of the Babcock forceps is laid down to retain the ovary in an elevated position. The site of contact with the abdominal wall is determined by palpation of the external abdominal wall while observing the peritoneum through the endoscope. Once the exact site has been determined, an ovariectomy hook is placed through the abdominal wall at the level of the top of the ovarian bursa to transfix the ovarian pedicle and hold the ovary in place. The point of the needle should pass immediately under the ovary and the point is then directed ventrally up and around the middle of the ovary and back towards the body wall. Once the needle has penetrated the abdominal wall it can be manipulated to a degree cranially, caudally, medially and laterally, as there is considerable laxity in the abdominal wall. The point of the ovariectomy hook can also be rotated cranially and caudally by rotating the handle to allow accurate placement below the ovary. The weight of the handle of this device means that the position of the needle within the abdomen is maintained when the handle is laid down on the patient. The Babcock forceps can then be removed and replaced with a bipolar cutting device (e.g. Robi® plus, LiNA PowerBlade™ or LigaSure™).

An alternative to using a percutaneous ovariectomy hook or suture needle is to use an EndoGrab™ device. This comprises a reusable, autoclavable applicator handle and a disposable spring-loaded organ retractor. Although designed for single use, the retractor can be gas sterilized, cold sterilized or autoclaved and reused many times. The retractor is deployed in the abdomen via the cranial port and the ovarian bursa is grasped with a blunt hook. The device is then released and the other end is picked up using the applicator handle. This allows a second sharp pincer to be deployed and attached to the ventral abdominal wall to elevate the ovary. The applicator is then released from the device and removed from the abdomen freeing the cranial port for the vessel sealer/cutter. Once the ovary has been dissected free, the applicator is reintroduced and attached to the sharp pincer, allowing the device to be removed from the abdominal wall. The device and ovary are placed adjacent to the caudal pole of the kidney, away from mesenteric fat, which could get caught in the hooks, and the device is released once again. The applicator is reattached to the blunt hook allowing the ovary to be dropped. The shaft is deployed to enclose the device and then the whole applicator and device are removed from the abdomen. The ovary can then be retrieved with Babcock forceps as below. This device has the advantage that it can be used to elevate an organ and attach it to the abdominal wall without the need for an additional port. Since a percutaneous needle is not used over the site of the ovary, clipping of the hair is kept to a minimum for a midline surgical approach.

Dissection should be as close to the ovary as possible to reduce the amount of fat surrounding the ovary once it is dissected free. This greatly facilitates removal of the ovary from the abdomen. In bitches with a lot of bursal fat, it is sometimes preferable to dissect the ovary from the bursa and leave the bursa and the ovarian and proper ligaments intact. However, this can be more challenging for

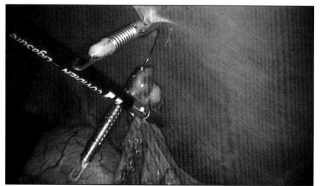

12.28 Ovary suspended against the abdominal wall with an EndoGrab™ device for dissection with a vessel sealer/divider.

the inexperienced laparoscopist, and usually the ovary and bursa are removed together. When an ovariectomy hook is used, the direction of dissection will vary with the position of the ovary on the hook. The ovarian vessels in the centre of the pedicle are sealed and sectioned first. If the ovary falls to one side of the hook, as invariably happens, dissection proceeds on that side to prevent the ovary falling from the hook before the dissection is complete. Care must be taken not to place inadvertent traction on the ovary during dissection, as this can pull it off the hook and require it to be repositioned.

Once the ovary has been dissected free, the uterine horn and remains of the pedicle are inspected for haemorrhage, and the bipolar device is removed from the abdomen and replaced by Babcock forceps. The ovary is grasped at one end with the forceps, being careful to avoid grasping only fat. The ovary is bean-shaped, so grasping it at the pole presents the smallest cross-section for removing it through the port site. As the poles are the site of attachment for the ovarian and proper ligaments, the tissue here is also more fibrous. The ovariectomy hook is removed, allowing the ovary to be retracted into the mouth of the cannula. The endoscope is withdrawn into the caudal cannula to prevent iatrogenic damage, and the patient is rotated back into dorsal recumbency. This realigns the incisions in the skin and linea alba and facilitates removal of the ovary. The ovary is removed from the abdomen either through the lumen of the cannula or, if it is too large, by removal of the cannula and direct traction through the body wall. It is usually best to gently remove the cannula and apply a gentle back-and-forth twisting motion to exteriorize the ovary enough to allow it to be grasped with artery forceps. These are then used to carefully tease the ovary out while maintaining a firm grip on it.

If ovarian fat has been grasped by mistake, the ovary may tear free when an attempt is made to remove it through the abdominal wall. If this happens, the cannula should be replaced, the ovary located within the abdomen and grasped firmly, and the removal procedure repeated. If the ovary cannot be easily located directly beneath the cranial port site, it may be stuck in the falciform fat near the abdominal wall. If this is the case, it can often be grasped percutaneously with artery forceps or pushed free to fall into the abdomen, where it can be grasped with Babcock forceps and retrieved. If the ovary is dropped back into the abdomen, the surgeon should not be tempted to roll the patient, as this will make locating it considerably more difficult.

Once the ovary has been successfully removed and examined for integrity, the cannula can then be replaced and the procedure repeated for the remaining ovary. Closed Babcock forceps placed through the cannula can be used as a blunt trocar to reintroduce the cannula. If necessary, closed haemostats can be used to locate the incision in the linea alba first. The patient is tilted to the right and the surgeon changes sides. The spleen may be overlying the kidney and ovary, and it is sometimes necessary to rotate the patient more than 45 degrees temporarily to allow gravity to move it out of the visual field.

If the cranial cannula has been placed to the right of the falciform ligament and the bitch is old or overweight, it may be difficult to pass instruments across to the left side of the abdomen directly, due to excessive falciform fat. If the tip of the cannula cannot be visualized easily on the left side of the abdomen, the endoscope should be withdrawn to the tip of the cannula and pointed cranially. Babcock forceps are then passed through the cranial cannula and directed caudally towards the ventral abdominal wall (i.e. directly towards the endoscope). In this way, the tips of the forceps can usually be seen and guided around the caudal edge of the falciform ligament where it attaches to the umbilicus (Video 12.1). Keeping the tips of the forceps near the ventral abdominal wall will prevent iatrogenic damage to the abdominal contents. Once the falciform ligament has been negotiated and the forceps are visible on the left side of the abdomen, the ovary can be grasped, dissected and removed as before.

At the end of the procedure, the cannulae are removed and the abdomen is desufflated. Following desufflation, closure is routine, with a single 2 metric (3/0 USP) polyglactin 910 suture and skin adhesive at each port site.

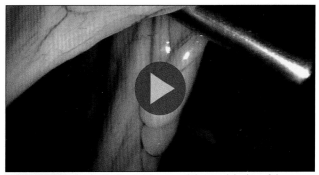

Video 12.1 Passing instruments around the caudal edge of the falciform fat.

Three-port ovariectomy

The three-port ovariectomy technique uses the same three ports as those described above for laparoscopic ovariohysterectomy. The caudal port is placed just cranial to the pelvic brim and Babcock forceps are inserted through it to grasp and elevate the ovary. The forceps are used in place of the ovariectomy hook in the two-port procedure, and the only purpose for utilizing this third port is to remove the need to clip hair on the lateral body wall, which is required when using the ovariectomy hook. While this is a perfectly usable approach, the author [PL] feels that it is somewhat counterintuitive to create an additional wound, increasing postoperative pain and discomfort, just to avoid clipping hair.

Ovarian remnant removal

Locating ovarian remnants during open surgery can be difficult and time-consuming. The magnification and illumination provided by laparoscopy greatly facilitates this procedure and results in considerably less trauma for the patient. Location of the remnant is often easier if the patient is in oestrus at the time of surgery, but this is not necessary.

Only two ports are required and the technique is the same as for laparoscopic ovariectomy. The ports are placed as described above and the patient is rolled to each side in turn to visualize the contralateral kidney. The area around and behind the kidney is inspected with the aid of a palpation probe. Location of the ovarian remnant is usually quite easy. The pedicle can be grasped directly with a bipolar vessel sealer/cutting instrument or, if necessary, can be transfixed with an ovariectomy hook or EndoGrab™ device before transection. In many cases, especially in cats, laparoscopic scissors attached to a monopolar electrosurgery unit are all that is required for transection (Figure 12.29). Following isolation of the remnant, the scissors or bipolar sealer/divider device are

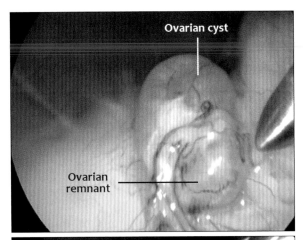

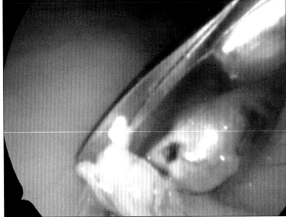

12.29 Removal of the ovarian remnant using monopolar scissors in a cat.

removed and replaced with grasping forceps, and the remnant is removed via the cannula. It is recommended to always inspect both sides, as bilateral remnants are not uncommon. It is also prudent to check the uterine stump to ensure there is no evidence of stump pyometra. The cannulae are then removed, the abdomen is desufflated and the ports are closed routinely.

Cryptorchid surgery and vasectomy

A testicle that is located in the abdominal cavity can be easily removed laparoscopically. This technique is simpler, quicker and less traumatic than open surgery, since the testicle is easily located by direct visualization and only a minimal incision is required for its removal. Laparoscopic vasectomy can also be performed on the normal scrotal testicle at the same time, if required.

The patient is placed in dorsal recumbency, in a 15-degree Trendelenburg position, rotated 45 degrees away from the affected side, and the abdomen is shaved, prepared and draped for surgery. Gravity will displace the abdominal organs towards the cranial abdomen, which will facilitate visualization of the internal inguinal canal. Two cannulae are adequate to perform the surgery. The abdomen is insufflated with a Veress needle placed at or close to the umbilicus on the midline, depending on the size of the patient. Care should be exercised to palpate the abdomen and direct the Veress needle and primary cannula away from the spleen. The Veress needle is removed from

the abdomen and a primary telescope port is introduced at the same site. The insufflation tubing is then transferred to the telescope port. The abdomen is inspected for iatrogenic damage and the testicle is usually easily located. A secondary port, preferably 11 mm with a 6 mm reducer to accommodate the instruments, is introduced under direct visualization directly over the testicle, just lateral to the rectus abdominis muscle. If the testicle is not visualized immediately, it may be necessary to place the second port and introduce a palpation probe to gently move the bladder laterally to visualize the vas deferens and trace it back to the testicle.

In unilateral cases, the normal side (usually the left) is examined first and the vas deferens and testicular vessels are traced to the inguinal ring, which is inspected for herniation. The inguinal ring on the affected side is then located and inspected. If the vas deferens and testicular vessels are seen entering the inguinal ring, then the testicle is located within the inguinal canal (Figure 12.30). In bilateral cases, both internal inguinal rings are inspected to determine the presence of the vas deferens and testicular arteries. If these structures are present, either the dog has already been castrated or the testicles are beyond the inguinal ring. The absence of the vas deferens and testicular artery in the inguinal canal means that the testicle is ectopic.

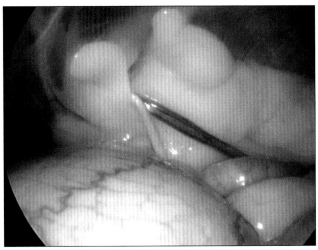

12.30 Normal inguinal canal showing the vas deferens and testicular vessels.

Once located, the ectopic testicle is grasped and pulled up to the mouth of the operating cannula. The cannula, forceps and testicle are then drawn out of the abdomen together (Figure 12.31). In small dogs, this does not require any further enlargement of the port incision. The vas deferens and spermatic vessels are ligated and the testicle is removed in a routine fashion. The ligated stump of the vas deferens and pampiniform plexus is returned to the abdomen. The abdomen is desufflated and the ports are closed routinely.

Alternatively, the ectopic testicle can be brought against the abdominal wall towards the midline and stabilized with a suture passed percutaneously through the abdominal wall. The vascular pedicle and the vas deferens are ligated with a pre-tied suture (Figure 12.32), staples or electrocautery. The pedicle is then transected and the testicle removed through one of the port incisions. In bilateral cryptorchid animals, the gubernaculum often prevents exteriorization of both testicles through the same port. In such cases it is often easiest to place the instrument port over

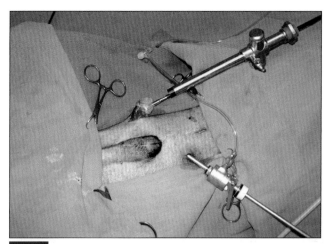

12.31 Removal of an ectopic testicle.

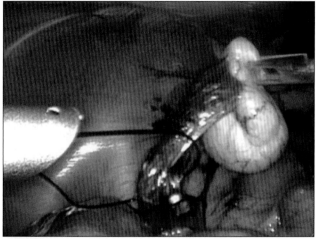

12.32 Right cryptorchid testicle cranial to the bladder. An Endoloop® has been placed around the pampiniform plexus.

one testicle and remove it directly through the port and then suspend the contralateral testicle as described above, dissect it free internally and then remove it through the same port.

Following removal of the ectopic testicle, often the remaining scrotal testicle is usually removed to prevent breeding and perpetuating the problem in future generations. However, some owners are reluctant to castrate their dog due to concerns about the animal developing weight problems or coat changes. As an alternative, it is relatively simple to perform a laparoscopic vasectomy. Before removing the ectopic testicle, a bipolar vessel sealer/cutting device is placed through the instrument port and a 1 cm section of the vas deferens is removed from the scrotal testicle. This is facilitated by rotating the patient 45 degrees away from the normal side. The section of vas deferens may then be sent for histological confirmation if required.

Laparoscopic-assisted cystotomy

Laparoscopic-assisted cystotomy is most commonly undertaken for the removal of cystic calculi, but can also enable exploration of the bladder and proximal urethra, biopsy or debulking of bladder masses and examination of the ureteral papillae (Rawlings *et al.*, 2003b; Rawlings, 2007; Pinel *et al.*, 2013). The advantages of laparoscopic-

assisted cystotomy include a smaller incision than is used for open cystotomy, better visualization of the mucosa of the bladder and urethra, and possibly less urinary contamination of the peritoneal cavity. Most dogs and cats with urinary calculi can be treated with laparoscopic-assisted cystoscopy. Animals with calculi that are too large to be removed by urohydropulsion (see Chapter 11 for a description of this technique) are suitable candidates, as are those where dissolution of the calculi by medical treatment is unlikely to be successful (i.e. animals with principally calcium oxalate stones).

Patient positioning and port placement

For a laparoscopic-assisted cystotomy (as described by Rawlings *et al.*, 2003b), the patient is placed in dorsal recumbency with or without Trendelenburg (head-down) positioning. A urinary catheter is placed and any urine is evacuated from the bladder. The bladder is then flushed with warm sterile saline and partially drained. The catheter is left in place for subsequent flushing. Following insufflation of the abdomen, a camera port is established in a subumbilical location (Figure 12.33). The caudal abdomen is inspected and a second (instrument) port is established under direct visualization on the ventral midline above the apex of the bladder. This usually lies approximately halfway between the camera port and the brim of the pubis. In male dogs, the instrument port is usually positioned at the cranial end of the prepuce.

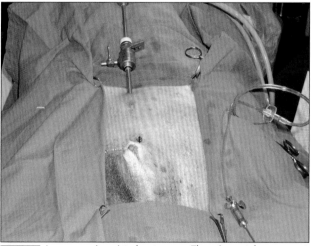

12.33 Laparoscopic-assisted cystoscopy. The primary telescope port is in place and a small skin incision has been made for insertion of the instrument port.

Surgical technique

Once the ports have been placed, the next step is exteriorization of a small area of the apex of the bladder in order to make the cystotomy incision. Laparoscopic Babcock forceps are placed into the instrument port and the apex of the bladder is grasped (Figure 12.34). The location at which the bladder is grasped is important because it will determine the ease with which the entire bladder can be visualized. If the cystotomy incision is made into an area of bladder nearer the trigone, full exploration of the entire bladder will be more challenging. As the apex is brought up towards the cannula, the instrument port incision is enlarged to approximately 2–4 cm, depending on the size of the animal and the calculi to be removed. The cannula and forceps are then removed together, while maintaining a firm grasp on the bladder.

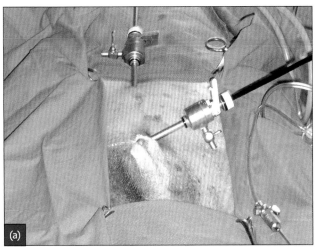

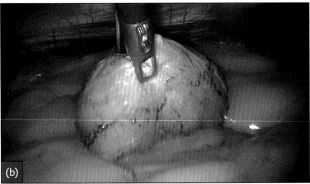

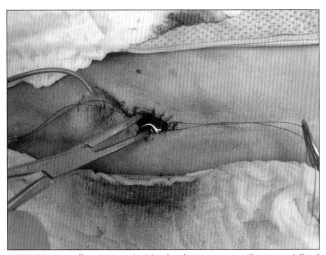

12.36 A small cystotomy incision has been temporarily marsupialized to the skin at the cranial margin of the prepuce in readiness for retrograde bladder flushing. Carmalt forceps are being used to open the incision to allow maximal fluid egress via the cystotomy site.

12.34 (a) Babcock forceps are placed in the instrument port to (b) grasp the apex of the bladder.

As soon as the bladder becomes visible externally, two stay sutures of 2 metric (3/0 USP) or 3 metric (2/0 USP) PDS are placed into the bladder wall to ensure that it does not slip back into the abdomen (Figure 12.35). At this point the pneumoperitoneum will be lost because of the size of the incision in the abdominal wall, and the telescope should be withdrawn from the camera port. While maintaining upward traction on the stay sutures to create a seal of the abdominal wall incision, a small cystotomy is made that is large enough to remove the largest calculus in the bladder (estimated from preoperative diagnostic imaging studies). Optionally, the edges of the cystotomy incision can be temporarily sutured to the border of the skin with a simple continuous pattern to allow marsupialization of the bladder (Figure 12.36). This will prevent contamination of the peritoneal cavity with urine or calculi.

Either a 2.7 mm, 30-degree endoscope can be placed into the cystotomy incision within a cystoscope sheath, or a traditional 5 mm laparoscope can be placed into the cystotomy with or without a cannula. A pressurized bag of sterile saline is attached to one of the ports on the cystoscope sheath and used to provide constant lavage of the bladder. This is essential to maintain good visualization during examination of the bladder and retrieval of the calculi. Alternatively, the saline can be flushed into the bladder retrograde through the urethral catheter.

Calculi can be retrieved in a variety of ways:

- A basket retrieval catheter can be placed down the working channel of the cystoscope to capture individual calculi. This technique works best with small numbers of calculi, but can become quite time-consuming in dogs with a large number of calculi. Other instruments, such as grasping or laparoscopic forceps, can also be placed alongside the cystoscope or laparoscope to help retrieve the calculi
- If a large amount of sandy debris or very small calculi are present, it can be helpful to flush large volumes of saline at high pressure through the urethral catheter into the bladder, allowing the calculi to pass out of the cystotomy incision under pressure. It is helpful to hold the cystotomy incision open with the jaws of Carmalt forceps (or a similar instrument) during flushing to allow an uninterrupted flow of saline and calculi to occur (Figure 12.36)
- Suction can also be used to remove very small calculi and sandy debris.

Once the calculi in the bladder have been removed, the urinary catheter is withdrawn slightly to allow endoscopic inspection of the urethra. In most male dogs, the urethra can be examined to the level of the prostatic urethra or even as far as the pelvic flexure (Figure 12.37). The urinary catheter is then flushed with sterile saline to push any urethral calculi into the bladder for removal. Once all the calculi have been removed, the bladder should be thoroughly inspected again and, if available, a small flexible bronchoscope or urethroscope should be passed along the entire length of the urethra to confirm that no calculi remain distally (see also Chapter 11).

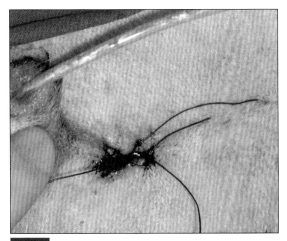

12.35 Bladder wall sutured to the abdominal incision.

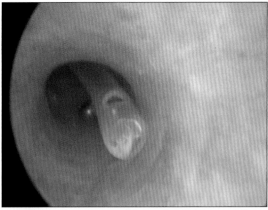

12.37 Endoscopic view of the urethra looking caudally towards the pelvic flexure.

Inspection of the bladder may reveal the presence of mass lesions which may be neoplastic or benign (e.g. polyps) (Figure 12.38). If these lesions are identified, a diode laser fibre can be inserted into the bladder to remove or ablate them (Figure 12.39; see also Chapter 16).

In all cases, the authors recommend that postoperative radiographs be obtained to document the absence of residual calculi within the bladder. After completion of the procedure, the cystotomy incision is closed routinely, usually with a single layer of simple interrupted appositional sutures of 1.5 metric (4/0 USP) to 3 metric (2/0 USP) PDS, depending on the size of the animal (Figure 12.40). The stay sutures or sutures between the skin and bladder wall are removed and closure is routine.

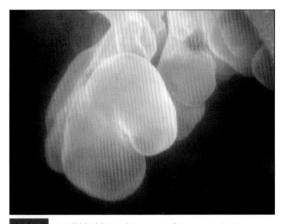

12.38 Small bladder polyp seen at laparoscopic cystoscopy.

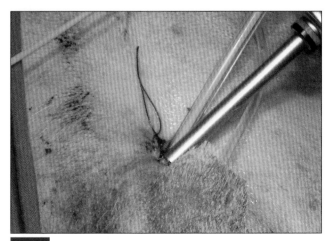

12.39 Telescope and laser fibre inserted into the bladder.

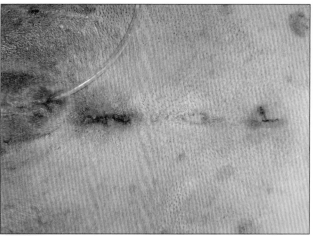

12.40 Postoperative appearance following wound closure after cystoscopy.

Percutaneous cystolithotomy

Percutaneous cystolithotomy is a modified laparoscopic-assisted cystotomy technique, where no insufflation is required and no subumbilical telescope port is placed (Runge et al., 2011). Before the procedure, the bladder is flushed, filled with saline and palpated to estimate the location of the apex. A small (1.5–2 cm) incision is made in this location on the ventral midline. Wound retractors are placed to expose the apex of the bladder, which is grasped with Babcock forceps. Three stay sutures are placed near the apex of the bladder in a triangular fashion to provide traction and stabilization.

A small incision is made with a No. 11 blade in the centre of the stay sutures and a 6 mm or 11 mm Ternamian ENDOTIP cannula is inserted into the bladder. A 2.7 mm, 30-degree endoscope in a cystoscope sheath or a ureteroscope is placed through the cannula and the calculi are removed using basket forceps placed through the instrument channel (Figure 12.41). At the end of the procedure, the cannula is removed, the incision in the bladder is closed using monofilament absorbable suture material and the abdomen is closed routinely. The advantage of this technique is that a closed system allows optimal distension and visualization of the bladder. The disadvantage is that larger calculi cannot be easily retrieved through the cannula.

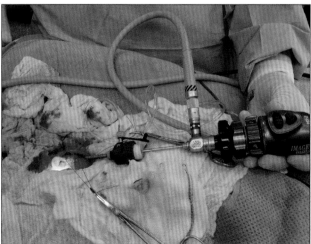

12.41 Placement of a laparoscopic cannula directly into the bladder. Calculi can be removed either through the side port of the cannula or by anterograde flushing of the calculi into a urethral catheter.

Splenectomy

Several reports in the veterinary literature document laparoscopic splenectomy in both healthy dogs and dogs with splenic lesions (Stedile *et al.*, 2009; Bakhtiari *et al.*, 2011; Shaver *et al.*, 2015; Wright *et al.*, 2016; Mayhew *et al.*, 2018), and there is one report describing the procedure in cats (O'Donnell *et al.*, 2013). In one study, healthy dogs undergoing laparoscopic splenectomy were found to be in less pain, had fewer wound complications and experienced less blood loss than those undergoing open surgery, although laparoscopic splenectomy was a longer surgical procedure than open splenectomy (Stedile *et al.*, 2009). The authors recommend laparoscopic splenectomy in dogs and cats with mild to moderate splenomegaly and modestly sized splenic masses. Suggested contraindications to laparoscopic splenectomy include severe splenomegaly, the presence of large splenic masses (>6–7 cm in diameter), the presence of a haemoabdomen and lack of surgical experience or appropriate equipment. Further studies are needed to refine these selection criteria.

A variety of approaches can be used, including totally laparoscopic (Stedile *et al.*, 2009; Bakhtiari *et al.*, 2011; Shaver *et al.*, 2015; Mayhew *et al.*, 2018) and laparoscopic-assisted (O'Donnell *et al.*, 2013; Wright *et al.*, 2016) techniques. In large-breed dogs, the totally laparoscopic technique becomes more challenging as the size of the spleen increases; this, coupled with the increased weight of the animal, makes manipulation difficult, and for these dogs the laparoscopic-assisted approach may be the better choice. Small dogs and cats can be treated using either a totally laparoscopic or a laparoscopic-assisted approach. A totally laparoscopic approach is relatively simple in this group of patients.

Patient positioning and port placement

The animal is placed in dorsal recumbency and following insufflation, a 5 mm camera port is established in a subumbilical location on the ventral midline. Two further ports are placed under direct visualization on the ventral midline, 3–8 cm cranial and 3–8 cm caudal to the subumbilical camera port (depending on the size of the patient). Alternatively, a single-port multiple-access device (e.g. the SILS™ port) can be placed at the umbilicus if a single-port laparoscopic splenectomy is to be performed (Mayhew *et al.*, 2018). For a laparoscopic-assisted splenectomy, two ports are placed initially to obtain liver biopsy samples, which are usually indicated in cases with potential splenic malignancy, followed by placement of a wound retractor device (e.g. an Alexis wound retractor) at the umbilicus.

Surgical technique

Totally laparoscopic approach

The spleen is manipulated with a blunt probe so that the hilar vessels become visible. Moving from the splenic tail towards the head of the spleen, the vessels and associated fat are sealed and divided using a vessel sealer. The most challenging aspect of the dissection is sectioning the splenic hilum (Figure 12.42) at the splenic head (and the short gastric vessels) due to its less mobile attachment to the greater curvature of the stomach. In cats, the close association of the splenic head with the left lobe of the pancreas increases the risk of iatrogenic damage to the pancreas. In most cases, as the splenic head is approached, dissection is facilitated by rotating the patient into a more lateral position with the left side upward. Once

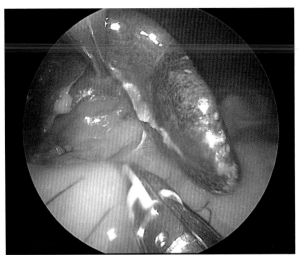

12.42 Progressive sealing of the splenic hilum with a vessel sealer in a totally laparoscopic splenectomy.

dissected free, the spleen should either be placed in a specimen retrieval bag or be exteriorized through a protected wound retractor. It will be necessary to enlarge one of the port incisions proportional to the size of the spleen or splenic lesion to be removed.

If a single-port laparoscopic splenectomy is to be performed using a SILS™ device, the dissection is similar but instrument interference makes the technique slightly more challenging, even when using articulating instruments. Following exteriorization of the single-port device, the incision created is often large enough for the spleen or splenic lesion to be exteriorized, or it can be enlarged as required.

Laparoscopic-assisted technique

A laparoscopic-assisted technique can also be used for splenectomy, and is technically less challenging than the totally laparoscopic procedure in most cases. If necessary, liver biopsy samples can be collected through two traditional ports; then, a wound retractor (e.g. an Alexis wound retractor) is placed at the umbilicus through an 'assist' incision. The size of this incision is dictated by the anticipated size of the spleen, as well as the available sizes of wound retractor. If a wound retractor is not available, then two Gelpi retractors placed at either end of the incision can be used to hold it open. After placement of the retractor(s), the spleen is gently grasped digitally by the surgeon and a vessel sealer is used to seal the splenic hilar vessels in a gradual fashion (Figure 12.43). The spleen

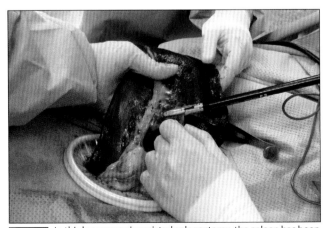

12.43 In this laparoscopic-assisted splenectomy, the spleen has been partially retracted through an 'assist' device and the splenic hilus is being serially sectioned using a vessel-sealing device.

is then progressively exteriorized through the wound retractor. If omental adhesions are present, they can also be sectioned with a vessel sealer as the spleen is exteriorized; however, if omental adhesion formation is extensive, this may preclude safe exteriorization and necessitate conversion to a traditional open coeliotomy. After removal of the spleen, the area is thoroughly inspected for any ongoing haemorrhage. The abdominal incision is closed in a routine fashion.

Cholecystectomy

Several important factors need to be taken into consideration by surgeons planning to offer laparoscopic cholecystectomy: obtaining the necessary equipment and advanced training to perform the procedure safely and efficiently, as well as the application of strict case selection criteria (Mayhew *et al.*, 2008; Jaffey *et al.*, 2018). Without these factors in place, little success can be expected and frequent conversion to an open approach is likely to be necessary.

In dogs and cats, conditions that can be treated by cholecystectomy include necrotizing cholecystitis, gall bladder trauma or neoplasia, symptomatic cholelithiasis and gall bladder mucocoele. Of these, uncomplicated gall bladder mucocoeles are probably the most suitable for laparoscopic cholecystectomy. Most authors agree that cholecystectomy is the treatment of choice for gall bladder mucocoeles, due to the significant morbidity and mortality associated with those cases that subsequently develop bile peritonitis or extrahepatic biliary obstruction (Scott *et al.*, 2016). Another possible, albeit uncommon, indication for laparoscopic cholecystectomy is symptomatic cholelithiasis without common bile duct stones or associated extrahepatic biliary obstruction. In these cases, care must be taken not to overlook stones that are residing in or mobile within the ductal system. Contraindications to laparoscopic cholecystectomy include uncontrolled coagulopathy, the presence of bile peritonitis, extrahepatic biliary obstruction, small body size (<3 kg) and the presence of conditions that will make the patient poorly tolerant of anaesthesia and pneumoperitoneum (e.g. severe cardiorespiratory disease, diaphragmatic hernia).

Patient positioning and port placement

A four-port approach has been described for laparoscopic cholecystectomy, although placement of a single-port device with an additional one or two instrument ports has also reportedly allowed a successful procedure. Following insufflation, a subumbilical telescope port is established and the abdomen is explored. Then, three further 6 mm instrument ports are placed under laparoscopic visual guidance. One port is placed 5–8 cm lateral and 3–5 cm cranial to the umbilicus in the left cranial quadrant, and two ports are placed 3–5 cm and 5–8 cm lateral to the umbilicus on the right side in a triangulated pattern around the anticipated location of the gall bladder (Figure 12.44). These general guidelines may be adapted to accommodate animals of different sizes.

Surgical technique

Good visualization of the area should be established to facilitate safe dissection around the cystic duct. Active retraction of the gall bladder and adjacent liver lobes will be necessary for an unobstructed view. This can be

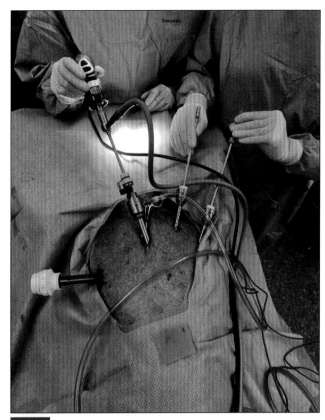

12.44 Port placement for laparoscopic cholecystectomy.

achieved with a 5 mm fan retractor (or other self-retaining retractor) placed through the instrument port on the left side. An assistant will be required to manipulate the retractor under the direction of the primary surgeon. Care should be taken not to damage the gall bladder (which will often be friable) and surrounding hepatic parenchyma.

The laparoscope is positioned in the port closer to the midline on the right side. Once adequate visualization is obtained, right-angled forceps (or articulating forceps, if available) can be used to dissect circumferentially around the cystic duct (Figure 12.45), ensuring that the dissection remains proximal to the entrance of the first hepatic duct to avoid iatrogenic damage. Some haemorrhage is likely but is typically minor. Intermittent suction, with or without saline flushing, should be used to remove the haemorrhage and maintain optimal visualization during the dissection. The

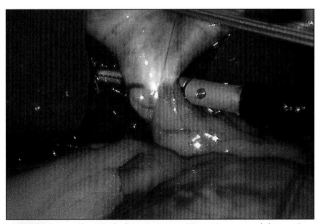

12.45 Laparoscopic cholecystectomy. Dissection around the cystic duct has been completed using articulating laparoscopic Kelly forceps. This instrument can greatly facilitate this challenging part of the procedure.

dissection is complete when the tips of the right-angled forceps are visible around the cystic duct. Any leakage of bile observed during dissection indicates iatrogenic penetration of the cystic duct, and in such cases conversion to an open approach should be considered.

The cystic duct can be ligated in a variety of ways (Figure 12.46). In the case of gall bladder mucocoeles, where there is often some thickening and mild distension of the duct, intracorporeally tied ligatures are recommended and provide good knot security, although laparoscopic needle holders and experience in intracorporeal suturing are necessary. Other options for cystic duct ligation include placement of extracorporeally tied ligatures and large haemoclips. If clips are used as the sole means of ligation, at least four clips should be applied to the duct before sectioning so that at least two clips remain on each side. Once the cystic duct has been transected, dissection of the gall bladder from the hepatic fossa can be completed. Upward traction on the gall bladder by manipulation of the end of the suture material or use of a blunt probe is helpful. Use of a vessel-sealing device or J-hook electrosurgical probe will aid in dissection of the gall bladder from the fossa. Once dissected free, the gall bladder should be placed in a specimen retrieval bag, which is introduced through the subumbilical port.

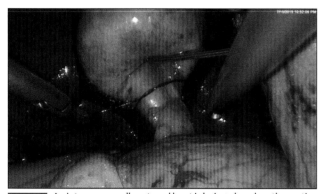

12.46 An intracorporeally sutured knot is being placed on the cystic duct during laparoscopic cholecystectomy in this patient. Laparoscopic needle holders are being used to tie the knot and a fan retractor is being used to retract the gall bladder.

To exteriorize the gall bladder, the entire cannula should be withdrawn from the port site with the first part of the retrieval bag. Tension is then placed on the retrieval bag until a small area of the gall bladder can be visualized and punctured with a No. 11 blade; care should be taken not to penetrate the retrieval bag during this process. The tip of the suction device is placed in the gall bladder, which is still located within the abdomen, and bile is suctioned from within the bag. Once the bile has been removed completely, the empty gall bladder within the specimen retrieval bag can be pulled through the telescope port. Alternatively, if a single-port device has been used, the incision created to accommodate the device may be large enough to pull the intact gall bladder through. The subumbilical port is closed, and the gall bladder fossa is lavaged followed by aspiration of the fluid using a suction/irrigation device. When the surgeon is satisfied that the haemorrhage has ceased, the abdomen is desufflated, the ports are removed and the incisions are closed in a routine manner. The gall bladder should be submitted for histopathology and culture of the contents.

In humans, the laparoscopic cholecystectomy procedure has been developed further to include adjunctive interventions such as intraoperative cholangiography and laparoscopic or endoscopic exploration of the common bile duct. These procedures might become commonplace in veterinary clinical patients in the future. Recently, laparoscopic flushing of the common bile duct was reported by Kanai *et al.* (2018) as an adjunctive therapy for dogs with gall bladder mucocoeles and suspected biliary sludge in the common bile duct.

Ureteronephrectomy

Ureteronephrectomy is most commonly indicated in dogs and cats with primary renal neoplasia, hydronephrosis, end-stage chronic renal failure with chronic infection, renal dysplasia, nephrolithiasis, renal trauma and idiopathic renal haematuria (Gookin *et al.*, 1996; Fossum, 2007). Before ureteronephrectomy, the function of the contralateral kidney should ideally be documented by measurement of the glomerular filtration rate. Case selection for laparoscopic ureteronephrectomy needs to be stringent, especially in the early part of a surgeon's learning curve, to avoid a high rate of conversion to open surgery and significant morbidity. Appropriate cases include modestly sized primary renal neoplasms, chronic renal failure with infection, renal dysplasia and idiopathic renal haematuria. However, it is imperative that less invasive nephron-sparing techniques that preserve kidney function be considered before opting to remove the kidney. Contraindications initially include large renal masses, including neoplasia, hydronephrosis and pyelonephritis with abscessation, and the presence of infection that extends beyond the renal capsule. Preoperative imaging with ultrasonography and, preferably, computed tomography (CT) (or magnetic resonance imaging (MRI)) is very helpful in ruling out conditions that might contraindicate a laparoscopic approach. These imaging modalities also allow assessment of the relationship between the kidney and the surrounding structures.

Patient positioning and port placement

A three-port technique with the patient placed in near lateral recumbency is used for ureteronephrectomy. Once a pneumoperitoneum has been established, a camera port is placed initially at a subumbilical location or a paramedian location more dorsal to the umbilicus; care should be taken not to place the camera port too dorsally. Two instrument ports are placed: one at a mid-abdominal level just caudal to the last rib, and one at the same level in the relevant caudal abdominal quadrant. In general, two ports are established using cannulae capable of accommodating 5 mm instrumentation and one is placed for use with 10 mm instrumentation.

Surgical technique

Initially, the surgeon should survey the kidney and the surrounding structures and optimize the patient's position to allow access to all the important anatomical landmarks. The ureter should be identified (Figure 12.47a), as well as the adrenal gland cranially. To initiate dissection, a vessel-sealing device or bipolar electrosurgical device is used to dissect the kidney from its retroperitoneal attachments. Next, the ureter is dissected free close to its insertion into the renal pelvis, but not transected. The ureter is then used as a 'handle' to suspend the kidney during dissection of the renal artery and vein (Figure 12.47b). The artery and vein should be ligated separately with three clips, using a laparoscopic clip applier, before being sectioned; alternatively,

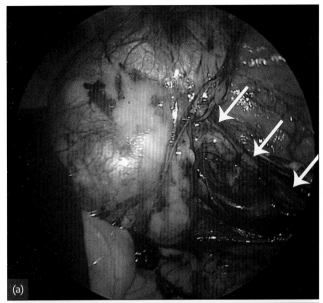

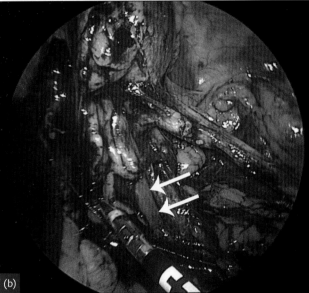

12.47 (a) Early isolation of the ureter (arrowed) during laparoscopic ureteronephrectomy can aid in elevation and dissection of the renal hilum. (b) Dissection of the renal hilum is being performed, with skeletonization of the renal artery and vein (arrowed) before ligation of these vessels.

intracorporeal suturing can be used to ligate the renal artery and vein separately. Placement of endoscopic staples across the renal hilum is also an option. In small dogs and cats, the renal artery and vein can be sealed and cut using a vessel-sealing device alone.

Once the renal artery and vein have been sectioned, the remaining attachments between the kidney and the surrounding retroperitoneum are dissected using a vessel sealer or monopolar electrosurgery. Once dissection of the kidney is complete, tension is placed on the proximal ureter. This facilitates dissection of the remaining section of the ureter down to its insertion into the bladder. Once close to the bladder, the ureter can be clipped with haemoclips or ligated and then sectioned. The resected kidney and ureter are removed from the abdomen using a specimen retrieval bag. The port sites are closed by placement of sutures in the muscular layers followed by placement of intradermal sutures (e.g. polyglactin 910). See also Mayhew et al. (2013a) and Kim et al. (2013) for further description of the surgical technique.

Hernia repair
Diaphragmatic hernia repair

There are few reports (Feranti et al., 2016) of minimally invasive diaphragmatic hernia repair in small animal patients in the veterinary literature, although one report of an experimental canine laparoscopic diaphragmatic hernia model has been published (de Souza et al., 2015). Several major challenges exist to the successful minimally invasive management of diaphragmatic hernia in small animal patients. First, in acute cases, patients are often systemically unstable due to associated trauma. If an approach is made from the abdomen, the induction of a pneumoperitoneum in the absence of an intact diaphragm will result in insufflation of the thoracic cavity, which is usually very poorly tolerated. At high intra-abdominal pressures, acute cardiovascular collapse should be expected in these situations, and so very low intra-abdominal pressures (2–4 mmHg) should be used, if at all. As the diaphragm is located cranially and largely under the rib cage, the rigidity of the caudal ribs creates some working space that may provide the surgeon with enough room to complete reduction of the herniated abdominal contents and close the defect. Working space can be supplemented with an abdominal lift technique with traction on stay sutures placed in the abdominal wall to lift it away from underlying viscera. Other challenges with these cases include: difficulty in safely reducing the organs back into the abdomen, especially in chronic cases where adhesions may be present; and the often small size of affected patients, which can make instrument manipulation and working space very limited. In one experimental study in dogs, liver entrapment was particularly challenging to reduce (de Souza et al., 2015). The authors recommend that diaphragmatic herniorrhaphy be attempted only by veterinary surgeons with considerable experience in both minimally invasive surgery and the associated anaesthetic challenges that this technique presents.

Patient positioning and port placement

The patient is placed in dorsal recumbency. It may be helpful to use a reverse Trendelenburg (head-up) position to encourage the reduction of organs back into the abdominal cavity. Following insufflation of the abdomen to a pressure of 3 mmHg, a subumbilical telescope port is established. Instrument ports are then placed in the right and left caudal quadrants of the abdomen in a triangulating pattern. A fourth port can be placed if extra traction is needed for organ reduction.

Surgical technique

The greatest challenge with this procedure is reduction of the hernia contents, which may be possible in some cases but not in others. Reduction of the small intestine is usually straightforward: gentle traction and a hand-over-hand technique can be used to gradually move the intestine back into the abdomen. Reduction of the spleen and liver may be more challenging due to their weight and propensity to bleed if forcefully manipulated. Manipulation with a blunt probe or the use of laparoscopic retractors may be beneficial for the reduction of these organs. Placement of one or two thoracic cannulae, to allow instruments to be introduced to push organs from the thoracic side of the diaphragm, may be useful in cases where manipulation from the abdominal ports alone is not successful.

If reduction is successful, then closure of the defect can begin with a simple continuous pattern of 2 metric (3/0 USP) or 3 metric (2/0 USP) monofilament absorbable or non-absorbable suture, starting at the dorsal margin of the defect and working ventrally. The use of barbed suture material (e.g. V-Loc™ suture) for this purpose greatly simplifies the procedure, as it maintains tension on the suture line as the closure progresses.

There are two options for the evacuation of air from the thorax:

- A red rubber catheter can be placed through one of the laparoscopic ports and into the thorax just before final closure of the defect. The thorax can then be evacuated just before tightening of the final knot closure, with the red rubber catheter being removed as this is performed
- A thoracic drain can be placed, which is evacuated at the time of final defect closure.

If the surgeon reaches the end of the defect and is satisfied that complete closure has been achieved, then the port sites can be closed routinely. A liberal policy of conversion to an open approach should be applied in these cases, as this is a challenging procedure.

Inguinal hernia repair

Although laparoscopic inguinal hernia repair is commonly performed in humans, it has not been widely reported in veterinary patients (see Chapter 17). This may be because inguinal hernia commonly occurs in many small breeds of dog and working space is limited in these cases. Challenges can also arise in these cases as a result of chronicity causing extensive formation of adhesions between the hernia contents and extra-abdominal tissues.

Patient positioning and port placement

Dogs (cats less commonly) are positioned in a Trendelenburg (head-down) position to encourage the reduction of the hernia contents back into the abdominal cavity. Following insufflation of the abdomen, a subumbilical telescope port is established. In small patients, the telescope port may be placed cranial to the umbilicus on the ventral midline to ensure that the instruments are not too close to the defect to be closed. For left-sided herniorrhaphy, an instrument port is placed in a paramedian location 3–5 cm lateral to the subumbilical port; for right-sided herniorrhaphy, the port is placed in the same location on the right side. A second instrument port is then placed more caudally on the ventral midline to ensure triangulation around the anticipated location of the hernia.

Surgical technique

The hernia is examined and an assessment made as to where the margins of the defect are located. Adhered fat may need to be dissected free in order to visualize the margins of the muscular defect. Organs that have herniated into the defect should be reduced back into the abdominal cavity by gentle traction (Figure 12.48). At this point the surgeon must decide whether there is satisfactory visualization and access to the margins of the defect to close the defect securely using suture traction alone. The use of barbed suture material (e.g. V-Loc™ suture) allows tension on the closure to be overcome due to the

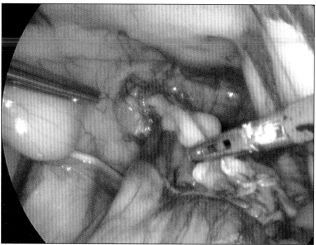

12.48 Inguinal hernia: organs are reduced back into the abdominal cavity by gentle traction.

friction created by the interaction of the suture barbs with the tissue. Suture bites are taken that engage the internal rectus fascia medially and the inguinal ligament laterally. The defect should be closed from cranial to caudal, leaving a small defect caudally that allows the pudendal vessels to pass through the inguinal ring unimpeded. Conversion to an open procedure should be considered in cases where the hernia contents cannot easily be reduced or if the surgeon feels that they do not have adequate visualization of the margins of the hernia to ensure that a secure closure can be achieved.

Hiatal hernia repair

Surgical techniques for the treatment of hiatal herniation in humans have been extensively studied and rigorously evaluated over the years in the medical literature. These techniques have not yet been developed and evaluated to the same extent in dogs. Of the group of gastro-oesophageal junction anomalies that are seen in the dog (which include sliding hiatal hernia, para-oesophageal hernia and gastro-oesophageal intussusception), sliding hiatal hernia is by far the most common. Medical management is aimed at the inhibition of normal gastric acid secretion to reduce its ulcerogenic effects on the oesophagus when gastro-oesophageal reflux occurs, and involves the administration of antacids or proton pump inhibitors and gastroprokinetic agents such as cisapride. However, medical management is not always successful and owner compliance can be a challenge as these cases are often diagnosed at a very young age. The most common approach is a combination of treatments, including diaphragmatic hiatal reduction (by phrenoplasty or crural apposition), oesophagopexy and left-sided gastropexy (Prymak et al., 1989). The results of a recent study documenting the outcomes of open surgery showed that in 80% of dogs for which pre- and postoperative clinical assessments were completed, postprandial regurgitation improved (Mayhew et al., 2017). Minimally invasive surgery is the standard of care for the treatment of hiatal hernia and gastro-oesophageal reflux disease in humans, and these techniques should be developed and evaluated for dogs with these conditions. The first report of laparoscopic hiatal hernia repair in dogs was recently published (Mayhew et al., 2016).

Patient positioning and port placement

Dogs are placed in dorsal recumbency for initial port placement so that the ventral midline can be draped into the surgical field in case conversion to an open approach becomes necessary. However, after port placement dogs are rotated into near right lateral recumbency. A three-port laparoscopic approach is used, with a sub-umbilical telescope port, an instrument port placed on the ventral midline 3–5 cm cranial to the umbilicus and a second instrument port in the left caudal quadrant of the abdomen.

Surgical technique

The procedure is initiated by incising the triangular ligament of the left lateral liver lobe to allow the left lobes of the liver to fall to the right side, thereby establishing a view of the oesophageal hiatus. Reconstruction is performed by placement of two to five interrupted sutures of 2 metric (3/0 USP) or 3 metric (2/0 USP) polypropylene suture material to plicate the hiatus (Figure 12.49). This plication is very subjective and the surgeon should be careful not to over-tighten the hiatus, which can lead to postoperative bloating. An oesophagopexy is then performed by placement of a simple continuous line of 2 metric (3/0 USP) or 3 metric (2/0 USP) barbed suture material (e.g. V-Loc™ suture), extending from the hiatus and incorporating bites of the crural musculature to the distal oesophagus and cardia to prevent axial motion of the stomach into the thorax (Figure 12.50). Finally, a left-sided intracorporeally sutured gastropexy is performed to prevent axial motion of the stomach into the thorax. The gastropexy is performed by initially creating an incision in the transversus abdominis using a monopolar J-hook probe and then scoring the seromuscular layer of the gastric fundus, again using the J-hook monopolar probe. Bites of the scored area of the gastric fundus are taken and apposed to the incision in the transversus abdominis using 2 metric (3/0 USP) or 3 metric (2/0 USP) barbed suture material in a simple continuous pattern. Once all the procedures are complete, the abdomen is desufflated and the laparoscopic ports are closed routinely.

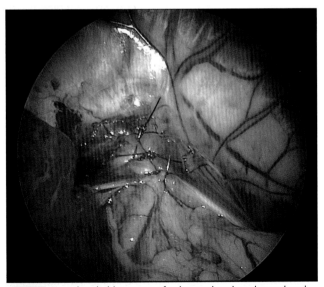

12.49 Non-absorbable sutures of polypropylene have been placed between the crural muscles that surround the ventral aspect of the oesophageal hiatus in this dog during laparoscopic hiatal herniorrhaphy.

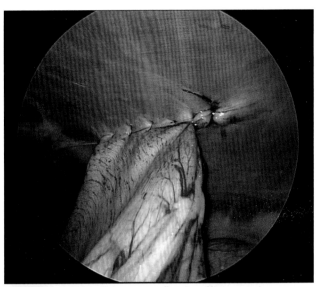

12.50 A completed intracorporeally sutured laparoscopic gastropexy has been performed using barbed suture.

Adrenalectomy

Laparoscopic adrenalectomy has been described in a number of veterinary patients (Jiménez Peláez *et al.*, 2008; Smith *et al.*, 2012; Naan *et al.*, 2013; Mayhew *et al.*, 2014; Pitt *et al.*, 2015; Mitchell *et al.*, 2017). This approach combines the best aspects of both the paracostal and ventral coeliotomy approaches. Positioning the animal in lateral, semi-sternal or sternal recumbency provides excellent visualization of the gland and its surrounding structures without the pain and morbidity associated with paramedian muscle incision. Unlike the coeliotomy approach, the laparoscopic approach does not require extensive retraction and compression of the surrounding organs. The most common indications for adrenalectomy in dogs are primary adrenal neoplasms, typically adrenocortical adenomas, adenocarcinomas and phaeochromocytomas. Functional adrenocortical tumours and aldosterone-secreting tumours occur in cats, but are less common.

Diagnostic imaging (Figure 12.51) is an important part of the preoperative investigation of adrenal masses and forms the basis for decision-making as to whether a laparoscopic approach might be feasible. The dimensions of the mass are important, as are its relationships to the surrounding organs and vascular structures. If detected preoperatively, vascular invasion should be considered an indication for an open approach. The authors recommend that all potential candidates for laparoscopic adrenalectomy undergo a CT scan, if possible, to rule out vascular invasion and evaluate the anatomical margins of the tumour (Schultz *et al.*, 2009).

Selection of suitable cases for laparoscopic adrenalectomy is the key to success, especially in the early part of the surgeon's learning curve. The author [PM] considers animals with functional tumours up to 5 cm in diameter that do not exhibit vascular invasion to be good candidates for laparoscopic adrenalectomy. Cases with vascular invasion of the mass into surrounding vessels, or large masses (>5 cm), are probably best treated by open adrenalectomy; however, the effect of tumour size on morbidity during laparoscopic adrenalectomy has not been properly evaluated in small animals.

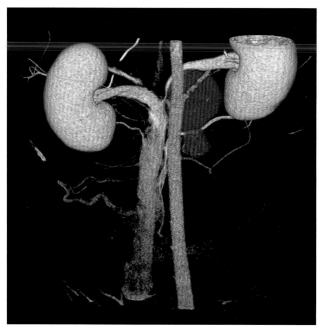

12.51 Three-dimensional CT reconstruction showing a left-sided adrenal mass with the surrounding vascular structures highlighted. These images can help considerably in planning laparoscopic adrenalectomy, which is a complex procedure.

Before surgery, the same preoperative management of adrenal neoplasms as would be used for animals scheduled to undergo an open adrenalectomy should be pursued. In the case of functional adrenocortical tumours, trilostane (2.5–5 mg/kg orally q12h) is administered for 2–3 weeks before surgery at the author's [PM] institution. Supplementation with corticosteroids before surgery to avoid an episode of hypoadrenocorticism in the recovery period is important. Suitable choices include dexamethasone (0.1–0.2 mg/kg i.v.), prednisolone sodium succinate (1–2 mg/kg i.v.) or hydrocortisone (2 mg/kg i.v.). In animals in which phaeochromocytoma is suspected, pre-treatment with an alpha-adrenergic blocker should be considered, such as phenoxybenzamine (increasing dose up to 1–1.5 mg/kg orally) for several weeks preoperatively until the animal is normotensive. This drug has been shown to improve the outcome in dogs undergoing adrenalectomy (Herrera et al., 2008). In cats with functional adrenocortical tumours, it has been suggested that treatment with trilostane should be instituted and continued until the skin abnormalities that accompany the condition in this species resolve. Cats with aldosterone-secreting tumours should have their metabolic and electrolyte disturbances corrected before surgery.

Patient positioning and port placement

The author's [PM] preference is to position the patient on the surgical table in a lateral or near-lateral position with the affected gland upward. The surgeon and surgical assistant (who will hold the laparoscope) should stand on the side of the table that faces the animal's ventral abdomen, with the endoscopic tower placed directly opposite the surgeon on the side facing the animal's back. Alternatively, the animal can be placed in sternal recumbency. The laparoscopic adrenalectomy procedure performed in sternal recumbency is described elsewhere (Naan et al., 2013). Proponents of sternal recumbency suggest that a less obscured view of the adrenal gland is obtained in this position, although studies comparing the two procedures have not yet been performed.

A three- or four-port technique can be used for laparoscopic adrenalectomy in dogs, depending on how much active retraction is necessary. The telescope port should be established 3–5 cm lateral to the umbilicus on the affected side for optimal visualization of the tumour. Instrument ports are placed in a triangulating pattern around the location of the adrenal gland. The ports should not be placed too close together to avoid instrument interference during dissection. For a lesion of the left adrenal gland, a trocar–cannula assembly suitable for the passage of 5 mm instrumentation should be placed 5–10 cm cranial to and 5–8 cm lateral to the subumbilical port on the left side in a location just caudal to the costal arch. It is important that the port is caudal to the last rib to avoid inadvertent penetration of the thoracic cavity. A second instrument port is placed 5–10 cm caudal and 5–8 cm lateral to the subumbilical port in the lower left quadrant. One of the three ports is usually established using a cannula suitable for the passage of 10 mm instrumentation. This allows passage of a specimen retrieval bag at the end of the procedure. If a right-sided adrenalectomy is being performed, the ports are placed at similar locations but on the right side of the animal.

Surgical technique

Obtaining good visualization of the lesion is the first challenge after port placement. During left-sided laparoscopic adrenalectomy, the spleen or stomach will often obscure visualization of the cranial pole of the adrenal gland, and the kidney will sometimes obscure visualization of the caudal margin of the gland. On the right side, the right lobes of the liver may obscure visualization and might need to be retracted cranially, although this is uncommon. The kidney may need to be retracted dorsally and caudally. Alternatively, a third (or further) instrument port(s) can be placed more dorsally over the kidney and a retractor used to move structures cranially or caudally during dissection as required.

In dogs, at least part of the adrenal gland is usually visible, allowing the surgeon to initiate dissection of the retroperitoneal space close to the gland. In obese dogs and in cats, the gland can be completely obscured by fat, in which case dissection through the fat to localize the gland may be necessary. A vessel-sealing device can be used to cut and coagulate the tissues around the gland. A blunt probe, Babcock forceps or Endo Peanut™ can be used to aid manipulation of the gland as the dissection progresses. Intermittent suctioning of small amounts of haemorrhage, as well as fat around the gland, helps with visualization, and the tip of the suction/irrigation device can be used as an aid to dissection.

The adrenal gland receives arterial blood supply from numerous small arteries and is drained principally by the adrenal vein, which on the right side enters directly into the caudal vena cava and on the left side enters the renal vein. These smaller vessels are difficult to visualize directly but result in haemorrhage from almost all planes of dissection if a vessel-sealing device or bipolar cautery is not used. The phrenicoabdominal vein and artery are large and must be identified and ligated. Vessel-sealing devices should reliably seal the phrenicoabdominal vessels of small to medium-sized dogs, if the vessels are less than 5–7 mm in diameter. In larger dogs, haemoclips can be placed on these vessels, but the author [PM] uses them only rarely.

In cats, laparoscopic adrenalectomy is more challenging, as all structures are much smaller and more delicate and there are often large deposits of fat perirenally within which the adrenal mass may be lying (Figure 12.52).

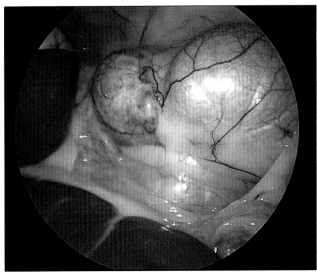

12.52 A large adrenal mass located just cranial to the left kidney in a cat. This mass was a phaeochromocytoma. Its close adherence to the left renal vein can be clearly seen.

In cats, 3 mm instrumentation is very helpful, as 5 mm instruments are challenging to pass into the small plane between the mass, the renal vessels and the vena cava. Although only small numbers of cases have been reported, conversion rates for laparoscopic adrenal-ectomy in cats may be higher than in dogs (Mitchell *et al.*, 2017).

As dissection of the adrenal gland progresses, Babcock forceps can sometimes be placed on the tissues surrounding the gland to aid retraction; however, care should be taken to avoid penetrating the capsule. The gland should be handled with blunt instruments to minimize the risk of penetrating the capsule and tumour seeding of the peritoneal cavity.

In order to minimize the risk of port-site metastases, it is important to place the mass in a specimen retrieval bag before removal (Figure 12.53). The inverted thumb of a large-sized surgical glove can be used as an inexpensive specimen retrieval device. The surgical site should be thoroughly lavaged with sterile saline and closely inspected for ongoing haemorrhage. The abdomen is desufflated, cannulae removed and wound closure is routine.

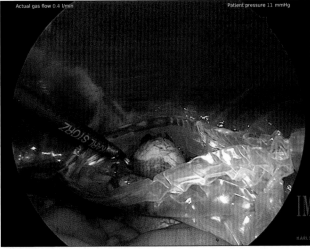

12.53 This adrenal tumour has been dissected and placed into a specimen retrieval bag for extraction through one of the port sites.

Cancer staging

As described above, several organs or masses can be biopsied via laparoscopy. Lymph nodes can be biopsied laparoscopically using 5 mm biopsy forceps, and can also be dissected and extracted. The mesenteric, gastric and external iliac lymph nodes are most commonly biopsied (Steffey *et al.*, 2015). Indocyanine green and near-infrared light have been used to highlight lymph nodes draining a tumour (Alander *et al.*, 2012).

Other potential surgical procedures

Other surgical procedures that can be performed using laparoscopy are:

- Vasopexy
- Cystopexy
- Colposuspension
- Nephrolith removal
- Ureteral transplantation in cases of ectopic ureter
- Extrahepatic portosystemic shunt attenuation.

Complications

Perioperative morbidity can occur following minimally invasive surgical procedures, just as it can in open surgery. Complications may be related to the surgeon's inexperience, and no procedure should be attempted unless the surgeon is experienced with laparoscopic surgery and is confident and competent with the respective open approach, as conversion may be required. Many complications are related to the procedure being performed rather than the surgical approach; however, certain characteristics of the minimally invasive approach can present unique challenges and complications. These include problems related to gaining access to the abdomen, the creation of a pneumoperitoneum or the technical aspects of completing a procedure. Some complications might also be more challenging to deal with when the surgeon has only port access to the site.

Potential complications

Potential laparoscopic complications may be related to various aspects of the procedure:

- Anaesthesia
- Veress needle/trocar insertion:
  - Injury to the abdominal wall
  - Penetration of organs
  - Perforation of a hollow viscus
- Insufflation:
  - Inappropriate
  - Subcutaneous emphysema
- Peritoneal tenting
- Pneumothorax
- Gas embolism
- Operative complications:
  - Bleeding
  - Tissue injury
- Technical problems:
  - Lack of experience
  - Equipment-related

Access-related complications

Obtaining safe access to the peritoneal cavity is the first step in completing any laparoscopic procedure in small animals. In humans, it has been shown that initial access to the peritoneal cavity is the most hazardous step in any laparoscopic procedure. Veress needle and Hasson (paediatric) techniques have similar rates of complications. Puncture of a solid organ (spleen or liver), a hollow organ (intestine or stomach) or a major blood vessel (vena cava or aorta) have been described with each entry technique in humans (Alkatout, 2017). One large study of 103,852 laparoscopic procedures in humans showed that 82% of vascular injuries and 75% of visceral injuries occurred at the time of the first trocar insertion (Champault et al., 1996). In dogs and cats, obtaining safe access is facilitated by the lack of subcutaneous fat at the subumbilical entry site. Whichever technique is used to gain peritoneal access, care should be taken not to traumatize organs inadvertently.

An air embolism, which can be fatal, can be induced if the Veress needle is inserted into the spleen and insufflation commenced. If air embolism is suspected, the patient should be placed in left lateral recumbency with the head down and ventilated with oxygen. This position moves the gas bubbles away from the right ventricular outflow tract to help alleviate the obstruction. CO_2 is readily soluble, and if the embolism is minor the gas should dissolve rapidly. Use of proper technique and careful positioning of the Veress needle should reduce the risks of air embolism considerably.

Splenic laceration is the most frequently reported access injury in cats and dogs, with incidences of 3–18% being reported in several small studies (Davidson et al., 2004; Mayhew and Brown, 2007; Dupré et al., 2009). In the majority of cases, splenic laceration occurs as a result of the initial insertion of a Veress needle or trocar. It is rare for splenic laceration to result in haemodynamically significant bleeding, and in most cases it is sufficient to simply observe until the bleeding ceases. In the rare cases where bleeding is severe, conversion to an open approach may be advisable. Correct needle/trocar placement technique greatly reduces the risk of splenic injury. Penetration of other visceral organs in small animal laparoscopy has rarely been reported.

Anaesthesia-related complications

Although laparoscopic procedures are generally well tolerated in small animals, there are several important physiological alterations specific to these interventions that should be taken into consideration. The establishment of a pneumoperitoneum is essential for most laparoscopic procedures, to create a working space in which to operate. Pneumoperitoneum is usually created by insufflation of the abdomen with CO_2. This gas has several favourable characteristics as an insufflating agent: it is inexpensive, non-flammable, colourless and rapidly excreted.

The physiological changes induced by CO_2 pneumoperitoneum are largely the result of two mechanisms: the rapid absorption of CO_2 across the peritoneal membrane and the compressive effect of the pneumoperitoneum on the diaphragm and posterior vena cava. Compression of the vena cava may reduce blood flow to the heart and consequently reduce cardiac output. Pressure on the diaphragm will increase pulmonary resistance and decrease tidal volume and effective ventilation, especially at higher pressures (>20 mmHg). Monitoring ventilation, by end-tidal capnography and/or blood gas analysis is therefore an essential component of anaesthetic monitoring during laparoscopy.

Positive-pressure ventilation with a mechanical ventilator is essential to control the ventilatory rate and to maintain tidal volume in animals undergoing long procedures or for those with pre-existing cardiopulmonary compromise. For short, elective procedures in healthy patients performed at low insufflation pressures, manual ventilation to provide an assisted breath every 1–2 minutes is usually sufficient. A very good working space can usually be obtained at intra-abdominal pressures of 6–10 mmHg or lower in dogs. A study in cats showed that the working space created at an intra-abdominal pressure of 4 mmHg is sufficient for some simpler procedures, and no detrimental cardiorespiratory changes were seen with pressures up to 8 mmHg (Mayhew et al., 2013b).

Intraoperative complications

There are many possible intraoperative complications that can be encountered during minimally invasive surgical procedures. In most cases, they are similar to the type of complications seen with open procedures, but the way in which they are managed is quite different. Most bleeding that occurs during laparoscopic procedures is 'nuisance' haemorrhage; this is where a haemodynamically insignificant amount of bleeding occurs, but it is nevertheless frustrating to clear and can significantly impair visualization. Most bleeding of this nature can be controlled with pressure from a palpation probe or grasping forceps, or it may even stop spontaneously. In addition, the higher intra-abdominal pressure resulting from insufflation compresses the capillaries and may reduce bleeding time. More severe bleeding from larger vessels obscures visualization but can also be haemodynamically significant.

In both cases, if appropriate equipment is available and the surgeon has sufficient experience, many intraoperative bleeds can be dealt with satisfactorily without conversion to an open procedure. In essence, most of the haemostatic tools available for use in open surgery are available to the surgeon performing a minimally invasive procedure, including the ability to ligate vessels with suture material, apply haemostatic clips, use vessel-sealing devices and apply topical haemostatic agents. If suction is available, then careful aspiration of blood followed by grasping and ligation of larger haemorrhaging vessels is often possible. However, decision-making in these cases should be rapid, and if haemostasis cannot be accomplished quickly conversion should be considered.

Penetration of the diaphragm by an instrument or biopsy needle will lead to pneumothorax, as can pre-existing diaphragmatic hernia. In such cases positive-pressure ventilation must be commenced immediately. It may be possible to proceed if the insufflation pressure is reduced to 3 mmHg, with appropriate monitoring as for an open chest surgery (see Diaphragmatic hernia repair, above). Otherwise, conversion to an open procedure will be required. A thoracic drain should be inserted at the end of the procedure in the normal fashion.

While endoscopic surgery usually provides the surgeon with a magnified view of the area of interest, it is sometimes difficult or even impossible to see organs peripheral to the lesion/organ being operated upon when the endoscope is focused on the site of interest. This can be a disadvantage, and iatrogenic damage to surrounding organs that are outside the field of vision can occur if great care is not taken, particularly when using monopolar electrosurgery (see Chapter 8). Maintaining cannulae so their tips are just inside the peritoneum not only maximizes the working space but also reduces blind spots considerably.

Subcutaneous emphysema can develop when CO_2 leaks between the port and the abdominal wall, especially if the incision in the linea alba is larger than the skin incision, which can occur if the incision is not made with a No. 11 blade. Usually, subcutaneous emphysema will resolve by itself over 24–48 hours.

Conversion

Conversion from a minimally invasive to an open approach may be necessary for a variety of different reasons, and conversion rates are often reported in studies describing various minimally invasive surgical procedures. Two types of conversion exist (Halpin and Soper, 2006):

- Emergent conversion – in which an intraoperative complication occurs that cannot be remedied without open access to the abdomen
- Elective conversion – where a complication has not occurred but the procedure cannot be completed by a minimally invasive surgical approach.

The conversion rates and risk factors for conversion have been reported for many different laparoscopic procedures in humans. General factors that may predispose to conversion of minimally invasive surgical procedures include a diagnosis of malignancy, higher patient bodyweight or body condition score, and surgeon experience (Halpin and Soper, 2006). More is being learned about conversion rates for specific procedures as data are published in the scientific literature, and this will aid in educating both veterinary surgeons and owners about the realistic expectations for minimally invasive surgical procedures. The decision to convert to an open approach should never be seen as a failure, but as good surgical judgement. Veterinary patients should be given the advantages that minimally invasive surgical procedures can provide, but without losing sight of the fact that if surgical principles have been compromised, the long-term outcome for the patient may be inferior to that achieved using an open approach.

Postoperative complications

Port-site complications following minimally invasive surgical procedures are generally associated with either seroma formation, surgical-site infection (SSI) or, rarely, herniation. Seroma formation is possible at any surgical site if dead space is not adequately eliminated (especially in laparoscopic-assisted gastropexy) and has been reported in dogs. Studies have reported that minimally invasive surgical procedures may have lower rates of SSI compared with open surgery in dogs and cats (Mayhew *et al.*, 2012; Charlesworth and Sanchez, 2019). Of the 558 patients in the study by Mayhew *et al.* (2012), the group that had open surgery had a rate of SSI of 5.5% compared with 1.7% in the group that underwent minimally invasive surgical procedures. However, care should be taken in interpreting this data, as the minimally invasive surgical approach was significantly associated with the SSI rate using simple analysis with only one variable.

Herniation of abdominal contents through port incisions is rare but has been reported with the use of port sites as small as 5 mm (Austin *et al.*, 2003). For this reason, it is advised to close the fascial sheath of the body wall in all port closures that involve incisions of 5 mm or larger.

Port-site metastasis is a potential complication when neoplastic lesions are resected and withdrawn through small port incisions. This process was initially considered to be a result of direct inoculation of neoplastic cells during traumatic removal of tissue through small port incisions. However, it is now known that the use of specimen retrieval bags to remove neoplastic or infected tissue, although highly recommended, does not completely prevent port-site metastasis. There is now general recognition that a complex interplay of factors such as the local immune response, pneumoperitoneum and surgical technique may play a role in the aetiopathogenesis of port-site metastasis (Castillo and Vitagliano, 2008).

References and further reading

Ahmad G, Baker J, Finnerty J *et al.* (2019) Laparoscopic entry techniques. *Cochrane Database of Systematic Reviews*, DOI: 10.1002/14651858

Alander JT, Kaartinen I, Laakso A *et al.* (2012) A review of indocyanine green fluorescent imaging in surgery. *International Journal of Biomedical Imaging*, 940585

Alkatout I (2017) Complications of laparoscopy in connection with entry techniques. *Journal of Gynecologic Surgery* **33**, 81–91

Austin B, Lanz OI, Hamilton SM *et al.* (2003) Laparoscopic ovariohysterectomy in nine dogs. *Journal of the American Animal Hospital Association* **39**, 391–396

Bakhtiari J, Tavakoli A, Khalaj A and Ghasempoor S (2011) Minimally invasive total splenectomy in dogs: a clinical report. *Iranian Journal of Veterinary Medicine* **5**, 9–12

Brandão F and Chamness C (2015) Imaging equipment and operating room setup. In: *Small Animal Laparoscopy and Thoracoscopy*, ed. BA Fransson and PD Mayhew, pp. 31–40. Wiley-Blackwell, Ames

Bufalari A, Short CE, Giannoni C *et al.* (1997) Evaluation of selected cardiopulmonary and cerebral responses during medetomidine, propofol, and halothane anesthesia for laparoscopy in dogs. *American Journal of Veterinary Research* **12**, 1443–1450

Case JB (2015) Diagnostic laparoscopy of the gastrointestinal tract. In: *Small Animal Laparoscopy and Thoracoscopy*, ed. BA Fransson and PD Mayhew, pp. 105–112. Wiley-Blackwell, Ames

Case JB, Marvel SJ, Boscan P and Monnet EL (2011) Surgical time and severity of postoperative pain in laparoscopic ovariectomy with one, two, or three instrument cannulas. *Journal of the American Veterinary Medical Association* **239**, 203–208

Castillo OA and Vitagliano G (2008) Port site metastasis and tumor seeding in oncologic laparoscopic urology. *Urology* **71**, 372–378

Champault G, Cazacu F and Taffinder N (1996) Serious trocar accidents in laparoscopic surgery: a French survey of 103,852 operations. *Surgical Laparoscopy & Endoscopy* **6**, 367–370

Charlesworth TM and Sanchez FT (2019) A comparison of the rates of postoperative complications between dogs undergoing laparoscopic and open ovariectomy. *Journal of Small Animal Practice* **60**, 218–222

Cole TC, Center SA, Flood SN *et al.* (2002) Diagnostic comparison of needle and wedge biopsy specimens of the liver in dogs and cats. *Journal of the American Animal Hospital Association* **220**, 1483–1490

Coleman KA, Adams S, Smeak DD and Monnet E (2016) Laparoscopic gastropexy using knotless unidirectional suture and an articulated endoscopic suturing device: seven cases. *Veterinary Surgery* **45**, O95–O101

Coleman KA and Monnet E (2017) Comparison of laparoscopic gastropexy performed via intracorporeal suturing with knotless unidirectional barbed suture using a needle driver *versus* a reticulated endoscopic suturing device: 30 cases. *Veterinary Surgery* **46**, 1002–1007

Culp WTN, Mayhew PD and Brown DC (2009) The effect of laparoscopic *versus* open ovariectomy on postsurgical activity in small dogs. *Veterinary Surgery* **38**, 811–817

Davidson EB, Moll HD and Payton ME (2004) Comparison of laparoscopic ovariohysterectomy and ovariohysterectomy in dogs. *Veterinary Surgery* **33**, 62–69

de Souza DB, Mariano CMA, de Andrade PSC Jr, Coelho GC and Abílio EJ (2015) Laparoscopic correction of experimentally induced diaphragmatic rupture in dogs. *Acta Cirurgica Brasileira* **30**, 537–541

Devitt CM, Cox RE and Hailey JJ (2005) Duration, complications, stress, and pain of open ovariohysterectomy *versus* a simple method of laparoscopic-assisted ovariohysterectomy in dogs. *Journal of the American Veterinary Medical Association* **227**, 921–927

Duke T, Steinacher SL and Remedios AM (1996) Cardiopulmonary effects of using carbon dioxide for laparoscopic surgery in dogs. *Veterinary Surgery* **1**, 77–82

Dupré G, Fiorbianco V, Skalicky M *et al.* (2009) Laparoscopic ovariectomy in dogs: comparison between single portal and two-portal access. *Veterinary Surgery* **38**, 818–824

Ewe K (1981) Bleeding after liver biopsy does not correlate with indices of peripheral coagulation. *Digestive Diseases and Sciences* **26**, 388–393

Feranti JPS, de Oliveira MT, Hartmann HF *et al.* (2016) Laparoscopic diaphragmatic hernioplasty in a dog. *Brazilian Journal of Veterinary Research and Animal Science* **53**, 103–106

Fossum TW (2007) Surgery of the kidney and ureter. In: *Small Animal Surgery, 3rd edn*, ed. TW Fossum, pp. 635–662. Mosby Elsevier, St Louis

Garry R (1999) Towards evidence-based laparoscopic entry techniques: clinical problems and dilemmas. *Gynaecological Endoscopy* **8**, 315–326

Gauthier O, Holopherne-Doran D, Gendarme T et al. (2015) Assessment of postoperative pain in cats after ovariectomy by laparoscopy, median celiotomy, or flank laparotomy. *Veterinary Surgery* **44**, O23–O30

Gilroy BA and Anson LW (1987) Fatal air embolism during anesthesia for laparoscopy in a dog. *Journal of the American Veterinary Medical Association* **5**, 552–554

Goethem BV, Schaefers-Okkens A and Kirpensteijn J (2006) Making a rational choice between ovariectomy and ovariohysterectomy in the dog: a discussion on the benefits of either technique. *Veterinary Surgery* **35**, 136–143

Gookin JL, Stone EA, Spaulding KA et al. (1996) Unilateral nephrectomy in dogs with renal disease: 30 cases (1985–1994). *Journal of the American Veterinary Medical Association* **208**, 2020–2026

Grauer G (1999) Laparoscopy of the urinary tract. In: *Small Animal Endoscopy, 2nd edn*, ed. TR Tams, pp. 427–430. Mosby, St Louis

Grauer GF, Twedt DC and Mero KN (1983) Evaluation of laparoscopy for obtaining renal biopsy specimens from dogs and cats. *Journal of the American Veterinary Medical Association* **183**, 677–679

Halpin VJ and Soper NJ (2006) Decision to convert to open methods. In: *The SAGES Manual of Perioperative Care in Minimally Invasive Surgery*, ed. RL Whelan, JW Fleshman and DL Fowler, pp. 296–303. Springer, New York

Hancock RB, Lanz OL, Waldron DR *et al.* (2004) Comparison of postoperative pain following ovariohysterectomy via harmonic scalpel-assisted laparoscopy *versus* traditional ovariohysterectomy in dogs. *Journal of the American Veterinary Medical Association* **224**, 75–78

Harmoinen J, Saari S, Rinkinen M and Westermarck E (2002) Evaluation of pancreatic forceps biopsy by laparoscopy in healthy beagles. *Veterinary Therapeutics* **3**, 31–36

Hasson HM (1984) Open laparoscopy. *Biomedical Bulletin* **5**, 1–6

Herrera MA, Mehl ML, Kass PH *et al.* (2008) Predictive factors and the effect of phenoxybenzamine on outcome in dogs undergoing adrenalectomy for pheochromocytoma. *Journal of Veterinary Internal Medicine* **22**, 1333–1339

Hewitt SA, Brisson BA, Sinclair MD *et al.* (2004) Evaluation of laparoscopic-assisted placement of jejunostomy feeding tubes in dogs. *Journal of the American Veterinary Medical Association* **225**, 65–71

Imhoff DJ, Cohen A and Monnet E (2015) Biomechanical analysis of laparoscopic incisional gastropexy with intracorporeal suturing using knotless polyglyconate. *Veterinary Surgery* **44(Suppl 1)**, 39–43

Jaffey JA, Graham A, VanEerde E *et al.* (2018) Gallbladder mucocele: variables associated with outcome and the utility of ultrasonography to identify gallbladder rupture in 219 dogs (2007–2016). *Journal of Veterinary Internal Medicine* **32**, 195–200

Jiménez Peláez M, Bouvy BM and Dupré GP (2008) Laparoscopic adrenalectomy for treatment of unilateral adrenocortical carcinomas: techniques, complications, and results in seven dogs. *Veterinary Surgery* **37**, 444–453

Johnson GF and Twedt DC (1977) Endoscopy and laparoscopy in the diagnosis and management of neoplasia in small animals. *Veterinary Clinics of North America* **7**, 77–92

Kanai H, Hagiwara K, Nukaya A, Kondo M and Aso T (2018) The short-term outcome of laparoscopic cholecystectomy in 76 dogs. *Veterinary Surgery* **47**, O112–O113

Kassir R, Blanc P, Lointier P *et al.* (2014) Laparoscopic entry techniques in obese patient: Veress needle, direct trocar insertion or open entry technique? *Obesity Surgery* **24**, 2193–2194

Kim YK, Park SJ, Lee SY *et al.* (2013) Laparoscopic nephrectomy in dogs: an initial experience of 16 experimental procedures. *Veterinary Journal* **98**, 513–517

Kimbrell L, Milovancev M, Olsen R and Lohr C (2018) Comparison of diagnostic accuracy of laparoscopic 3 mm and 5 mm cup biopsies to wedge biopsies of canine livers. *Journal of Veterinary Internal Medicine* **32**, 701–706

Kolata RJ and Freeman LJ (1999) Access, portal placement and basic endosurgical skills. In: *Veterinary Endosurgery*, ed. LJ Freeman, pp. 44–60. Mosby, St Louis

Krishnakumar S and Tambe P (2009) Entry complications in laparoscopic surgery. *Journal of Gynecological Endoscopy and Surgery* **1**, 4–11

Kroft J, Aneja A, Tyrwhitt J *et al.* (2009) Laparoscopic peritoneal entry preferences among Canadian gynaecologists. *Journal of Obstetrics and Gynaecology Canada* **31**, 641–648

Magne ML and Tams TR (1999) Laparoscopy: instrumentation and technique. In: *Small Animal Endoscopy, 2nd edn*, ed. TR Tams, pp. 397–408. Mosby, St Louis

Manasnayakorn S, Cuschieri A and Hanna GB (2008) Ideal manipulation angle and instrument length in hand-assisted laparoscopic surgery. *Surgical Endoscopy* **22**, 924–929

Manassero M, Leperlier D, Vallefuoco R and Viateau V (2012) Laparoscopic ovariectomy in dogs using a single-port multiple-access device. *Veterinary Record* **171**, 69

Mayhew PD and Brown DC (2007) Comparison of three techniques for ovarian pedicle hemostasis during laparoscopic-assisted ovariohysterectomy. *Veterinary Surgery* **36**, 541–547

Mayhew PD and Brown DC (2009) Prospective evaluation of two intracorporeally sutured prophylactic laparoscopic gastropexy techniques compared with laparoscopic-assisted gastropexy in dogs. *Veterinary Surgery* **38**, 738–746

Mayhew PD, Culp WTN, Hunt GB *et al.* (2014) Comparison of perioperative morbidity and mortality rates in dogs with non-invasive adrenocortical masses undergoing laparoscopic *versus* open adrenalectomy. *Journal of the American Veterinary Medical Association* **245**, 1028–1035

Mayhew PD, Freeman L, Kwan T and Brown DC (2012) Comparison of surgical site infection rates in clean and clean-contaminated wounds in dogs and cats after minimally invasive *versus* open surgery: 179 cases (2007–2008). *Journal of the American Veterinary Medical Association* **240**, 193–198

Mayhew PD, Marks SL, Pollard R *et al.* (2016) Prospective evaluation of laparoscopic treatment of type 1 sliding hiatal hernia and gastroesophageal reflux in four dogs. *Veterinary Surgery* **45**, O124–O125

Mayhew PD, Marks SL, Pollard R, Culp WTN and Kass PH (2017) Prospective evaluation of surgical management of sliding hiatal hernia and gastroesophageal reflux in dogs. *Veterinary Surgery* **46**, 1098–1109

Mayhew PD, Mehler SJ, Mayhew KN *et al.* (2013a) Experimental and clinical evaluation of transperitoneal laparoscopic ureteronephrectomy in dogs. *Veterinary Surgery* **42**, 565–571

Mayhew PD, Mehler SJ and Radhakrishnan A (2008) Laparoscopic cholecystectomy of uncomplicated gall bladder mucocele in six dogs. *Veterinary Surgery* **37**, 625–630

Mayhew PD, Pascoe PJ, Kass PH *et al.* (2013b) Effects of pneumoperitoneum induced at various pressures on cardiorespiratory function and working space during laparoscopy in cats. *American Journal of Veterinary Research* **74**, 1340–1346

Mayhew PD, Sutton JS, Singh A *et al.* (2018) Complications and short-term outcomes associated with single-port laparoscopic splenectomy in dogs. *Veterinary Surgery* **47**, O67–O74

McGill DG (1981) Predicting hemorrhage after liver biopsy. *Digestive Diseases and Sciences* **26**, 385–387

Minami S, Okamoto Y, Eguchi H and Kato K (1997) Successful laparoscopy assisted ovariohysterectomy in two dogs with pyometra. *Journal of Veterinary Medical Science* **9**, 845–847

Mitchell JM, Mayhew PD, Culp WTN *et al.* (2017) Outcome of laparoscopic adrenalectomy for resection of unilateral noninvasive adrenocortical tumors in 11 cats. *Veterinary Surgery* **46**, 714–721

Murphy SM, Rodriguez JD and McAnulty JF (2007) Minimally invasive cholecystostomy in the dog: evaluation of placement techniques and use in extrahepatic biliary obstruction. *Veterinary Surgery* **36**, 675–683

Naan EC, Kirpensteijn J, Dupré GP, Galac S and Radlinsky MG (2013) Innovative approach to laparoscopic adrenalectomy for treatment of unilateral adrenal gland tumors in dogs. *Veterinary Surgery* **42**, 710–715

O'Donnell E, Mayhew P, Culp W and Mayhew K (2013) Laparoscopic splenectomy: operative technique and outcome in three cats. *Journal of Feline Medicine and Surgery* **15**, 48–52

Peña FJ, Anel L, Domínguez JC et al. (1998) Laparoscopic surgery in a clinical case of seminoma in a cryptorchid dog. *Veterinary Record* **142**, 671–672

Pinel CB, Monnet E and Reems MR (2013) Laparoscopic-assisted cystotomy for urolith removal in dogs and cats – 23 cases. *Canadian Veterinary Journal* **54**, 36–41

Pitt KA, Mayhew PD, Steffey MA *et al.* (2015) Laparoscopic adrenalectomy for removal of unilateral non-invasive pheochromocytomas in 10 dogs. *Veterinary Surgery* **45**, O70–O76

Pope JFA and Knowles TG (2014) Retrospective analysis of the learning curve associated with laparoscopic ovariectomy in dogs and associated perioperative complication rates. *Veterinary Surgery* **43**, 668–677

Prymak C, Saunders HM and Washabau RJ (1989) Hiatal hernia repair by restoration and stabilization of normal anatomy. An evaluation in four dogs and one cat. *Veterinary Surgery* **18**, 386–391

Rawlings CA (2002) Laparoscopic-assisted gastropexy. *Journal of the American Animal Hospital Association* **38**, 15–19

Rawlings CA (2007) Resection of inflammatory polyps in dogs using laparoscopic-assisted cystoscopy. *Journal of the American Animal Hospital Association* **43**, 342–346

Rawlings CA, Diamond H, Howerth EW *et al.* (2003a) Diagnostic quality of percutaneous kidney biopsy specimens obtained with laparoscopy *versus* ultrasound guidance in dogs. *Journal of the American Veterinary Medical Association* **223**, 317–321

Rawlings CA, Foutz TL, Mahaffey MB *et al.* (2001) A rapid and strong laparoscopic-assisted gastropexy in dogs. *American Journal of Veterinary Research* **6**, 871–875

Rawlings CA, Howerth EW, Bement S and Canalis C (2002) Laparoscopic-assisted enterostomy tube placement and full-thickness biopsy of the jejunum with serosal patching in dogs. *American Journal of Veterinary Research* **63**, 1313–1319

Rawlings CA, Mahaffey MB, Barsanti JA *et al.* (2003b) Use of laparoscopic-assisted cystoscopy for removal of urinary calculi in dogs. *Journal of the American Veterinary Medical Association* **222**, 759–762

Richter KP (2001) Laparoscopy in dogs and cats. *Veterinary Clinics of North America: Small Animal Practice* **31**, 707–727

Rothuizen J (1985) Laparoscopy in small animal medicine. *Veterinary Quarterly* **3**, 225–228

Rothuizen J and Twedt DC (2009) Liver biopsy techniques. *Veterinary Clinics of North America: Small Animal Practice* **39**, 469–480

Runge JJ, Berent AC, Mayhew PD *et al.* (2011) Transvesicular percutaneous cystolithotomy for the retrieval of cystic and urethral calculi in dogs and cats: 27 cases (2006–2008). *Journal of the American Veterinary Medical Association* **239**, 344–349

Schultz RM, Wisner ER, Johnson EG *et al.* (2009) Contrast-enhanced computed tomography as a preoperative indicator of vascular invasion from adrenal masses in dogs. *Veterinary Radiology & Ultrasound* **50**, 625–629

Scott J, Singh A, Mayhew PD *et al.* (2016) Perioperative complications and outcome of laparoscopic cholecystectomy in 20 dogs. *Veterinary Surgery* **45**, O49–O59

Shaver SL, Mayhew PD, Steffey MA *et al.* (2015) Short-term outcome of multiple port laparoscopic splenectomy in 10 dogs. *Veterinary Surgery* **44**, 71–75

Smith RR, Mayhew PD and Berent AC (2012) Laparoscopic adrenalectomy for management of an aldosterone-secreting tumor in a cat. *Journal of the American Veterinary Medical Association* **241**, 368–372

Spah CE, Elkins AD, Wehrenberg A *et al.* (2013) Evaluation of two novel self-anchoring barbed sutures in a prophylactic laparoscopic gastropexy compared with intracorporeal tied knots. *Veterinary Surgery* **42**, 932–942

Stedile R, Beck CA, Schiochet F *et al.* (2009) Laparoscopic *versus* open splenectomy in dogs. *Pesquisa Veterinária Brasileira* **29**, 653–660

Steffey MA, Daniel L, Mayhew PD *et al.* (2015) Laparoscopic extirpation of the medial iliac lymph nodes in normal dogs. *Veterinary Surgery* **44 (Suppl 1)**, 59–65

Takacs JD, Singh A, Case JB *et al.* (2017) Total laparoscopic gastropexy using 1 simple continuous barbed suture line in 63 dogs. *Veterinary Surgery* **46**, 233–241

Ternamian AM, Vilos GA, Vilos AG *et al.* (2010) Laparoscopic peritoneal entry with the reusable threaded visual cannula. *Journal of Minimally Invasive Gynecology* **17**, 461–467

Toro A, Mannino M, Cappello G, Di Stefano A and Di Carlo I (2012) Comparison of two entry methods for laparoscopic port entry: technical point of view. *Diagnostic and Therapeutic Endoscopy*, 305428

Twedt DC (1999) Laparoscopy of the liver and pancreas. In: *Small Animal Endoscopy, 2nd edn*, ed. TR Tams, pp. 44–60. Mosby, St Louis

Twedt DC and Johnson GF (1977) Laparoscopy in the evaluation of liver disease in small animals. *American Journal of Digestive Disease* **22**, 571–580

Twedt DC and Monnet E (2005) Laparoscopy: technique and clinical experience. In: *Veterinary Endoscopy for the Small Animal Practitioner*, ed. TC McCarthy, pp. 357–386. Elsevier, Philadelphia

Vilos GA (2006) The ABCs of a safer laparoscopic entry. *Journal of Minimally Invasive Gynecology* **13**, 249–251

Vilos GA, Ternamian A, Dempster J *et al.* (2007) Laparoscopic entry: a review of techniques, technologies, and complications. *Journal of Obstetrics and Gynaecology Canada* **29**, 433–465

Wildt DE (1980) Laparoscopy in the dog and cat. In: *Animal Laparoscopy*, ed. RM Harrison and DE Wildt, pp. 31–72. Williams & Wilkins, Baltimore

Wildt DE and Lawler DF (1985) Laparoscopic sterilization of the bitch and queen by uterine horn occlusion. *American Journal of Veterinary Research* **46**, 864–869

Wright T, Singh A, Mayhew PD *et al.* (2016) Laparoscopic-assisted splenectomy in dogs: 18 cases (2012–2014). *Journal of the American Veterinary Medical Association* **248**, 916–922

Video extra

● **Video 12.1 Passing instruments around the caudal edge of the falciform fat**

Access via QR code or: bsavalibrary.com/endoscopy2e_12

Chapter 13

Rigid endoscopy: thoracoscopy

Philipp D. Mayhew

Introduction

Thoracoscopic surgery, otherwise known as video-assisted thoracoscopic surgery (VATS), offers a minimally invasive approach for the treatment of a variety of thoracic disease processes. In humans, the suggested advantages of VATS approaches include a reduced volume of thoracic drainage, less postoperative pain, a shorter stay in hospital and a more rapid return to normal function (Stammberger et al., 2000; Chetty et al., 2004). Few objective comparisons of traditional 'open' versus VATS procedures have been reported in the veterinary literature, but similar advantages are likely to exist for canine and feline patients (Walsh et al., 1999).

Before the veterinary surgeon (veterinarian) performs a thoracoscopic procedure, it is important to inform the owners of the possible need to convert the procedure to an open approach. It is also essential to have the instrumentation for open surgery available on the operating room table ready for use if conversion to open surgery becomes necessary. Having experience in open thoracic surgery and advanced training in minimally invasive surgical techniques, as well as carefully selecting patients on the basis of their suitability for thoracoscopic procedures, will help to ensure a high level of success and a low rate of conversion to open surgery.

Indications

Several thoracoscopic procedures have been described in small animals, including the creation of pericardial windows (Jackson et al., 1999; Dupre et al., 2001; Case et al., 2013), subphrenic pericardiectomy (Mayhew et al., 2009; Case et al., 2013), resection of cranial mediastinal masses (Mayhew and Friedberg, 2008; MacIver et al., 2017), ligation of patent ductus arteriosus (Borenstein et al., 2004) and vascular ring anomalies (MacPhail et al., 2001; Townsend et al., 2016), thoracic duct ligation (Allman et al., 2010; Mayhew et al., 2018) and pulmonary lobe resection (Lansdowne et al., 2005; Mayhew et al., 2013), as well as various diagnostic procedures (Kovak et al., 2002). As is the case for laparoscopic approaches, careful selection of patients for thoracoscopy is imperative to achieve success, especially for surgeons who are in the early part of the learning curve for these procedures. Larger dogs are ideal patients early on, as it is easier to work in the larger working space in the thorax of these animals.

Smaller dogs and cats can be technically more challenging. In the case of neoplastic lesions of the lung or mediastinum, ideal early cases are smaller lesions or those that are located peripherally in the lung parenchyma. For each procedure detailed in this chapter, a discussion of case selection for that specific intervention will be included to help guide the decision-making of prospective thoracoscopic surgeons.

Instrumentation

In common with other types of flexible and rigid endoscopy, thoracoscopy requires the use of components that are usually housed on an endoscopic tower. These include a medical grade monitor, a camera, a light source, and a data-recording device. A mechanical insufflator, which is frequently used for creating a pneumoperitoneum during laparoscopic procedures (see Chapter 12), is not necessary for most thoracoscopic interventions unless carbon dioxide insufflation is being used, because the ribs form a rigid frame that maintains a working space in which the surgeon can manipulate organs and operate instruments.

Telescopes

Rigid telescopes used for thoracoscopy come in a range of diameters and tip angulations. The most frequently used telescope diameters are 5 and 10 mm. The 5 mm telescope is suitable for cats and dogs of almost all sizes, although 10 mm telescopes (the principal size used in human endosurgery) are often available to veterinary surgeons and are perfectly adequate for most sizes of patient if a 5 mm telescope is not available. A 3 mm diameter, 14 cm telescope exists that provides excellent visualization within the thoracic cavity of very small dogs (<10 kg bodyweight) and cats. Telescopes 2.7 mm in diameter that are sometimes used for arthroscopy can also be used for thoracoscopy in smaller patients. However, arthroscopes that are smaller than 2.7 mm in diameter may not provide adequate illumination of the thoracic cavity in larger dogs. The 2.7 mm, 30-degree multipurpose endoscope is longer than the arthroscope and is commonly used for thoracoscopy in cats and small dogs, as well as for urethrocystoscopy, rhinoscopy and laparoscopy. The angulation of the tip of the telescope dictates the direction of the field of view. A 0-degree telescope provides an image of what lies directly in front of the telescope tip. In the thorax, a telescope with a tip angle of 30 degrees is recommended (Figure 13.1). Although these telescopes are somewhat more difficult to manipulate initially, rotation of the light post (and therefore the telescope) allows a greater field of view compared with a 0-degree telescope. In addition, angled telescopes allow the operator to view spaces that might be difficult to manoeuvre the telescope into, such as around lung lobes or the heart. As well as the angle-tipped telescopes, a variety of deflectable telescopes are available. The EndoCAMeleon® (Karl Storz Endoscopy) is available with a diameter of 4 mm or 10 mm and has a rotating lens at the distal tip that can deflect up to 120 degrees, allowing the operator to view more inaccessible areas and around corners.

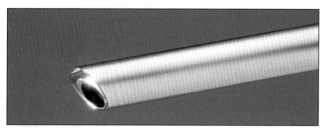

13.1 A 30-degree angled telescope is very useful for thoracoscopy as rotation of the light post allows a great field of view and the possibility of looking around organs in the thorax.

Thoracic trocar–cannula assemblies

The choice of trocar–cannula assemblies for thoracoscopic procedures is based on somewhat different considerations than those for laparoscopy. During thoracoscopy, because insufflation is generally not used, cannulae are not essential because there is no need for an airtight seal. In theory, the telescope and instruments can be passed through incisions in the chest wall without cannulae. However, the use of thoracic cannulae is still recommended, as iatrogenic damage to the body wall (especially the intercostal arteries and veins) or lungs is more likely when instruments are repeatedly inserted and withdrawn through unprotected thoracic wall incisions. Additionally, it can be difficult to pass the telescope through an unprotected port incision without contaminating the lens with blood, which results in loss of optimal visualization. Thoracic cannulae can be simple in design because they do not need to incorporate a one-way valve to prevent loss of insufflated gas. Disposable (Figure 13.2) and non-disposable (Figure 13.3) cannulae are available. Thoracic cannulae with threaded shafts are especially helpful, as they prevent dislodgement of the cannula during instrument exchanges. Thought should always be given to the size of the instruments necessary to complete any given procedure while planning the procedure, so that cannulae of corresponding sizes can be selected.

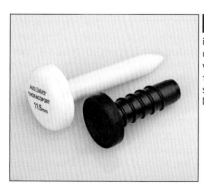

13.2 A Thoracoport™ (Medtronic Inc.) is a simple disposable port used for thoracoscopy that will accommodate the 12 mm endoscopic staplers sometimes used for lung lobectomy procedures.

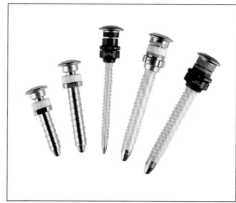

13.3 A variety of non-disposable thoracic cannulae are available for use in thoracoscopy. The use of threaded cannulae is encouraged to reduce cannula pull-out during instrument exchanges.

Thoracoscopic instrumentation

A routine set of minimally invasive instruments for thoracoscopy usually includes Metzenbaum scissors, hook scissors (for cutting suture material), a blunt probe, Kelly or Blakesley dissection forceps, Babcock forceps, a biopsy punch and/or cup forceps and a knot pusher (if extracorporeal knot tying is anticipated). Other more specialized instruments that might be necessary for certain procedures include right-angled dissection forceps, a fan or other type of minimally invasive retractor and needle holders (if intracorporeal suturing is anticipated).

Haemostasis

Haemostasis within the thoracic cavity can be achieved using haemoclips, pre-tied suture loops (e.g. Endoloop®, Ethicon, Johnson & Johnson), extra- or intracorporeally tied sutures or vessel-sealing devices. The LigaSure™ device (Medtronic Inc.), the Enseal® (Ethicon, Johnson & Johnson) and the Caiman® (B Braun) are three bipolar vessel-sealing devices that are indicated to seal arteries and veins up to 7 mm in diameter. These devices can be used effectively within the thoracic cavity to provide haemostasis and to section the mediastinum, perform pericardiectomies and aid in the dissection of pulmonary or mediastinal masses. When using vessel-sealing devices, care should always be taken not to cause thermal damage to the surrounding organs. The devices mentioned have a lateral thermal spread of 1–3 mm (Harold *et al.*, 2003). Another option that is also extremely effective is the HARMONIC® scalpel (Ethicon, Johnson & Johnson), which is also suitable for sealing vessels up to 7 mm in diameter. This device creates a seal using ultrasonic rather than bipolar energy. Other vessel sealer/dividers are available from various manufacturers. Single-use devices should be gas sterilized. Autoclavable devices such as the Robi® plus and VetSeal may also be used; the Robi® plus will work with most bipolar energy sources, whereas the VetSeal requires its own bespoke generator.

Surgical staplers

The use of endoscopic stapling is mandatory for certain thoracoscopic procedures. The most commonly used staplers are the Endo GIA™ (Medtronic Inc., Figure 13.4) and the Echelon Flex™ (Ethicon, Johnson & Johnson), both of which must be passed down a cannula 12 mm in diameter or larger. These staplers place two triple rows of

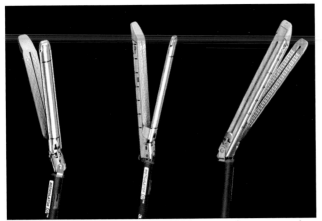

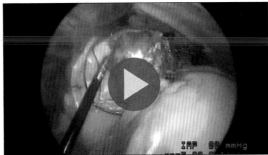

13.4 Endoscopic staplers such as the Endo GIA™ (Medtronic Inc.) discharge six rows of staggered staples and incorporate a cutting blade between the third and fourth rows of staples. These staplers must be passed through a 12 mm or larger cannula.

Video 13.1 Resection of a cranial mediastinal mass and removal from the thorax in a specimen retrieval bag.

staggered staples that are separated by a cutting blade, thus allowing secure sealing on each side of the cut and preventing back-bleeding or spillage of contaminated material into the surgical field. Cartridges for the staplers are generally available in lengths of 30–60 mm depending on the brand used. The staples come in a variety of sizes (2.0, 2.5, 3.5 and 4.8 mm) to accommodate different types of tissue, and surgeons should familiarize themselves with the recommendations for each size before use. The most frequently used cartridge for lung lobectomy in dogs is 30–60 mm in length with a 3.5 mm staple leg length (Lansdowne *et al.*, 2005; Mayhew *et al.*, 2013). Pre-tied (Endoloop®) or extracorporeally tied ligature loops can also be used to ligate small, peripheral areas of lung tissue when a biopsy of the lung only is indicated.

Miscellaneous instrumentation

A suction/irrigation device can be very helpful when performing thoracoscopic procedures. Disposable single-use suction/irrigation catheters come pre-attached to tubing that hooks into motorized fluid pumps or fluid bags that can be placed in pressure cuffs, thus allowing rapid large-volume irrigation of surgical sites followed by aspiration. These catheters are also very useful for aspiration of haemorrhage that may obscure the surgical field. Non-disposable devices have the advantage of being significantly cheaper than disposable suction irrigators because they can be resterilized and reused. The author routinely uses the trumpet valve (Karl Storz Endoscopy) attachment for a non-disposable suction/irrigation wand, which allows fine control over suction.

Specimen retrieval bags are used to assist in withdrawing tissue specimens through port-site incisions. Commercially manufactured bags are available from various medical device companies. For small samples, the thumb of a surgical glove can be used as a cheaper substitute. Specimen retrieval bags should be used when tissue that could be neoplastic or infected is to be removed through a small port incision. The sample is placed in the bag before being withdrawn through the incision (Video 13.1). The use of specimen retrieval bags helps to minimize the risk of port-site metastases by preventing seeding of tumour cells from the specimen into the thoracic wall during removal. They also allow large tissue samples to be withdrawn through much smaller incisions than would otherwise be necessary, due to the significant traction that can be applied when using them.

Patient preparation

When a thoracoscopic approach is chosen for a procedure in a dog or cat, significant thought needs to be given to the position of the equipment in the operating room, as well as that of the patient, to ensure that there is optimal access to the target organ or lesion throughout the procedure. Because traditional manual retraction of organs is not possible in the absence of a thoracotomy incision, the surgeon needs to optimize the patient's positioning to aid gravity-assisted retraction of organs. The judicious use of internal retraction using a variety of thoracoscopic instruments and retractors is also possible. For procedures traditionally performed by open intercostal thoracotomy, an intercostal port placement technique is likely to be used, with the patient positioned in the relevant lateral recumbency. For procedures that would otherwise be performed through a median sternotomy, a subxiphoid approach is used. Wide clipping of the hair coat and aseptic preparation of the entire lateral thorax from the dorsal to the ventral midline is routinely used for any thoracoscopic procedure performed in lateral recumbency in case conversion to an open thoracotomy becomes necessary during the procedure. For procedures performed in dorsal recumbency, wide clipping and aseptic skin preparation of the whole ventrum of the thorax and the cranial half of the abdomen is performed to ensure that sterile technique is maintained and conversion to a median sternotomy can be performed if necessary.

Anaesthetic considerations

For certain thoracoscopic interventions, such as the creation of a pericardial window, thoracic duct ligation and lung biopsy, the pneumothorax that forms within the chest when the first cannula is placed and air is allowed to enter the pleural cavity will provide adequate working space for the procedure to be completed safely in most cases. For these procedures, anaesthetic concerns are similar to those for any open thoracotomy. Intravenous access should be established and, if possible, an indwelling arterial catheter should be placed for direct measurement of arterial blood pressure. Variables that should be monitored during the procedure include the heart rate and rhythm (via electrocardiography), oxygen saturation by pulse oximetry, end-tidal capnography and/or intermittent blood gas analysis and continuous arterial pressure. Positive-pressure ventilation, preferably with a mechanical ventilator, is mandatory for anaesthetic maintenance, just as it is for open thoracic surgery.

Several techniques can be used to increase the working space in the thoracic cavity during more advanced thoracoscopic procedures. Intermittent ventilation can be used for shorter procedures and is tolerated to a variable extent by animals under anaesthesia: animals with normal pulmonary parenchyma may tolerate long breaks between ventilation, but those with cardiorespiratory disease may tolerate only short breaks. Intermittent ventilation is also generally frustrating when performing more complex procedures where intermittent inflation of the lung fields obscures visualization, making iatrogenic trauma to the pulmonary parenchyma during instrument exchanges more likely and generally prolonging the procedure.

Thoracic insufflation

If thoracic cannulae with one-way valves are used, it is possible to insufflate the thorax to increase the working space, in the same way as is done for laparoscopic surgery. Carbon dioxide is used for thoracic insufflation. The advantages of thoracic insufflation are that it is very easy to institute and can significantly increase the volume of the working space. The disadvantage is that the thoracic cavity is poorly tolerant of positive-pressure insufflation, due principally to the many thin-walled, low-pressure vascular compartments within it, which include the right side of the heart, the cranial and caudal vena cava and the pulmonary veins. Even at low insufflation pressures (3 mmHg) significant cardiopulmonary depression has been shown to occur (Daly et al., 2002). Although initial studies warned largely against the use of thoracic insufflation, the use of insufflation at low pressures (3 mmHg) for limited periods may be helpful in some cases where it is difficult to achieve adequate visualization. The intervention appears to be particularly well tolerated in cats (Mayhew et al., 2019b).

One-lung ventilation

One-lung ventilation (OLV) is generally considered to be the preferred technique for improving working space during more advanced thoracoscopic interventions. Whenever OLV is used, significant physiological changes must be anticipated, as a significant ventilation/perfusion mismatch occurs as a result of the non-ventilated lung remaining perfused. However, studies have shown that OLV does not have a large effect on oxygen delivery in healthy dogs (Kudnig et al., 2003). It should be remembered that tidal volume must be reduced, usually by a factor of 30–50%, to avoid barotrauma and, to compensate, the respiratory rate is usually increased by approximately 20%. In most dogs without significant cardiopulmonary disease, OLV is very well tolerated. Positive end-expiratory pressure (PEEP) of 5 cm H_2O can be helpful during OLV and has been shown to increase the arterial partial pressure of oxygen (P_aO_2) and decrease shunt fraction without having a detrimental effect on cardiac output (Kudnig et al., 2006). However, the author has noted subjectively that PEEP usually significantly impairs visualization within the thorax of smaller or flat-chested dogs, where even small amounts of residual inflation during ventilatory cycles can reduce the visualization of organs.

Various techniques can be used to create OLV, including the use of selective intubation, endobronchial blockers (EBBs) or double-lumen endobronchial intubation. All of these devices usually require bronchoscopic-assisted placement, although blind thoracoscopic-assisted placement of double-lumen endobronchial tubes (DLTs) has

been described (Mayhew et al., 2012) and is feasible in certain breeds of dog; fluoroscopic-guided placement has also recently been investigated by the author's group (Mayhew et al., 2019a). Selective intubation involves the placement of a smaller diameter long endotracheal tube into one mainstem bronchus. A bronchoscope is placed down the lumen of the tube and the tube is guided into either the left or right mainstem bronchus depending on which side requires ventilating (the contralateral lung field to the side with the lesion). Selective intubation is used principally for very large dogs in which DLTs are usually too short and in which the balloon on the tip of the EBB is not always large enough to completely occlude the lumen of the mainstem bronchus.

EBBs are relatively easy to place and consist of an endotracheal tube with a small-diameter balloon-tipped catheter either attached to the end of the tube or running within the lumen of the tube. In the model used most commonly (Arndt Endobronchial Blocker, Cook Medical), the bronchoscope is passed through a suture loop on the tip of the EBB as it is passed down the lumen of the endotracheal tube. This allows the balloon-tipped catheter to be guided by the bronchoscope into the left or right mainstem bronchus so that when the balloon is inflated, fresh gas inflow is prevented from entering the now-obstructed bronchus. The technique for placement of an EBB is illustrated in Video 13.2. EBBs are available in 5, 7 and 9 Fr sizes with either spherical or ellipsoid/barrel-shaped balloons. These devices work well, although in very large dogs the balloons of even the largest EBBs may not inflate to a large enough diameter to completely occlude a mainstem bronchial lumen. The 5 Fr EBB is probably the best option for induction of OLV in smaller patients, as DLTs cannot be used in dogs smaller than approximately 10 kg bodyweight. A newer variant of the EBB is the EZ-blocker™ (Teleflex Inc.), which has a Y-shaped tip (Figure 13.5). The bifurcated tip usually positions itself within the right and left mainstem bronchi, from where separate balloons can be inflated to achieve either right- or left-sided blockade. Because these devices are designed for the human tracheobronchial anatomy, the author has found that after resting the Y-piece on the carina the blocker needs to be slowly withdrawn 1–3 cm in order to achieve successful blockade of the cranial lobar bronchi (Mayhew et al., 2019a).

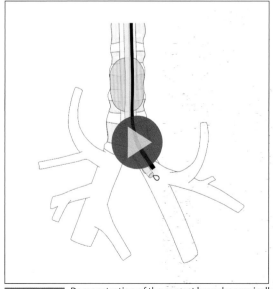

Video 13.2 Demonstration of the correct bronchoscopically guided placement of an endobronchial blocker.

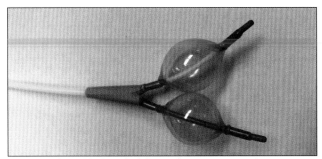

13.5 The EZ-blocker™ (Teleflex Inc.) is a newer type of endobronchial blocker that has a bifurcated tip and two balloons, each of which can be inflated in a mainstem bronchus depending on which side needs to be blocked.

DLTs are slightly more challenging to place, but dogs with right cranial lobe lesions can benefit from the use of a left-sided DLT, as the tube can be placed into the left mainstem bronchus and ventilation through the bronchial lumen will prevent inflation of the right cranial lung lobe; this is difficult to achieve with either an EBB or selective intubation due to the very cranially located entrance of the right cranial lobar bronchus. DLTs come in a variety of designs but Robertshaw left-sided tubes (Figure 13.6) are preferred (Mayhew *et al.*, 2012). The major disadvantage of DLTs is their relatively short length, which means that they can generally be used only in dogs <30 kg.

In all cases, whether selective intubation, endobronchial blockade or DLTs are used, it is essential that anaesthesia is monitored very carefully. The most significant clinical problem is tube displacement intraoperatively. Most commonly this results in loss of OLV intraoperatively, impairing the surgeon's ability to proceed with the procedure. Less commonly, if an EBB or DLT slips cranially out of the mainstem bronchus into the trachea an acute airway obstruction may occur, resulting in total cessation of ventilation. This must be noticed immediately and the tube repositioned. Placing the OLV tube with the patient in the operating room rather than the anaesthesia preparation area will minimize movement of the patient once the tube is placed and so minimize the risk of initial displacement. After placement, every effort should be made by the surgeon and anaesthetist to minimize movement of the patient.

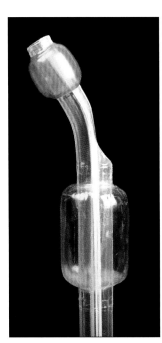

13.6 The double-lumen endobronchial tube is helpful, especially when the right lung needs to be blocked, as ventilation through the left-sided bronchial tip can allow left-sided ventilation without the need for direct obstruction of the very cranially located right mainstem bronchus.

Thoracoscopic access and port placement

The major difference between minimally invasive procedures in the thoracic and peritoneal cavities is that thoracoscopy does not usually require insufflation because the ribs form a rigid frame that maintains a working space. For the same reason, there is no need to maintain a tight seal around cannulae placed into the thoracic cavity. To allow pneumothorax to develop, access to the thoracic cavity can be initiated using either an open technique or an optical entry technique. These techniques can be used to gain initial thoracic access via a subxiphoid or an intercostal location depending on the procedure to be performed.

Establishment of the initial telescope port
Open technique

The traditional open technique is similar to the Hasson technique used for laparoscopy: a small skin incision is made, after which dissection down through the deeper tissue layers is continued until the parietal pleura is penetrated. Dissection can be pursued either using a combination of blunt and sharp dissection or with the aid of monopolar electrosurgery. Many surgeons prefer to perform the deeper dissection by blunt dissection with a mosquito haemostat. Penetration of the pleura itself with electrosurgery is avoided, to prevent iatrogenic injury to the lung tissue beneath, and blunt penetration with forceps or blunt scissors is preferred. Once penetration of the pleura has been accomplished, the incision is widened to allow passage of the cannula. Correct placement of the cannula can be confirmed by passing the telescope down the cannula to visualize the intrathoracic structures. If a subxiphoid telescope port is being placed, final penetration of the cannula into the pleural cavity is usually performed at least partially with the trocar–cannula assembly, as penetration through the most ventral part of the diaphragm is challenging with surgical instruments due to its deep location. Alternatively, pneumothorax may be initiated with a Veress needle placed intercostally lateral to the sternum before placement of the paraxiphoid port.

Optical entry

Optical entry uses the telescope to visualize the penetration of the thoracic wall tissues as cannula placement is being performed. This procedure necessitates the use of either a trocarless cannula (e.g. ENDOTIP cannula, Karl Storz Endoscopy) (Video 13.3) or a specialized disposable optical entry cannula (e.g. Versaport™ Bladeless Optical Trocar, Medtronic Inc., or Kii® Fios First Entry,

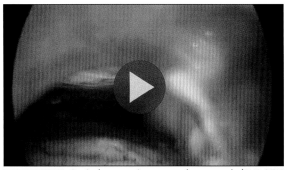

Video 13.3 Optical entry using a trocarless cannula (ENDOTIP, Karl Storz Endoscopy).

Applied Medical). Optical entry is gaining widespread use in the human field and is usually performed using specialized disposable cannulae that incorporate a translucent trocar with a lumen that can accommodate the telescope. An initial 1–1.5 cm incision is made in the desired location of the port. The subcutaneous tissues can be incised, although penetration into the deeper layers is achieved by advancement of the trocar–cannula assembly during placement. Placement of the cannula is initiated just until it starts to become 'seated' in the deeper tissues. Once this has occurred, the telescope is placed into the cannula (or trocar–cannula assembly in the case of disposable versions) and the cannula is advanced into the thorax by using firm pressure combined with a twisting motion around the telescope. This method of entry can be used for both subxiphoid and intercostal cannula placement. During the procedure the telescope allows visualization of the penetration of the deeper muscle layers as it occurs, and penetration of the visceral pleura is seen as soon as it happens, preventing excessively deep cannula placement.

Establishment of instrument ports

Once access to the thoracic cavity has been obtained, instrument ports are generally placed in a triangulating pattern around the area of interest, under direct visualization. The port positions are dictated by the specific surgical technique being performed and, to some extent, by the surgeon's preference. When establishing instrument ports for thoracoscopy, it can be helpful to make a small skin incision with a scalpel blade and then use mosquito or Kelly forceps to bluntly dissect a small hole that penetrates the pleural cavity, before passing the instrument cannula under direct visualization. The size of each cannula needs to be chosen on the basis of the size of the instruments that are anticipated to be passed through it; for example, if surgical staplers (most of which are 12 mm diameter devices) are to be used, cannulae accommodating 12 mm instruments need to be placed.

In procedures that are performed with the patient in dorsal recumbency, the first step after establishing access to the thoracic cavity is to section the ventral mediastinal attachments if access to both hemithoraces is required. These are usually thin 'curtains' of tissue that hang down from the sternum; they are generally poorly vascular but are best sectioned using a vessel-sealing device or electrosurgical unit. Once this tissue has been sectioned, access to both hemithoraces is established and the surgical procedure can begin.

Thoracoscopic placement of thoracic drains

After most surgical procedures within the thorax, placement of a thoracic drain is indicated, to monitor for postoperative bleeding and air leakage and to drain any ongoing pleural effusion. With thoracoscopic procedures, placement of a thoracic drain is performed before final removal of the telescope port and is generally facilitated by direct visualization of the drain as it enters the thoracic cavity, which can reduce the risk of iatrogenic penetration of intrathoracic structures. Penetration of the thoracic drain through the deep subcutaneous tissues and muscle of the intercostal space can be facilitated by blunt dissection initially. The drain should tunnel under the skin for two intercostal spaces before being directed into the thoracic cavity, to help prevent leakage of air on withdrawal. The pleura is then penetrated, and finally the drain is advanced into the cranioventral aspect of the thoracic cavity before being secured to the skin using a Chinese finger-trap suture. More recently, the use of Seldinger catheter-over-guidewire thoracic drains (e.g. MILA International Inc.) has gained popularity; these drains obviate the need for significant pressure to be placed on the thoracic wall during drain placement.

Surgical procedures
Thoracoscopic pericardiectomy

Creation of a pericardial window has traditionally been considered the best treatment to palliate clinical signs of idiopathic or neoplasia-associated pericardial effusion (Jackson et al., 1999; Dupre et al., 2001; Case et al., 2013). Subphrenic pericardiectomy (SPP) is the treatment of choice for constrictive pericarditis and has also been recommended as an adjunctive therapy in patients with idiopathic chylothorax (Mayhew et al., 2009; Case et al., 2013; Mayhew et al., 2018). However, a recent report has questioned whether a pericardial window provides lasting relief from signs of cardiac tamponade, and SPP may provide longer-term palliation, especially in dogs with idiopathic pericardial effusion (Case et al., 2013).

Anaesthesia

For the thoracoscopic creation of a pericardial window, generally no increase in working space is required during the procedure, except perhaps in dogs with very low thoracic depth-to-width ratios (flat-chested dogs such as English Bulldogs) where very little working space exists. For SPP, the pericardium must be resected from both sides of the heart, necessitating visualization of the two sides sequentially. In some deep-chested breeds of dog this may be possible without OLV (Dupre et al., 2001); another option is the use of DLTs that can allow alternating OLV during the procedure (Mayhew et al., 2009).

Patient positioning and port placement

The patient is positioned in dorsal recumbency on a tilting table. The viewing monitor and endoscopic tower are positioned at the head of the patient on the left side. A three-port technique is used for both pericardial window creation and SPP. Thoracoscopic access is achieved by placement of a subxiphoid telescope port. An instrument port is established at the 4th to 6th intercostal space ventral to the costochondral junction on the side corresponding to the side the telescope port has entered. The ventral mediastinal attachments to the sternum are removed with laparoscopic scissors or a vessel-sealing device. Once both hemithoraces can be visualized via the telescope, a second instrument port is established at the 4th to 6th intercostal space on the contralateral side in the same fashion as the first, or further caudally, at the 8th or 9th intercostal space. Alternatively, both ports may be placed on the same side, one in the 4th to 6th and the other in the 9th or 10th intercostal space. When creating a pericardial window, the patient is generally not tilted in any direction during the procedure. For SPP, it can be helpful to tilt the patient away from the side of the heart that is being operated on, to allow the heart to move in that direction to optimize visualization of the phrenic nerves.

Thoracoscopic technique for pericardial window creation

Once good visualization has been established, the pericardium over the apex of the heart is incised. This can be the most challenging part of the procedure, as care needs to be taken not to damage the underlying epicardium or coronary vessels. If a significant pericardial effusion is present, incision into the pericardium is usually easier and safer, as the fluid will act as a protective barrier that helps to avoid iatrogenic damage to the underlying structures. However, for patients with significant cardiac tamponade, pericardiocentesis should be carried out before anaesthesia to minimize tamponade-related anaesthetic complications. The pericardium is elevated using a Kelly or Babcock forceps and laparoscopic scissors are used to incise the pericardial sac (Figure 13.7). Once the pericardium is penetrated, any effusion present will pour out. The edges of the pericardial incision are elevated with forceps (Figure 13.8). Laparoscopic scissors or, preferably, a vessel-sealing device is then used to excise a window of pericardium approximately 4 x 4 cm in size over the apex of the heart (Figure 13.9). Whichever device is used to create the window, care must be taken to avoid damaging the underlying coronary vessels and epicardium.

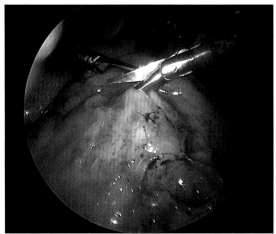

13.7 The initial incision into the pericardium during thoracoscopic pericardiectomy is one of the most challenging parts of the procedure and is best made by taking small bites with sharp laparoscopic scissors.
(© Karl Storz SE & Co. KG)

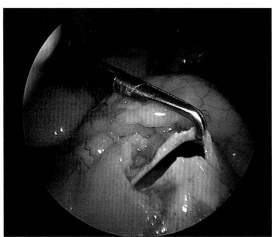

13.8 Once penetration into the pericardial sac has been established, forceps are used to elevate the pericardium from the epicardium to facilitate further dissection.
(© Karl Storz SE & Co. KG)

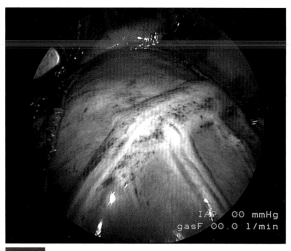

13.9 A completed pericardial window in a dog.

Resected pericardial tissue should be removed from the thoracic cavity either through one of the cannulae or in a specimen retrieval bag. Port-site metastasis has been reported in a dog with pericardial mesothelioma where the pericardial tissue was not removed using a retrieval bag (Brisson *et al.*, 2006).

Thoracoscopic technique for SPP

To initiate SPP, an incision is made into the pericardium similar to that performed for pericardial window creation. Once this incision has been made, a vessel-sealing device is used to continue sectioning the pericardium in a caudolateral direction down to the level of the phrenic nerve. At this point the table is tilted away from the side of the pericardium initially being operated on. If visualization is poor, OLV can be initiated, with blockade of whichever side is to be operated on first (Mayhew *et al.*, 2019a). Once dissection down to the level of the caudodorsal pericardium close to the phrenic nerve is complete, the thoracoscope is removed from the subxiphoid port and placed into the ipsilateral instrument port. The vessel-sealing device is then placed in the subxiphoid port. Babcock forceps are placed into the contralateral instrument port to allow the cut edge of the pericardium to be retracted medially, thus improving visualization of the phrenic nerve. The pericardium is then sectioned along a line parallel to the phrenic nerve in a caudal to cranial direction. Care should be taken to identify the atrial appendages, which generally come into view during this part of the dissection, especially if they are associated with a neoplastic process.

Once the dissection is complete, the previously collapsed lung is reinflated (if OLV has been used) and the contralateral lung is collapsed if necessary. The table is tilted to the opposite side and the pericardial dissection procedure is repeated on that side until only a small cranial attachment of the pericardium remains. The thoracoscope is replaced into the subxiphoid port and Babcock forceps are placed into one instrument port with the vessel-sealing device placed into the other, so that final sectioning of the remaining cranial attachment of the pericardium can be accomplished (Figure 13.10). The excised pericardial tissue with associated fat is placed into a specimen retrieval bag and removed through one of the port incisions. The collapsed lung is reinflated, and reinflation of both lungs is visually verified after termination of the procedure. A chest tube is placed to evacuate the pneumothorax, and the ports are closed routinely.

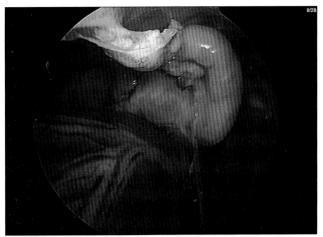

13.10 During a subphrenic pericardiectomy, all the pericardium below the phrenic nerves is removed. In this image, all that remains attached is the cranial portion of the pericardium, which will be sectioned before removal of the pericardial tissue in a specimen retrieval bag.

Modified thoracoscopic technique for SPP

Recently, a technique has been described that may offer similar advantages to the SPP technique described above while being less technically challenging (Barbur *et al.*, 2018). In this technique a pericardial window is initially created, which is subsequently followed by the creation of three or four deep incisions in the pericardium that extend to the phrenic nerves, but without removal of the incised tissue. The incisions are sometimes termed 'banana skin incisions'.

Complications

Iatrogenic damage to the phrenic nerve is possible. This is unlikely to cause clinical signs in a dog if the damage is unilateral, but hypoventilation may be apparent if the damage is bilateral, or in animals with pre-existing respiratory compromise. In dogs with constrictive pericarditis, adherence between the pericardium and epicardium may occur, making SPP more challenging or even impossible. Epicardial stripping can be performed, but has rarely been described in dogs and is likely to be associated with a high rate of complications. Profuse haemorrhage from a bleeding cardiac mass is possible after the creation of a pericardial window, as in some cases the pericardium probably causes some degree of tamponade to the underlying bleeding lesion. Therefore, owners should always be advised about the possibility of fatal haemorrhage after the creation of a pericardial window for palliation of pericardial effusion secondary to cardiac neoplasia.

Right auricular mass resection

Most right auricular masses are haemangiosarcomas. Most of these tumours have metastasized by the time of diagnosis, so it is questionable whether resection of these masses will make a significant difference to the patient's survival. However, if they are removed the potential for haemorrhage may be diminished and the risk of secondary pericardial effusion and cardiac tamponade may be reduced, at least for a period of time. Thoracoscopic resection of auricular masses is likely to be possible only in larger breeds of dog, as the endoscopic staplers used will be challenging to deploy in small-breed dogs.

Anaesthesia

Similar anaesthetic concerns as those noted above for pericardiectomy apply to patients where auricular mass resection is being considered.

Patient positioning and port placement

The patient is positioned in dorsal recumbency initially, but lateral tilting may be helpful depending on the location and size of the mass. A subxiphoid telescope port is placed first and then instrument ports are added at the 5th to 7th intercostal spaces on both sides of the thorax. An endoscopic stapler must be introduced sufficiently far from the location of the right auricle to allow enough room for the stapler to be opened. To achieve this, the stapler is introduced through a 12 mm cannula placed at the 9th or 10th intercostal space in a ventral location close to the sternum.

Surgical technique

It is important to note that the decision to resect an auricular mass depends on its size and location. Case selection for this procedure is challenging, as preoperative diagnostic imaging generally does not provide an accurate enough assessment of whether the mass can be resected. Ideal cases are small and very peripherally located lesions. Larger lesions, or those that erode into the deeper aspects of the auricle and atrium, are probably not good candidates for thoracoscopic resection and may be better approached through an open thoracotomy or treated solely by the creation of a pericardial window or SPP without resection of the mass.

A pericardial window is created initially to allow an assessment of whether resection of the auricular mass is feasible. Once the window has been completed, the rim of the incised pericardium is elevated and the pericardium and epicardium are visualized (pericardioscopy) to inspect the auricular mass closely. If the mass is located peripherally and the surgeon feels that there is a good trajectory to place an endoscopic stapler across the base of the mass, the thoracoscopic resection can proceed. Through the 12 mm instrument port that has been established, a 45–60 mm, 2.5 or 3.5 mm leg length endoscopic linear stapler is introduced and positioned across the base of the auricular appendage (Figure 13.11). The ability to articulate the tip of the endoscopic stapler is essential in most cases,

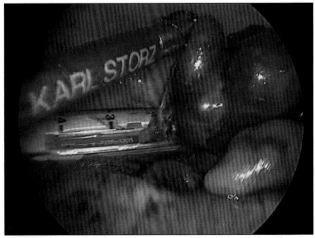

13.11 Placement of an endoscopic stapler at the base of a right auricular mass before resection.
(Courtesy of Dr J. Brad Case)

to ensure that the correct trajectory is achieved. If the stapler can be seated in a location that will allow complete removal of all macroscopic tumour, then the stapler cartridge is fired. If incomplete resection of the tissue occurs, a second cartridge can be used to complete the resection. After the resection is completed, the staple line is inspected for ongoing haemorrhage and the tissue is placed in a specimen retrieval bag, removed and submitted for histopathological evaluation.

Complications

The most important complications of auricular mass resection are haemorrhage and arrhythmias resulting from stimulation of the pericardium and epicardium. In one retrospective study of nine dogs that underwent auricular mass resection, rupture of the staple line occurred in one dog, resulting in fatal haemorrhage, and three dogs experienced ventricular arrhythmias, which were treated with lidocaine (Ployart *et al.*, 2013). In this population of dogs, the median survival of eight dogs with haemangiosarcoma was only 90 days (range 0–251 days), reinforcing the point that most dogs with auricular haemangiosarcoma will die of metastatic disease and auricular mass resection may not prolong life in all cases.

Thoracoscopic cranial mediastinal mass resection

Cranial mediastinal masses in dogs are most frequently diagnosed as either thymoma or lymphoma, with ectopic thyroid carcinoma, branchial cysts and chemodectomas seen less commonly. Of these, thymoma is generally the most amenable to thoracoscopic resection, and if diagnosed, surgical resection is usually recommended. Complete excision of the tumour, without penetration of the capsule, is the critical technical element in successful surgical treatment. The most common paraneoplastic syndrome associated with thymoma in both dogs and humans is myasthenia gravis, and the presence of myasthenia preoperatively may worsen the prognosis for dogs undergoing thoracoscopic thymectomy (MacIver *et al.*, 2017).

Many thymomas will be too large to be removed by a thoracoscopic approach, although those that are up to 5–8 cm in diameter (Figure 13.12) in medium-sized to large-breed dogs and that have not invaded the

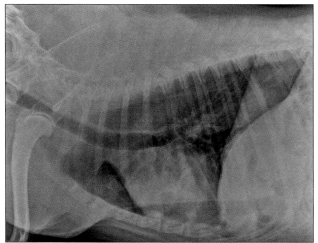

13.12 Lateral radiograph showing a modestly sized cranial mediastinal mass in a 12-year-old Labrador Retriever. The mass was diagnosed as a thymoma. This case is an excellent candidate for thoracoscopic thymoma resection.

surrounding organs may be amenable to thoracoscopic resection (Mayhew and Friedberg 2008; MacIver *et al.*, 2017). One case of thoracoscopic resection of a thymoma in a cat has been described (Griffin *et al.*, 2016), although most cases in cats are diagnosed too late to be amenable to this approach. The surgical anatomy of these masses is quite variable and so preoperative computed tomography (CT) can be very helpful for clinical decision-making. The CT images can be used to rule out vascular invasion and aid in planning appropriate placement of the ports in relation to the location of the mass.

Anaesthesia

OLV may be very helpful during the procedure to maximize visualization and potentially reduce iatrogenic damage to the pulmonary parenchyma during dissection, although it may be possible to complete the procedure without OLV in many larger, deep-chested dogs. The smaller thymomas that have been resected in the author's practice have generally been located from the midline towards the left cranial quadrant of the thoracic cavity, but the anatomy of these tumours can vary widely. If a DLT is used, OLV can be alternated between the left and right lung depending on which side of the tumour is being dissected at any given time (Mayhew and Friedberg, 2008). OLV can also be achieved with placement of an EBB, although intraoperative repositioning of the blocker may be required depending on the type used. If OLV cannot be instituted, reduction of the tidal volume to the minimal tolerable amount may be helpful, or carbon dioxide insufflation at a very low pressure (2–3 mmHg) can be used for the most critical parts of the procedure.

Patient positioning and port placement

It may be possible to resect cranial mediastinal masses with the patient in lateral or dorsal recumbency, but the author favours dorsal recumbency. Dorsal recumbency often results in the mass being 'suspended' within the cranial mediastinal root and often provides good visualization of its relationship to surrounding structures (especially the internal thoracic arteries). A telescope port is established in a subxiphoid location. Instrument port placement can be variable and depends on the nature of the lesion and the surgeon's level of experience with this procedure. An instrument port is usually placed on the right side at the 6th to 9th intercostal space in the ventral third of the thoracic cavity, and another is placed on the left side caudally, at the level of the 9th or 10th intercostal space. The surgeon should not hesitate to place extra instrument ports if necessary to facilitate surgical dissection of the mass.

Surgical technique

Once all the ports are in place, a blunt grasping instrument or blunt probe is used to manipulate the mass to assess whether resection is likely to be possible. Masses that are somewhat mobile and do not appear to be firmly attached to vital surrounding structures are the best candidates for thoracoscopic resection (Figure 13.13). A vessel-sealing device is used to initiate the dissection of the mass from the surrounding tissue planes. In some cases, the mass may be attached to the internal thoracic artery, and careful dissection is required to separate these two structures. The author initially leaves the thymoma attached to the ventral mediastinal attachments (if the thymoma is located

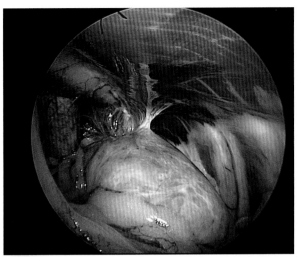

13.13 A large thymoma can be seen in the cranial mediastinum of this dog. The mass was mobile and resectable in this case.

within the cranial mediastinum) as this causes the thymoma to 'hang' up in the mediastinum, which sometimes facilitates dissection of the more dorsal attachments adjacent to the pericardium. Every effort should be made to resect the mass without penetrating the tumour capsule. Once completely dissected, the mass is placed into a specimen retrieval bag and removed through a modest enlargement of one of the instrument port incisions.

Preoperative assessment of the sternal and mediastinal lymph nodes by CT and/or intraoperative visualization of these nodes should be performed to assess for metastasis. Removal of the sternal lymph node should be possible through the same ports if there is a suspicion of metastatic spread.

Complications

A number of complications can arise during thoracoscopic cranial resection of a mediastinal mass. These include inadequate visualization due to the inability to achieve OLV, intraoperative loss of OLV, or inadequate room for dissection if the mass is too large or the patient too small. Conversion to an open approach is always reasonable in these situations if the problem cannot be resolved otherwise. Major haemorrhage can occur and must be controlled using either a vessel-sealing device or haemostatic clips. Port-site metastasis has been noted by the author in one dog with a thymoma where the capsule of the mass was penetrated during dissection (Alwen *et al.*, 2015). An inability to dissect the tumour free without disrupting the capsule is probably in itself a reasonable criterion for conversion to an open approach. Preservation of the capsule, along with careful use of a specimen retrieval bag, might help to minimize the occurrence of port-site metastases in these patients.

Thoracoscopic lung lobectomy

Lung lobectomy is indicated for the treatment of primary or metastatic lung neoplasia, bulla/bleb formation with or without secondary pneumothorax, chronic consolidation, major trauma, pulmonary abscessation or lung lobe torsion. However, only a proportion of cases will be appropriate for thoracoscopic approaches. The use of thoracoscopic approaches for pulmonary surgery has been historically limited by the availability of OLV and the size of the instrumentation available, principally the endoscopic

staplers. However, as the technology advances some of these challenges are being overcome, and thoracoscopic pulmonary surgery is likely to become increasingly popular.

A thoracoscopic-assisted technique may be used in cases where a thoracic mass is modestly sized and located distant from the pulmonary hilum; this technique has the advantage of potentially not requiring OLV to improve visualization (Laksito *et al.*, 2010; Wormser *et al.*, 2014). Fully thoracoscopic approaches are more complex and will require OLV as well as endoscopic staplers, but probably allow lesions of a wider range of sizes and at a wider range of locations to be resected (Lansdowne *et al.*, 2005; Mayhew *et al.*, 2013; Bleakley *et al.*, 2015).

CT of the thorax is generally recommended in cases being considered for VATS lobectomy, to evaluate the relationship of the mass to surrounding structures such as the pulmonary hilum, to evaluate the tracheobronchial lymph nodes more closely and to rule out metastatic disease elsewhere in the lungs (Figure 13.14). Generally, lung masses up to 6–8 cm in size may be resected thoracoscopically in dogs >30 kg. In dogs weighing 15–30 kg, the author would probably approach lung masses thoracoscopically only if they were <5 cm in diameter. Few dogs <15 kg or cats have undergone surgery with a fully thoracoscopic approach, but these smaller patients may be very amenable to a thoracoscopic-assisted approach. Dogs with spontaneous pneumothorax have undergone thoracoscopic procedures, although caution is warranted with these cases as early published experience reported a high rate of conversion to an open approach and several dogs that experienced ongoing pneumothorax (Case *et al.*, 2015).

Anaesthesia

In order to offer thoracoscopic lung lobectomy on a routine basis, the veterinary surgeon will have to master the ability to increase the working space using OLV. Carbon dioxide insufflation or intermittent ventilation are other options to enhance working space, but neither induces pulmonary atelectasis as OLV does, making the necessary visualization and manipulation a challenge in most cases when these techniques are used.

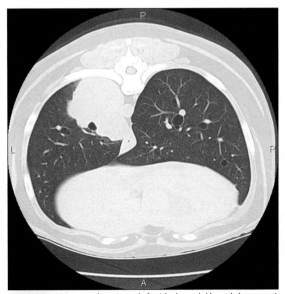

13.14 CT image showing a left-sided caudal lung lobe mass in a Labrador Retriever that was large but still a good candidate for lung lobectomy. CT is a valuable part of case selection for thoracoscopic lung lobectomy.

Patient positioning and port placement

The patient's position and port positioning for lung lobectomy will depend on the nature and location of the disease process. If a lung mass is present and its location is known, lateral recumbency is recommended, and all ports will be placed intercostally. In cases where exploration of the entire thoracic cavity is indicated, for example, patients with spontaneous pneumothorax, dorsal recumbency may be chosen, although evaluation of the most dorsal aspects of the lung fields may be challenging with the patient in dorsal recumbency. With either approach at least one 12 mm cannula should be placed to accommodate an endoscopic stapler if this technique is to be used to seal the lung tissue.

In general, if the patient is positioned in lateral recumbency the ports should be placed as far away from the pulmonary hilum to be resected as is possible. For resection of a caudal lung lobe, instrument ports could be placed in a triangulating pattern at the 4th to 6th intercostal spaces, although some surgeons prefer to place all three cannulae in one intercostal space. For cranial lobe resection, the ports will be established in the 8th to 10th intercostal spaces. It is important to place instrument ports sufficiently far from the lung lobe to be resected to allow opening of the endoscopic stapler at the correct location within the thorax. Placement of additional ports to allow the procedure to be completed in a safe and efficient manner is encouraged.

For patients placed in dorsal recumbency, the telescope is placed through a subxiphoid port, and instrument ports are placed at positions appropriate to the specific lobe to be resected.

Surgical technique

Once the cannulae are in position and OLV has been established, an attempt should be made to visualize the lesion. Most pulmonary masses are grossly obvious (Figure 13.15) but some may be buried within the pulmonary parenchyma. Use of an endoscopic stapler facilitates sectioning of the pulmonary artery, vein and bronchus. For lung lobectomy in dogs the use of 60 mm cartridges with 3.5 mm leg length staples is generally recommended (Lansdowne *et al.*, 2005; Mayhew *et al.*, 2013; Bleakley *et al.*, 2015). As well as straight linear forms, most endoscopic staplers are available as articulating forms in which

the tip of the cartridge can be moved from side to side at an angle to the shaft. This is a very useful feature when attempting to manoeuvre the stapler into position around the base of the pulmonary hilum and to maintain a position as close to the hilum as possible.

The endoscopic stapler must be passed through a 12 mm instrument port. If a partial lung lobectomy is to be performed, the tips of the stapler cartridge are opened and the stapler is positioned across the lung lobe to be resected. For a complete lung lobectomy, the cartridge is placed across the pulmonary, artery, vein and bronchus together, as close to the hilum as possible (Video 13.4). Once in the correct position, the cartridge tips are closed, the staples are dispensed, and the cartridge is reopened and carefully pulled back and out of the cannula. Care should be taken during this manoeuvre, as the cartridge will often adhere slightly to the stapled tissue, making abrupt removal potentially traumatic to the lung tissue. If the stapler cartridge used was not long enough to section the entire length of the lung lobe (as is often the case in larger dogs) a second cartridge can be used to complete the transection (Figure 13.16). Alternatively, if a small piece of lung remains attached an Endoloop® or intracorporeally

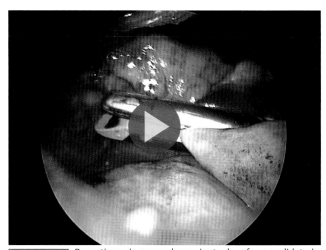

Video 13.4 Resection using an endoscopic stapler of a consolidated lung lobe in a dog secondary to pneumonia associated with chronic grass awn migration.

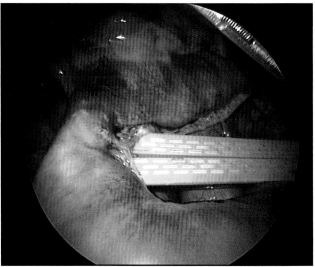

13.16 The Endo GIA™ stapler (Medtronic Inc.) can be seen having just been deployed across the hilus of a caudal lung lobe during thoracoscopic lung lobectomy. Note that the stapler has not transected the full length of the lung lobe and a second cartridge will be required to complete the resection.

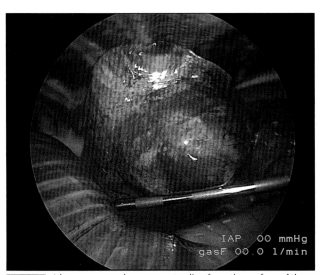

13.15 A large mass can be seen protruding from the surface of the lung lobe.

tied ligature can be used. When a lung mass is present, the author almost always performs a complete lung lobectomy to ensure a maximal margin of resection. Complete lung lobectomy may also be associated with a smaller risk of air leakage, as the bronchus is sealed directly.

Once the lung lobectomy has been completed, the cut surface of the pulmonary hilum is examined closely for haemorrhage or air leakage. The resected lung lobe should be placed in a specimen retrieval bag and the bag removed through one of the port incisions; this may require enlargement of the incision.

Thoracoscopic-assisted lung lobectomy

In cases where totally thoracoscopic lung lobectomy is not possible, for example, because OLV cannot be instituted or because the patient is small, making the use of the endoscopic stapler more challenging, thoracoscopic-assisted lung lobectomy is a good option. With this technique, the lung lobe containing the lesion is exteriorized under thoracoscopic guidance and the resection takes place externally or through an 'assist' incision (Figure 13.17). An initial 3–5 cm assist incision is usually made in a similar location to the incision that would be made for a traditional thoracotomy, that is, centred over the anticipated location of the hilum of the lung lobe to be resected. In the case of caudal or accessory lobes, before exteriorizing the lobe, thoracoscopic instruments are used to incise the pulmonary ligament to facilitate exteriorization. It is helpful, although not essential, to place a wound retractor in the assist incision to facilitate exteriorization and subsequent resection of the lung lobe. Once exteriorized, the lung lobe can be resected using a thoracoabdominal stapler or, if available, an endoscopic stapler can be used. A thoracic drain is then placed and the assist incisions and other port sites are closed routinely.

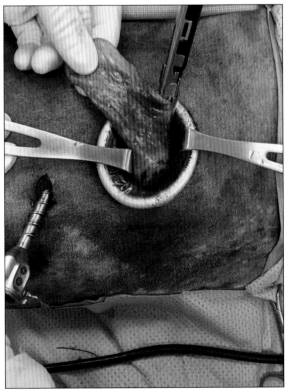

13.17 Thoracoscopic-assisted lung lobectomy. The lung lobe has been partially exteriorized through an assist incision. In this case, an endoscopic stapler is being placed across the hilus of the lung lobe through the assist incision to complete the resection.

Complications

Several important intra- and postoperative complications may occur with VATS lung lobectomy. Haemorrhage from intercostal vessels has been reported to cause significant postoperative haemorrhage. Haemorrhage or air leakage from the pulmonary hilum can also occur if the endoscopic stapler was placed incorrectly or did not function correctly to seal the tissue properly. Iatrogenic damage to surrounding structures can occur; great care should therefore be taken when passing instruments through thoracic cannulae to avoid damaging the pulmonary parenchyma. The most common reasons for conversion of a thoracoscopic lung lobectomy to an open procedure are failure of OLV and haemorrhage.

Thoracoscopic management of chylothorax

Idiopathic chylothorax in dogs is a complex and incompletely understood disorder that results in the accumulation of chyle within the pleural space, resulting in respiratory distress and, in some cases, restrictive pleuritis. While some medical therapies have been attempted, it is generally accepted that idiopathic chylothorax requires surgical treatment in most cases. Early reports of surgical management of idiopathic chylothorax in dogs were not always highly encouraging and generally focused on the outcomes of thoracic duct ligation (TDL). More recent work has provided a much better understanding of the natural variation of the lymphatic drainage patterns in cats and dogs, and improvements in diagnostic imaging techniques have enhanced veterinary surgeons' ability to accurately identify the lymphatic anatomy in an individual patient. This in turn has improved pre- and intraoperative decision-making for existing surgical management techniques, as well as spurring the development of new techniques. The intraoperative use of contrast agents such as methylene blue, as well as lymphangiographic techniques using intraoperative fluoroscopy or preoperative percutaneous CT lymphangiography (Figure 13.18), have been described (Esterline *et al.*, 2005; Johnson *et al.*, 2009). These techniques have enhanced the surgeon's ability to make sure that all branches of the thoracic duct are ligated during surgery. The most recent advance in this area is the use of intraoperative near-infrared fluorescence imaging for the

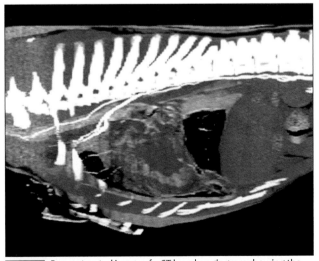

13.18 Reconstructed image of a CT lymphangiogram showing the lymphatic anatomy before thoracic duct ligation. These studies help greatly in preoperative planning for patients that will undergo thoracoscopic thoracic duct ligation.

detection of lymphatic channels in the mediastinum (Steffey and Mayhew, 2018). Early clinical studies of thoracoscopic TDL in dogs with idiopathic chylothorax reported promising results (Allman *et al.*, 2010), and recently a much larger study of 39 dogs reported the resolution of pleural effusion in 95% of dogs, with 6% suffering a late recurrence (Mayhew *et al.*, 2018).

Anaesthesia

OLV is not usually necessary for TDL in dogs as the caudal mediastinum can usually be satisfactorily accessed with both lung fields ventilated. It is sometimes necessary to decrease the tidal volume to prevent the lungs from interfering with the surgical field; good communication with the anaesthetist is essential to optimize working space for TDL. If SPP is to be performed in conjunction with TDL, OLV is not usually necessary, but can be helpful in very flat-chested dogs.

Patient positioning and port placement

The patient can be positioned in either lateral or sternal recumbency for thoracoscopic TDL. Sternal recumbency may provide improved visualization of the caudal mediastinal area during TDL. In dogs, thoracic ports are established in the dorsal third of the right 8th, 9th and 10th intercostal spaces. In cats, classically the ports would be placed at similar locations but on the left side, although in practice the side used in cats is usually decided after a CT lymphangiogram has been obtained; the author has seen several cats with right-sided thoracic duct branches.

Surgical technique

Dissection through the mediastinal root dorsal to the aorta is initiated, being careful not to rupture the segmental vertebral branches from the aorta. Sterile methylene blue dye, diluted 1:1 with sterile saline and administered at no more than 1.5 mg/kg, is then slowly infused either into a mesenteric lymph node (via a small paracostal incision made into the abdomen) or into a popliteal lymph node that has been surgically approached. Within 1–2 minutes the dye will usually be visualized passing through the thoracic duct(s) in the caudal mediastinum. In the author's experience, when popliteal lymph node injection is chosen the opacification of the thoracic ducts with methylene blue is much more variable and generally slower to arrive at the ducts in the caudal mediastinum than with injection into a mesenteric lymph node. Further dissection is performed to isolate all the ducts that are visualized with the dye, and they are then ligated with laparoscopic haemoclips (Figure 13.19; Video 13.5) or by intracorporeal suturing. Further injection of methylene blue into the lymph node after duct ligation often produces a visible bulging of the duct caudal to the ligation site if complete ductal occlusion has been achieved, although this does not occur in every case.

An alternative technique, known as 'en bloc' ligation, involves mass ligation of all the mediastinal tissues from ventral to the aorta to the level of the sympathetic trunks. Theoretically, this approach may achieve the ligation of small branches of the thoracic duct that may not be obvious on preoperative or intraoperative imaging, but care needs to be taken with this approach to make sure that the principal ducts, which can be firmly adhered to the aortic wall, are not missed.

After the TDL has been completed, the thoracic cannulae are removed and the incisions are closed routinely. If

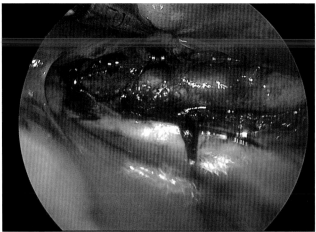

13.19 Intraoperative view of a thoracic duct ligation. The haemoclips can be seen in position on the thoracic ducts dorsal to the aorta.

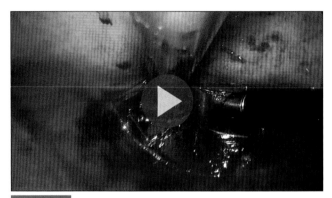

Video 13.5 Thoracic duct ligation with haemoclips.

the patient is to undergo a concurrent SPP the animal is then repositioned into dorsal recumbency and the procedure follows as described above. A minimally invasive approach to the cisterna chyli has also been recently documented in a clinical study of dogs with chylothorax, with good results (Morris *et al.*, 2019).

Complications

The most significant complication of thoracoscopic TDL is likely to be persistence of a chylous pleural effusion leading to the clinical signs persisting postoperatively. Because of the incomplete understanding of the pathophysiology of this condition, it may be difficult to identify the underlying reason for treatment failures. In some cases, failure to ligate all the thoracic duct branches may result in ongoing effusion. When treatment failures occur, other described techniques, such as cisterna chyli ablation, pleural port placement or thoracic duct embolization, can be attempted. Other complications that have been described during thoracoscopic TDL include leakage of chyle during dissection and iatrogenic lung laceration (Mayhew *et al.*, 2018).

Thoracoscopic division of a persistent right aortic arch

Although a large number of different vascular ring anomalies have been identified in dogs, over 90% of them are due to a left ligamentum arteriosum compressing the oesophagus, associated with persistence of the right fourth aortic arch (PRAA). This is the only type of vascular ring anomaly that has been treated by a thoracoscopic technique (Townsend *et al.*, 2016; Nucci *et al.*, 2018). Preoperative diagnosis of a PRAA is made by the radiographic finding of oesophageal dilatation cranial to the heart base with a focal left-sided deviation of the trachea at the cranial aspect of the heart. It is important to correctly identify all the vascular anomalies in these patients. Because of this, in the author's institution CT angiography is routinely performed to confirm the diagnosis and rule out the presence of intercurrent abnormalities such as a retro-oesophageal left subclavian artery, which is present in about one-third of dogs that have a PRAA but does not always require treatment if it is not compressive.

Anaesthesia

It is possible to perform thoracoscopic identification and resection of a PRAA without OLV, by decreasing the tidal volume as much as possible and retracting the cranial lung lobe with a blunt probe or fan retractor. However, patients undergoing PRAA correction are often very small, so working space is limited. The author therefore prefers to use OLV with these cases to allow maximal exposure and visualization of the PRAA. In very small patients there are few options for OLV, but the 5 Fr Arndt Endobronchial Blocker may be small enough to place in the left mainstem bronchus and provide right-sided OLV in patients <10 kg.

Patient position and port placement

Dogs and cats are placed in lateral recumbency with the left side uppermost. A small sandbag or towel can be placed under the epaxial muscles to provide improved access to the dorsal aspect of the cranial thoracic cavity. The telescope and instrument ports are placed quite caudal in the thoracic cavity to provide enough working space during dissection; the telescope is usually placed at the mid-thoracic level in the left 8th or 9th intercostal space, with instrument ports placed in a triangulating pattern also at the 8th or 9th intercostal space. If a further instrument port is required for the placement of a blunt probe or retractor, as is often the case, it can be placed more ventrally in the 6th or 7th intercostal space.

Surgical technique

It is very helpful to pass a flexible endoscope down the oesophagus during thoracoscopic PRAA surgery to ensure that the oesophageal wall, which transilluminates easily, can be visualized at all times. Oesophagoscopy also allows the aortic pulsation on the right side of the oesophagus, which is a typical finding in dogs with a PRAA, to be recognized. If an endoscope is not available to use for this purpose, a stomach tube can be passed down to the point of the oesophageal constriction.

Dissection begins by probing the area caudal to the oesophageal dilatation, which can also be identified by placing the endoscope at the level of the oesophageal narrowing and probing the area to localize the narrowing. At this point, it is also important to identify and protect the vagus nerve, which courses over the ligamentum. Dissection with dissecting forceps should then be initiated at that site to try to identify one or more bands of tissue that are constricting the oesophagus (Figure 13.20). In some cases, this tissue appears as one thick, obvious band, whereas in other cases the author has encountered multiple smaller, less obvious bands causing constriction.

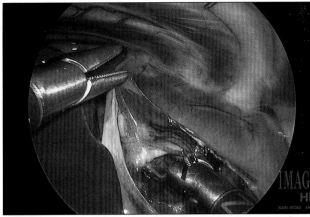

13.20 Persistent right aortic arch in a dog. The ligamentum can be seen as the white band of tissue being elevated by the right-angled forceps. The ligamentum was subsequently sectioned and released.
(© Karl Storz SE & Co. KG)

The bands of tissue are dissected and elevated until a vessel-sealing device can be placed safely around the tissue without being in contact with the oesophageal wall below. The HARMONIC ACE® (Ethicon Johnson & Johnson), if available, is very useful here, as it creates less collateral thermal damage than bipolar vessel-sealing devices and can be used to gently incise tissues as well as to seal vessels. It is important to remember that the ligamentum may be patent. Ideally, this will be known from preoperative diagnostic imaging or the presence of a murmur on physical examination, but care needs to be taken when dividing the ligamentum, as profuse haemorrhage can result if the ligamentum is patent and is simply cut by sharp dissection. The oesophagus in these (usually young) patients is very thin and lateral thermal spread from vessel-sealing devices could burn a hole in the oesophageal wall if they are not used with care. The surgeon must ensure that such devices are not in contact with the oesophageal wall when they are activated.

Once the constricting bands have been severed, the endoscope or stomach tube is used to try to dilate the oesophagus and ensure that no remaining bands are present. Alternatively, a Foley catheter with a polypropylene catheter (dog urinary catheter) passed down the lumen to give it rigidity can be used to dilate the oesophagus and to identify any remaining bands of tissue by moving it up and down the oesophagus. If other bands are continuing to constrict the oesophagus they should also be incised. Once the procedure is complete, a thoracic drain is placed and the ports are closed routinely.

Complications

A thoracoscopic approach for PRAA resection is an advanced procedure and should be performed only by experienced surgeons. Complications can include profuse haemorrhage from a patent ligamentum or surrounding vascular structures (Nucci *et al.*, 2018). Oesophageal perforation can also be a complication in these patients and can be fatal in some cases (Townsend *et al.*, 2016). Postoperative chylothorax may be profuse and can necessitate re-exploration, but is usually treated conservatively at first as it can be self-limiting (Nucci *et al.*, 2018) Clinical signs of regurgitation and poor weight gain, which are typical of dogs with PRAA, usually improve but can persist in at least a residual form in many cases. Early treatment of these patients may help to decrease the severity of megaoesophagus and improve the long-term outcome. It may be beneficial to feed these patients in an upright position for several weeks postoperatively until an improvement in oesophageal function occurs (see the *BSAVA Manual of Canine and Feline Gastroenterology*).

Thoracoscopic management of pyothorax

Pyothorax in dogs can be caused by a variety of underlying disease processes that include the migration of foreign bodies, lung abscesses, trauma or haematogenous spread of infection. Patients with pyothorax should always undergo a thorough diagnostic evaluation to look for underlying causes. Whether surgical management is warranted in these cases is sometimes controversial depending on the severity and extent of disease, and so it is perhaps not surprising that the decision whether to pursue a minimally invasive approach or an open thoracic exploration is equally challenging in many cases. Generally speaking, if a patient is diagnosed with pyothorax and found to have obvious focal disease in the thorax, or if bacteria are present that are often associated with vegetal migration (i.e. filamentous organisms), or if grass awns (Figure 13.21) are identified by diagnostic imaging or bronchoscopy, surgery is generally considered to be warranted. In one study, surgical management of pyothorax was shown to be more likely to result in resolution of clinical signs 1 year later compared with medical management (Rooney and Monnet, 2001).

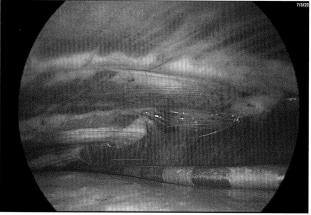

13.21 A grass awn can be seen located at the diaphragmatic reflection in the very most caudal aspect of the pleural cavity. This is a common site for grass awns that have migrated through the lung lobe out into the pleural space and become lodged there.

The author recommends a relatively conservative approach to the thoracoscopic management of pyothorax in dogs, especially in geographical areas where grass awn migrations are common, such as the Mediterranean parts of Europe and the west coast of the USA. In these cases, and in cases of very long-standing pyothorax, extensive mediastinitis and pleuritis or extensive adhesion formation, thoracoscopic exploration may be difficult. In these cases, it may be better to use an open thoracic approach or to begin with a thoracoscopic approach and be ready to convert to an open approach if visualization is a problem or if migrating grass awns that are suspected to be present cannot be found. However, in cases where the clinical signs are more acute, where the majority of the lung fields appear healthy and where there is focal disease or a suspicion of well circumscribed disease that may be the cause of the problem, it may be reasonable to try a thoracoscopic approach. Generally, a preoperative CT

scan of these patients should be performed to try to evaluate the extent of the disease and the location and size of any focal lesions. In cases where grass awn migration is suspected, a thorough preoperative bronchoscopic examination is warranted to rule out the presence of other grass awns in other airways.

Anaesthesia

Patients with pyothorax should be carefully evaluated for systemic disease and treated as necessary in order to reduce the risk of anaesthesia as far as possible. The specific anaesthetic needs of the individual patient will depend on the interventions to be performed, as dictated by the nature of the disease. Patients requiring lung lobectomy as part of their treatment may require OLV. In cases where lung lobectomy is not required, anaesthetic concerns will be similar to those for other surgical procedures in the thorax.

Patient position and port placement

In cases of pyothorax, the patient's position and the placement of instrument ports will generally be dictated by the location and extent of the disease. If a general exploration of the thorax is to be undertaken, the patient is probably best positioned in dorsal recumbency, but it is prudent to clip the hair coat very widely and drape the patient in such a manner as to allow intercostal ports to be placed in case the findings of the exploration indicate that a lung lobectomy in lateral recumbency is needed. In cases where a focal pulmonary lesion has been detected that is suspected to be the inciting cause of the pyothorax, patient positioning and port placement may be planned to optimize access to that specific lesion. In these cases, lateral recumbency may be the position of choice, especially if a complete lung lobectomy is anticipated or if the very caudal aspects of the pleural cavity at the diaphragmatic recesses need to be explored for suspected migrating grass awns.

Surgical technique

The specific procedures that will be performed during thoracoscopic management of pyothorax will depend on the underlying aetiology in the individual patient and the findings at surgery. In the case of foreign body migration, any damage to the lung from transpulmonary migration needs to be inspected and a decision made as to whether the damaged lobe should be resected. In cases of ongoing pneumothorax associated with leakage of air from the foreign body's migration tract, resection is probably warranted. In less seriously affected cases, a more conservative approach can be taken if there is little evidence of foreign material remaining in the lobe. In cases where a bronchoscopic evaluation has detected migrating grass awns in the terminal bronchi (see Chapter 7) but removal was not possible bronchoscopically, there may be reasonable grounds for thoracoscopic lung lobe resection to avoid further migration of the foreign body with possible subsequent development of pneumothorax or pyothorax in the future.

In cases of pyothorax where no evidence of foreign body migration can be found, thorough pleural lavage, with mediastinal debridement if deemed necessary, may be warranted. Similarly, removal or biopsy of masses, lymph nodes, pleura or pericardium may be warranted to rule out neoplastic or inflammatory/infectious disease;

these procedures can all be accomplished thoracoscopically in cases where disease is not so advanced that visualization of the normal anatomy is obscured. In all cases, microbial culture and sensitivity testing should be performed on the tissue and foreign material obtained during surgery, followed by treatment with antimicrobials chosen on the basis of the results.

Complications

Failure of the pyothorax to resolve, or recurrence, can be considered a complication and can occur after thoracoscopic management of the problem. However, in the one report of 14 dogs with pyothorax managed thoracoscopically, clinical signs resolved in all dogs, and only one dog had a recurrence of pyothorax and required a second surgery (Scott *et al.*, 2017). Other complications may be associated with additional interventions performed to treat specific findings in each case.

Thoracoscopy for oncological staging

Intrathoracic neoplasia can take several forms, including primary or metastatic lung tumours, cranial mediastinal neoplasms, mesothelioma (which can affect the pericardium and pleural surfaces) and, less commonly, primary or metastatic cardiac neoplasms. In all of these cases, staging of the disease may involve diagnostic imaging as well as sampling of any draining lymph nodes. In the case of lung tumours, it is known that dogs with primary lung tumours that have evidence of metastatic spread to the tracheobronchial lymph nodes (TBLNs) have a significantly poorer prognosis than dogs with no evidence of metastatic disease. It is therefore currently recommended that dogs undergoing lung lobectomy for resection of primary lung tumours also have the draining TBLNs sampled or excised to assess for metastatic disease.

The pulmonary lymphatics drain into three principal TBLNs located around the tracheal bifurcation. These lymph nodes are the primary site of lymphatic metastasis of pulmonary neoplasms. The right TBLN lies just caudal to the insertion of the azygous vein into the cranial vena cava; it is sometimes somewhat obscured by the base of the right cranial lung lobe but may be the easiest lymph node to dissect. The left TBLN lies just ventral to the aorta on the left side and is somewhat more challenging to dissect. The central TBLN is generally bilobed, with a narrow isthmus connecting the two sides; it is accessible from the right side but not the left, and is ventral to the azygous vein, more caudal to the right node and just dorsal to the caudal lobar bronchus. The sternal and mediastinal lymph nodes are sometimes also resected thoracoscopically if preoperative diagnostic imaging suggests that these lymph nodes are abnormal.

Other forms of thoracoscopic staging of intrathoracic disease include pericardiectomy to gain access to the pericardial sac during the investigation of pericardial effusion. Visualization of the pericardial tissue, the epicardial surface, the margins of the auricular appendages and any masses at the heart base are facilitated by pericardial evaluation and pericardioscopy (Carvajal *et al.*, 2019). Pleural or mediastinal biopsies can also easily be performed thoracoscopically, and examination of biopsy samples may provide vital diagnostic information regarding the presence of mesothelioma or other pleural metastatic lesions.

Surgical excision of TBLNs

In general, OLV will be required for lymph node resection, but in any case OLV is usually required for lobectomy of the lung lobe containing the primary tumour. Dogs are placed in either sternal or lateral recumbency, with the position being somewhat dependent on the other techniques to be performed concurrently.

Three cannulae are placed into the thorax at the mid-thoracic level in the 4th, 5th and 6th intercostal spaces on the right or left side depending on which node(s) is/are to be resected (Steffey *et al.*, 2015). The telescope is generally placed in the middle of the three ports to allow maximal triangulation of instruments in the other two ports. A vessel-sealing device is placed into one instrument port and grasping forceps are placed into the other instrument port. The TBLN is identified either grossly or by injection of a contrast dye such as methylene blue. When methylene blue is injected near the primary tumour, the surgeon will sometimes observe the draining lymph node becoming stained with the dye, making its identification easier. The capsule of the node is gently grasped, and careful dissection around the node is commenced, using either the tip of the vessel-sealing device or laparoscopic right-angled forceps. Sometimes the tissue of the lymph node is very friable and piecemeal resection may be necessary; however, the author always tries to resect the node *en bloc* if possible. The vessel-sealing device or a J- or L-hook monopolar probe is used to seal any bleeding vessels that are seen during the dissection.

Surgical excision of sternal lymph nodes

Sternal lymph nodes may be resected in conjunction with another procedure, which might dictate port placement to some extent. However, if sternal lymph node resection is the only procedure being performed, OLV is usually not necessary and the patient is placed in dorsal recumbency. A subxiphoid telescope port is used and two instrument ports are placed in the ventral aspects of the 6th and 8th intercostal spaces. These ports will usually provide easy access to the sternal lymph nodes that are located just cranial to the internal thoracic artery and vein. Blunt dissection into the area cranial to those vessels will usually reveal the nodes if they are not immediately visualized.

Pleural and mediastinal biopsy

Biopsy of the pleura will often be added on to other procedures being performed. Therefore, no 'typical' port placement is described. Pleural biopsy simply involves the use of sharp cup biopsy forceps that are inserted deeply into the pleural lining, being careful to avoid the intercostal vascular bundles located on the caudal aspect of each rib. The cups are then closed, followed by a twisting and pulling action that will sever a small piece of the pleural lining that can be withdrawn and submitted for diagnostic pathology. Biopsy of the mediastinum can be performed similarly by using cup biopsy forceps or a vessel-sealing device to excise a portion of the mediastinum.

Complications

Access-related complications

The first step in any thoracoscopic procedure is to gain safe access into the pleural cavity. During the initial port placement, iatrogenic damage to intracavitary structures must be avoided. Injuries during paraxiphoid port placement have not been reported in small animals, possibly because of the lack of large vascular structures close to this entry site. When the first cannula is inserted in an intercostal location or, indeed, when further instrument ports are placed intercostally after placement of the telescope port, it is imperative to perform the initial incision in the middle of the intercostal space to avoid iatrogenic damage to the intercostal artery and vein, which run parallel and caudal to each rib. Bleeding from intercostal vessels can be profuse and will generally not cease spontaneously. If bleeding does occur, placement of a circumcostal suture proximal and distal to the bleeding vessel is usually necessary to achieve haemostasis. During intercostal cannula placement, contact with lung tissue is unlikely to cause iatrogenic damage as the blunt tip of the trocar–cannula assembly will usually push the lobe away rather than penetrate it. However, in cases where unrecognized adhesions of the lung lobes to the thoracic wall exist, iatrogenic lung damage can occur even when blunt trocars are used. For intercostal trocar insertion, the use of blunt dissection through the thoracic wall before insertion of the trocar–cannula assembly may help to reduce iatrogenic damage to blood vessels and the lung parenchyma during insertion.

Postoperative complications

The most commonly observed complications after thoracoscopic surgery in humans are prolonged air leakage, bleeding and wound infection. Air leakage can arise from staple lines placed across pulmonary tissue if the tissue is not completely sealed by the staples, or from iatrogenic damage to the surface of the pulmonary parenchyma by instruments, cannulae or thoracic drains. Although this complication is not commonly described in the veterinary literature, it has been reported (Lansdowne et al., 2005). It is difficult to identify the origin of these air leaks, but it is suspected that they are usually the result of minor damage to the surface of the lung that occurs during the procedure or from over-zealous aspiration via a chest tube in the postoperative period. Treatment of persistent mild to moderate air leaks is usually conservative for the first few days, using continuous (e.g. the Pleur-evac® device, Teleflex Inc.) or intermittent suction through a thoracic drain. If the air leak resolves, no further treatment may be required. With more substantial or more persistent air leaks, re-exploration of the thoracic cavity may be necessary.

Port-site complications after thoracoscopic procedures are generally associated with either seroma formation, surgical-site infection or subcutaneous emphysema. Seroma formation is relatively common with intercostal ports, as it is challenging to appose the deeper layers of the thoracic wall closely without causing iatrogenic damage to the lungs during passage of the needle. These seromas almost always resolve spontaneously, and rarely require drainage. Herniation of thoracic contents through incompletely closed port incisions is possible but probably much less likely than the herniation of abdominal organs through laparoscopic port incisions, due to the less mobile nature of most thoracic viscera. This complication has not been reported to date in veterinary patients.

Port-site metastasis can occur when neoplastic lesions are resected and withdrawn through small port incisions. Metastasis of a pericardial mesothelioma to a port site after thoracoscopic creation of a pericardial window has been described in the veterinary literature (Brisson et al.,

2006), as has port-site metastasis after thoracoscopic resection of a thymoma (Alwen et al., 2015). This process was initially considered to be a result of direct inoculation ('seeding') of neoplastic cells during traumatic extirpation of tumour tissue through small port incisions. However, it is now known that the use of specimen retrieval bags to remove neoplastic tissue, although highly recommended, does not completely prevent port-site metastasis. It is now generally recognized that a more complex interplay of factors such as the local immune response, pneumoperitoneum and surgical technique may all play a role in the aetiopathogenesis of port-site metastasis (Castillo and Vitagliano, 2008).

References and further reading

Allman DA, Radlinsky MG, Ralph AG and Rawlings CA (2010) Thoracoscopic thoracic duct ligation and pericardectomy for treatment of chylothorax in dogs. *Veterinary Surgery* **39**, 21–27

Alwen SG, Culp WT, Szivek A, Mayhew PD and Eckstrand CD (2015) Portal site metastasis after thoracoscopic resection of a cranial mediastinal mass in a dog. *Journal of the American Veterinary Medical Association* **247**, 793–800

Barbur LA, Rawlings CA and Radlinsky MG (2018) Epicardial exposure provided by a novel thoracoscopic pericardectomy technique compared to standard pericardial window. *Veterinary Surgery* **47**, 146–152

Bleakley S, Duncan CG and Monnet E (2015) Thoracoscopic lung lobectomy for primary lung tumors in 13 dogs. *Veterinary Surgery* **44**, 1029–1035

Borenstein N, Behr L, Chetboul V *et al.* (2004) Minimally invasive patent ductus arteriosus occlusion in 5 dogs. *Veterinary Surgery* **33**, 309–311

Brisson BA, Reggeti F and Bienzle D (2006) Portal site metastasis of invasive mesothelioma after diagnostic thoracoscopy in a dog. *Journal of the American Veterinary Medical Association* **229**, 980–983

Carvajal JL, Case JB, Mayhew PD *et al.* (2019) Outcome in dogs with presumptive idiopathic pericardial effusion after thoracoscopic pericardectomy and pericardioscopy. *Veterinary Surgery* **48**, O105–O111

Case JB, Maxwell M, Aman A and Monnet EL (2013) Outcome evaluation of a thoracoscopic pericardial window procedure or subtotal pericardectomy via thoracotomy for the treatment of pericardial effusion in dogs. *Journal of the American Veterinary Medical Association* **242**, 493–498

Case JB, Mayhew PD and Singh A (2015) Evaluation of video-assisted thoracic surgery for treatment of spontaneous pneumothorax and pulmonary bullae in dogs. *Veterinary Surgery* **44(S1)**, 31–38

Castillo OA and Vitagliano G (2008) Port site metastasis and tumor seeding in oncologic laparoscopic urology. *Urology* **71**, 372–378

Chetty GK, Khan OA, Onyeaka CV *et al.* (2004) Experience with video-assisted surgery for suspected mediastinal tumours. *European Journal of Cancer Surgery* **30**, 776–780

Daly CM, Swalec-Tobias K, Tobias AH and Ehrhart N (2002) Cardiopulmonary effects of intrathoracic insufflation in dogs. *Journal of the American Animal Hospital Association* **38**, 515–520

Dupre GP, Corlouer JP and Bouvy B (2001) Thoracoscopic pericardectomy performed without pulmonary exclusion in 9 dogs. *Veterinary Surgery* **30**, 21–27

Esterline ML, Radlinsky MG, Biller DS *et al.* (2005) Comparison of radiographic and computed tomography lymphangiography for identification of the canine thoracic duct. *Veterinary Radiology and Ultrasound* **46**, 391–395

Griffin MA, Sutton JS, Hunt GB, Pypendop BH and Mayhew PD (2016) Video-assisted thoracoscopic resection of a noninvasive thymoma in a cat with myasthenia gravis using low-pressure carbon dioxide insufflation. *Veterinary Surgery* **45**, O28–O33

Hall EJ, Williams DA and Kathrani A (2019) *BSAVA Manual of Canine and Feline Gastroenterology, 3rd edn*. BSAVA Publications, Gloucester

Harold KL, Pollinger H, Matthews BD *et al.* (2003) Comparison of ultrasonic energy, bipolar thermal energy and vascular clips for the hemostasis of small-, medium- and large-sized arteries. *Surgical Endoscopy* **17**, 1228–1230

Jackson J, Richter KP and Launer DP (1999) Thoracoscopic partial pericardiectomy in 13 dogs. *Journal of Veterinary Internal Medicine* **13**, 529–533

Johnson EG, Wisner ER, Kyles A, Koehler C and Marks SL (2009) Computed tomographic lymphography of the thoracic duct by mesenteric lymph node injection. *Veterinary Surgery* **38**, 361–367

Kovak JR, Ludwig LL, Bergman PJ, Baer KE and Noone KE (2002) Use of thoracoscopy to determine the etiology of pleural effusion in dogs and cats: 18 cases (1998–2001). *Journal of the American Veterinary Medical Association* **221**, 990–994

Kudnig ST, Monnet E, Riquelme M *et al.* (2003) Effect of one-lung ventilation on oxygen delivery in anesthetized dogs with an open thoracic cavity. *American Journal of Veterinary Research* **64**, 443–448

Kudnig ST, Monnet E, Riquelme M *et al.* (2006) Effect of positive end-expiratory pressure on oxygen delivery during 1-lung ventilation for thoracoscopy in normal dogs. *Veterinary Surgery* **35**, 534–542

Laksito MA, Chambers BA and Yates GD (2010) Thoracoscopic-assisted lung lobectomy in the dog: report of two cases. *Australian Veterinary Journal* **88**, 263–267

Lansdowne JL, Monnet E, Twedt DC and Dernell WS (2005) Thoracoscopic lung lobectomy for treatment of lung tumors in dogs. *Veterinary Surgery* **34**, 530–535

MacIver M, Case JB, Monnet E *et al.* (2017) Video-assisted extirpation of cranial mediastinal masses in dogs: 18 cases (2009–2014). *Journal of the American Veterinary Medical Association* **250**, 1283–1290

MacPhail CM, Monnet E and Twedt DC (2001) Thoracoscopic correction of a persistent right aortic arch in a dog. *Journal of the American Animal Hospital Association* **37**, 577–581

Mayhew KN, Mayhew PD, Sorrell-Raschi L and Brown DC (2009) Thoracoscopic sub-phrenic pericardectomy using double-lumen endobronchial intubation for alternating one-lung ventilation. *Veterinary Surgery* **38**, 961–966

Mayhew PD, Chohan A, Hardy B *et al.* (2019a) Evaluation of fluoroscopic-assisted placement of one-lung ventilation devices for video-assisted thoracoscopic surgery in large-breed dogs. *Veterinary Surgery* **48**, O143–O152

Mayhew PD, Culp WTN, Pascoe PJ, Kass PH and Johnson LR (2012) Evaluation of blind thoracoscopic-assisted placement of three double-lumen endobronchial tube designs for one-lung ventilation in dogs. *Veterinary Surgery* **41**, 664–670

Mayhew PD and Friedberg JS (2008) Video-assisted thoracoscopic resection of non-invasive thymomas using single-lung ventilation in two dogs. *Veterinary Surgery* **37**, 756–762

Mayhew PD, Hunt BG, Steffey MA *et al.* (2013) Evaluation of short-term outcome after lung lobectomy for resection of primary lung tumors via video-assisted thoracoscopic surgery or open thoracotomy in medium- to large-breed dogs. *Journal of the American Veterinary Medical Association* **243**, 681–688

Mayhew PD, Pascoe PJ, Giuffrida MA *et al.* (2019b) Cardiorespiratory effects of variable pressure thoracic insufflation in cats undergoing video-assisted thoracic surgery. *Veterinary Surgery* **48**, O130–O137

Mayhew PD, Steffey MA, Fransson BA *et al.* (2018) Long-term outcome of video-assisted thoracoscopic thoracic duct ligation and pericardectomy in dogs with chylothorax: A multi-institutional study of 39 cases. *Veterinary Surgery* **48**, O112–O120

Morris KP, Singh A, Holt DE *et al.* (2019) Hybrid single-port laparoscopic cisterna chyli ablation for the adjunct treatment of chylothorax disease in dogs. *Veterinary Surgery* **48**, O121–O129

Nucci DJ, Hurst KC and Monnet E (2018) Retrospective comparison of short-term outcomes following thoracoscopy *versus* thoracotomy for surgical correction of persistent right aortic arch in dogs. *Journal of the American Veterinary Medical Association* **253**, 444–451

Ployart S, Liebermann S, Doran I, Bomassi E and Monnet E (2013) Thoracoscopic resection of right auricular masses in dogs: 9 cases (2003–2011). *Journal of the American Veterinary Medical Association* **242**, 237–241

Rooney MB and Monnet E (2001) Medical and surgical treatment of pyothorax in dogs: 26 cases (1991–2001). *Journal of the American Veterinary Medical Association* **221**, 86–92

Scott J, Singh A, Monnet E *et al.* (2017) Video-assisted thoracic surgery for the management of pyothorax in dogs: 14 cases. *Veterinary Surgery* **46**, 722–730

Stammberger U, Steinacher C, Hillinger S *et al.* (2000) Early and long-term complaints following video-assisted thoracoscopic surgery: evaluation in 173 patients. *European Journal of Cardiothoracic Surgery* **18**, 7–11

Steffey MA, Daniel L, Mayhew PD *et al.* (2015) Video-assisted thoracoscopic extirpation of the tracheobronchial lymph nodes in dogs. *Veterinary Surgery* **44(S1)**, 50–58

Steffey MA and Mayhew PD (2018) Use of direct near-infrared fluorescent lymphography for thoracoscopic thoracic duct identification in 15 dogs with chylothorax. *Veterinary Surgery* **47**, 267–276

Townsend S, Oblak ML, Singh A, Steffey MA and Runge JJ (2016) Thoracoscopy with concurrent esophagoscopy for persistent right aortic arch in 9 dogs. *Veterinary Surgery* **45**, O111–O118

Walsh PJ, Remedios AM, Ferguson JF *et al.* (1999) Thoracoscopic *versus* open partial pericardectomy in dogs: Comparison of post-operative pain and morbidity. *Veterinary Surgery* **28**, 472–479

Wormser C, Singhal S, Holt DE and Runge JJ (2014) Thoracoscopic-assisted pulmonary surgery for partial and complete lung lobectomy in dogs and cats: 11 cases (2008–2013). *Journal of the American Veterinary Medical Association* **245**, 1036–1041

 Video extras

- **Video 13.1** Resection of a cranial mediastinal mass and removal from the thorax in a specimen retrieval bag
- **Video 13.2** Demonstration of the correct bronchoscopically guided placement of an endobronchial blocker
- **Video 13.3** Optical entry using a trocarless cannula (ENDOTIP, Karl Storz Endoscopy)
- **Video 13.4** Resection using an endoscopic stapler of a consolidated lung lobe in a dog secondary to pneumonia associated with chronic grass awn migration
- **Video 13.5** Thoracic duct ligation with haemoclips

Access via QR code or: bsavalibrary.com/endoscopy2e_13

Chapter 14

Rigid endoscopy: arthroscopy

Rob Pettitt and John F. Innes

Introduction

The use of rigid endoscopy for joint surgery has been the standard in human and equine orthopaedics for over three decades. The use of arthroscopy in small animals for the treatment and diagnosis of joint disease has increased dramatically in the past 15–20 years due to advances in equipment and techniques. Numerous benefits of arthroscopy have been cited, including improved viewing and magnification of lesions, decreased operative time, minimal joint trauma and lower patient morbidity compared with conventional 'open' techniques. There is, however, a considerable learning curve, and these advantages can be achieved only through training, practice and an understanding of and correct selection of arthroscopic equipment. This chapter provides an introduction to small animal arthroscopy and discusses its indications, ancillary procedures, instrumentation and current applications.

Indications

Although arthroscopy is a minimally invasive surgical modality, it allows a thorough and detailed investigation of the major appendicular joints of the dog and the larger joints of the cat. The ability to perform comprehensive and detailed joint inspection and the magnification of intra-articular structures and pathological lesions, combined with the increased field of view achieved by moving the arthroscope through the joint, increases the diagnostic value of the technique. Arthroscopy can reveal early or very discrete lesions when other modalities, such as radiography, fail to demonstrate evidence of pathology. Second-look arthroscopy permits the surgeon to assess the efficacy of previous surgery and/or the progression of disease, and to determine whether further clinical interventions are necessary. However, the high diagnostic sensitivity of arthroscopy means that there is often some contention surrounding the significance of the lesions noted.

The advantages of arthroscopy significantly outweigh the disadvantages. Decreased postoperative pain with arthroscopically assisted surgery in human beings is well documented, and the same appears to be true for small animals (Hoelzler *et al.*, 2004). Small instruments passing through inflamed capsular tissue will transect fewer nerve endings compared with a standard arthrotomy. This leads to reduced postoperative morbidity, increased use of the limb and, hence, an improved recovery.

Even though the advantages of arthroscopy outweigh the disadvantages, the latter are worthy of comment. The major disadvantage is the long learning curve associated with arthroscopically assisted surgery. Coordination is required to manoeuvre the arthroscope and instruments through the joint while viewing the instruments on a monitor; this is compounded by the relatively small size of canine and feline joints. Skill and training are required to manipulate the instruments within the joint without causing iatrogenic damage to the articular surfaces. This skill can be learned by attending suitable arthroscopy training courses, especially those that involve practical sessions on cadavers. Continued practice using cadavers will facilitate learning and should be continued until the veterinary surgeon (veterinarian) can easily establish the required portals and evaluate the whole joint competently. In the early stages of gaining experience with live patients, it is preferable to restrict arthroscopy to the joints that are more accessible, and the surgeon should always be prepared to convert the arthroscopic procedure to an open arthrotomy if needed. Initially, arthroscopy may be used only as a diagnostic aid but, as the operator's skill improves, therapeutic arthroscopy can be performed. Invariably, arthroscopic surgery initially takes longer to perform than a conventional arthrotomy, but as the surgeon's proficiency increases arthroscopic procedures often take less time than conventional surgery.

Although feasible, arthroscopy in the cat is performed only occasionally, and little is known about the arthroscopic management of feline joint disease. The main focus of this chapter is therefore arthroscopy in the dog.

Instrumentation

Good arthroscopy is reliant on the correct selection and understanding of equipment and instrumentation. The quality of the optical system is paramount in obtaining high-quality images for diagnosis. Good, accurate inspection of the joint structures is possible only with appropriate fluid flow through the joint during the examination. This requires the correct establishment and maintenance of ingress and egress portals and the administration of fluids either by gravity or, preferably, with a fluid pressure system. Successful therapeutic and exploratory arthroscopy may also rely on the correct selection and use of specialized hand, powered or radiofrequency instruments. A more complete discussion of endoscopic instrumentation is provided in Chapter 2.

Optical system

The optical system consists of a monitor, a light source and cable, a camera, the arthroscope and (optionally) a data capture system. A suitable heavy-duty cart is essential for storage of the equipment and to facilitate its use, although a ceiling-mounted, multi-arm equipment pendant in a bespoke endoscopic theatre (Figure 14.1) is a desirable option, in that cables are not left trailing on the floor but are routed through pendant arms and ceiling ducts.

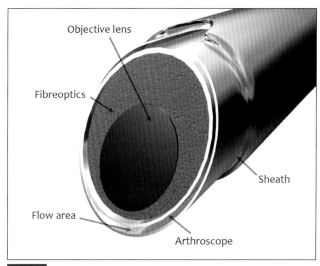

14.2 Arthroscope tip, showing the arrangement of components.

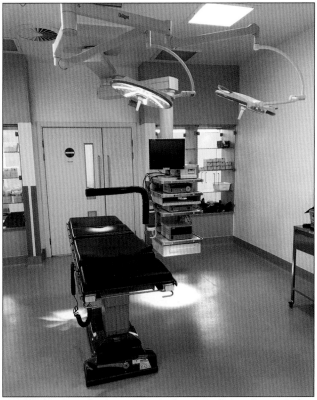

14.1 Dedicated arthroscopic suite for minimally invasive surgical techniques.

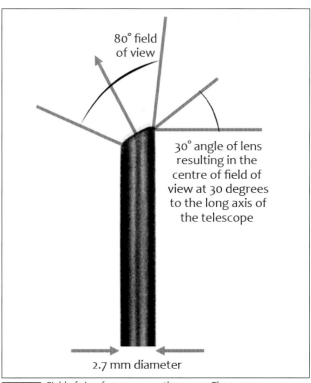

14.3 Arthroscopes of different sizes. Top to bottom: 1.9 mm, 2.4 mm and 2.7 mm.

Arthroscopes

An arthroscope is made up of a central series of lenses, to allow transmission of an image to the eyepiece, surrounded by optical fibres. The optical fibres transmit light from the light post adjacent to the eyepiece along the shaft to the tip of the arthroscope to provide illumination (Figure 14.2). Arthroscopes are classified based on the length and diameter of the shaft and the angle of the lens.

It should be noted that the diameter measurement is that of the outside diameter of the arthroscope itself, without the accompanying sleeve. Arthroscopes used in small animals typically have a diameter of 4.0, 2.7, 2.4 or 1.9 mm (Figure 14.3); 1.9 mm arthroscopes are very fragile and should not be used by inexperienced surgeons as they are prone to breakage. The larger the diameter of the arthroscope, the greater the field of view (Figure 14.4) and the brighter the transmitted light. Typically, a 2.7 mm arthroscope has a field of view of 80 degrees, compared with 65 degrees for a 1.9 mm arthroscope. The advantages of choosing a narrower arthroscope are minimization of joint trauma combined with increased mobility within the joint, especially in the elbow, carpus, hip and tarsus. These advantages must be balanced against the fragility and the smaller field of view of the narrower arthroscopes. The

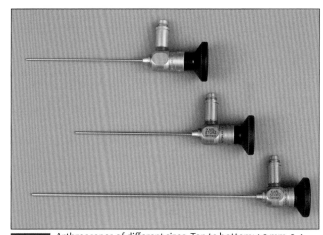

14.4 Field of view for a 2.7 mm arthroscope. The 2.4 mm arthroscope has a similar field of view.

larger arthroscopes have increased durability due to their resistance to bending but have a higher risk of causing iatrogenic trauma.

Lens angle refers to the angle between the long axis of the shaft and the face of the lens. This can be 0, 30 or 70 degrees; 30 degrees is the angle most commonly employed in canine arthroscopy. This angle provides a compromise between the field of view and the amount of image distortion. A 0-degree arthroscope has no image distortion but the working field of view is small. Conversely, a 70-degree arthroscope has a much larger working field of view when it is rotated around its long axis, but the image is distorted.

With an angled lens, the operator needs to be aware of the direction in which the arthroscope is pointing. The direction of viewing is opposite to the position of the light post. On some arthroscopes there is a notch on the projected image on the monitor to indicate this direction. With angled lenses, rotation of the endoscope along its long axis allows inspection of a larger area of the joint with minimal movement of the arthroscope, thereby reducing the risk of damage to the articular surface.

The length of the arthroscope refers to its long axis and is usually designated as 'long' or 'short'. Long arthroscopes have a larger depth of field than short arthroscopes of similar diameter, but short arthroscopes are easier to handle in small joints and are less susceptible to damage from bending.

Each arthroscope requires a dedicated sheath or sleeve for use within the joint, to protect it from bending and to deliver fluid (see also Chapter 2). At the proximal end of the cannula is an attachment for a fluid line with a stopcock. High-flow cannulae are now available for the smaller arthroscopes and these are preferable. Sleeves and accompanying obturators or trocars are introduced into the joint via a small stab incision. A blunt obturator (Figure 14.5) is preferable to a trocar in that it is less likely to cause injury to the joint tissues.

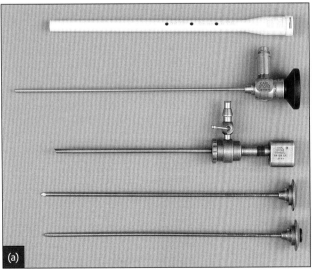

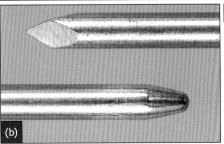

14.5 (a) A 2.7 mm arthroscope plus protective cover, cannula and obturators. (b) Sharp and blunt obturator tips.

Accessory instruments

There is a very wide range of instruments available to the surgeon for use in arthroscopy, and initially the selection of appropriate ones may seem daunting. Hand instruments for use in small animal arthroscopy must be small in diameter to minimize iatrogenic trauma and manufactured to high standards for maximum reliability. Some basic instruments are essential: these include probes, grasping forceps, cannulae and milling drills (see below). It is advisable to have a separate basic surgical kit that has been modified for use in arthroscopic procedures. In addition to surgical instruments, suitably sized sterile hypodermic needles, syringes, scalpel blades, forceps and needle holders can be added when required. An example of a suitable basic kit used by the authors is shown in Figure 14.6.

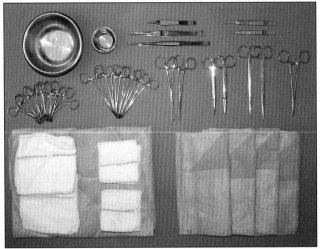

14.6 A basic instrument kit used in addition to bespoke arthroscopy instruments.

Instrument cannulae

Visual inspection of the intra-articular structures may not be sufficient to evaluate a joint fully, and it is advisable – and often necessary – to palpate the soft tissue structures and the articular surface. Instruments can be introduced either through a cannula or directly through a stab incision in the periarticular soft tissues. Cannulae are generally used for joints with greater soft tissue coverage (e.g. the shoulder and hip) and are optional for more superficial joints. Instrument cannulae are available in a range of sizes and facilitate ease of instrument introduction and switching. Cannulae may be reusable or single-use disposable. Suitable sizes for use in canine arthroscopy are between 2.3 and 3.5 mm, with lengths of 3–5 cm.

Small joint cannula systems are commercially available. These consist of a series of cannulae and a 'switching stick' to permit serial dilation of portals to facilitate the insertion of larger instruments (Figure 14.7a). After triangulation using a hypodermic needle, the switching stick is introduced through a small stab incision in the periarticular tissues. Once the switching stick is in the field of view, a cannula can be introduced over the switching stick, which is subsequently removed. If a larger cannula is needed, the switching stick is reintroduced and the cannulae are exchanged.

The disadvantage of using a cannula system is the relatively restricted diameter of instruments that can be inserted (or fragments of tissue removed) and the limited mobility of the instruments when in the joint. It is also relatively easy to displace the cannula from the joint, which may lead to extravasation of fluid and compress the joint. This problem can be minimized by using cannulae that possess external threads such that they can be 'screwed' into the joint capsule.

A range of more flexible, reusable cannulae are now available (Figure 14.7bc). These offer the advantages of having a larger bore than metal cannulae but, due to the softer materials used, cause less iatrogenic damage to the joint surfaces. Threads or flanges on the cannulae also reduce the likelihood of accidentally pulling the cannula from the joint.

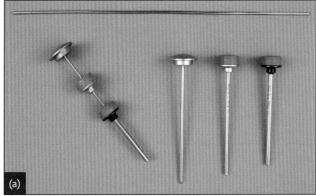

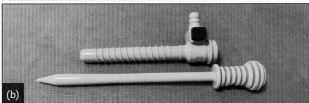

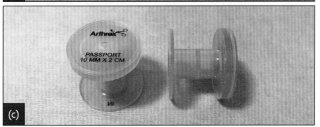

14.7 (a) Instrument cannulae for elbow and shoulder arthroscopy, with switching stick (top). (b) Plastic cannula for use as an egress or instrument portal in the stifle or shoulder. (c) Rubber 'passport' cannulae with low-profile flanges that seat flush to the skin and minimize accidental pull-out when removing instruments.

Hand instruments

Hand instruments are required to explore and palpate intra-articular structures. A minimum of two pairs of grasping forceps, a probe, a milling drill and a curette are recommended. Instrument sets are available that consist of a single handle with interchangeable tips.

Probes (Figure 14.8) are usually right-angled and approximately 2 mm across at the tip. They are used to palpate articular surfaces, to move soft tissue structures to improve the view, or to elevate meniscal or cartilage defects.

Grasping forceps (Figure 14.9) are available in a range of sizes; the grasping surfaces are available as locking or non-locking types. Most have an internal operating mechanism that avoids any interference with the surrounding structures. They need to be small enough to fit into the joint but strong enough to remove osteochondral lesions. Modern instruments are fitted with an overload protection device that prevents breakage of the pin in the forceps when excessive force is applied. Smaller (e.g. 2 mm) forceps are particularly prone to breakage. A range of tips are available, depending on the required purpose of the forceps.

A hand milling drill or burr (Figure 14.10) is a useful tool for curettage and abrasion of the subchondral surface following fragment removal. The 2 mm tip of the instrument is easily inserted into a joint and a high degree of accuracy can be achieved by using controlled delicate movements. Large lesions can take a long time to be milled using a hand drill, and in such cases it may be more suitable to use a power shaver.

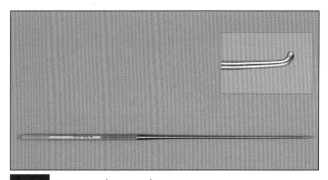

14.8 A 2 mm 90-degree probe.

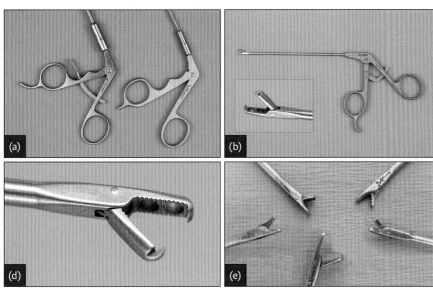

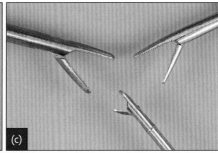

14.9 Grasping forceps. (a) Locking (left) and non-locking (right) handles; (b) locking forceps with grasping teeth for large fragment removal; (c) a variety of tips; (d) close-up of rat-toothed tip; (e) close-up of meniscal punch tips.

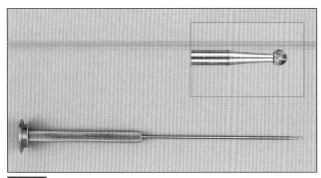

14.10 A 2.0 mm hand burr for curettage of cartilage and bone.

Arthroscopic knives are available in forward- or back-cutting designs (Figure 14.11). They may be straight, curved or hooked, and the selection of a suitable knife is dependent on the procedure being performed. They are particularly useful for removing meniscal lesions and transecting soft tissue attachments to bony structures (e.g. the annular ligament attachment to a fragmented coronoid process lesion). Disposable versions are preferable as the knives blunt very quickly.

A range of curettes is available and these are useful for removing defective articular cartilage and bony fragments. The tip may be open (eye) or closed (cup); the open type is better for cartilage debridement. Straight curettes are easier to insert through a cannula and usually suffice, but a curved curette may be more useful for working at awkward angles.

Awls, used for microfracture of subchondral bone, are available for use in canine arthroscopy. An alternative is to use a small (1.1 mm) Kirschner wire secured in a Jacob's chuck or power drill.

Arthroscopic punches and scissors can be used to cut pieces of tissue within the joint. These can be straight or angled (left or right). Such instruments are useful for manual debridement or cutting of synovium, meniscus or tendon.

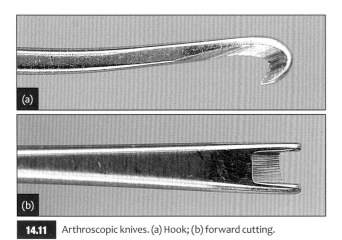

14.11 Arthroscopic knives. (a) Hook; (b) forward cutting.

Power shavers

Power shavers have advanced considerably in the past decade and a vast array of different shaver heads is now available. Most of the available tools are designed specifically for humans, especially for the shoulder or knee, but a number are suitable for canine arthroscopy. Although these are not essential, in certain situations they may expedite surgeries, especially the removal of hyperplastic

synovium and fat pad, the treatment of large articular cartilage lesions or the management of meniscal disease. A small joint shaver is required for all canine joints except for the stifle of medium- and large-breed dogs, where the 'standard' handpieces are suitable and more efficient.

The shaving unit (see Figure 2.43) can be operated in forward, reverse or oscillating modes, depending upon the procedure being performed. Foot or hand controls are used to control the direction and speed of the shaver. For debridement of soft tissue structures, such as the infrapatellar fat pad, it is best to use the shaver in oscillating mode to effectively 'suck' the tissue into the shaver head in the pause between forward and reverse revolutions. For harder structures, forward or reverse mode is more suitable. Speed control is important because different tissues require different speeds to optimize their removal. For example, slower speeds are more useful when removing the fat pad. A range of shaving heads is available (Figure 14.12), designed for the removal of either bone or soft tissue. Tips used for soft tissue removal tend to be larger and have more aggressive cutting teeth. Most handpieces come with a suction device. This has the benefit of removing the debrided material from the joint but also draws the soft tissues into the tip to facilitate further removal.

The disadvantages of using power shavers are the initial costs of acquiring and setting up the equipment and the increased risk of iatrogenic damage. Extreme care must be taken when using these instruments to minimize this damage. Most shaver units come with a protective shroud in which the oscillating part of the shaver sits. The user should carefully locate the shroud against the tissues they wish to protect in order to minimize any iatrogenic damage. There are few situations in canine arthroscopy where it is essential to have a power shaver, which means that the high cost of purchasing a unit does not need to be incurred by those starting out in arthroscopy.

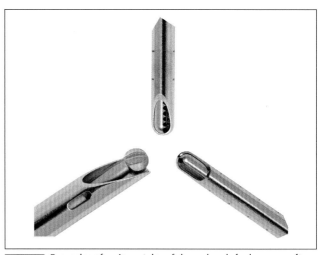

14.12 Examples of various styles of shaver heads for bone or soft tissue removal.
(Courtesy of Arthrex GmbH)

Fluid management systems

Good-quality arthroscopy is reliant upon well controlled fluid flow through the joint. Fluid flow is essential:

- To distend the joint before insertion of the obturator and sleeve, in order to minimize the risk of iatrogenic articular damage. The stifle and carpus are two joints where prior distension may not be required

- For removal of debris and blood to increase the clarity of the view
- For joint lavage to remove inflammatory mediators
- To stop/minimize intraoperative haemorrhage through fluid pressure.

Fluid control requires the establishment and maintenance of ingress and egress portals. Failure to maintain fluid control will result in a poor view of the joint and/or extravasation of the fluid into the adjacent soft tissues. The joint will then collapse, hindering the procedure.

Lactated Ringer's solution (also known as Hartmann's solution) is the fluid of choice. It can be provided under gravity or by pressurized systems. Gravity-fed systems supply fluid via a normal fluid administration set attached to the arthroscope cannula. The pressure can be increased by enclosing the fluid bag in an infusion pressure jacket (Figure 14.13a). These systems are cheap, easy to set up and maintain and require little space, but they offer poor control of pressure and require closer attention than automatic fluid pumps to prevent excessive pressure drops. Fluid pumps (Figure 14.13b) are able to provide consistent pressure over longer periods of time but may be expensive to purchase and require dedicated tubing. The more advanced units are able to maintain a constant intra-articular pressure by controlling fluid flow into and out of the joint.

Systems that use a two-piece tubing system are available; these can reduce costs and set-up time when performing several arthroscopic procedures in one day. The main tubing can be used for multiple procedures during the day as the pump's backflow valves prevent contaminated fluid reaching this tubing. For each procedure, new extension tubing is used to maintain sterility; this is more economical than having to replace all of the tubing.

Aiming device

The aiming device (Figure 14.14) facilitates the triangulation of instruments into the viewing window and may be useful to the inexperienced arthroscopist, especially for the shoulder joint. The device is attached to the arthroscope sleeve (there are specific devices designed for 2.4 and 2.7 mm arthroscopes). A Kirschner wire is placed into the device and advanced through the soft tissues and joint capsule until it is visible via the arthroscope. The aiming device can then be removed and the procedure continued as normal using the Kirschner wire as a switching stick.

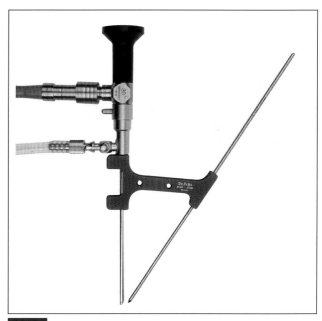

14.14   Dr Fritz aiming device for triangulation of instruments.

| **14.13** | (a) Hand pressure infusion cuff. |

(b) Arthroscopy fluid pump.

Patient preparation and positioning

Irrespective of which joint is to be examined arthroscopically, the patient is clipped and prepared as if for a standard open arthrotomy. This allows the arthroscopy to be readily converted to arthrotomy if needed; this occurs most commonly during the surgeon's learning phase. As the surgeon's competence, conversion will be required less often, minimizing the anaesthetic duration and increasing the aesthetic appearance postoperatively.

There are several ways of draping the surgical field and these are used at the discretion of the surgeon. The draping technique chosen should allow for suitable mobility of the limb. For maximum manoeuvrability, a hanging limb preparation with four-quarter draping (Figure 14.15a) is recommended for joints such as the stifle. A further large drape is then placed over the dog, leaving only the relevant limb exposed. This technique is also advised where the surgeon is inexperienced and conversion to an open arthrotomy may be needed. Where mobility of the joint is less important, a single adherent operating drape with a translucent window can be used. Whatever technique is employed, it is important that the uppermost layer of drapes is impermeable to fluids, to prevent strikethrough and breakdown of asepsis (Figure 14.15b).

Careful positioning of the patient, surgeon and equipment is essential to minimize the technical difficulty of arthroscopy. The exact position of the animal depends on the joint being investigated and the approach required. It can be difficult to orientate around a limb when the patient is draped, so use should be made of ties and sandbags to secure the position of the patient. A sandbag can also be used to act as a fulcrum, especially in the elbow, to widen the joint and minimize iatrogenic damage. Custom braces are available (Figure 14.16) and may be useful for supporting the limb in fixed positions. Distraction devices are used widely in human arthroscopic surgery but less commonly in small animal arthroscopy, probably due to the wide variety in size of veterinary patients requiring a large number of distraction devices.

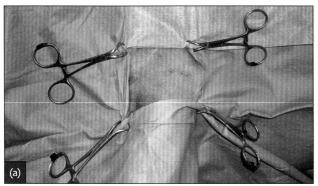

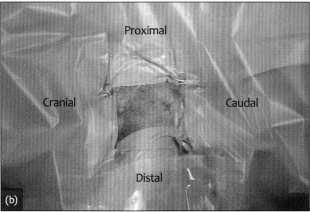

14.15 (a) Four-quarter draping of the right elbow for arthroscopy. For routine elbow arthroscopy, a hanging limb is used for preparation only. The limb is then laid parallel to the table for the arthroscopic procedure. (b) Impermeable drape used to prevent strikethrough.

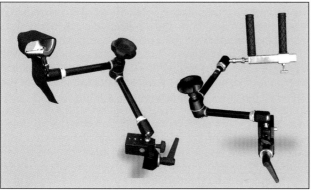

14.16 Multiarm positional aid and stifle brace for multiarm attachment. (Courtesy of Veterinary Instrumentation, Sheffield)

Analgesia

Pre-emptive and continuous multimodal analgesia is essential for all animals undergoing arthroscopy. Drug groups that can be used include opioids, non-steroidal anti-inflammatory drugs (NSAIDs), α2-adrenergic agonists, ketamine, nitrous oxide and local anaesthetics.

Intra-articular analgesia, in particular using local anaesthetics, is very useful in arthroscopy. Bupivacaine (1 mg/kg) is commonly used, as it has a duration of action of 6–8 hours. Mu (μ) receptors in the synovium are upregulated in cases of chronic inflammation and therefore intra-articular morphine (0.1 mg/kg) is beneficial in animals with more chronic disease.

Other local anaesthesia techniques can be employed, including brachial plexus blocks in the thoracic limb (for the elbow and distal limb) and extradural (epidural) analgesia for pelvic limb procedures. These techniques are not normally used by the authors for arthroscopic procedures alone but are employed when arthroscopy is performed before performing more invasive procedures, for example, treatment of a cranial cruciate ligament (CCL) rupture.

Postoperative care

Postoperatively, analgesia is continued using opioids and NSAIDs. Cold therapy may also be employed. Arthroscopy does facilitate day-case surgery, but some surgeons prefer to hospitalize patients overnight in cases where some form of therapeutic arthroscopy has been performed, in order to continue postoperative opioid analgesia for up to 24 hours. NSAIDs are recommended postoperatively to provide ongoing analgesia.

Antibiotics

Unless arthroscopy is being used to investigate a joint before a further planned procedure, such as a tibial plateau levelling osteotomy, antibiotic treatment is not indicated either perioperatively or postoperatively. The continuous flushing of the joint with fluid during arthroscopy means that there is a very low risk of surgical site infection.

The shoulder joint

Arthroscopy is providing new insights into articular disorders of small animals, and this is particularly the case in the shoulder. Increasing awareness of the potential for arthroscopically assisted surgery and the continued advancement in technology have led to many areas of progress.

Anatomical considerations

The shoulder is a diarthrodial ball and socket joint (Figure 14.17) that is capable of a wide range of motion – primarily flexion and extension, but also abduction, adduction, and internal and external rotation. The canine shoulder joint is not an intrinsically stable socket joint; normal joint motion is limited by capsular, muscular, ligamentous and bony restraints. Passive mechanisms contributing to shoulder joint stability include the medial glenohumeral ligament

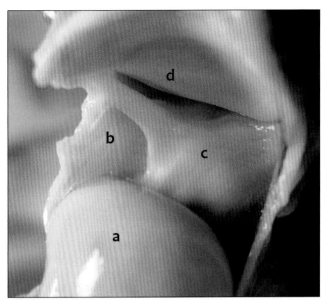

14.17 Shoulder joint. a = humeral head; b = subscapularis tendon; c = medial glenohumeral ligament; d = glenoid cavity.

(MGHL), the lateral glenohumeral ligament (LGHL), the joint capsule, joint conformity, and finite joint fluid and adhesion/cohesion mechanisms. Active mechanisms have been hypothesized to contribute to shoulder joint stability through the action of the 'cuff' muscles (supraspinatus, infraspinatus, subscapularis and teres minor muscles) and the biceps brachii. Selective contraction of these muscles increases glenohumeral compression and thus resists the displacing forces acting on the joint. In humans, the active and passive mechanisms are proposed to act in unison, with the active stabilizers being more important when humeral head displacement is small and the passive stabilizers being more important when displacement is large.

Indications

The shoulder is a common site of lameness in dogs but before the advent of arthroscopy it was difficult to diagnose the cause of the lameness accurately. Arthroscopy provides an excellent view and permits palpation of the intra-articular structures of the shoulder with minimal trauma (Van Ryssen *et al.*, 1993b). Osteochondritis dissecans (OCD) is probably the most common indication for surgical arthroscopy of the shoulder, but diagnostic arthroscopy can be considered in all cases of lameness attributable to the shoulder. This is particularly important considering the number of ligamentous and soft tissue injuries that can occur around the shoulder. Conditions that are readily diagnosed by arthroscopy include:

- OCD of the caudal humeral head
- Medial shoulder instability (MSI) (subscapularis tendon tears, MGHL tears)
- LGHL tears
- Incomplete ossification/osteochondral fragmentation of the caudal glenoid
- Partial or complete rupture of the biceps brachii tendon of origin
- Synovitis.

Instrumentation

A long 2.7 mm, 30-degree oblique arthroscope is most commonly used in the shoulder, although a 1.9 or 2.4 mm

arthroscope should be considered in small dogs and in cats. If diagnostic arthroscopy is all that is required, two portals can be used. It is advisable to palpate all the intra-articular structures of the shoulder, and so ideally an instrument portal should also be established. The minimum selection of instruments required for arthroscopy of the shoulder includes probes, cannulae (and switching stick), large grasping forceps (for OCD lesions), a milling drill, a curette and an aiming device.

Patient preparation and positioning

The patient is placed in lateral recumbency with the affected limb uppermost. The limb should be held horizontal to the table or slightly adducted. The limb can be draped either as a hanging limb preparation or with a single drape placed laterally; the latter still allows manoeuvrability of the limb.

Procedure
Portal placement

The traditional portal for shoulder arthroscopy is the lateral portal. Usually the egress cannula is established craniolaterally, with the instrument portal caudolaterally (Figure 14.18). However, when primarily interested in the biceps tendon and sheath, the authors prefer to use a craniolateral arthroscope portal, and when particularly interested in the LGHL, the authors place the lateral portal slightly caudal to the acromion. Use of a craniomedial portal has also been reported (see later).

The egress portal is established first, using a 20 G, 40–50 mm (1.5–2 inch) needle. The needle is introduced midway along the craniocaudal border of the superior ridge of the greater tubercle. It is directed caudally and medially, at 70 degrees to the vertical, in order to enter the joint. Aspiration of synovial fluid is usually possible after correct introduction of the needle; 10–12 ml of lactated Ringer's solution can then be introduced to distend the joint. If synovial fluid cannot be aspirated but the surgeon is confident that the needle is placed correctly in the joint, then fluid can still be injected. Fluid should be injectable

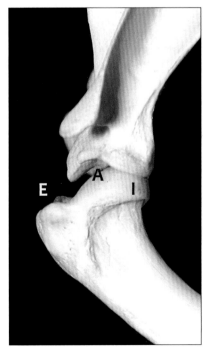

14.18 Model demonstrating the position of portals for shoulder arthroscopy. A = arthroscope portal; E = egress portal; I = instrument portal.

with minimal pressure initially. As the intra-articular pressure increases, back pressure will be felt on the syringe. The syringe is usually left in place initially and pressure is maintained by an assistant. Care should be taken not to inject fluid extra-articularly as this will collapse the joint, making the arthroscopy difficult.

The arthroscope portal is established next. A second hypodermic needle is introduced approximately 1 cm distal to the acromion. Correct placement of the needle will result in fluid flow through the needle due to the pressure maintained on the syringe. A No. 11 scalpel blade is then used to make a small incision through the skin and periarticular soft tissues. The blade should not pass through the synovium, as this will lead to extravasation of fluid. The arthroscope cannula, with an attached blunt obturator, is then introduced parallel to the needle until it is felt to enter the joint. The limb should be held parallel to the table when introducing the cannula, with the assistant placing a distal distraction force on the limb to widen the joint space; this minimizes the risk of iatrogenic trauma. Confirmation of correct placement of the cannula is achieved by opening the fluid stopcock on the cannula and observing fluid egress. The obturator is then removed and the arthroscope is inserted into the sleeve. The camera, fluid line and light cable can then be attached and the optical equipment switched on.

If required, an instrument portal is established next. For the treatment of OCD, this is usually created approximately 2 cm caudal to and slightly distal to the acromion. The portal is created in the same way as for the arthroscope portal. The use of a cannula is recommended for the instrument portal in the shoulder due to the depth of the periarticular musculature.

The initial view from the lateral portal is usually cranial to the dome of the humeral head. It is not uncommon for the arthroscope to be initially more medial than required and it may need to be carefully retracted until the articular surfaces of the humeral head and glenoid are visible. It is possible to retract the arthroscope too far and pull it out of the joint, so care should be exercised. Once the articular surfaces are visualized, spatial awareness becomes easier. The initial view consists of, from top to bottom of the image (proximal to distal in the joint), the glenoid, MGHL, subscapularis muscle tendon of insertion and the humeral head (Figure 14.19).

Examining the joint

It is important for the surgeon to develop their own pattern of examining each joint. There are no right or wrong ways as long as the examination is thorough and methodical. The pattern used by the authors is described here.

From the initial starting position, the camera should be held still and the light post moved ventrally to view the articular surface of the medial glenoid. The light post is then rotated into the 9 o'clock position and the camera head moved cranially in order to view the caudal humeral head (Figure 14.20). With minor alterations to the position of the light post and camera, it is possible to examine the medial gutter, consisting of the caudomedial joint capsule and the medial humeral head (Figure 14.21). Advancement of the arthroscope in a caudomedial direction will facilitate visualization of the gutter.

The camera is then returned to the neutral position and the light post is rotated to the 3 o'clock position to view the cranial compartment. From this position, the craniomedial joint capsule and biceps tendon are visible (Figure 14.22). The tendon can be seen coursing distally through the bicipital groove. Flexion of the elbow at this point increases the length of the tendon that is visible. The light post is then moved clockwise, to the 4 o'clock position, to view the origin of the biceps tendon and the supraglenoid

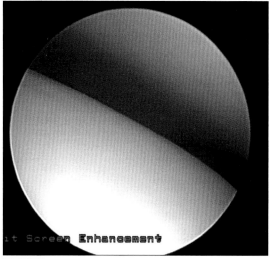

14.20 Normal caudal humeral head.

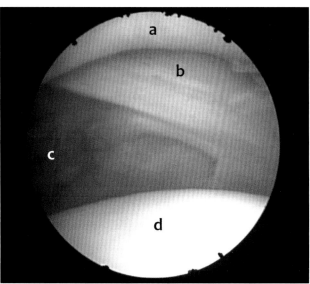

14.19 Normal arthroscopic anatomy of the medial shoulder joint. a = glenoid; b = MGHL; c = subscapularis tendon; d = humeral head.

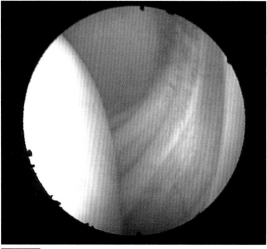

14.21 Normal caudomedial gutter.

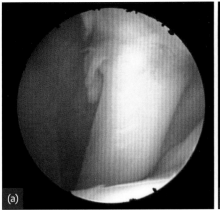
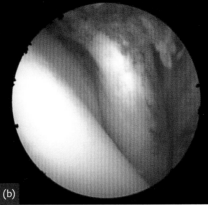
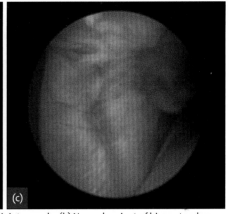

14.22 Cranial compartment of the shoulder joint. (a) Normal origin of biceps tendon and cranial joint capsule. (b) Normal variant of biceps tendon. (c) Bipartite biceps tendon.

tuberosity. By advancing the arthroscope at this point the cranial aspect of the joint capsule can be examined lying cranial to the biceps tendon.

The final part of the joint to be inspected is the lateral compartment (Figure 14.23). Care must be taken when examining this region, as it is easy for the arthroscope to 'pop' out of the joint, causing extravasation of fluid; for this reason, this compartment is inspected last. The camera is moved further caudally and the light source is rotated to the 4–5 o'clock position to view the craniolateral compartment. The camera is then moved cranially, and the light post clockwise to the 7–8 o'clock position, to view the caudolateral joint capsule.

Suspended limb arthroscopy

In contrast to the human shoulder, the shoulder of the dog does not have a histologically distinct labrum and therefore, although reported in the literature, tears of the labrum (so-called Bankart tears in humans) cannot exist. One possible reason for the confusion lies in the fact that it is difficult to view the medial and lateral restraints or the rotator cuff muscles accurately from a standard lateral portal. A craniomedial portal is preferred for viewing these structures and is best established with the limb in a suspended position (Figure 14.24). A standard lateral portal is established with the limb suspended. Slight adduction should be placed on the limb and the table lowered until the weight of the dog is suspended through the shoulder; this

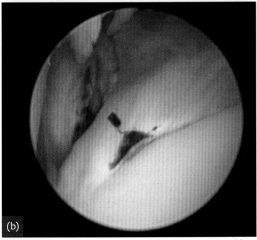

14.23 Lateral compartment of the shoulder joint. (a) Origin of lateral glenohumeral ligament. (b) Normal variant.

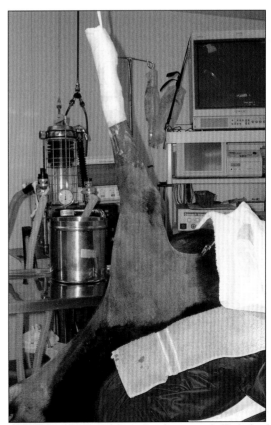

14.24 Positioning of the patient for suspended limb shoulder arthroscopy. Note the position of the head to facilitate easy access to the craniomedial aspect of the shoulder.
(Courtesy of C Deintt)

will help to distract the limb. The joint should be examined thoroughly from the lateral portal before establishment of the craniomedial portal. This can be achieved directly (from the outside in) or indirectly (from the inside out).

Direct technique: With the arthroscope viewing the craniomedial joint capsule, a 20 G needle is inserted into the joint between the biceps tendon and the subscapularis tendon. The light source can usually be seen through the skin at this point, which will help with triangulation. With the aid of a switching stick, a craniomedial portal is established in the normal manner.

Indirect (push-through) technique: The arthroscope is advanced until it rests in the desired position against the craniomedial compartment of the shoulder. The arthroscope is then removed from its cannula and replaced with a switching stick, which is pushed through the joint capsule and soft tissues until the skin tents. A small stab incision is made through the skin and the switching stick is exited through this incision. The arthroscope cannula is then removed from the lateral portal and replaced craniomedially.

Once the arthroscope is in position in the craniomedial portal, the medial glenoid recess and lateral compartment can be assessed.

Pathological conditions
Osteochondritis dissecans

Osteochondrosis is a failure of endochondral ossification and, in the shoulder, is most commonly seen on the caudal third of the humeral head, although occasionally the caudal glenoid may be affected (see below). The classic lesion is an under-run cartilage flap on the caudal humeral head. The flap may remain *in situ* (Figure 14.25) or break off and float around the joint (a so-called joint mouse); it may also be reabsorbed or mineralize.

Although medical management is an option for shoulder OCD, surgery is the treatment of choice (Person, 1989a; Van Ryssen *et al.*, 1993a). The disease is often bilateral, and with the use of arthroscopy both shoulders can be treated during one surgical session if necessary. The area should be clipped widely to facilitate conversion to an open arthrotomy, should the need arise, although with practice this is very unlikely. A hanging limb preparation offers the greatest freedom of movement of the limb, with the dog positioned in lateral recumbency. A standard

lateral arthroscope portal, using a 2.7 mm, 30-degree oblique arthroscope, and a craniolateral egress portal are used. The instrument portal is established caudolaterally unless the OCD lesion has been displaced. With a displaced lesion, the instrument portal may be placed craniolaterally or caudolaterally depending on the location of the lesion (see below).

After a complete joint inspection, grasping forceps are introduced through the instrument portal. If the flap is still well attached (typically medially), it is better to elevate it using a probe or fragment elevator to facilitate grasping. The OCD lesion is grasped and gently rolled (Figure 14.26). *In situ* fragments may roll up, which aids their removal. The surgeon can choose to grasp, twist and remove small pieces of the flap or, using larger forceps, grasp the whole flap, twist and remove it in one piece. Although the latter technique is potentially very fast, it is dependent on appropriately sized forceps and runs the risk that the flap may become loose within the joint if removal is unsuccessful. If the flap is grasped whole, it is often too large to pass through the cannula, and extreme care must be taken not to lose the flap in the joint. A loose cartilage flap within the joint can be frustrating to grasp again because it will usually lodge in the medial gutter and be relatively inaccessible. The soft tissue surrounding the cannula can be gently widened using mosquito forceps and the flap, forceps and cannula removed as one. The instrument cannula can then be re-established using a switching stick.

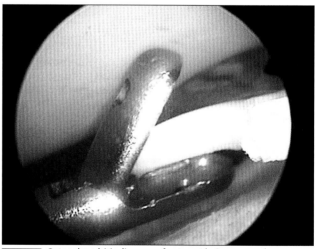

14.26 Osteochondritis dissecans fragment being grasped. (Courtesy of B Van Ryssen)

After complete removal of the flap, the remaining edges of articular cartilage are curetted back to healthy cartilage. Ideally, the edges of the cartilage lesion should be vertical in order to allow inflow of the surrounding cartilage matrix. The subchondral bone surface is then milled using a hand drill or power shaver. The surface is abraded until it readily bleeds, although overzealous curettage should be avoided. If the flow rate of irrigation fluid is high then haemorrhage may not be observed. Temporary cessation of fluid flow will readily highlight the presence of subchondral bone bleeding. Microfracture techniques can be employed to release mesenchymal stem cells and promote the healing process: 1–2 mm deep holes, 4 mm apart, are created in the subchondral bed using a micropick and mallet (or a 1.1 mm Kirschner wire secured in a Jacob's chuck) (Person, 1989). On completion of this procedure, the joint should be flushed for 5 minutes at a high rate in order to remove as much debris as possible. The portals are then sutured using non-absorbable fine suture material or a skin stapler.

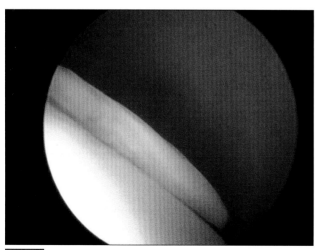

14.25 Osteochondritis dissecans: *in situ* lesion.

Occasionally the OCD lesion is no longer attached to the humeral head and is free within the joint. The lesion most commonly displaces to the caudal joint recess, where it may cause no pain, and lameness may resolve. However, occasionally the flap may lodge in the bicipital groove or, rarely, between the MGHL and the joint capsule. These latter positions may result in continued lameness and require intervention to remove the flap. For cases where the fragment is behind the biceps tendon, a cranio-lateral instrument portal should be used. For cases where the lesion is in the medial position, the instrument cannula is positioned caudolaterally. The fragment can sometimes be drawn towards the egress cannula by the direction of fluid flow; grasping forceps can then be introduced to capture the fragment. Displaced fragments are often less flexible due to mineralization, and therefore do not roll up. Care must therefore be taken to ensure that the opening in the joint capsule is large enough to accommodate the fragment during removal.

The prognosis for shoulder OCD is generally good, with 75% of dogs regaining full limb function (Rudd *et al.*, 1990). Most dogs should have restricted exercise for 6–8 weeks while the defect fills with fibrocartilage. Normal exercise can usually be started approximately 12 weeks after surgery.

Incomplete ossification/osteochondral fragmentation of the caudal glenoid

Lesions of the caudal glenoid are uncommon. Occasionally, in young dogs, a separate centre of ossification is noted on the caudal glenoid on plain radiographs; this normal variant has a smooth, non-displaced appearance and should not be interpreted as a pathological lesion. Arthroscopy can be used to identify true lesions and assess the stability of the fragment (Figure 14.27). Mobile lesions and those that have failed to respond to conservative management should be resected (Olivieri *et al.*, 2004).

Medial shoulder instability

The medial aspect of the glenohumeral joint consists of the subscapularis muscle tendon of insertion and the MGHL (Cook *et al.*, 2005a). All cases of MSI should undergo arthroscopic examination in order to determine the cause of the instability, as radiography is often unrewarding. Tears to the subscapularis muscle tendon of insertion (Figure 14.28) and the cranial arm of the MGHL can result in MSI.

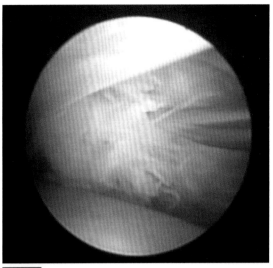
14.28 Subscapularis tear.

Concurrent capsular tears are sometimes evident. Treatment options can be either arthroscopic or via an open approach and placement of a medial prosthesis (Fitch *et al.*, 2001; Pettitt *et al.*, 2007; Penelas *et al.*, 2018).

Thermal capsulorrhaphy has been reported in dogs as a treatment for MSI (O'Neill and Innes, 2004; Cook *et al.*, 2005b), although the procedure has fallen out of favour due to very mixed long-term outcomes.

Lateral glenohumeral ligament tears

Diagnosing LGHL tears is more difficult than MGHL tears due to the difficulty of viewing this area from a lateral portal. If there is any doubt regarding the integrity of the lateral capsule, a craniomedial portal should be established. Indeed, if arthroscopic surgery to stabilize lateral shoulder instability is being considered, then a cranio-medial portal is recommended. The LGHL is usually taut when the limb is held neutrally or in slight adduction and lax when the limb is abducted. As for the medial structures, the LGHL should be assessed for complete or partial tears (Figure 14.29), fraying or inflammation. Probing the ligament is difficult but should be attempted. Instability should be suspected if the ligament is lax in the neutral or adducted position or if pathology is evident on inspection and probing.

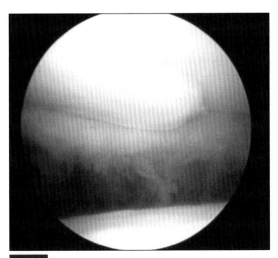
14.27 Incomplete ossification of the caudal glenoid.

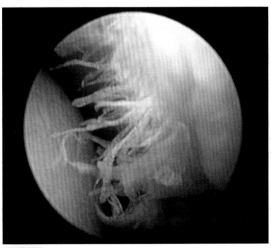
14.29 Lateral glenohumeral ligament tear.

Treatment options for tears of the LGHL are similar to those for MGHL tears. Complete tears of the ligament can be reconstructed either using an open arthrotomy (Mitchell and Innes, 2000) or arthroscopically, using suture anchors. Two reports of the arthroscopic management of LGHL rupture exist in the literature. In the first of these (Pettitt and Innes, 2008), using a hanging limb position and a craniomedial arthroscopic portal, a suture anchor loaded with Fiberwire® suture was inserted into the craniolateral scapula just proximal to the glenoid, via a craniolateral portal (Figure 14.30). Using a caudolateral portal

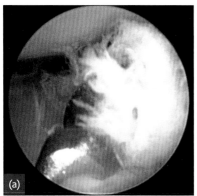
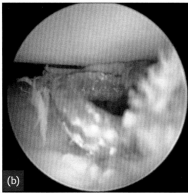
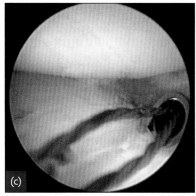
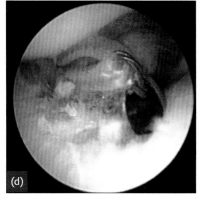

14.30 Arthroscopic repair of a lateral glenohumeral ligament tear. (a) Placement of the suture anchor. (b) Advancement of the suture material into the joint, to ensure adequate visualization. (c, d) A lasso is used to extract the suture through the capsular tissue.

and an arthroscopic lasso instrument, each strand of the suture was shuttled separately through the ligamentocapsular tissue before being returned to the craniolateral portal and tied using an arthroscopic knot pusher. Ridge *et al.* (2014) described a modification of this technique that utilized two suture anchors, which could be placed through a single, enlarged lateral portal.

The prognosis for shoulder instability is fair to good. Imbrication or thermal capsulorrhaphy is usually successful, at least in the short term, but postoperative management of these cases is critical and may be prolonged. It is common for lameness to resolve but the condition may recur.

Bicipital tenosynovitis

Before the advent of arthroscopy, bicipital tenosynovitis (BTS) was a commonly diagnosed shoulder injury. The diagnosis was usually based on the history, clinical findings and results of radiography or arthrography. Only rarely was the diagnosis based on a visual assessment or histopathology. BTS is a poorly defined condition that is difficult to diagnose accurately and, in the authors' opinion, is uncommon or rare. Ultrasonography has also been shown to detect pathology of the biceps tendon parenchyma reliably (Figure 14.31).

Standard lateral portal arthroscopy allows inspection of the biceps brachii tendon of origin. The normal tendon appears as a smooth white structure with variable amounts of vasculature and some fat and synovial folds proximally. Changes that occur with this disease include thickening and/or discoloration of the tendon, and synovitis (Figure 14.32) and adhesions of the tendon sheath. Care must

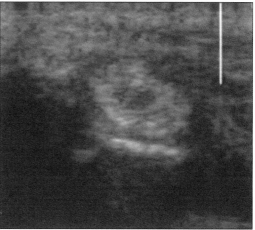

14.31 Transverse ultrasound image of the biceps tendon, showing a hypoechoic 'core' lesion.

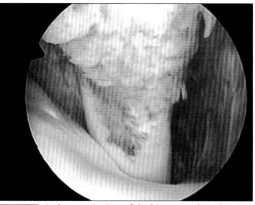

14.32 Arthroscopic view of the biceps tendon, showing severe synovial hyperaemia.

be taken in interpreting these findings as primary BTS because synovial hyperplasia may occur secondary to other pathological processes in the shoulder, such as OCD or MSI. Treatment of the primary cause will often resolve the changes seen on the tendon and, in the authors' opinion, synovitis of the tendon sheath is most likely an extension of generalized synovitis of the shoulder due to pathology other than BTS.

Conservative management, involving strict rest and analgesia, is recommended for at least 4–6 weeks. At the end of arthroscopy, a long-acting corticosteroid (e.g. 1.33 mg/kg methylprednisolone) may be injected intra-articularly. It is reported that approximately 50% of painful shoulders in adult dogs treated in this way will respond (Butterworth, 2003). In cases where this treatment fails to resolve the lameness, tenodesis/tenotomy is recommended. This can be performed either arthroscopically or via an open arthrotomy. The authors' preference is to perform an arthroscopic tenotomy without reattaching the tendon to the proximal humerus. Although a tenodesis can be performed by arthroscopic guidance, it is technically more demanding and may be unnecessary. An arthroscopic tenotomy is a relatively straightforward procedure (Holsworth et al., 2002) and seems to produce results comparable to those of tenodesis. A lateral arthroscope portal is used, with the instrument portal placed cranio-laterally. Alternatively, the instrument portal can be created in a craniomedial position, just over the proximal bicipital groove. The tenotomy is performed using an arthroscopic hook knife, scissors or a radiofrequency probe. It has been shown that sharp transection is quicker than radiofrequency tenotomy, but haemorrhage may be a problem due to bleeding from the small vessels in the centre of the tendon.

Biceps tendon rupture

Partial or complete ruptures of the biceps tendon occur occasionally. Complete rupture of the biceps tendon can be confirmed clinically by observing hyperextension of the elbow when the shoulder is fully flexed (Figure 14.33). Pain during this manoeuvre may indicate partial rupture of the biceps tendon, but this is not a specific test. Diagnostic arthroscopy is indicated in cases of complete rupture to ensure that no other shoulder pathology requiring treatment is present.

Partial ruptures may be treated by arthroscopic tenotomy (Figure 14.34). In cases where rupture is suspected but not conclusive, it is important that the tendon is palpated carefully using a small joint probe. In the normal tendon, the probe should be able to pass around the complete tendon. The prognosis for partial biceps tendon ruptures treated by tenotomy, or for complete rupture, appears to be good, with most dogs returning to normal function after 6–10 weeks.

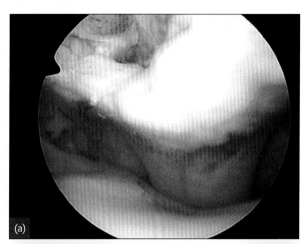

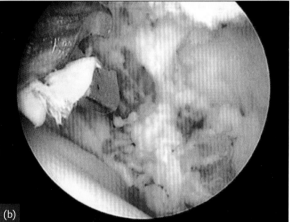

14.34 (a) Partial rupture of the biceps tendon. (b) Tenotomy using arthroscopic scissors.
(Courtesy of B Van Ryssen)

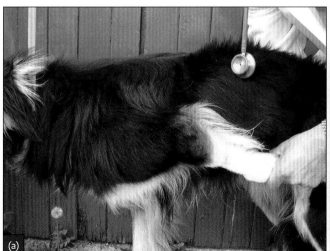

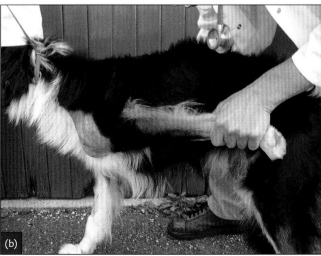

14.33 (a) Normal biceps tendon: with the shoulder in full flexion, the elbow cannot fully be extended. (b) Ruptured biceps tendon: the elbow can be fully extended.

The elbow joint

Arthroscopy is a useful modality for the diagnosis of elbow pain in young dogs. Radiography is insensitive to pathology of the elbow joint, and commonly produces false-negative results. Computed tomography (CT) and magnetic resonance imaging (MRI) have better sensitivity and specificity than radiography. These cross-sectional imaging modalities allow the evaluation of structures beyond the articular space (e.g. subchondral bone of the medial coronoid process) and in many ways are complementary to arthroscopy, which allows detailed inspection of the articular surfaces and joint capsule.

The elbow is the most common site of thoracic limb lameness, especially in young medium-sized to large dogs. Arthroscopy provides an excellent view and allows palpation of the intra-articular structures of the elbow with minimal trauma. The elbow joint is potentially the easiest joint of the dog to examine arthroscopically due to its superficial position and readily identifiable landmarks. Arthroscopy of the elbow allows a much better view of pathology than an open arthrotomy. Treatment of pathology within the joint is relatively straightforward, especially as the surgeon becomes more proficient at handling and using the instrumentation.

Indications

Indications for arthroscopy of the elbow include:

- Diagnosis and treatment of elbow dysplasia: fragmented coronoid process (FCP), OCD, ununited anconeal process (UAP)
- Diagnosis and management of elbow osteoarthritis
- Surgical management of septic arthritis
- Diagnosis of humeral intracondylar fissure (HIF) where the fissure extends to the articular surface.

Instrumentation

A 2.4 mm, 30-degree oblique arthroscope is most commonly used in the elbow of medium-sized to large dogs; a 1.9 mm arthroscope should be considered in small breeds. Three portals should be used (egress, arthroscope and instrument) as it is advisable to palpate all the intra-articular structures. Some lesions associated with elbow dysplasia and HIF are not obvious until the cartilage is carefully probed. Instruments required for arthroscopy of the elbow include probes, cannulae (and switching stick), various grasping forceps, a milling drill, a curette and elevators. The use of a power shaver is optional. Other instruments are discussed under the relevant procedures.

Patient preparation and positioning

The patient should be clipped as for an open arthrotomy. As the surgeon increases in experience, a small clip on the medial aspect of the limb is all that is required. The patient is placed in lateral recumbency with the affected limb down. A sandbag is placed under the elbow to act as a fulcrum. The limb can be draped either as a hanging limb preparation or with a single drape placed medially. If bilateral arthroscopy is to be performed the dog can be placed in either lateral or dorsal recumbency. Lateral recumbency requires the dog to be rolled when changing from one elbow to the other but makes viewing the joint easier, especially in more complex cases. Dorsal recumbency does not require the animal to be moved but does require a larger clip, and the procedure can be more difficult technically.

Procedure

Various portals for inspecting the elbow have been described, including medial, craniolateral and caudal portals. The authors prefer the medial portal (Figure 14.35) for inspection and treatment of lesions associated with elbow dysplasia. The craniolateral portal is useful for assessing incongruency, especially that associated with short radius syndrome, and for reduction of humeral condylar fractures. The value of the caudal portal remains unclear to date.

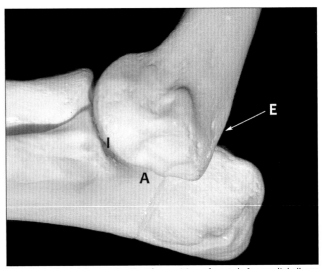

14.35 Model demonstrating the position of portals for medial elbow arthroscopy. A = arthroscope portal; E = egress portal; I = instrument portal.

Medial portal

A 20 G hypodermic needle, with an attached 10 ml syringe, is inserted into the proximocaudomedial joint capsule between the anconeal process and the medial supracondylar ridge. Joint fluid is usually aspirated when negative pressure is applied to the attached syringe; 6–10 ml of saline or lactated Ringer's solution is then injected intra-articularly. Correct placement of the needle allows easy injection of the fluid and the joint capsule is seen to bulge. Surgeons with minimal experience of arthroscopy should identify the medial epicondyle (used for location of the arthroscope portal) before injecting the fluid. Palpation of the epicondyle may be difficult after the fluid has been injected. The fluid line is then connected to the needle to prevent fluid loss.

In some cases, joint fluid is not aspirated from the needle. The surgeon has two choices in this situation. If they feel that the needle is placed correctly in the joint, then they can start to inject fluid; if the needle is intra-articular, the fluid should enter under minimal pressure. Care must be taken to ensure that the fluid is not entering the peri-articular tissues, as this will cause collapse of the joint capsule and subsequently may prevent introduction of the arthroscope cannula without causing iatrogenic damage. An alternative is to inject the fluid via another portal. Another 20 G hypodermic needle is placed perpendicular to the skin, approximately 1.5 cm distal to the medial epicondyle. Slight adjustment of the direction of the needle may be needed to enter the joint. Aspiration of synovial fluid from this portal ensures correct placement of the needle. The authors will often adjust the proximo-caudomedial needle when injecting fluid to ensure its correct placement. A small stab incision is made through the skin adjacent to the second needle and the arthroscope cannula is introduced. A coned obturator is always used, to minimize damage to the articular cartilage. Internal rotation and flexion over a fulcrum will widen the joint space and help introduction of the cannula.

Inspection of the joint from the medial portal allows observation of the following structures:

- Anconeal process
- Caudal joint recess
- Medial humeral condyle
- Lateral humeral condyle
- Lateral coronoid process
- Lateral joint capsule
- Medial coronoid process
- Radial head
- Craniomedial joint capsule
- Annular ligament
- Medial collateral ligament.

Inspection of the elbow should follow a logical, standardized order (Figure 14.36). The authors' recommended starting position is with the endoscope aiming towards the olecranon (for the right elbow this would be with the light post in the 9 o'clock position, and for the left elbow 3 o'clock) so that the anconeal process is visualized. The light post is then rotated through 180 degrees as the medial trochlear ridge of the ulna and medial condyle of the humerus are inspected. It is not uncommon to see a region of the central trochlear notch that is devoid of cartilage. This is a normal finding and probably reflects the lack of loading of this region; the underlying subchondral bone appears normal. This is known as a synovial fossa. To inspect the lateral capsule and lateral coronoid process, the arthroscope is carefully advanced while rotating the light post slowly in a clockwise direction. External rotation of the elbow may help at this point. From this position, the light post is rotated to the 2–3 o'clock position for the right elbow (and 10–11 o'clock for the left elbow) in order to observe the radial head. In some cases, the camera needs to be moved caudoproximally to allow the radius to enter

the field of view. Further leaning of the camera head allows the medial coronoid process to be examined. Advancing the arthroscope from this position allows a more complete inspection of the central and cranial aspects of the medial coronoid process.

After careful examination of the elbow, an instrument portal should be established cranial to the arthroscope. The light post should be rotated so that the craniomedial portion of the joint can be seen. A 20 G needle is inserted approximately 1–1.5 cm cranial to the arthroscope. The needle should be almost parallel to the arthroscope portal to prevent 'crossing over' of the needle with respect to the arthroscope cannula within the joint. It is easier to observe the instruments rather than the monitor when trying to triangulate. A useful indicator for placement of the needle in most canine elbows is to observe the light under the skin. This is often visible due to the minimal soft tissue overlying the joint on the medial aspect of the elbow and is a good marker for needle placement. Once the needle is seen on the monitor, a small stab incision is made in the skin, taking care not to inadvertently penetrate the joint capsule. A switching stick is then introduced parallel to the needle until it enters the joint. The use of an instrument cannula is at the discretion of the surgeon. A large clean open portal may be preferable to an instrument cannula as a cannula can sometimes inhibit the use of instruments such as grasping forceps.

Careful palpation of the joint, especially the articular cartilage, using a 2 mm right-angled probe, is paramount. Some cases of FCP have normal cartilage overlying large subchondral defects.

Pathological conditions
Fragmented coronoid process

FCP of the ulna is the most common cause of elbow lameness in young, rapidly growing, medium-sized to large dogs, and leads to osteoarthritis. Many breeds are affected but the Labrador Retriever, Rottweiler and Bernese Mountain Dog are over-represented. FCP often occurs bilaterally,

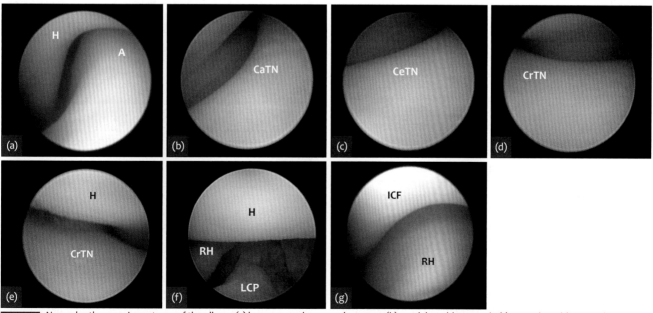

14.36 Normal arthroscopic anatomy of the elbow: (a) humerus and anconeal process; (b) caudal trochlear notch; (c) central trochlear notch; (d, e) cranial trochlear notch; (f) lateral coronoid process and radial head; (g) radial head and intercondylar fossa. A = anconeal process; CaTN = caudal trochlear notch; CeTN = central trochlear notch; CrTN = cranial trochlear notch; H = humerus; ICF = intercondylar fossa; LCP = lateral coronoid process; RH = radial head.

although most presentations are for unilateral thoracic limb lameness. The aetiology of the disease is not fully understood and many theories exist, including radioulnar incongruency, humeroulnar incongruency and osteochondrosis. The reader is referred to the *BSAVA Manual of Canine and Feline Musculoskeletal Disorders* for further detail.

A complete orthopaedic examination is required to rule out other juvenile orthopaedic conditions, such as panosteitis, metaphyseal osteopathy and septic arthritis. Diagnosis of FCP is not straightforward due to the difficulty in visualizing the lesions with radiography. An inference can be made based upon the signalment, history, clinical findings, presence of secondary osteoarthritic changes on radiographs and the elimination of other known causes of arthritis. The earliest change on radiographs is sclerosis of the trochlear notch. As the disease progresses, osteophytosis of the joint is evident. This is initially noted on the proximal border of the anconeus. It is uncommon to see an FCP lesion directly on radiographs because of the superimposition of the coronoid on the adjacent radius. Elbow dysplasia should still be suspected in these cases on the basis of the signalment, history and clinical signs. It is not uncommon for significant intra-articular pathology to be present in cases where no radiographic changes are evident. Arthroscopy allows a minimally invasive examination of the elbow to be performed and can be used as a diagnostic tool. Arthrocentesis of the joint may reveal an effusion, with cell counts in the range 2000–5000 cells/μl. CT allows observation of FCP lesions that may not be evident on plain radiographs, and may demonstrate fissuring of the subchondral bone that may not be evident on arthroscopic examination. If CT is not performed, this fissuring may be missed at the time of surgery, which explains why careful probing of the articular surface is needed. CT is now becoming more widely available but is not absolutely necessary to justify arthroscopic examination.

Both medical management and surgery are treatment options for FCP. The disease is often bilateral and, with the use of arthroscopy, both elbows can be treated in one session. A hanging limb preparation offers a greater range of movement of the limb, although the authors' current preference is to examine one elbow in a standard lateral position before re-draping in the contralateral recumbency.

Positioning of the patient is as described above for arthroscopic examination of the elbow. Arthroscopy for FCP (and other causes of elbow dysplasia) is performed through a medial portal. After placement of the egress needle and injection of fluid into the joint, the arthroscope portal is established. A visual examination of the whole joint is performed initially and the degree of cartilage integrity is graded using the modified Outerbridge scale (Figure 14.37). Other lesions within the elbow that may be identified in conjunction with FCP include osteoarthritis of the medial compartment, OCD and UAP. These other pathologies occur frequently and their management is described separately.

FCP lesions vary in severity from chondromalacia (abnormal softening of the cartilage) to large displaced fragments (Figure 14.38). Once the visual examination is complete, an instrument portal is established in order to probe the articular cartilage and facilitate removal of FCP lesions. The instrument portal is established as described above. The coronoid region is carefully probed to assess the integrity of the articular cartilage. If chondromalacia is present, it appears as a soft, fragile surface. More severely diseased cartilage is readily elevated and the yellow avascular subchondral bone is evident beneath (Figure 14.39). Fragments are often visible and may remain *in situ* or become displaced.

Outerbridge score	Outerbridge descriptors (original)	Modified Outerbridge descriptors
0	Normal	Normal
1	Cartilage softening and swelling	Chondromalacia or cartilage softening assessed by probing
2	Partial thickness defect with surface fissures that are <15 mm in diameter or do not reach subchondral bone	Partial thickness fibrillation
3	Fissures >15 mm diameter or reach the subchondral bone	Deep fibrillation
4	Exposed subchondral bone	Full thickness cartilage loss
5	n/a	Subchondral bone eburnation

14.37 The Outerbridge and modified Outerbridge classification scoring systems used to classify the severity of articular cartilage damage.
(Reproduced from the *BSAVA Manual of Canine and Feline Musculoskeletal Disorders, 2nd edn*)

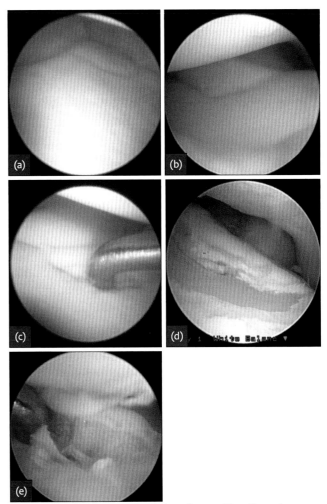

14.38 Varying degrees of pathology, from cartilage fissure to complete displacement of the fragment, seen with fragmentation of the coronoid process. (a) Fissuring of the apical region of the medial coronoid process (MCP). (b) Non-displaced fragment of the MCP. (c) Probing of a non-displaced fragment to assess stability. (d) Non-displaced fragment of the MCP with adjacent Outerbridge Grade 3 lesions on the adjacent ulna and Grade 2 on the humerus. (e) Elevation of a fragment exposing the yellow necrotic subchondral bone.

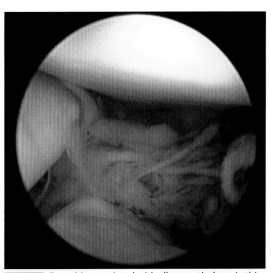

14.39 Synovitis associated with elbow pathology, in this case a displaced fragmented coronoid visible below the inflamed synovium. The yellow discoloration of the bone is caused by necrosis.

Removal of these fragments can sometimes be technically challenging. Often, they are quite large, and the small size of the elbow joint means that it is not possible to pass sufficiently large forceps into the joint to grasp them. The fragments are necrotic and tend to disintegrate when grasped; this is usually not a problem as they can be removed in a number of pieces, although care should be taken not to displace any sizeable fragments into inaccessible areas of the joint. If this does occur, the fluid flow should be increased to try to flush the fragment back towards the instrument portal. Placement of a cannula may facilitate this. Alternatively, an arthroscopic curette can be pushed past the fragment and used to guide it back into the working field. The annular ligament attaches to the medial and the lateral coronoid. Some fragments are well adhered to this ligament and sharp dissection may be needed to remove the lesion. Alternatively, the lesion can be grasped and rotated several times in order to tear away the soft tissues. Non-displaced fragments may need to be elevated using a curette or arthroscopic elevator before they are free enough to be removed. Very occasionally, displaced fragments may continue to grow and can become very large. These can sometimes be removed in one piece, although it is often easier to break them down. A power shaver is useful in these situations to burr the lesions rapidly; the debris is then removed through the suction channel. Hand milling can be performed but is sometimes a laborious and lengthy process. These procedures occasionally need to be converted to an open arthrotomy when the surgeon is relatively inexperienced with arthroscopy.

After removal of any fragments or diseased cartilage, the remaining cartilage and subchondral bone needs to be treated. The remaining edges of articular cartilage are curetted back to healthy cartilage. Ideally, the edges of the cartilage lesion should be vertical in order to allow inflow of the surrounding cartilage matrix. The subchondral bone surface is then milled using a hand drill. The surface is abraded until it readily bleeds, which can be easily observed if fluid ingress is temporarily stopped.

After complete removal of the fragments and treatment of the subchondral bone, the joint is lavaged under pressure (40–100 mmHg) for several minutes to remove any debris. Closure is then routine, using non-absorbable monofilament suture material.

The prognosis for FCP varies considerably and is probably dependent upon the severity of the disease at the time of presentation and the postoperative management of the dog. In one study, approximately 60% of dogs treated arthroscopically returned to normal function (Meyer-Lindenberg et al., 2003) without the use of analgesia, although some (25–30%) remained lame and showed progressive lameness. A more recent study by Farrell et al. (2014) showed an association between the degree of radiographic arthrosis and cartilage pathology. Elbows with severe radiographic changes were significantly more likely to have severe cartilage changes compared with elbows with a lower radiographic score. These findings can be used to determine the benefit or otherwise of arthroscopy, as the grading of cartilage alone is beneficial only if it influences the surgeon's decision about the therapeutic approach to the case. Elbow osteoarthritis may require lifelong treatment and, in very severe cases, salvage procedures may be required.

Osteochondritis dissecans

The aetiology and pathogenesis of elbow OCD is poorly understood but the condition is believed to be due to necrosis around the vascular channels in the articular–epiphyseal region, which leads to a fissure in the articular cartilage (see above). The lesion often occurs bilaterally and is seen on the weight-bearing outer surface of the centromedial portion of the humerus. OCD may be seen concurrently with FCP and/or osteoarthritis.

The presentation and diagnosis are similar to that of FCP, with radiographs demonstrating secondary osteoarthritic changes. On the craniocaudal view of the elbow, there may be a radiolucent region in the subchondral bone of the medial humeral condyle; the radiograph sometimes needs to be taken as a craniolateral–caudomedial oblique view in order to see this. The lesions seen radiographically can be subtle and, once proficiency with arthroscopy is achieved, it may be prudent to examine both elbows in one session to obtain more diagnostic information. In chronic cases, the lesion may become mineralized or be displaced and lodge in the caudomedial aspect of the joint. Occasionally, displaced bone can continue to grow, forming a linear osteochondral ossicle. Although CT is well reported to define the extent of OCD lesions, it is not necessary for diagnosis.

The dog should be positioned in lateral recumbency with the affected limb nearest the table. The authors use the same position for bilateral elbow arthroscopies and roll the dog over to the other side between examining the first and the second elbow. An alternative is to place the animal in dorsal recumbency, from which position both elbows can be examined arthroscopically. A standard medial portal, as described above, is used to examine the elbow joint and visualize the lesion. If an OCD lesion is observed (Figure 14.40) it is often adjacent to the arthroscope portal. These lesions are often large and so it is advisable to create a new arthroscope portal 1–1.5 cm caudally in these cases to see the whole lesion. Lesions may appear as a softened region of cartilage or an obvious flap.

Basic instrumentation is required to treat elbow OCD and should include a curette, a milling drill, a probe and grasping forceps. An instrument portal can be established through the original arthroscope portal using a switching stick. The authors prefer not to use an instrument cannula for cases of OCD as they can be difficult to maintain. An open portal is sufficient for the therapeutic management of elbow OCD. If the lesion is *in situ*, forceps can be

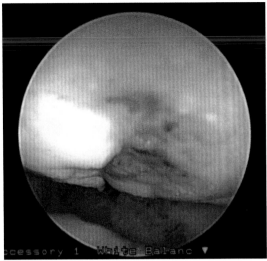

14.40 Non-displaced osteochondritis dissecans lesion of the medial humeral head of the humerus.

introduced through the instrument portal to grasp the flap. A second instrument, such as a probe or small curette, can be introduced at the same time and used to elevate the periphery of the lesion gently. Normal cartilage is difficult to remove, so minimal further damage is caused by gentle application of this technique. Once released, the flap can be removed through the portal. Some OCD lesions can be up to 15 mm across and so may need to be broken into several pieces for removal, or the portal may need to be enlarged. After removal of the fragment, the underlying subchondral bone is treated as discussed above for OCD of the shoulder. Concomitant lesions (e.g. FCP) should then be treated. The joint is lavaged for 5 minutes before closure.

The prognosis for elbow OCD, as for other causes of elbow disease, depends on the severity of the lesion. Cartilage pathology is often more severe than that seen with FCP, although the underlying subchondral bone often bleeds much more readily. This releases mesenchymal cells from the bone, and the lesions readily fill with fibrocartilage. The osteoarthritis will continue to progress despite the treatment and is often the cause of lameness seen in older animals that have undergone previous surgery. Other treatment modalities, such as autogenous osteochondral grafting, can be used in conjunction with arthroscopy for the management of this disease (Fitzpatrick *et al.*, 2009).

Ununited anconeal process

UAP is predominantly seen in German Shepherd Dogs and is also prevalent in Bloodhounds and Basset Hounds. A secondary centre of ossification exists in these three breeds, which should unite with the proximal ulna by 20 weeks of age. The use of arthroscopy for direct treatment of UAP has been described (Meyer-Lindenberg *et al.*, 2006), although its main indication is to assess the stability of the anconeus and to inspect the joint for the presence of concomitant lesions (e.g. FCP).

UAP is readily diagnosable from a flexed mediolateral radiograph of the elbow (Figure 14.41). Animals should be at least 20 weeks old before a definitive diagnosis can be made. A radiolucent line is seen between the proximal ulna and the anconeus, and there are often signs of secondary osteoarthritic changes. Arthrocentesis may reveal an effusion similar to that seen in other causes of elbow dysplasia, that is, an increased volume of fluid with low

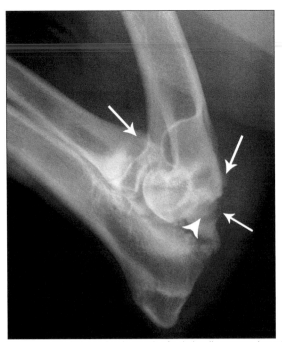

14.41 Mediolateral radiograph of a skeletally mature dog with ununited anconeal process (arrowhead) and secondary osteoarthritis. Osteophytes are denoted by the arrows.

viscosity. Cell counts are approximately 2000–5000 cells/µl and there is a predominance of mononuclear cells.

Medical and surgical options exist for the treatment of UAP, although medical treatment is often unsuccessful. Surgical options include proximal ulnar osteotomy (PUO) (Sjöström *et al.*, 1995) with or without an intramedullary pin (Turner *et al.*, 1998), PUO combined with lag screw fixation of the anconeus (Krotscheck *et al.*, 2000) or fragment removal (Guthrie, 1989). Lag screw fixation of the anconeal process can be via arthrotomy or arthroscopy. Lag screw fixation in conjunction with a PUO has been shown to achieve radiographic evidence of union of the anconeal process to the ulna in 84% of dogs (Pettitt *et al.*, 2009). Arthroscopy can be used to view the fragment (Figure 14.42) during tightening of the compression screw, but its other role is to diagnose and treat concomitant lesions.

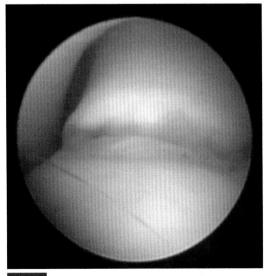

14.42 A non-displaced ununited anconeal process.

The portal sites for surgical exploration and treatment of UAP are as for other causes of elbow dysplasia. In most cases a 2.4 mm, 30-degree oblique arthroscope is suitable. A full exploration of the joint is performed initially and the authors prefer to treat any other lesions first. After this, the UAP is palpated to assess its stability, using a caudal instrument portal. This is established approximately 1 cm caudal to the arthroscope portal in the same way as described previously for other portals. The authors usually leave the egress needle caudal as well, although if this interferes with the procedure the egress portal can easily be re-established cranially.

For arthroscopic placement of the lag screw, a small Kirschner wire is initially placed from the caudal ulna through the fibrous tissue and into the anconeal process, until it is visualized exiting the process. This is very important to ensure the subsequent correct placement of the lag screw. It is very easy for the Kirschner wire to exit the fragment laterally and not be seen. It is preferable to over-drill the Kirschner wire with a 2.5 mm cannulated drill bit to ensure the same track is followed. If a cannulated bit is not available, a second Kirschner wire should be placed parallel to the first one but 5 mm caudally. The initial wire can then be removed and a 2.0 mm drill bit used to create the pilot hole for the screw. The authors prefer to use a 3.5 mm cortical screw, placed in lag fashion. Following screw placement, a PUO is performed. This last procedure is recommended if a lag screw has been placed, to prevent breakage of the screw due to shearing forces.

Distal ulnar osteotomy has been reported as an alternative to PUO. Placement of the pin to stabilize the osteotomy is at the discretion of the surgeon; it does reduce the morbidity of the surgery in the short term but is associated with complications of its own.

The prognosis for UAP is better than that for OCD/FCP provided the condition is treated early. In one study of 20 dogs (22 joints), 70% of cases had an excellent outcome (Sjöström et al., 1995). Secondary osteoarthritis will continue to progress and may result in lameness as the dog ages.

Elbow osteoarthritis

Arthroscopy is a useful tool for the staging of osteoarthritis (Figure 14.43). The modified Outerbridge scale can be used to grade the severity of articular cartilage loss and this can be useful in formulating a treatment plan.

The use of arthroscopy for the management of osteoarthritis has been a controversial subject for many years. Arthroscopic debridement involves using instruments to remove damaged cartilage or bone combined with lavage or 'washout'. Outcome studies in canine osteoarthritis are not available, but in recent years randomized controlled trials have been performed in human medicine that show that arthroscopic debridement does not provide positive benefits for knee osteoarthritis. In a Cochrane review, Laupattarakasem et al. (2008) conclude that there is 'gold' level evidence that arthroscopic debridement provides no benefit for osteoarthritis resulting from mechanical or inflammatory causes. Therefore, at the current time, the authors do not recommend arthroscopic debridement for the management of canine elbow osteoarthritis.

Humeral intracondylar fissure

HIF, also known as incomplete ossification of the humeral condyle, is predominantly reported in spaniels (Marcellin-Little et al., 1994; Butterworth and Innes, 2001) and Labrador Retrievers, although many other breeds may be affected. Although initially proposed as a failure of the two centres of the humeral condyle to fuse, recent reports of fissures appearing in previously intact humeral condyles, as observed by CT, have cast doubt on this hypothesis. The term 'humeral intracondylar fissure' is a more neutral description of the lesion. Although the failure of ossification is still a possible explanation for some cases, fatigue fracture of the humeral condyle is another possible aetiology.

Diagnosis is possible with a craniocaudal radiograph of the elbow, although multiple slightly angled views may be needed before observation of the radiolucent defect is possible. A slight increase in the kV setting is often necessary. On plain radiography, care must be taken not to confuse HIF with the Mac Band that is often seen in rotated craniocaudal views of the elbow joint. CT is more sensitive for identifying HIF. The lesion is evident as an articular cartilage defect that traverses the central region of the humeral condyle (Figure 14.44). Careful palpation of this region is very important, especially in cases where HIF is suspected but not evident arthroscopically. Occasionally, the surface of the cartilage appears normal but palpation exposes a defect that would otherwise be overlooked.

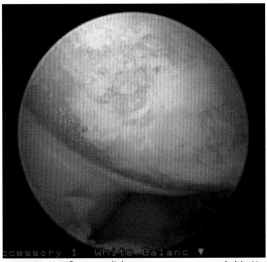

14.43 Significant medial compartment osteoarthritis. Note the distinct demarcation between the medial and lateral compartments of the joint.

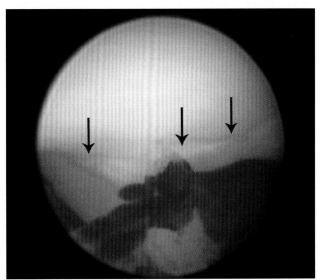

14.44 Humeral intracondylar fissure. A circumferential cartilage defect (arrowed) can be seen clearly in the centre of the humeral condyle.

Arthroscopy is also used in cases of HIF to assess for concomitant lesions and can be used for intraoperative assessment of screw placement to confirm that the screw is not placed intra-articularly. Fluoroscopy provides an alternative intraoperative technique to confirm implant placement, and aiming devices are also useful to help place the screw accurately.

As described previously, a medial portal is used to examine the elbow joint and treat any obvious lesions. If arthroscopy is used for intraoperative assessment the arthroscope can be left *in situ* while another surgeon places the transcondylar screw, or it can be removed from the joint and then replaced after the screw has been inserted to assess screw placement.

The antebrachiocarpal joint

The carpus is a three-level hinge (ginglymus) joint. Only the antebrachiocarpal joint is accessible to arthroscopic inspection; the other joints are low-motion joints with insufficient space for arthroscopy. Carpal arthroscopy is performed infrequently, but the radiocarpal joint is amenable to arthroscopic examination and there are occasions when arthroscopic examination may be beneficial for patient management. These include the assessment of intra-articular fractures, such as radiocarpal bone fracture (Li *et al.*, 2000), assessment of soft tissue injuries, grading of arthritis and synovial biopsy. Diagnosis of carpal ligamentous injuries in racing Greyhounds is another potential indication for arthroscopy. Because the carpus is often involved in inflammatory joint disease, it is a good location for performing arthroscopic synovial biopsy if required.

Instrumentation

For medium-sized and large dogs a 2.4 mm, 30-degree oblique arthroscope is preferred. For small dogs and cats, a 1.9 mm arthroscope is mandatory. Small instrumentation is required for all patients.

Patient preparation and positioning

The limb is clipped from just proximal to the main pad to the mid-antebrachium. The foot is covered in an impervious barrier, such as a plastic bag or surgical glove, which is taped in place. The patient is positioned in dorsal recumbency with the limb suspended. The limb is free draped to allow it to be manipulated intraoperatively.

Procedure

The arthroscope portal is placed between the common digital extensor tendon laterally and the extensor carpi radialis tendon medially (Figure 14.45, site A1). The egress portal can be placed lateral to the common digital extensor tendon (Figure 14.45, site A2). Because there is limited working space in the carpus, if instruments are required, they are placed at the egress portal site.

The procedure is started with the placement of a hypodermic needle at the arthroscope portal site, with the carpus in full flexion to open the antebrachiocarpal joint space. The needle should enter the radiocarpal joint space easily. The joint is inflated with 2–5 ml of lactated Ringer's solution and the needle is withdrawn. A stab incision is made with a No. 11 scalpel blade at the arthroscope portal site and should be extended to enter the joint capsule. The blade should be oriented vertically

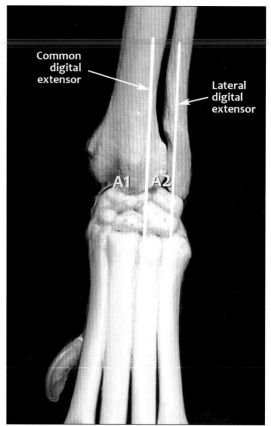

14.45 Model demonstrating the position of portals for carpal arthroscopy. A1 and A2 represent alternative suggested arthroscope portal sites.

to avoid damage to the tendinous structures either side of the portal. The arthroscope sleeve is inserted with a blunt obturator in place. The obturator is then removed and the arthroscope inserted.

Arthroscopic anatomy

Upon entering the joint, the radial articular surface is seen at 12 o'clock, with the radiocarpal bone at 6 o'clock (Figure 14.46). The arthroscope may be moved left or right to inspect the joint surfaces. If the joint is extended slightly and the arthroscope inserted further, the palmar joint capsule can be observed.

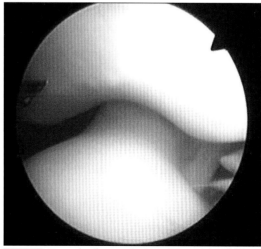

14.46 Normal arthroscopic view of the antebrachial carpal joint. The radius is at the top, with the radiocarpal bone below.

Pathological conditions

The carpus is a complex hinge joint, stabilized medially and laterally by collateral ligaments. Palmar stability is provided by flexor tendons, the palmar radiocarpal and ulnocarpal ligaments and the palmar fibrocartilage. This latter structure is critical and failure results in a palmigrade stance. The radiocarpal bone develops as two separate centres of ossification and there can occasionally be incomplete ossification of this bone, resulting in susceptibility to fracture. This is noted particularly in Boxers (Li *et al.*, 2000). Figures 14.47 and 14.48 illustrate some pathological conditions of the carpal joint.

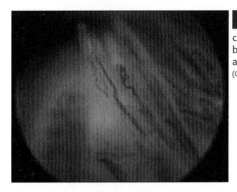

14.47 Cases of severe carpal synovitis can be investigated arthroscopically. (Courtesy of J Cook)

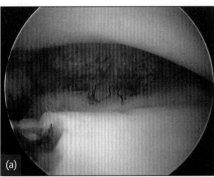

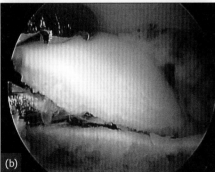

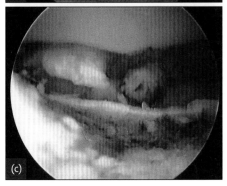

14.48 Carpal chip fracture. (a) Fracture *in situ*. (b) Fragment being removed using 2.7 mm grasping forceps. (c) The carpal defect in the subchondral bone following debridement with a power shaver. (Courtesy of J Cook)

The hip joint

Arthroscopy of the hip is not performed commonly but is very achievable for the experienced arthroscopist. The hip is a common site of lameness in dogs, with hip dysplasia and osteoarthritis being particularly common. Hip dysplasia is usually diagnosed using a combination of clinical and radiographic examinations, as is osteoarthritis. While arthroscopy of the hip can be used to stage osteoarthritis accurately, currently this is not usually performed. However, there is no doubt that arthroscopy is a more sensitive method for identifying the early changes associated with osteoarthritis, such as chondropathy and synovitis.

Indications

Indications for hip arthroscopy include:

- Idiopathic hip pain in the absence of radiographic changes
- Biopsy of the synovium
- Staging of osteoarthritis, e.g. during decision-making for triple pelvic osteotomy (TPO)
- Diagnosis and treatment of infective arthritis of the hip.

Instrumentation

The choice of arthroscope is dependent on patient size. In large dogs, a long 2.7 mm, 30-degree oblique arthroscope is used. A 2.4 mm arthroscope should be considered in small-breed dogs. Although a 1.9 mm arthroscope could also be used in small dogs, this arthroscope is very fragile and the operator must be very careful not to damage it through bending it in the soft tissues between the skin and the joint. Instruments required for arthroscopy of the hip include probes, cannulae, a switching stick and synovial biopsy forceps.

Patient preparation and positioning

The dog is placed in lateral recumbency, with the affected limb uppermost. To facilitate movement of the joint and limb during arthroscopy, a hanging limb preparation is recommended. The lower limb is covered with a sterile impervious drape.

Procedure

Portal placement

Portals for the hip were originally described by Person (1989b). If one considers the hip as a clock face, for the right hip, the egress cannula is placed at 5 o'clock and the arthroscope portal at 12 o'clock. Should an instrument portal be required, this is placed at 2 o'clock (Figure 14.49). For the left hip, these portal positions are mirrored: the egress cannula is placed at 7 o'clock, the arthroscope portal at 12 o'clock and the instrument portal at 10 o'clock.

The egress portal is established with a 20 G, 40–50 mm hypodermic needle, depending on patient size. The needle is placed immediately cranial to the greater trochanter in a similar position to that used for arthrocentesis. Often the surgeon will feel the needle puncture the joint capsule. Aspiration may produce some synovial fluid but there is often minimal joint fluid in the hip. The joint is then distended with lactated Ringer's solution (typically 4–8 ml is used).

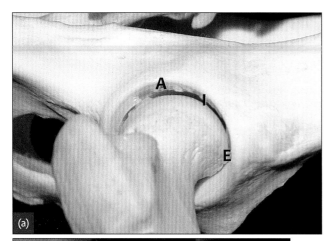

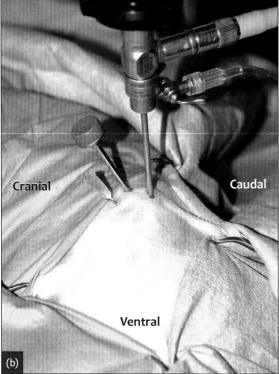

14.49 (a) Model demonstrating the position of portals for right hip arthroscopy. A = arthroscope portal; E = egress portal; I = instrument portal. (b) Clinical arthroscopy of the left hip (dorsal surface is uppermost; head is to the left).

femur. The teres (round) ligament of the femoral head can also be viewed as it emerges from the acetabular fossa and inserts on the femoral head. The acetabulum is otherwise covered in hyaline cartilage and also has a fibrocartilage extension dorsally, called the labrum. The joint capsule extends from the margins of the acetabulum to the femoral neck. Normal anatomy is depicted in Figure 14.50.

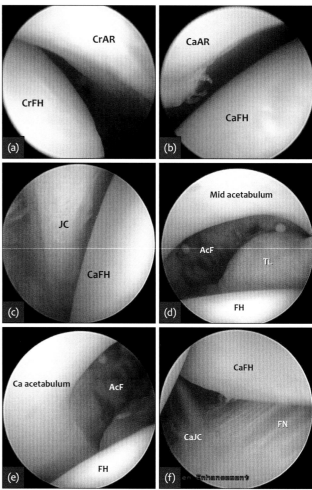

14.50 Normal arthroscopic anatomy of the right coxofemoral joint. (a) Normal cranial aspect of the femoral head and acetabulum on the abaxial side. (b) Normal caudal aspect of the femoral head and acetabulum on the abaxial side. (c) Normal joint capsule and caudal femoral head. (d) Normal Teres ligament insertion into the acetabular fossa. (e) Normal caudal femoral head and acetabulum on the axial side. (f) Normal joint capsule as it inserts caudally on the femoral neck. AcF = acetabular fossa; CaAR = caudal acetabular rim; CaFH = caudal femoral head; CaJC = Caudal joint capsule; CrAR = cranial acetabular rim; CrFH = cranial femoral head; FH = femoral head; FN = femoral neck; JC = joint capsule; TL = teres (round) ligament.

The arthroscope portal is then established. A 20 G, 40–50 mm hypodermic needle is used to locate the correct position for the portal, using a 'trial and error' approach, making sure that the selected location will allow movement of the arthroscope circumferentially from 9 o'clock to 3 o'clock. Once the desired location is found, a No. 11 blade is placed alongside the needle and used to make a stab incision down to the joint capsule. The arthroscope sleeve, with a blunt obturator in place, is then inserted into the capsule. The obturator is removed and the surgeon should observe fluid egress from the open sleeve, confirming the intra-articular position of the end of the sleeve. The arthroscope is then inserted.

Arthroscopic anatomy

The hip is a ball and socket joint. External and internal rotation of the femoral head during arthroscopy can allow inspection of the majority of the articular surface of the

Pathological conditions
Hip dysplasia

It is not currently widespread practice to evaluate the hip joints of dogs with hip dysplasia arthroscopically. Holsworth et al. (2005) reported the use of arthroscopy to evaluate young dogs with hip laxity and pain, which were being considered for procedures such as TPO; traditional opinion has indicated that dogs with pre-existing osteoarthritis should not be considered for TPO. The results of this study indicate that arthroscopy is more sensitive than radiography for the detection of intra-articular pathology. However, the significance of the arthroscopically identified lesions with respect to the outcome of TPO is not known. Nevertheless, this study indicated that arthroscopy is a sensitive method for evaluation of the hip joint.

Idiopathic hip pain

Occasionally a dog will present with apparent hip pain but the hip joints appear normal on radiography. The authors have seen a few patients with this presentation and have used arthroscopy for further evaluation. In a proportion of these dogs, chondropathy and synovitis have been identified. This again illustrates the sensitivity of arthroscopy for the detection of intra-articular pathology and indicates that a small number of dogs may develop osteoarthritic changes in the hip without apparent osteophytosis on plain radiographs. However, this scenario appears to be unusual and less common than in the elbow joint.

Radiographically silent hip pain

Minimally displaced acetabular fractures or soft tissue injuries of the hip may also be diagnosed using arthroscopy (Figure 14.51).

Other uses

Occasionally the clinician may need to biopsy the synovium of the hip joint (e.g. in cases of suspected infective or immune-mediated arthritis, suspected neoplasia and osteochondromatosis), and this can be done arthroscopically. However, the need for such a procedure is very uncommon.

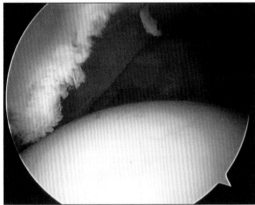

14.51 Mildly displaced acetabular fracture with concomitant labral tear.
(Courtesy of J Cook)

The stifle joint

Arthroscopy of the knee is the most common orthopaedic intervention in human surgery. However, the canine stifle is a challenging joint for the inexperienced arthroscopist, as it is relatively small and dogs are prone to proliferative synovitis once the stifle becomes diseased. This hyperplastic synovium (Figure 14.52) obscures the surgeon's view and can be problematical and frustrating. The infrapatellar fat pad can also obscure the viewing window. For these reasons, inexperienced arthroscopists are advised to master their skills in the shoulder and elbow before attempting stifle arthroscopy. That said, stifle arthroscopy is now established as a standard procedure for many orthopaedic surgeons.

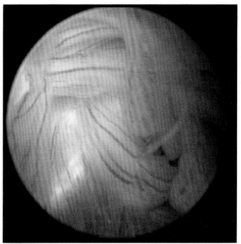

14.52 Hyperplastic synovium. This may need to be removed in order to visualize the intra-articular structures.

Indications

The stifle is the most common site of lameness in dogs. Many conditions of the stifle can be diagnosed arthroscopically, and a growing number can also be treated using arthroscopic techniques. Conditions that can be diagnosed arthroscopically include:

* CCL injury
* Medial meniscal injury
* Lateral meniscal injury
* Osteoarthritis and chondropathy
* OCD
* Patellar luxation
* Long digital extensor tendon avulsion
* Caudal cruciate ligament injury
* Popliteal tendon avulsion.

Instrumentation

For very small dogs and cats a 1.9 mm arthroscope is used, and for small dogs a 2.4 mm arthroscope works well. However, for the majority of patients, which are medium-sized to large dogs, a 2.7 mm arthroscope is used. In large and giant breeds some surgeons use a 4 mm arthroscope. The larger arthroscopes have the advantage of a greater depth of field and the ability to provide greater irrigation, both of which are important in stifle arthroscopy.

It is very useful to have a fluid pump for stifle arthroscopy because the volumes of fluid used can be large and positive pressure can facilitate a clear viewing window. An egress cannula is also very useful. In larger dogs, the authors prefer to use disposable plastic cannulae with a threaded exterior surface (Figure 14.53). These cannulae are atraumatic and retain their position in the joint even during flexion and extension. They also have side holes in the tip, which avoid blockage by soft tissues, and an on/off switch to allow joint distension under increased pressure. Smooth-surfaced cannulae tend to displace from the joint during manipulation. The cannula should be attached to a suction tube to collect fluid.

Some surgeons find a power shaver system very useful in the stifle joint to debride the infrapatellar fat pad and hyperplastic synovium. An aggressive full-radius cutting blade of an appropriate size is used in oscillating mode at 3000 rpm. Suction tubing is connected to the shaver handpiece to facilitate entry of synovial tissue into the blade tip during the pause between oscillations.

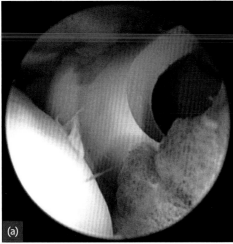

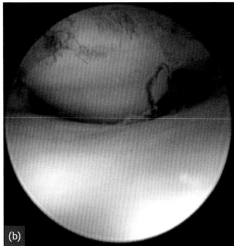

14.53 (a) Placement of a disposable plastic egress cannula into the proximolateral pouch of the stifle. (b) Femoropatellar joint space with the patella above. The egress cannula can just be seen on the left side of the image.

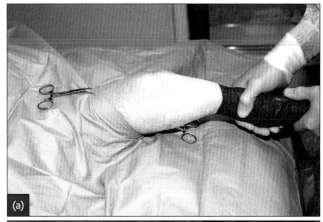

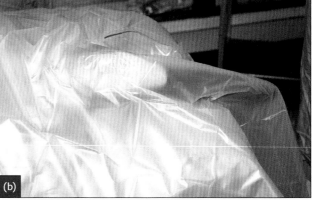

14.54 (a) Stifle prepared and draped for arthroscopy. (b) Impermeable plastic drape used to prevent breakdown of asepsis.

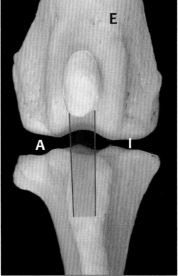

14.55 Model demonstrating the position of portals for stifle arthroscopy.
A = arthroscope portal;
E = egress portal;
I = instrument portal.

Particular additional hand instruments can be useful in the stifle joint. Small joint punches can be useful for removing synovium, fat pad, cruciate ligament remnants and meniscal tissue. Some models also have a suction portal to facilitate the removal of resected tissue.

A bipolar or monopolar radiofrequency unit can also be very useful in the stifle joint, but must be used with caution. The probe can be used to remove hyperplastic synovium and has the advantage of simultaneous haemostasis during use. Some surgeons use an electrosurgery unit for haemostasis. Other probe heads can be used to cut or remove meniscal tissue or debride a torn CCL.

Patient preparation and positioning

The operative limb is clipped from the level of the proximal crus to just above the tarsus. The foot and distal limb are covered with an impervious barrier (Figure 14.54) and the limb is suspended for aseptic preparation. The patient is positioned in dorsal recumbency, with the limb upwards.

Procedure

Portal placement

The main portals for the stifle joint are craniomedial and craniolateral either side of the patellar ligament (Figure 14.55). Some surgeons prefer to create these portals at the

distal end of the patellar ligament, but the authors prefer to site the portals at the midpoint of the patellar ligament. The portal placement can have a significant effect on the immediate viewing window for the surgeon, with lower portal sites necessitating more resection of the fat pad. The egress portal is placed either proximolaterally or proximomedially, using a push-through technique.

The procedure is started by distending the joint with 5–20 ml of lactated Ringer's solution using a hypodermic needle and syringe. For the craniomedial portal, a stab incision is made using a No. 11 scalpel blade. The blade is oriented vertically to avoid damage to the patellar ligament.

A switching stick is placed into the portal and into the joint space. With the joint in full extension, the switching stick is pushed through the femoropatellar joint space to exit the joint capsule proximolaterally. The stick is pushed so that it protrudes and causes the skin to tent. A scalpel blade is then used to cut down on the stick, and the stick is pushed through the incision to exit the skin. The egress cannula is then placed over the stick and pushed into the joint. Once the cannula tip is in the joint, the stick is removed to leave the cannula in place. The cannula can then be positioned in the lateral joint space adjacent to the lateral femoral condyle and the long digital extensor tendon of origin.

The arthroscope sleeve, with a blunt obturator in place, is then inserted into the craniomedial portal. Once in the joint, the obturator is removed and the arthroscope is inserted.

A craniolateral portal is also established as an instrument portal. This is achieved with a stab incision made using a No. 11 blade. The arthroscope and instrument portals are interchangeable, and it is common for the surgeon to swap back and forth during a procedure to obtain the optimal positions for the arthroscope and instruments.

Arthroscopic anatomy

The stifle is a complex hinge joint. Although it acts primarily as a hinge joint, the menisci allow the femoral condyle to glide during movement so that the axis of rotation varies with the degree of flexion. The femoropatellar joint space is best viewed with the joint in extension because this releases tension on the quadriceps mechanism. The femorotibial joint is best viewed in flexion. The stifle has several significant soft tissue structures, including the CCL, the caudal cruciate ligament, the menisci and the origin of the long digital extensor tendon (Figure 14.56).

The CCL (Figure 14.57) originates on the caudolateral intercondylar region of the femur and runs distally, cranially and medially to insert on the craniomedial tibial plateau. The caudal cruciate ligament originates on the craniolateral intercondylar region of the femur and runs distally, caudally and laterally to insert on the caudolateral tibial plateau.

The menisci are attached to each other by the cranial intermeniscal ligament, and each meniscus is attached to the tibia by the cranial and caudal meniscotibial ligaments. The medial meniscus (Figure 14.58) has an additional attachment to the medial collateral ligament.

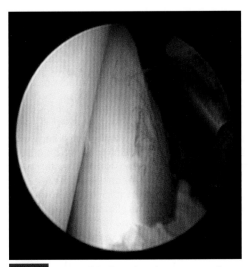

14.56 Origin of the long digital extensor tendon.

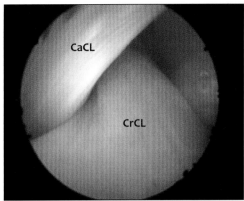

14.57 Normal cruciate ligament. CaCL = caudal cruciate ligament; CrCL = cranial cruciate ligament.

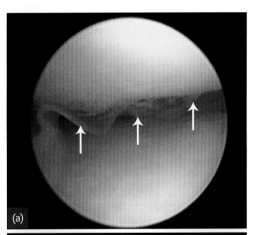

(a)

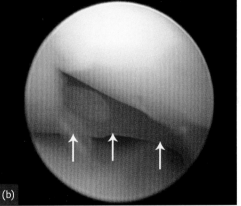

(b)

14.58 (a) Flounce of the normal medial meniscus (arrowed). (b) Normal medial meniscus (arrowed).

Pathological conditions
Cranial cruciate ligament injury

CCL injury is the most common pathology of the stifle joint and probably the most common orthopaedic problem of dogs that requires surgical intervention. The CCL has three functions: to limit internal rotation of the tibia with respect to the femur, to limit cranial translation of the tibia and to limit hyperextension of the stifle joint. While many cases of CCL injury result in overt instability of the stifle joint with a positive cranial drawer test, a considerable number involve either partial tearing of the CCL or insidious pathology that can be compensated for by periarticular fibrosis. Therefore, there may not be an obvious cranial drawer sign and the clinician may require confirmation of CCL rupture.

Although some other imaging modalities, such as MRI and ultrasonography, can help in this respect, arthroscopy probably has the highest sensitivity and specificity for CCL injury. The CCL is readily inspected arthroscopically but should also be probed with a blunt hooked probe to ensure torn fibres are not missed.

Following CCL injury, particularly complete rupture, the menisci are at risk from degeneration and tearing. The medial meniscus is torn in 40–60% of stifle joints with complete CCL rupture. The lateral meniscus rarely sustains clinically important injury, although minor injuries are common.

The medial meniscus may sustain a variety of types of tear (Bennett and May, 1991), some of which appear to be more important than others in terms of the pain caused to the patient. The most important medial meniscal pathology seems to be a fold of the caudal horn of the medial meniscus (Figure 14.59). In reality, this is a bucket handle tear in which the majority of the caudal horn of the medial meniscus forms the 'bucket handle' and a small peripheral portion of the caudal horn remains *in situ*. The caudal horn injury allows a significant section of meniscal tissue to be mobile within the joint. During the stance phase of the gait cycle this meniscal tissue can become displaced and trapped, causing pain.

Arthroscopic inspection of the menisci requires some practice. The arthroscope is positioned in the medial or lateral femorotibial joint space and the light post is oriented medially or laterally, respectively. The joint is flexed to bring the menisci into view. The menisci should be probed, paying particular attention to the caudal horn of the medial meniscus to ensure that it is secure and not torn (Pozzi *et al.*, 2008). In addition, flexion and extension of the joint while inspecting the menisci can be useful to check meniscal stability.

A caudal horn tear of the medial meniscus can be removed under arthroscopic guidance. The authors use a variety of techniques to achieve this, depending on the exact pathology and the size of the patient. In larger joints, the loose meniscal tissue can be grasped with forceps while small hook and push knives are used to transect each limb of the 'bucket handle'. Alternatively, small punches can be used to resect meniscal tissue in 'bite-sized' pieces. In smaller patients, forceps can be used to remove small pieces of meniscal tissue by grasping and rotating the forceps; repeating this manoeuvre several times can remove the desired amount of tissue. Alternatively, a power shaver can be used to remove meniscal tissue, although care must be taken to avoid iatrogenic damage to the surrounding tissues. Smaller axial tears can be treated using arthroscopic forceps, a punch or a shaver.

Arthroscopic medial meniscal transection

Some surgeons prefer to perform medial meniscal transection in conjunction with surgical treatment for CCL injury. This technique can reduce the incidence of subsequent meniscal injury, but it does destroy meniscal function and means that the dog will inevitably develop more osteoarthritis. Nevertheless, there may be instances when the procedure can be justifiable, such as in an older dog where the client wishes to avoid the future risk of meniscal tearing but is not as concerned the about longer-term consequences of loss of meniscal function. It is possible to perform this technique by inserting a hypodermic needle into the medial joint immediately caudal to the medial collateral ligament under arthroscopic guidance. Once the hypodermic needle is in the desired location, a No. 11 scalpel blade is guided alongside this needle, oriented in a proximodistal direction to avoid medial collateral ligament damage. The blade can be viewed arthroscopically as it enters the joint, and the medial meniscus is then sectioned.

Osteochondritis dissecans

OCD occurs in the stifle in medium-sized to large dogs, but is uncommon. The lesion is usually located on either the medial (Figure 14.60) or the lateral femoral condyle. Dogs with stifle OCD typically present with lameness at 4–6 months of age, with associated stifle joint effusion. Flattening of the femoral condyle is usually visible radiographically. Arthroscopic confirmation of the diagnosis is usually straightforward, although some cases have extreme synovial hyperplasia, which can limit the viewing window. The use of a power shaver or radiofrequency unit to remove excessive synovium may assist the surgeon to obtain a suitable viewing window.

Arthroscopic treatment of OCD lesions is achieved through a combination of craniomedial and craniolateral portals, with the arthroscope and instruments positioned in the respective portals to suit the location of the lesion.

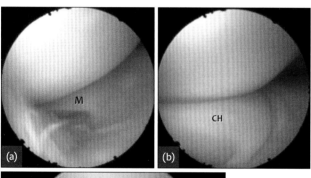
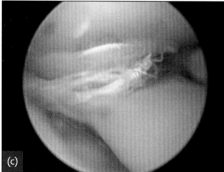
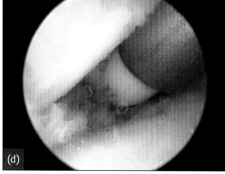

14.59 Medial meniscal caudal horn fold. (a) The meniscus (M) appears normal until the joint is flexed. (b) After the stifle is flexed, the caudal horn (CH) is folded cranially. (c,d) Treatment with radiofrequency ablation.

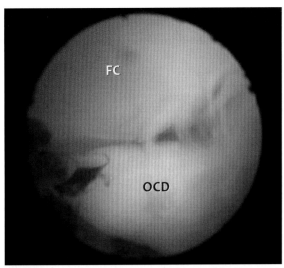

14.60 *In situ* stifle osteochondritis dissecans (OCD) lesion of the medial trochlear ridge. FC = femoral condyle.

The cartilage flap is removed either as a single piece or in smaller pieces, using suitably sized grasping forceps. Following removal of the flap, the subchondral defect is subjected to light curettage of the margins and/or forage (subchondral drilling) of the defect base. The latter is aimed at allowing migration of pluripotent mesenchymal cells through the subchondral bed to form fibrocartilaginous repair tissue in the defect. This can be achieved by a micropick technique or by drilling small holes with a Kirschner wire (e.g. 0.9–1.1 mm); either technique can be performed under arthroscopic guidance.

Arthroscopically assisted CCL surgery

Arthroscopic treatment of CCL rupture has not yet become widely established in veterinary surgery. In humans, a common technique is to use either a graft of bone–patellar ligament–bone (B–PL–B) taken from the middle third of the patellar ligament or a hamstring tendon graft, and to place this in a minimally invasive fashion under arthroscopic guidance. The smaller size of dogs has limited such an approach, although B–PL–B allografts have been used and placed arthroscopically.

Arthroscopically assisted suture stabilization has been reported for the treatment of canine CCL injury. The technique appears to have acceptable results, from the limited published information, and the authors have used this technique in small, medium-sized and large dogs. However, the arthroscopic part of the surgery is the inspection of the joint and the diagnosis and treatment of meniscal lesions, before a lateral suture stabilization performed through limited incisions but without the need for arthroscopic assistance.

The talocrural joint (tarsus)

The tarsus is a composite multiple joint consisting of four separate joints. Only the talocrural joint is accessible to arthroscopic inspection, and this allows a slightly limited examination of the articular surfaces of the tibia, fibula and talus. In addition, part of the calcaneus and deep digital flexor tendon can be viewed.

Indications
Indications for talocrural arthroscopy include:

- OCD of the medial talar ridge
- OCD of the lateral talar ridge
- OCD of the distal tibia
- Infective arthritis
- Synovial biopsy.

Instrumentation
The talocrural joint is a small and rather superficial space and thus a small arthroscope (1.9 or 2.4 mm) is required. Small hand instruments are also required for any operative arthroscopy.

Patient preparation and positioning
The limb is clipped from the mid-tibia to just above the main pad. The foot is covered in an impervious layer and a hanging limb preparation is performed. Bilateral talocrural arthroscopy is possible and may be indicated in some patients (e.g. those with bilateral talar OCD). Positioning of the patient depends on the portal selection. The patient may be positioned in ventral (with plantar portals) or dorsal (with dorsal portals) recumbency, or occasionally a hanging limb position (with all portals) may be utilized.

Procedure
There are four traditional portals for the talocrural joint: dorsolateral, dorsomedial, plantarolateral and plantaromedial (Figure 14.61). These can be used in combination, although rarely all at once. Portal selection is dependent on the suspected lesion and is often directed by the results of preoperative imaging. For example, plain radiographs or CT scans may reveal that an OCD lesion is located more dorsally on the medial ridge of the talus; in such a case, the dorsal portals are utilized. However, if the lesion is more plantar, the plantar portals are selected.

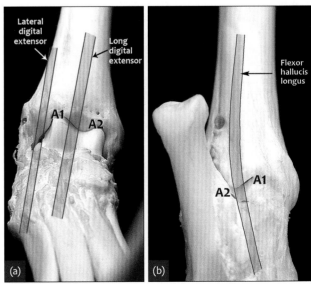

14.61 Models demonstrating portals for tarsal arthroscopy. (a) Dorsal tarsal portals; (b) plantar tarsal portals. A1 and A2 represent alternative suggested arthroscope portal sites.

Dorsal portals

The patient is placed in dorsal recumbency with the pelvic limb extended caudally. The talocrural joint space is located dorsally by palpation and 'trial and error' use of a 23 G hypodermic needle. Once the joint space is located optimally, synovial fluid is aspirated and submitted for analysis if required. The joint is inflated with 3–8 ml of lactated Ringer's solution. A No. 11 scalpel blade is then used to make a proximodistally oriented stab incision at the location of the hypodermic needle. The arthroscope sleeve, with a blunt obturator in place, is inserted into the joint and the obturator is then removed and the arthroscope inserted.

An instrument portal is established in the opposing dorsal portal position. A narrow-gauge hypodermic needle is used initially to locate the optimal portal location before making a proximodistally oriented stab incision to the depth of the capsule. Only small instruments can be used and a cannula is not recommended in such a superficial joint cavity.

Plantar portals

The patient is placed in ventral recumbency with the pelvic limb extended caudally. The patient needs to be supported with several sandbags or a cradle to allow the joint to be oriented such that the os calcis is directed towards the ceiling.

The talocrural joint space is located from a plantar direction (medially or laterally depending on which portal is required for the arthroscope) by palpation and 'trial and error' use of a 23 G hypodermic needle. Once the joint space is located optimally, synovial fluid is aspirated and submitted for analysis if required. The joint is then inflated with 3–8 ml of lactated Ringer's solution. A No. 11 scalpel blade is then used to make a proximodistally oriented stab incision at the location of the hypodermic needle. The arthroscope sleeve, with a blunt obturator in place, is inserted into the joint and the obturator is then removed before insertion of the arthroscope.

An instrument portal is established in the opposing plantar portal position. A narrow-gauge hypodermic needle is used initially to locate the optimal portal location before a proximodistally oriented stab incision is made to the depth of the capsule.

> **WARNING**
>
> One of the major problems of talocrural arthroscopy is the small articular space and the superficial nature of the joint cavity. It is very easy for the arthroscope to slip out of the joint cavity and cause leakage of extracapsular fluid and consequent joint collapse

Arthroscopic anatomy

The talocrural joint may be viewed from a plantar or dorsal perspective but both give only a limited view of the articular surfaces. Little more than the articular surfaces can be inspected because of the tightness and congruity of the joint. Some parts of the joint capsule can also be seen and, from the plantaromedial portal, a portion of the deep digital flexor tendon can be seen.

Pathological conditions
Osteochondritis dissecans of the medial talar ridge

Careful evaluation of radiographs or CT scans is a prerequisite to arthroscopy of the talocrural joint for OCD of the talus. The location of the lesion in a dorsoplantar direction will guide the surgeon's selection of portals and patient positioning.

For dorsally located lesions, the dorsal portals are selected. The arthroscope is placed dorsolaterally and used to inspect the joint dorsally before settling on a view of the medially located lesion. A dorsomedial instrument portal is established, and small grasping forceps are used to grasp pieces of the loose cartilage and bone. For more plantar lesions, the plantar portals are selected but the general approach is similar.

In cases of talar OCD, the lesions can contain a significant amount of bone and can be relatively large (Figure 14.62). Although the bone is often necrotic and therefore rather soft, it can still be difficult to grasp with small forceps, or the forceps may be placed under excessive strain, risking damage to or breakage of the pin within the instrument. It is sometimes necessary to perform a limited arthrotomy to remove such large fragments.

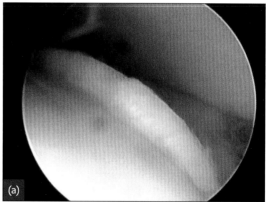

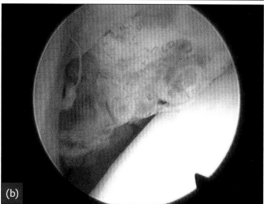

14.62 (a) *In situ* osteochondritis dissecans (OCD) lesion on the lateral trochlear ridge. (b) Synovitis secondary to an OCD lesion. The deep digital flexor tendon is to the left and the lateral trochlear ridge is to the right.
(Courtesy of B Van Ryssen)

Osteochondritis dissecans of the lateral talar ridge

This is an uncommon condition that is noted very occasionally, particularly in the Rottweiler (Gielen *et al.*, 2005). The approach to arthroscopic inspection and treatment is as for medially located lesions, although the positions of the arthroscope and instrument portals are reversed.

Synovial biopsy

Synovial biopsy can be performed using any of the portals, although the authors prefer the plantar portals as they provide greater access to synovial tissue. Tarsal osteoarthritis is a sequela to primary tarsal pathology. Arthroscopy allows this to be graded and also allows cartilage debridement when indicated (Figure 14.63).

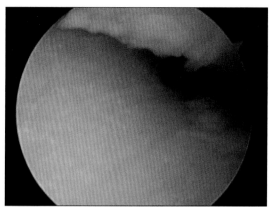

14.63 Tarsal osteoarthritis with full-thickness cartilage loss and two visible wear lines.

Other conditions

In addition to the uses described above, arthroscopy can be useful as an adjunct to treating other conditions.

Sepsis

In cases of non-responsive septic arthritis (Figure 14.64) it is possible to flush a joint with a significant volume of fluid in a relatively short period of time, using a fast flow system under high pressure. Synovial biopsy specimens can be taken at the same time and then submitted for culture.

Fractures

It is possible, although sometimes impractical, to use arthroscopy to assess fracture alignment. In cases of humeral condylar fractures (or the treatment of HIF) where the joint may have been examined arthroscopically before fracture repair, it is feasible to examine the joint again at the time of screw placement to ensure that the articular surface is not displaced.

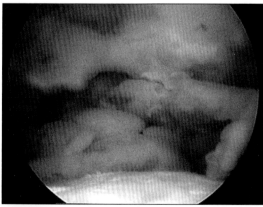

14.64 Septic arthritis in the hip of a dog presented for total hip replacement.
(Courtesy of J Cook)

Acknowledgements

The authors are indebted to Mr Alan Bannister of the Faculty of Veterinary Science, University of Liverpool, for his valuable assistance with the preparation of many of the figures in this chapter.

References and further reading

Arthurs G, Brown G and Pettitt R (2018) *BSAVA Manual of Canine and Feline Musculoskeletal Disorders, 2nd edn*. BSAVA Publications, Gloucester

Bennett D and May C (1991) Meniscal damage associated with cruciate disease in the dog. *Journal of Small Animal Practice* **32**, 111–117

Butterworth SJ (2003) The use of intra-articular methylprednisolone in the management of shoulder lameness in the dog. *Proceedings of the 46th Annual BSAVA Congress*. Birmingham, April 3–6, 2003. p 598

Butterworth SJ and Innes JF (2001) Incomplete humeral condylar fractures in the dog. *Journal of Small Animal Practice* **42**, 394–398

Cook JL, Renfro DC, Tomlinson JL and Sorensen JE (2005a) Measurement of angles of abduction for diagnosis of shoulder instability in dogs using goniometry and digital image analysis. *Veterinary Surgery* **34**, 463–468

Cook JL, Tomlinson JL, Fox DB, Kenter K and Cook CR (2005b) Treatment of dogs diagnosed with medial shoulder instability using radiofrequency-induced thermal capsulorrhaphy. *Veterinary Surgery* **34**, 469–475

Danielson KC, Fitzpatrick N, Muir P and Manley PA (2006) Histomorphometry of fragmented medial coronoid process in dogs: a comparison of affected and normal coronoid processes. *Veterinary Surgery* **35**, 501–509

Farrell M, Heller J, Solano M et al. (2014) Does radiographic arthrosis correlate with cartilage pathology in Labrador retrievers affected by medial coronoid process disease? *Veterinary Surgery* **43**, 155–165

Fitch RB, Breshears L, Staatz A and Kudnig S (2001) Clinical evaluation of prosthetic medial glenohumeral ligament repair in the dog (ten cases). *Veterinary and Comparative Orthopaedics and Traumatology* **14**, 222–228

Fitzpatrick N, Yeadon R and Smith TJ (2009) Early clinical experience with osteochondral autograft transfer for treatment of osteochondritis dissecans of the medial humeral condyle in dogs. *Veterinary Surgery* **38**, 246–260

Frostick SP, Sinopidis C, Al Maskari S et al. (2003) Arthroscopic capsular shrinkage of the shoulder for the treatment of patients with multidirectional instability: minimum 2-year follow-up. *Arthroscopy* **19**, 227–233

Gielen I, van Ryssen B and van Bree H (2005) Computerized tomography compared with radiography in the diagnosis of lateral trochlear ridge talar osteochondritis dissecans in dogs. *Veterinary and Comparative Orthopaedics and Traumatology* **18**, 77–82

Guthrie S (1989) Some radiographic and clinical aspects of ununited anconeal process. *Veterinary Record* **124**, 661–662

Guthrie S, Plummer JM and Vaughan LC (1992) Post natal development of the canine elbow joint: a light and electron microscopical study. *Research in Veterinary Science* **52**, 67–71

Hoelzler MG, Millis DL, Francis DA and Weigel JP (2004) Results of arthroscopic versus open arthrotomy for surgical management of cranial cruciate ligament deficiency in dogs. *Veterinary Surgery* **33**, 146–153

Holsworth IG, Schulz KS and Ingel K (2002) Cadaveric evaluation of canine arthroscopic bicipital tenotomy. *Veterinary and Comparative Orthopaedics and Traumatology* **15**, 215–222

Holsworth IG, Schulz KS, Kass PH et al. (2005) Comparison of arthroscopic and radiographic abnormalities in the hip joints of juvenile dogs with hip dysplasia. *Journal of the American Veterinary Medical Association* **227**, 1091–1094

Innes JF (2005) Laboratory evaluation of joint disease. In: *BSAVA Manual of Canine and Feline Clinical Pathology, 2nd edn*, ed. E Villiers and L Blackwood, pp. 355–363. BSAVA Publications, Gloucester

Kirberger RM and McEvoy FJ (2016) *BSAVA Manual of Canine and Feline Musculoskeletal Imaging, 2nd edn*. BSAVA Publications, Gloucester

Krotscheck U, Hulse DA, Bahr A and Jerram RM (2000) Ununited anconeal process: lag screw fixation with proximal ulnar osteotomy. *Veterinary and Comparative Orthopaedics and Traumatology* **13**, 212–216

Laupattarakasem W, Laopaiboon M, Laupattarakasem P and Sumananont C (2008) Arthroscopic debridement for knee osteoarthritis. *Cochrane Database of Systematic Reviews* **1**, CD005118

Li A, Bennett D, Gibbs G et al. (2000) Radial carpal bone fractures in 15 dogs. *Journal of Small Animal Practice* **41**, 74–79

Marcellin-Little DJ, De Young DJ, Ferris KK and Berry CM (1994) Incomplete ossification of the humeral condyle in spaniels. *Veterinary Surgery* **23**, 475–477

Meyer-Lindenberg A, Fehr M and Nolte I (2006) Co-existence of ununited anconeal process and fragmented medial coronoid process of the ulna in the dog. *Journal of Small Animal Practice* **47**, 61–65

Meyer-Lindenberg A, Langhann A, Fehr M and Nolte I (2003) Arthrotomy versus arthroscopy in the treatment of the fragmented medial coronoid process of the ulna (FCP) in 421 dogs. *Veterinary and Comparative Orthopaedics and Traumatology* **16**, 204–210

Mitchell RAS and Innes JF (2000). Lateral glenohumeral ligament rupture in three dogs. *Journal of Small Animal Practice* **41**, 511–514

Olivieri M, Piras A, Marcellin-Little DJ *et al.* (2004) Accessory caudal glenoid ossification centre as possible cause of lameness in nine dogs. *Veterinary and Comparative Orthopaedics and Traumatology* **17**, 131–135

O'Neill, T and Innes JF (2004) Treatment of shoulder instability caused by medial glenohumeral ligament rupture with thermal capsulorrhaphy. *Journal of Small Animal Practice* **45**, 521–524

Penelas A, Gutbrod A, Kuhn K and Pozzi A (2018) Feasibility and safety of arthroscopic medial glenohumeral ligament and subscapularis tendon repair with knotless anchors: a cadaveric study in dogs. *Veterinary Surgery* **47**, 817–826

Person MW (1986) Arthroscopy of the canine shoulder joint. *Compendium on Continuing Education for the Practicing Veterinarian* **8**, 537

Person MW (1989a) Arthroscopic treatment of osteochondritis dissecans in the canine shoulder. *Veterinary Surgery* **18**, 175–189

Person MW (1989b) Arthroscopy of the canine coxofemoral joint. *Compendium on Continuing Education for the Practicing Veterinarian* **11**, 930–935

Pettitt RA, Clements DN and Guilliard MJ (2007) Stabilisation of medial shoulder instability by imbrication of the subscapularis muscle tendon of insertion. *Journal of Small Animal Practice* **48**, 625–630

Pettitt RA and Innes JF (2008) Arthroscopic management of a lateral glenohumeral ligament rupture in two dogs. *Veterinary and Comparative Orthopaedics and Traumatology* **21**, 302–306

Pettitt RA, Tattersall J, Gemmill T *et al.* (2009) Effect of surgical technique on radiographic fusion of the anconeus in the treatment of ununited anconeal process. *Journal of Small Animal Practice* **50**, 545–548

Pozzi A, Hildreth BE and Rajala-Schultz PJ (2008) Comparison of arthroscopy and arthrotomy for diagnosis of medial meniscal pathology: an *ex vivo* study. *Veterinary Surgery* **37**, 749–755

Ridge PA, Cook JL and Cook CR (2014) Arthroscopically assisted treatment of injury to the lateral glenohumeral ligament in dogs. *Veterinary Surgery* **43**, 558–562

Rudd RG, Whitehair JG and Margolis JH (1990) Results of management of osteochondritis dissecans of the humeral head in dogs: 44 cases (1982–1987). *Journal of the American Animal Hospital Association* **26**, 173–178

Scholz J, Kuhling T and Turczynsky T (1992) The advantages of arthroscopic knee surgery. *Biomedizinische Technik* **37**, 11–13

Schulz KS, Holsworth IG and Hornof WJ (2004) Self-retaining braces for canine arthroscopy. *Veterinary Surgery* **33**, 77–82

Sjöström L, Kasström H and Kallberg M (1995) Ununited anconeal process in the dog. Pathogenesis and treatment by osteotomy of the ulna. *Veterinary and Comparative Orthopaedics and Traumatology* **8**, 170–176

Turner BM, Abercromby RH, Innes J, McKee WM and Ness MG (1998) Dynamic proximal ulnar osteotomy for the treatment of ununited anconeal process in 17 dogs. *Veterinary and Comparative Orthopaedics and Traumatology* **11**, 76–79

Van Ryssen B and van Bree H (1997) Arthroscopic findings in 100 dogs with elbow lameness. *Veterinary Record* **140**, 360–362

Van Ryssen B, van Bree H and Missinne S (1993a) Successful arthroscopic treatment of shoulder osteochondrosis in the dog. *Journal of Small Animal Practice* **34**, 521–528

Van Ryssen B, van Bree H and Vyt P (1993b) Arthroscopy of the shoulder joint in the dog. *Journal of the American Animal Hospital Association* **29**, 101–105

Wolschrijn CF, Gruys E and Weijs WA (2005) Microcomputed tomography and histology of a fragmented medial coronoid process in a 20-week-old Golden Retriever. *Veterinary Record* **157**, 383–386

Chapter 15

Interventional endoscopy and radiology

Gerard McLauchlan

Introduction

Interventional radiology and interventional endoscopy involve the combined use of imaging modalities such as fluoroscopy, bronchoscopy and cystoscopy to undertake minimally invasive procedures. Using primarily a combination of percutaneous access and natural orifices, the veterinary surgeon (veterinarian) can target the required organ to carry out the desired intervention (e.g. placing a stent to relieve an obstruction or delivering targeted drug therapy such as intra-arterial chemotherapy). The main advantages of interventional endoscopy and radiology are the shorter recovery time, reduced rate of complications and lower mortality compared with many of the 'traditional' surgical options. In addition, with many of the commonly performed techniques discussed in this chapter a good traditional treatment for the underlying condition may simply not exist. The techniques are technically challenging and the veterinary surgeon will require access to advanced equipment and training to undertake them. As such referral to a specialist centre would often be most appropriate.

Equipment

A C-Arm fluoroscopy unit (Figure 15.1) is ideal for most interventional radiology/endoscopy procedures. It allows real-time imaging during the procedure, will obtain various rotational views without the need to move the patient and can be used at the same time as bronchoscopy, gastrointestinal endoscopy or cystoscopy. In addition, an ability to perform digital subtraction angiography is preferable. This allows an initial non-contrast image to be subtracted from the subsequent serial images obtained following an injection of contrast medium into the target vessels, thus significantly improving the contrast resolution of the images. Some of the techniques described in this chapter, including placement of a tracheal stent or a subcutaneous ureteral bypass (SUB) device, have been reported with the guidance of other imaging modalities such as digital radiography or ultrasonography. However, the author does not recommend the use of these imaging techniques as they do not allow the continuous, real-time imaging required for the procedures that is possible with fluoroscopy. Various flexible and rigid endoscopes are required to obtain an image of the organ of interest for display on a monitor, and the reader is referred to other chapters in the Manual for further details of this equipment. Other

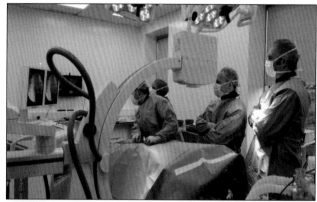

15.1 A traditional fluoroscopic C-Arm X-ray system and monitor. The operator and assistants should wear personal protective equipment including lead gowns and thyroid shields as a minimum during all procedures using this machine.

specialist equipment for interventional endoscopy and radiology commonly includes but is not limited to:

- Guidewires (Figure 15.2) – these are used to facilitate the placement of catheters in various target sites. They are available in different sizes and configurations. Guidewires have many differing characteristics, including surface coating, tip angle and rigidity, each of which have advantages when it comes to vessel selection/superselection and providing support for the catheter being advanced (superselection referring to selection of tiny feeding vessels). The most commonly used guidewire in veterinary interventions is a 0.035 inch (0.9 mm) hydrophilic angle-tipped Weasel Wire® (Infiniti Medical). Hydrophilic guidewires should be flushed with sterile saline before use and frequently during the procedure to ensure they pass with minimal friction. When performing an intervention through a flexible endoscope, is it important to use a guidewire at least double the length of the endoscope
- Introducer sheaths (Figure 15.3) – these are thin-walled catheters that are advanced over a guidewire to allow placement of angiographic catheters or other devices. They are placed with a vascular dilator to allow smooth atraumatic access to a vessel; the dilator is a thick-walled stiffer tube with a tapered leading end. The dilator/sheath combination is commonly placed into vessels for vascular interventions or into the urethra for urinary tract interventions. Once access is achieved,

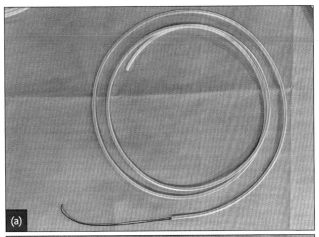

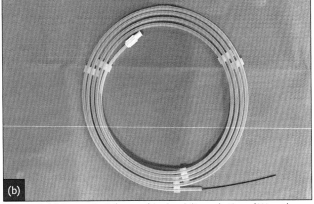

the dilator is removed, leaving the sheath in place. Introducer sheaths are named after their inner diameter whereas catheters after their outer diameter (e.g. a 4 Fr sheath can accommodate a 4 Fr catheter). They have a side port to allow procedures such as contrast imaging, sampling or pressure measurements to be performed, and a haemostatic valve to allow exchange of wires and catheters without blood loss or air embolization occurring. The sheath also allows repeat access to a vessel while minimizing trauma to the vascular wall

- Angiographic catheters (Figure 15.4) – these are flexible catheters that allow contrast medium to be administered to perform a fluoroscopic study or drugs to be delivered in a targeted fashion. Catheters are measured by their outer diameter and the most commonly used are 4 Fr or 5 Fr. Various catheters are available in different lengths and with different tip configurations, which allow the clinician to access different target vessels. The most commonly used in veterinary interventions are the Berenstein catheter and Cobra catheter of between 65 and 100 cm in length. A straight radiographic marker catheter is also commonly used – this has radiographic marks placed every 1cm that allow accurate sizing for stent placement

- Stents (Figure 15.5) – these are most commonly placed to relieve luminal obstructions. In veterinary medicine they are used in cases of tracheal collapse, nasopharyngeal stenosis (NPS), ureteral or urethral

15.2 (a) A 0.035 inch (0.9 mm) hydrophilic angle-tipped Weasel Wire®. This is the most commonly used wire in interventional procedures. (b) A 0.035 inch (0.9 mm) straight-tipped Bentson wire.

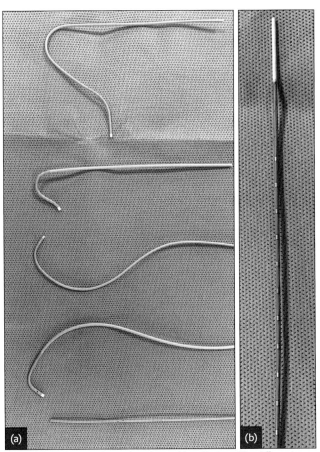

15.4 (a) Commonly used angiographic catheters. The different shapes of the catheter ends allow access to various vessels depending on the procedure being performed. (b) A straight angiographic marker catheter. The metallic marks indicate 1 cm from the back of one mark to the back of the next, allowing accurate measurement during fluoroscopic procedures where magnification of the image occurs.

15.3 (a) An introducer sheath with a side arm to allow flushing and blood sampling (left). The vascular dilator (right) should be flushed before insertion into the sheath. (b) The introducer sheath with the vascular dilator in place.

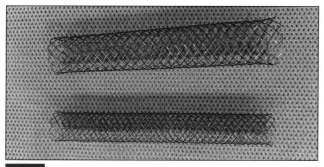

15.5 Two deployed nitinol (nickel–titanium) tracheal stents.

obstruction, blood vessel occlusion due to thromboembolic disease and in coil embolization of intrahepatic portosystemic shunts (PSSs). In veterinary medicine, the most commonly used tracheal and vascular stents are composed of nitinol (a nickel–titanium alloy) and ureteral stents are typically double-pigtailed, multi-fenestrated and made of polyurethane. Metallic stents are either self-expanding or balloon expandable and can be covered or uncovered. The vast majority of stents placed in veterinary patients are self-expanding metallic stents. The author generally prefers to use uncovered stents; however, a covered stent can be considered for refractory obstructions, recurrent tracheal granulation tissue and complete imperforate NPS. Each stent has a specific deployment system (e.g. reconstrainable *versus* non-reconstrainable) and the clinician should ensure they are aware of these details before attempting stent placement
- Balloon dilation catheters (Figure 15.6) – balloons are used to dilate strictures in various locations, including the oesophagus, nasopharynx, colon and urethra. They should be placed over a guidewire to avoid trauma to the surrounding tissue. The author recommends that any balloon dilation be monitored with a combination of endoscopy and fluoroscopy

- Coils (Figure 15.7) – these are placed to achieve thrombosis of vessels. In veterinary medicine, coils are most commonly placed during transjugular coil embolization of an intrahepatic PSS. Coils of various sizes are commercially available. They are typically made of platinum, although other options are also available
- Embolics (Figure 15.8) – the use of polyvinyl alcohol beads and cyanoacrylate glue has been reported in various cases, including non-resectable hepatocellular carcinoma, prostatic neoplasia, nasal tumours, hepatic arteriovenous malformations and refractory epistaxis. It is essential to avoid non-target embolization and, therefore, these procedures should be performed only by a veterinary surgeon with intricate knowledge of the vascular anatomy.

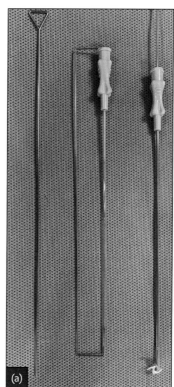

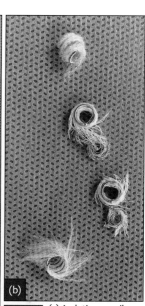

15.7 (a) A platinum coil within its delivery system (centre), the coil pusher (left) and a partially deployed coil (right). (b) Multiple deployed coils.

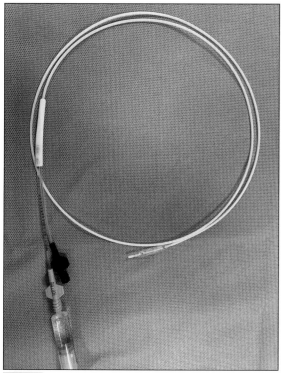

15.6 A balloon dilator catheter.

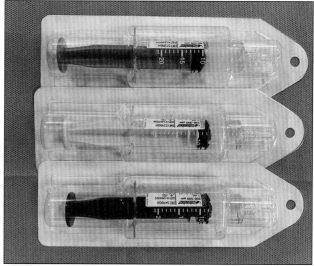

15.8 Polyvinyl alcohol beads of various sizes for use in embolization procedures.

Respiratory conditions

Tracheal collapse

Tracheal collapse is a progressive and debilitating disease that primarily affects middle-aged, small-breed dogs, with Yorkshire Terriers and Pomeranians being particularly over-represented among cases. This condition arises as a result of degeneration of the tracheal cartilage combined with reduced glycosaminoglycan content in the cartilage and loss of elastic fibres in the tracheal membrane, which leads to dorsoventral flattening of the trachea. Tracheal collapse causes repeated luminal contact of the tracheal mucosa during respiration, which results in a vicious cycle of inflammation and coughing. While tracheal collapse is initially focal, due to its progressive nature, many cases progress to become diffuse and can eventually involve the entire trachea and lower airways. Clinically, the disease is characterized by a classic 'goose honking' cough (often induced by exercise or excitement) and sometimes periods of cyanosis. The presence of a more 'traditional' cough may indicate concurrent bronchial collapse or a pulmonary parenchymal disease. The location of the tracheal collapse, any concurrent bronchial collapse and the presence of other respiratory diseases will influence the findings on physical examination. If the collapse is restricted to the cervical trachea, the dog will present with inspiratory noise; if the disease involves the thoracic trachea alone, then clinical signs are most apparent during expiration; and if the thoracic inlet is collapsing, the patient can show both inspiratory and expiratory signs.

Diagnosis can be made by three-view thoracic radiography (ideally, expiratory and inspiratory views should be obtained); however, as the collapse is dynamic, radiographs lack sensitivity. Fluoroscopy is the ideal method for diagnosing tracheal collapse, but it is likely to be available only in referral settings, which limits its accessibility and therefore its utility. A study showed that the location of tracheal collapse was misdiagnosed in 44% of dogs and that the collapse was missed entirely in 8% of cases examined via radiography compared with fluoroscopy (Macready *et al.*, 2007). Tracheal collapse can also be diagnosed by tracheobronchoscopy; this allows grading of the tracheal collapse from I to IV based on the degree of luminal obstruction (Grade I being 25% luminal obstruction by the collapsing membrane, Grade II 50% obstruction, Grade III 75% obstruction and Grade IV 100%), identification of a tracheal malformation (a fixed obstruction most commonly recognized in Yorkshire Terriers resulting from a ventrodorsal narrowing of the tracheal rings rather than the traditional dorsoventral collapse of the membrane; this fixed obstruction requires balloon dilating of any stent placed to ensure adequate apposition the to the tracheal wall) and an assessment of any bronchial collapse to be performed at the same time, as well as bronchoalveolar lavage, in order to identify any concurrent pneumonia. However, tracheobronchoscopy requires general anaesthesia, and clinicians should be aware that recovery of a patient with tracheal collapse can be complicated and that emergency stenting may be required in this situation.

While medical management with a combination of antitussives, anti-inflammatory steroids, bronchodilators and anxiolytics can initially be successful, some dogs require interventional procedures as the disease progresses; in one study, the median duration of successful medical management exceeded 200 days (Weisse and Berent, 2015). The options for managing tracheal collapse that is no longer responding to medication alone are the placement of tracheal rings or intraluminal stenting. Clients should be informed that both of these options are considered salvage procedures, neither has been shown to slow the progression of the disease and patients are likely to require ongoing medical management after either procedure (Weisse and Berent 2015). For information on tracheal ring placement, see the References and further reading at the end of chapter and Chapter 7.

Tracheal stenting is ideally performed using a combination of bronchoscopy and fluoroscopy. While there are reports of the procedure being performed using digital radiographic guidance, this is not recommended, as it does not allow continuous real-time imaging during the deployment of the stent as fluoroscopy does. The author performs a full tracheobronchoscopy once the patient is under anaesthesia and obtains a sample via bronchoalveolar lavage to submit for cytology and culture. Following these procedures, under the same anaesthetic, the patient is placed in right lateral recumbency and a radiographic marker catheter is placed down the oesophagus over a guidewire to allow accurate measurement of the maximal tracheal diameter under positive-pressure ventilation (20 cmH$_2$O) and the tracheal length; the marker catheter is used to account for any magnification produced by the fluoroscopy unit. Measurements of tracheal diameter are made at several points in the thoracic and cervical trachea, and if significant variation (>15%) is noted between the two regions, then placement of a Duality Vet Stent® (Infiniti Medical) can be considered. This may result in fewer complications, such as stent fracture, granulation tissue or chronic infections due to poor apposition of the stent. A Duality Vet Stent® is a custom-made stent with a variable diameter to closely match the tracheal diameter at all points. These stents are up to 400% stronger than traditional stents when placed in a variable diameter environment.

Tracheal stents (Figure 15.9) are composed of nitinol and various self-expanding and balloon-expandable stents are commercially available. Although tracheal collapse can be focal (most commonly seen at the thoracic inlet), if it is diagnosed early, due to its progressive nature it is recommended that the entire length of the trachea, from 1 cm caudal to the larynx to 1 cm cranial to the carina, be stented. Accurate stent sizing is essential to reduce the risk of complications such as stent shortening or

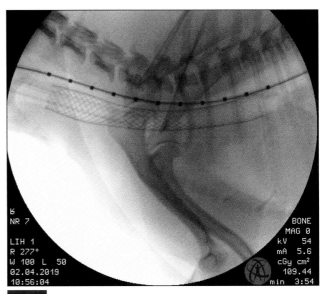

15.9 A fluoroscopic image of a deployed tracheal stent.

migration, and for this reason, tracheal stenting should be performed only by veterinary surgeons properly trained in the technique. Placement of the stent into either mainstem bronchus or the larynx should be avoided, as this may result in significant coughing (if placed in the larynx) or mucus entrapment and infection (if placed in a bronchus). Use of a stent with too small a diameter may result in complications such as stent migration or fracture; the current recommendation is that the stent placed should be 15–20% larger than the maximal tracheal diameter (Raske et al., 2018). The other significant complication that has been reported is the formation of granulation tissue, which is seen in around 20% of cases (Weisse et al., 2019).

Although tracheal stents generally result in a significant improvement in clinical signs immediately after placement, the owner should be made aware that ongoing medical management will be required, along with frequent radiographic monitoring to assess the location and integrity of the stent and for the occurrence of significant granulation tissue; the author recommends 3-monthly thoracic radiographs with the animal's limbs pulled cranially and then caudally to evaluate the entire length of the stent. A recent report suggests that around 40% of cases may require placement of a second stent at some point in their lifetime (Weisse et al., 2019). Overall, clinical improvement and owner satisfaction rates after placement of a tracheal stent are considered excellent. Tracheal stenting in cats has been reported in a small number of cases and is most commonly performed following trauma associated with endotracheal tube placement.

Bronchial collapse

Bronchial collapse may occur in conjunction with tracheal collapse, as an isolated disease, in animals with brachycephalic obstructive airway syndrome or secondary to cardiomegaly. Bronchial collapse can be static or dynamic. It may involve only the mainstem bronchi but it is much more common for secondary and tertiary bronchi to also be affected. The role of bronchial stenting in the management of bronchial collapse is the subject of much debate; patients with only mainstem bronchial collapse may be candidates for stenting. In a case report of bronchial collapse secondary to cardiomegaly, the dog developed acute pulmonary oedema following the stenting procedure (Dengate et al., 2014). The value of bronchial stenting in cases of diffuse bronchial collapse is unclear. In cases with concurrent tracheal and bronchial collapse, the author recommends that the patient undergo tracheal stenting and that the effect this has on airway dynamics and bronchial collapse be evaluated before considering bronchial stenting. It is important to warn owners that in a small number of cases tracheal stenting may result in a worsening of bronchial collapse and its associated clinical signs due to the alteration in airway dynamics.

Nasopharyngeal stenosis

NPS is a narrowing within the nasopharynx caudal to the choanae. It can be seen in both dogs and cats as a congenital abnormality (choanal atresia) but most commonly occurs following aspiration rhinitis as a complication of general anaesthesia (with clinical signs developing within a few days of the event) or chronic rhinitis in cats. Clinical signs associated with NPS include both inspiratory and expiratory stertor along with recurrent nasal discharge and/or infection. Obligate mouth-breathing is seen in cases of complete obstruction.

Surgical options for NPS include transpalatal resection, dilation with vascular forceps and laser ablation, which may be associated with high recurrence rates in both dogs and cats. A recent publication reported an excellent outcome in cats treated with extended palatoplasty (Sériot et al., 2019). The use of topical medications, such as mitomycin C and triamcinolone, may improve postsurgical outcomes; however, they were not associated with an improved outcome in the largest single study evaluating nasopharyngeal stenting (Burdick et al., 2018).

Endoscopic interventional options for NPS include balloon dilation or placement of a metallic stent. NPS stents include balloon-expandable and self-expanding stents. The stents can be covered or uncovered; covered stents are stronger but carry an increased risk of migration and chronic infection, as they do not become incorporated into the nasopharyngeal mucosa. A covered retrievable stent has recently become available and is the author's preferred choice for the treatment of NPS; these stents are removed only if complications develop (see below).

Ideally, a contrast computed tomography (CT) scan of the area should be performed to allow accurate measurement of the stenosis before balloon dilation or stent placement; however, if finances are limited then a contrast fluoroscopic nasopharyngeogram with a marker catheter spanning both sides of the stenosis can be used for the purposes of measurement. The stenosis is most commonly located at the junction of the hard and soft palate but can occur both rostral and caudal to this location. In cats with a very thin stenosis (<0.5 cm), multiple balloon dilations alone may be successful in up to 50% of cases (Burdick et al., 2018). For stenoses longer than 0.5 cm, recurrent lesions or cases of complete stenosis, balloon dilation alone is unlikely to be successful and placement of a nasopharyngeal stent will probably be required.

Both balloon dilation (Figure 15.10ab) and nasopharyngeal stenting (Figure 15.10c) are performed with the patient in lateral recumbency, using a combination of endoscopy and fluoroscopy. This ensures accurate identification of the location of the stricture and placement of the stent across the stenosis. Under fluoroscopic guidance, a 0.035 inch (0.9 mm) guidewire is directed into the ventral meatus, through the stenosis and into the oesophagus. If complete stenosis is present, then an introducer is advanced over the wire to the level of the stenosis and a needle is directed through this under fluoroscopic and endoscopic visualization to puncture an opening through the stenosis before the guidewire is directed into the oesophagus. An appropriately sized balloon is then advanced over the guidewire to span the stricture and inflated with a combination of saline and contrast medium under fluoroscopic visualization until the 'waist' of the structure is fully removed; the maximal inflation pressure of each individual balloon is listed on the balloon. The author then holds the balloon inflated for 1–2 minutes through the effaced stricture.

Ideally, the required balloon size is calculated from a pre-procedural CT scan, but if this is not available, the balloon size can be determined by performing a dual-contrast fluoroscopic study, where contrast medium is injected via the introducer cranial to the stenosis and via the endoscope located in the nasopharynx caudal to the stenosis. Balloon dilation should be performed using an inflation device rather than manually, as it is difficult to generate enough pressure manually to fully dilate the stricture. Following balloon dilation, a stent can be placed across the region of the stricture; if a covered stent is used, it is often toggled in place to avoid migration. Correct placement is essential to avoid the stent being situated too

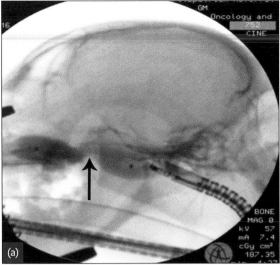

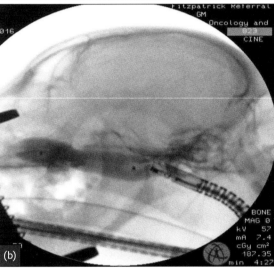

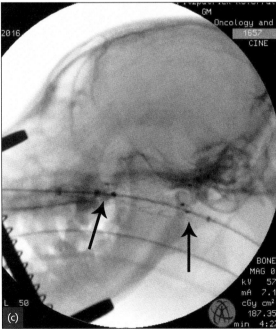

15.10 (a) Fluoroscopic image of a nasopharyngeal stenosis (arrowed) being treated by balloon dilation. (b) Fluoroscopic image from later in the same balloon dilation procedure. The area of stenosis visible in (a) is no longer present. (c) Fluoroscopic image of a nasopharyngeal stent deployed over a hydrophilic guidewire. The arrows highlight the radiodense markers at the cranial and caudal aspects of the stent.

far cranially in one of the nasal passages, as this can result in excessive accumulation of mucus, or too far caudally in the nasopharynx, as this can result in irritation and reflux. Accumulation of hair ingested during grooming within a caudally positioned stent has also been reported in cats.

Complications associated with NPS stenting are rare but include re-stenosis following stent removal, stent compression, stent migration, chronic infection and development of an oronasal fistula. The prognosis for dogs and cats with NPS is considered good to excellent, although owners should be warned about the possible need for repeat procedures.

Gastrointestinal conditions

Oesophageal strictures

Oesophageal strictures occur in both dogs and cats and are associated with clinical signs including regurgitation, hypersalivation and dysphagia. In dogs, they most commonly occur following anaesthesia that has resulted in severe gastroesophageal reflux, leading to circumferential scar tissue formation and luminal narrowing. In cats, certain medications (in particular doxycycline and clindamycin) have been associated with the development of strictures, and care should be taken to administer these drugs either with, or followed by, food or water to ensure rapid passage to the stomach (German *et al.*, 2005). Current options for managing oesophageal strictures include balloon dilation, bougienage and stenting. In general, surgery for oesophageal strictures is not recommended because of the associated high morbidity and mortality.

The author's preferred treatment for oesophageal strictures is balloon dilation guided by a combination of fluoroscopy and endoscopy. The maximal oesophageal diameter is determined fluoroscopically by insufflating the oesophagus with air delivered via the endoscope. A marker catheter is placed over a guidewire and introduced into the oesophagus to account for any fluoroscopic magnification. The length of the stricture is measured by performing a contrast oesophagogram through the marker catheter under fluoroscopy using iodinated contrast medium. With many oesophageal strictures there is a muscular component to the fibrosis, and endoscopy can be used to monitor mucosal/submucosal tearing as a result of balloon dilation, while fluoroscopy can be performed to determine whether the entire stricture 'belt' has torn (Figure 15.11). Although it is generally recommended to start with a balloon 2–4 mm larger than the stricture diameter and gradually increase the size of balloon used by 2–4 mm until the maximal oesophageal diameter is achieved and the stricture 'belt' is completely effaced, the author has often started with a balloon of the maximal oesophageal diameter without complication, thus resulting in significant financial savings for the client.

Once the stricture has been dilated, the author prefers to leave the balloon in place and inflated for 3–5 minutes and, to date, has not encountered any complications with this technique. Before performing balloon dilation, some clinicians may consider injecting triamcinolone into the stricture, which may help limit stricture recurrence (see Chapter 4). The number of balloon dilations required is on average between two and four; however, significantly more procedures may be needed with severely refractory strictures. There is currently no standard recommendation regarding

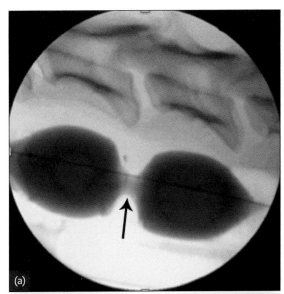

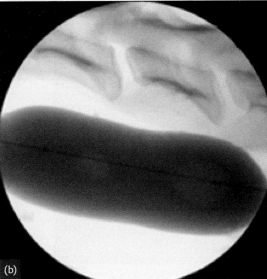

15.11 (a) Fluoroscopic image of an oesophageal stricture during a balloon dilation procedure. The arrow highlights the stricture 'belt' that must be fully effaced during the procedure. (b) Complete effacement of the stricture shown in (a).

the interval that should be left between balloon dilations but, in general, 7 days would be considered appropriate. Postoperatively, the author recommends oral feeding as soon as possible, with a gradual increase in the volume and consistency of the feed over the following 24–48 hours. Following the procedure, the author also recommends a 5-day course of proton pump inhibitors and broad-spectrum antibiotics.

In cases of refractory oesophageal strictures, consideration should be given to the placement of an indwelling balloon oesophageal tube. This tube is placed under fluoroscopic guidance and should remain in place for 6 weeks. The tube allows the owners to inflate the balloon twice daily at home to prevent stricture reformation. The tube also allows assisted feeding, although oral feeding should be encouraged.

Oesophageal stenting has been investigated as a possible single-stage treatment for strictures. Although this procedure improved short-term dysphagia in dogs, a study reported that seven out of nine dogs (78%) experienced major complications after stent placement (Lam *et al.*, 2013), and therefore oesophageal stenting cannot be currently recommended.

Colonic obstructions

Balloon dilation of colonic obstructions and the placement of colonic stents have both been reported in the veterinary literature. Colorectal stenting has been extensively described in human medicine for the treatment of both benign and malignant strictures; however, reports in veterinary patients have been limited to the treatment of malignancy. In one case of a dog with a rectal carcinoma, a survival time of 238 days after placement of a stent was reported (Culp *et al.*, 2011). In two cats with colonic adenocarcinoma in which a stent was placed, survival times of 19 days and 274 days were reported (Hume *et al.*, 2006).

Vascular interventions

Interventional oncology

Interventional oncology is regarded as the fourth pillar of human oncology alongside medical, surgical and radiation oncology. Interventional oncology can be used as a primary treatment, to palliate clinical signs or in an attempt to shrink a tumour to make surgical removal possible. In veterinary medicine, interventional oncology primarily involves transarterial therapy (i.e. the intra-arterial administration of a chemotherapeutic drug or embolic agent) or ablative therapy (either thermal, e.g. microwave ablation, or chemical, e.g. ethanol ablation).

There has been increasing interest in targeted intra-arterial chemotherapy in veterinary patients in recent years. Most research and clinical work in this area has focused on non-resectable hepatocellular carcinomas (HCCs) and urinary tract neoplasms (urothelial cell carcinomas and prostatic carcinoma). Intra-arterial chemotherapy normally involves vascular access being obtained via the femoral or carotid artery. Using fluoroscopic guidance, the veterinary surgeon then selectively delivers the cytotoxic agent directly to the tumour via its arterial supply. The intra-arterial administration of chemotherapeutic agents is not associated with an increase in the severity of drug-associated side effects, and in one recent study of dogs with lower urinary tract neoplasia systemic side effects occurred significantly less commonly following intra-arterial administration compared with intravenous administration (Culp *et al.*, 2015). The effect of intra-arterial chemotherapy on disease-free interval and survival compared with intravenous administration of the same agent(s) remains contentious.

With regard to urinary tract tumours, various studies have shown higher local concentrations of chemotherapeutic agents and superior remission rates in laboratory animals that received chemotherapy via the intra-arterial route *versus* traditional intravenous administration (Hoshi *et al.*, 1997). A study in research Beagles documented that it was possible to achieve a greater than eight-fold increase in the concentration of the chemotherapeutic agent pirarubicin in the bladder, as well as higher concentrations in the prostate and regional lymph nodes, following intra-arterial administration, compared with the concentrations in the respective tissues in dogs receiving the drug via the traditional intravenous route (Sumiyoshi *et al.*, 1991). Intra-arterial chemotherapy has been shown to result in higher concentrations of the drug in the tumour and may therefore achieve greater efficacy. In dogs with naturally occurring prostatic carcinoma, the use of intra-arterial carboplatin was found to result in significantly more dogs entering clinical remission (as judged by a modification of the Response Evaluation Criteria in Solid Tumours (RECIST) criteria for assessing the response of solid tumours to treatment) but significantly fewer showing chemotherapy-associated side effects (anaemia, lethargy and anorexia) compared with dogs receiving intravenous carboplatin (Culp *et al.*, 2015). The author has commonly treated bladder, urethral and prostatic neoplasia with intra-arterial chemotherapy (Figure 15.12) alongside other modalities including surgery, intravenous chemotherapy and radiotherapy, with a positive response. Embolization of the prostatic artery has recently been presented (unpublished) and shows promising results (Figure 15.13) including reduction in prostatic volume greater than 40% and statistically significant improvement in clinical signs including stranguria and faecal tenesmus. Following targeted intra-arterial therapy (either chemotherapy or embolization), systemic chemotherapy should be administered to treat any metastatic disease.

Solitary HCCs should be regarded as a surgical disease in dogs, and a median survival time of greater than 3 years has been achieved following complete excision (Liptak *et al.*, 2004). In patients in which the neoplasm is considered non-resectable, is diffusely infiltrating the liver, or for which the owners decline surgery, there is the option of transarterial chemoembolization. This technique has been used for several years in such cases. HCCs receive almost their entire blood supply from the hepatic artery, whereas the normal liver receives most of its supply from the hepatic portal vein; this makes HCCs particularly susceptible to arterial chemoembolization. Access is gained via the femoral artery and, using fluoroscopic guidance, this is followed by selection of the coeliac and then common hepatic artery. After this, superselection of the specific arterial branches supplying the tumour is achieved to ensure that minimal non-target embolization occurs. Particular care must be taken to avoid embolization of the gastroduodenal artery, as this may result in significant morbidity, notably pancreatitis. The combined chemotherapy and embolization agent (generally, either cyanoacrylate glue mixed with lipiodol or polyvinyl alcohol particles) is administered into the feeding arteries and a repeat contrast fluoroscopy study is performed to confirm vascular stasis within the tumour. Following chemoembolization, an HCC does not generally significantly reduce in

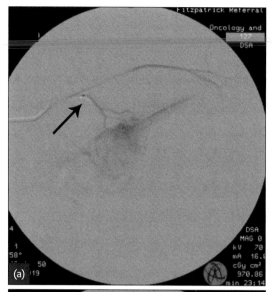

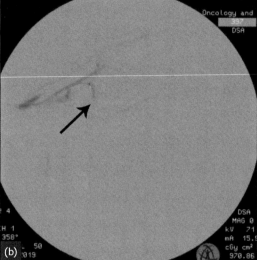

15.13 Embolization of the prostatic artery. (a) With the patient in lateral recumbency, a digital subtraction image highlights the prostatic artery (arrowed). (b) Digital subtraction image following prostatic embolization. Note the blunt end of the prostatic artery (arrowed).

volume (reductions of 10–30% occur); however, repeat CT angiography 6–8 weeks after embolization will often show marked changes in the attenuation of the mass, indicating significant tumour necrosis. The aim should be 'stable disease' and owners should be made aware that the procedure may need to be repeated every 3–6 months to limit tumour growth.

Intrahepatic shunt embolization

Congenital PSSs are suspected on the basis of appropriate clinical signs (failure of growth, hepatic encephalopathy, urinary tract signs), routine haematology and serum chemistry (mild non-regenerative microcytic anaemia, reduction in urea, cholesterol, glucose and albumin, and mild elevation in hepatic markers), urinalysis (hyposthenuria/isosthenuria and ammonia biurate crystals) and specific assessment of hepatic function (elevation in ammonia and bile acids). Confirmation of a congenital PSS is best achieved via dual-phase contrast CT; compared with ultrasonography, CT is significantly more sensitive (96% *versus* 68%) for PSS diagnosis and 5.5 times as likely to correctly identify the anatomy of the PSS (Kim *et al.*, 2013).

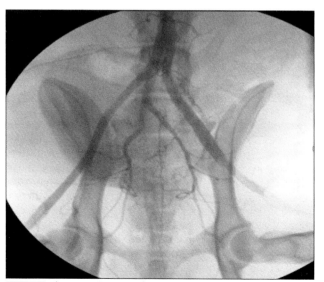

15.12 Fluoroscopic image of an intra-arterial approach to the bladder. Access was via the carotid artery. Contrast agent has been injected to highlight both the external and internal iliac arteries.

Surgical correction of an extrahepatic PSS is generally recognized as being preferable to medical management with regard to long-term outcome (Greenhalgh *et al.*, 2010). However, the technical difficulties, perioperative complications and mortality associated with surgical correction of an intrahepatic PSS have led to the development of an alternative technique, percutaneous transvenous embolization (PTE).

As with surgical correction of extrahepatic PSSs, patients with an intrahepatic PSS should be medically managed with a combination of diet, antibiotics and lactulose for at least 2–4 weeks before PTE. The author also starts treatment with levetiracetam (20 mg/kg orally q8h) 72 hours before any procedure to correct an intrahepatic or extrahepatic PSS in an attempt to reduce the occurrence of post-attenuation neurological complications such as seizures, although the effectiveness of this treatment remains debatable (Fryer *et al.*, 2011; Mullins *et al.*, 2019). Advanced imaging by dual-phase contrast CT is mandatory before PTE in order to measure the maximal caval diameter (to enable calculation of the desired stent diameter) and the length of the shunt opening (and therefore the length of stent to use). Advanced imaging may also identify the presence of multiple intrahepatic shunts, which can be seen in up to 10% of cases.

PTE is typically started by accessing the right jugular vein and placing a 12 Fr vascular sheath. A guidewire and angiographic catheter are then advanced under fluoroscopic guidance via the caudal vena cava into the shunt and, if possible, into the portal vein. At this point, resting portal and caval (central venous) pressures are measured by connecting the angiographic catheter to a pressure transducer that has been zeroed to the level of the heart. The transducer is then connected to the anaesthetic monitor so that real-time caval and portal pressures can be monitored throughout the procedure. Following this, the laser-cut stent is deployed within the vena cava across the shunt entrance. In general, a stent around 20% larger than the pre-measured maximal caval diameter is placed. Care must be taken to monitor the caval and portal pressures at all times to ensure portal hypertension does not develop. Following placement of the stent, a hydrophilic guidewire and catheter combination is used to access the shunt vessel through the interstices of the stent and deploy stainless steel coils (typically around 12 per case; in a recent study, a range of 1–18 was reported (Culp *et al.*, 2018)) (Figure 15.14). During coil deployment, the veterinary surgeon must continually monitor the portal pressure to ensure that there is an increase of no more than 8 mmHg from baseline (i.e. to a maximum of 18–20 mmHg). The coils are thrombogenic, which will result in gradual further occlusion of the shunt over the following weeks and should therefore allow staggered withdrawal of any medical and dietary management.

The major complication following PTE is the development of neurological signs including seizures (reported in 6% of cases) (Culp *et al.*, 2018). Around 15–20% of patients may require additional coils to be placed during a second procedure if there are ongoing clinical signs and/or failure of biochemical markers to improve. A recent study (Culp *et al.*, 2018) evaluating the efficacy of PTE indicated that an improvement of greater than 50% in urea, cholesterol and albumin values would be expected following successful PTE. In addition, whilst a reduction in pre- and postprandial bile acids following the procedure was seen in 52% and 29% of dogs, respectively, these values still remained higher than normal in 76% and 94% of dogs (Culp *et al.*, 2018).

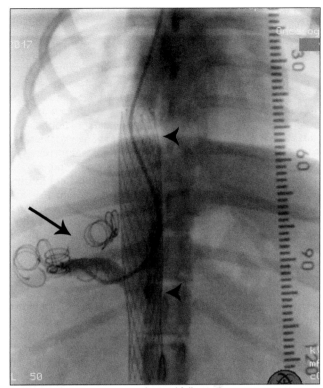

15.14 Fluoroscopic image obtained following percutaneous transvenous embolization of an intrahepatic portosystemic shunt. A stent has been placed within the caudal vena cava (arrowheads) and multiple platinum coils have been deployed within the shunting vessel (arrowed).

In summary, PTE is a safe, fast and effective technique when performed by a clinician who has undertaken appropriate training. It offers a similar long-term outcome to traditional surgical options for intrahepatic PSS, but with lower morbidity and mortality.

Urinary tract conditions

Ectopic ureter

Ectopic ureter is a congenital abnormality that results in the ureteral opening being located distal to the trigone of the bladder. The vast majority of cases (85–90% in some studies (Holt and Moore, *et al.*, 1995) are intramural, meaning that the ureter enters the bladder in a normal location but then tunnels within the submucosa and opens in the urethra, or in some cases the vagina or vestibule. It is most commonly identified in female animals (>90% of cases) and is the most common cause of juvenile incontinence in dogs. The majority of cases are unilateral, with the left and right ureter being affected with equal prevalence. Golden Retrievers, Huskies and Labrador Retrievers are overrepresented among cases. Ectopic ureters are typically identified in bitches younger than 6 months of age; these animals are normally presented to the veterinary surgeon because the owner perceives that they cannot be house trained. The incontinence caused by ectopic ureters is usually continuous in nature, and concurrent urinary tract infection is common (seen in 80% of cases). The ability of the patient to also pass a normal stream of urine may indicate that the ectopic ureter is unilateral rather than bilateral, although the author has seen many cases where the ability to urinate normally is not predictive. Ectopic ureters are less commonly associated with incontinence in male dogs as there is usually a stenosis at the distal ureter, meaning that these cases are typically identified much later in life and are found to have marked hydroureter and hydronephrosis on ultrasonographic examination. Concurrent urinary tract disorders are common and include urinary tract infections (>60% of females), renal dysplasia/agenesis, persistent paramesonephric remnant (90% of females), congenital urethral sphincter mechanism incompetence (USMI) (80% of females) and bladder hypoplasia.

Diagnosis of an ectopic ureter is best achieved via contrast CT or cystoscopy, both of which have been shown to have significantly greater sensitivity than either contrast radiography or ultrasonography. The author prefers to perform a focused ultrasonographic examination of the urinary tract in all cases to detect any concurrent upper urinary tract structural abnormalities, such as renal dysplasia, and then moves to cystoscopy for confirmation of the ectopic ureter, thus saving the client the cost of a CT scan and allowing cystoscopic laser ablation (CLA) to be performed at the time of cystoscopy.

Traditional surgical reimplantation of ectopic ureters is associated with various complications, which include but are not limited to stricture formation and the development of uroabdomen; reported complication rates are around 25%. The rate of urinary continence following surgical reimplantation is between 39% and 75% and increases with additional medical management (Holt and Moore, et al., 1995; Reichler et al., 2012). CLA of ectopic ureters is a minimally invasive alternative treatment that can be used in both male and female animals; in males, the procedure is performed via fluoroscopically guided perineal access. CLA allows the diagnosis and treatment of intramural ectopic ureters within a single procedure, while avoiding the vast majority of the complications associated with traditional surgical treatment via a coeliotomy. The author prefers to use a diode laser (980 nm) (Figure 15.15) for CLA of ectopic ureters, rather than a holmium:YAG laser, as the diode laser provides

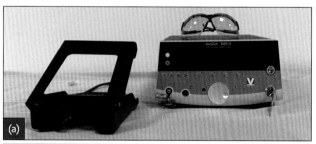

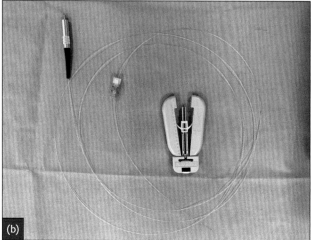

15.15 (a) A surgical diode laser and safety goggles for use when operating the laser. (b) Diode laser fibre and scissors used to trim the fibre.

coagulation as well as ablation of tissue, so the surgeon's view is not compromised by bleeding; however, the use of both types of laser has been reported in the literature. The procedure is performed on an outpatient basis. In unilateral disease, CLA involves ablation of the medial wall of the ectopic ureter until it is at the same level as the normal ureter. In cases of bilateral disease, both ureters are corrected to open within the bladder. A study of 30 dogs undergoing CLA (Berent et al., 2012) showed that 70% were continent immediately following the procedure, but the rate of continence decreased to 57% after 6 weeks. CLA is therefore associated with a similar improvement in continence to that achieved with surgical reimplantation. If the patient is not completely continent after CLA then medication for concurrent USMI, injectable urethral bulking agents and hydraulic occluders can be considered. At the same time as CLA, the author also performs laser correction of any paramesonephric remnant that is present, as this may contribute to ongoing incontinence or recurrent infections (see also Chapters 11 and 16 for further discussion of laser surgery to correct ectopic ureters).

Ureteral obstructions

Ureteral obstructions in dogs and cats can be caused by both benign and malignant disease. They are more commonly seen in cats but are likely to be underdiagnosed in both species. Ureteral obstruction is primarily seen in cats with calcium oxalate ureterolithiasis but can also occur in dogs and cats secondary to other stone types, strictures, neoplasia, dried solidified bloodstones or circumcaval ureters, among other causes. Around 15–20% of ureteral obstructions in cats are bilateral and the clinical presentation varies from acute renal failure to more insidious signs, such as weight loss, reduced appetite and lethargy. Given that around 70% of renal function must be lost for the development of an azotaemia, it is possible that many animals with unilateral ureteral obstruction may not show increased blood creatinine. More often than not, however, azotaemia is present. The importance of performing an ultrasonographic examination of the urinary tract to identify any dilatation of the renal pelvis or proximal ureter in all patients with increased blood creatinine cannot be overstated. Any dilatation of the renal pelvis or proximal ureter should raise concern for ureteral obstruction. One study (D'Anjou et al., 2011) identified any dilatation of the renal pelvis to greater than 7 mm as being highly likely to indicate an obstruction, and a more recent paper (Fages et al., 2018) identified obstruction in patients with a renal pelvis smaller than 4 mm. Experimental studies in research animals have shown that, following complete ureteral ligation, there is an irreversible loss of up to 40% of renal function after 7 days (Wilson, 1977). Thus, while the majority of cases of ureterolithiasis result in partial obstruction, timely intervention is still essential.

Medical management of an obstructive ureterolith should be attempted in all cases for a finite period of time (in the author's opinion, no longer than 48 hours). Careful attention must also be paid to potassium levels and acid–base disturbances in patients whose urine output is compromised. Intravenous fluid therapy forms part of the medical management of these cases but care must be taken to avoid volume overload, as cats in particular may have subclinical cardiomyopathies, and congestive heart failure as a consequence of aggressive fluid therapy is possible. In patients with anuric renal failure due to bilateral ureteral obstruction, extra care must be taken to avoid the risk of volume overload, and the author commonly does not recommend fluid rates above 2–4 ml/kg/h in the majority of cases once volume replacement has taken place. Various medical regimens have been suggested to promote stone propulsion, including the use of mannitol, amitriptyline and prazosin; all have limited success, with some reports showing that less than 10% of obstructive nephroliths are successfully managed in this way.

Traditional ureteral surgery is challenging to perform and is associated with high mortality (20–25%) and complication rates (16% of surgical cases develop uroabdomen and up to 40% develop ureteral strictures). For these reasons, alternative methods have been investigated for managing ureteral obstructions.

Ureteral stents (Figures 15.16 and 15.17) are, in the author's opinion, the method of choice for treating ureteral obstructions in dogs. Stents can be placed cystoscopically using a 2.7 mm rigid cystoscope in bitches and via a perineal approach, which allows rigid cystoscopy, in male dogs. Ureteral stents are generally not well tolerated in cats and can result in significant dysuria due to the stent irritating the trigone of the bladder. The mortality rate associated with stent placement is around 15%, which is significantly lower than that reported following ureteral surgery. Around 50% of humans who have a ureteral stent placed can experience discomfort, but this does not appear to be a problem in dogs. Ureteral stents have been used successfully in dogs and cats to alleviate both benign and malignant obstructions.

Ureteral obstructions in cats are best addressed by placement of a SUB device (Figure 15.18). The SUB device consists of a subcutaneous port attached to two catheters, one placed directly into the renal pelvis and the other placed directly into the bladder. Placement of the device therefore does not involve any manipulation of the ureter, and the device provides a bypass for urine flow. The procedure is performed via an open abdominal approach using fluoroscopic guidance (successful ultrasound-guided placement has also been reported; Livet et al., 2017). Placement of a SUB device is associated with significantly lower mortality than traditional ureteral surgery (around 6%) when performed by a surgeon who has been appropriately trained in the technique. The major complication associated with SUB placement is obstruction of the device with encrustation, which occurs in around 25% of cases (Berent et al., 2018). Of these cases, however, only half require device exchange, as in the remainder of cases the previous ureteral obstruction has resolved by

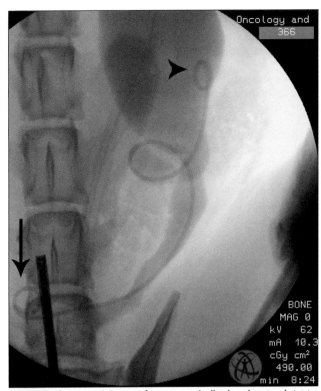

15.17 Fluoroscopic image of a cystoscopically placed ureteral stent. The cranial aspect of the stent (arrowed) is in the dilated proximal ureter and the distal aspect (arrowhead) is within the bladder.

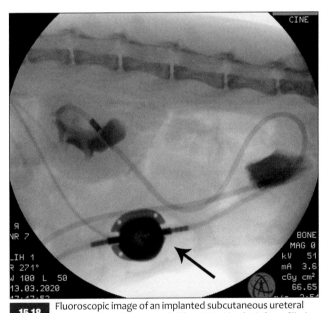

15.18 Fluoroscopic image of an implanted subcutaneous ureteral bypass device. The kidney (left) and bladder (right) are filled with contrast agent. The port used for flushing and sampling is highlighted with an arrow.

the time device obstruction is identified. It is recommended that the SUB device be flushed via the subcutaneous port under ultrasonographic guidance every 3 months. Recently, an EDTA-containing flush has become commercially available that may reduce the occurrence of mineralization of the device. The underlying cause of the ureteral obstruction should be addressed by appropriate medical and dietary management. SUB devices have also been placed in a number of dogs in which ureteral stent placement was not possible; however, the complication rate in dogs is higher than that reported in cats.

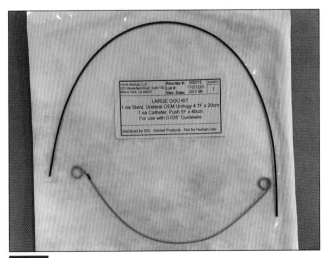

15.16 A canine double-pigtail ureteral stent and pusher catheter.

Urethral obstructions

Malignant urethral obstructions occur much more commonly in dogs than cats. They are primarily due to neoplastic disease of the bladder, urethra or prostate, most commonly a urothelial/transitional cell carcinoma or a prostatic adenocarcinoma. Placement of urethral stents has been reported in veterinary patients with obstruction due to both malignant and benign (strictures, uroliths and proliferative urethritis) disease.

If bladder tumours are located at the apex of the bladder, then at the author's hospital they are often managed with surgical resection and systemic chemotherapy; a median survival time of 772 days following partial cystectomy has been reported (Marvel *et al.*, 2017). However, the majority of bladder tumours are located at the trigone and these are rarely considered surgical candidates. Repeated palliative laser ablation can be considered; however, reported complications can be high and recurrence quick. Such laser ablation of malignant urethral obstructions should only be undertaken by someone with considerable experience (Cerf and Lindquist, *et al.*, 2012; see Chapter 16). Tumours of the trigone, urethra and prostate can all result in obstruction of the urine outflow tract. These tumours can also be seen to result in bilateral ureteral obstruction if growth of the tumour involves the ureterovesicular junction, and such cases require concurrent ureteral and urethral stent placement. Urethral stenting is best performed using a combination of fluoroscopy and cystoscopy, and the vast majority of these procedures can be done on an outpatient basis. It is important to determine whether the patient's clinical signs are caused by a urethral obstruction or are due to infiltration of the urinary tissue by the tumour, as both can result in dysuria/pollakiuria; this is best done by ultrasonographic examination of the bladder. In the author's opinion, urethral stents should be placed only when the patient is showing clinical signs of partial to complete urinary obstruction, as they are unlikely to relieve signs of dysuria secondary to tumour tissue infiltration alone. Urethral stents can be placed quickly and result in immediate relief of the obstruction and accompanying clinical signs.

The major complication following urethral stent placement is incontinence (seen in approximately 25% of cases in both dogs and cats). The location, length and diameter of the stent were not associated with the development of incontinence in one study (Blackburn *et al.*, 2013); however, where possible, the author avoids crossing the trigone with the stent. In cases with malignant obstructions the mean survival time following stent placement in dogs receiving concurrent chemotherapy was 270 days (Blackburn *et al.*, 2013).

Refractory urethral sphincter mechanism incompetence

Cystoscopic injections of collagen into the proximal urethra have been reported in dogs with USMI that was refractory to medical therapy. While this treatment is an attractive option compared with the various surgical techniques due to its minimally invasive nature, its efficacy decreases over time, and the treatment may need to be repeated every 6–12 months.

Idiopathic renal haematuria

Idiopathic renal haematuria is a diagnosis of exclusion. It has been reported in only a small number of case series, primarily in young large-breed dogs. Medical therapy with an angiotensin converting enzyme inhibitor or the Chinese herb Yunnan Baiyao has been reported to be successful in some cases (Bazelle and Foale *et al.*, 2011; Adelman *et al.*, 2017). In cases that are refractory to medical therapy, those that develop anaemia or those that develop an obstruction due to the formation of blood clots, the option to perform fluoroscopy-assisted sclerotherapy (with povidone–iodine/silver nitrate) with concurrent ureteral stenting is available. This procedure has been reported in six dogs, with resolution of the condition seen in four cases and improvement in two (Berent *et al.*, 2013).

References and further reading

Adelman LB, Olin S, Egger CM and Stokes JE (2017) Effect of oral Yunnan Baiyao on periprocedural hemorrhage and coagulation in dogs undergoing nasal biopsy. *Proceedings of the 2017 ACVIM Forum*. National Harbor, Maryland, USA, June 8–9, 2017

Bazelle J and Foale R (2011) The successful treatment of idiopathic renal haemorrhage with benazepril in four dogs. *Proceedings of the BSAVA Congress 2011*. Birmingham, April 5–8, 2001

Berent AC, Weisse CW, Bagley DH and Lamb K (2018) Use of a subcutaneous ureteral bypass device for treatment of benign ureteral obstruction in cats: 174 ureters in 134 cats (2009–2015). *Journal of the American Veterinary Medicine Association* **253**, 1309–1327

Berent AC, Weisse CW, Branter E *et al.* (2013) Endoscopic-guided sclerotherapy for renal-sparing treatment of idiopathic renal hematuria in dogs: 6 cases (2010–2012). *Journal of the American Veterinary Medical Association* **242**, 1556–1563

Berent AC, Weisse C, Mayhew PD *et al.* (2012) Evaluation of cystoscopic-guided laser ablation of intramural ectopic ureters in female dogs. *Journal of the American Veterinary Medical Association* **240**, 716–725

Blackburn AL, Berent AC, Weisse CW and Brown DC (2013) Evaluation of outcome following urethral stent placement for the treatment of obstructive carcinoma of the urethra in dogs: 42 cases (2004–2008). *Journal of the American Veterinary Medical Association* **242**, 59–68

Burdick S, Berent AC, Weisse C *et al.* (2018) Interventional treatment of benign nasopharyngeal stenosis and imperforate nasopharynx in dogs and cats: 46 cases (2005–2013). *Journal of the American Veterinary Medical Association* **253**, 1300–1308

Cerf DJ and Lindquist EC (2012) Palliative ultrasound-guided endoscopic diode laser ablation of transitional cell carcinomas of the lower urinary tract in dogs. *Journal of the American Veterinary Medical Association* **240**, 51–60

Culp WTN, MacPhail CM, Perry JA and Jensen TD (2011) Use of a nitinol stent to palliate a colorectal neoplastic obstruction in a dog. *Journal of the American Veterinary Medical Association* **239**, 222–227

Culp W, Weisse C, Berent A *et al.* (2015) Early tumor response to intraarterial or intravenous administration of carboplatin to treat naturally occurring lower urinary tract carcinoma in dogs. *Journal of Veterinary Internal Medicine* **29**, 900–907

Culp WTN, Zwingenberger AL, Giuffrida MA *et al.* (2018) Prospective evaluation of outcome of dogs with intrahepatic portosystemic shunts treated via percutaneous transvenous coil embolization. *Veterinary Surgery* **47**, 74–85

D'Anjou MA, Bédard A, Dunn ME (2011) Clinical significance of renal pelvic dilatation on ultrasound in dogs and cats. *Veterinary Radiology and Ultrasound* **52**, 88–94

Dengate A, Culvenor JA, Graham K *et al.* (2014) Bronchial stent placement in a dog with bronchomalacia and left atrial enlargement. *Journal of Small Animal Practice* **55**, 225–228

Fages J, Dunn M, Specchi S and Pey P (2018) Ultrasound evaluation of the renal pelvis in cats with ureteral obstruction treated with a subcutaneous ureteral bypass: a retrospective study of 27 cases (2010–2015). *Journal of Feline Medicine and Surgery* **2**, 875–883

Fryer K, Levine J, Peycke L, Thompson J and Cohen N (2011) Incidence of postoperative seizures with and without levetiracetam pretreatment in dogs undergoing portosystemic shunt attenuation. *Journal of Veterinary Internal Medicine* **25**, 1379–1384

German AJ, Cannon MJ, Dye C *et al.* (2005) Oesophageal strictures in cats associated with doxycycline therapy. *Journal of Feline Medicine and Surgery* **7**, 33–41

Greenhalgh SN, Dunning MD, McKinley TJ *et al.* (2010) Comparison of survival after surgical or medical treatment in dogs with a congenital portosystemic shunt. *Journal of the American Veterinary Medical Association* **236**, 1215–1220

Holt PE and Moore AH (1995) Canine ureteral ectopia: an analysis of 175 cases and comparison of surgical treatments. *Veterinary Record* **136**, 345–349

Hoshi S, Mao H, Takahash T *et al.* (1997) Internal iliac arterial infusion chemotherapy for rabbit invasive bladder cancer. *International Journal of Urology* **4**, 493–499

Hume DZ, Solomon JA and Weisse CW (2006) Palliative use of a stent for colonic obstruction caused by adenocarcinoma in two cats. *Journal of the American Veterinary Medical Association* **228**, 392–396

Kim SE, Giglio RF, Reese DJ *et al.* (2013) Comparison of computed tomographic angiography and ultrasonography for the detection and characterization of portosystemic shunts in dogs. *Veterinary Radiology and Ultrasound* **54**, 569–574

Lam N, Weisse C, Berent A *et al.* (2013) Esophageal stenting for treatment of refractory benign esophageal strictures in dogs. *Journal of Veterinary Internal Medicine* **27**, 1064–1070

Liptak JM, Dernell WS, Monnet E *et al.* (2004) Massive hepatocellular carcinoma in dogs: 48 cases (1992–2002). *Journal of the American Veterinary Medicine Association* **225**, 1225–1230

Livet V, Pillard P, Goy-Thollot I *et al.* (2017) Placement of subcutaneous ureteral bypasses without fluoroscopic guidance in cats with ureteral obstruction: 19 cases (2014–2016). *Journal of Feline Medicine and Surgery* **19**, 1030–1039

Macready DM, Johnson LR and Pollard RE (2007) Fluoroscopic and radiographic evaluation of tracheal collapse in dogs: 62 cases (2001–2006). *Journal of the American Veterinary Medical Association* **230**, 1870–1876

Marvel SJ, Séguin B, Dailey DD and Thamm DH (2017) Clinical outcome of partial cystectomy for transitional cell carcinoma of the canine bladder. *Veterinary and Comparative Oncology* **15,** 1417–1427

Mullins RA, Sanchez Villamil C, de Rooster H *et al.* (2019) Effect of prophylactic treatment with levetiracetam on the incidence of postattenuation seizures in dogs undergoing surgical management of single congenital extrahepatic portosystemic shunts. *Veterinary Surgery* **48**, 164–172

Raske M, Weisse C, Berent AC *et al.* (2018) Immediate, short-, and long-term changes in tracheal stent diameter, length, and positioning after placement in dogs with tracheal collapse syndrome. *Journal of Veterinary Internal Medicine* **32**, 782–791

Reichler IM, Eckrich Specker C, Hubler M *et al.* (2012) Ectopic ureters in dogs: clinical features, surgical techniques and outcome. *Veterinary Surgery* **41**, 515–522

Sériot P, Gibert S, Poujol L *et al.* (2019) Extended palatoplasty as surgical treatment for nasopharyngeal stenosis in six cats. *Journal of Small Animal Practice* **60**, 559–564

Sumiyoshi Y, Yokota K, Akiyama M, Kawaoto H and Kosugi I (1991) Tissue levels of pirarubicin (THP) in dogs following intra-arterial infusion. *Gan To Kagaku Ryoho* **18**, 1621–1626 (in Japanese)

Weisse C and Berent A (2015) *Veterinary Image-Guided Interventions*. Wiley-Blackwell, Ames

Weisse C, Berent A, Violette N *et al.* (2019) Short-, intermediate-, and long-term results for endoluminal stent placement in dogs with tracheal collapse. *Journal of the American Veterinary Medical Association* **254**, 380–392

Wilson DR (1977) Renal function during and following obstruction. *Annual Review of Medicine* **28**, 329–339

Chapter 16

An introduction to laser endosurgery

David Sobel, Jody Lulich and Maurici Batalla

Introduction

In recent decades, the combination of minimally invasive surgery and surgical lasers has provided veterinary surgeons (veterinarians) the opportunity to perform interventions in anatomical locations that were previously inaccessible. It is now possible to perform all but the most invasive of surgical procedures using endosurgical techniques. Lasers utilizing a fibreoptic delivery system, at certain wavelengths, are a valuable complement to endosurgery.

Having invested in the basic equipment required for minimally invasive surgical procedures, it makes sense for the veterinary practice to provide as many clinically appropriate uses for the equipment as possible. The addition of lasers to the surgeon's armamentarium improves the quality of surgical interventions and provides a significant value-added component for veterinary practices that are already making use of endoscopy and endosurgery.

Laser physics

Although the optical physics of lasers is beyond the scope of this chapter, a basic understanding of the underlying principles of lasers and how light interacts with biological tissue is important for the veterinary surgeon using this technology. In-depth information on the physics and biology of lasers can be found elsewhere.

The word 'laser' is an acronym for **L**ight **A**mplification by the **S**timulated **E**mission of **R**adiation. The theoretical concepts of lasers can be credited to Max Planck, amongst others. The theory of quantum electrodynamics allows the concurrent understanding and application of light conceptualized as both particulate (photon theory) and a wave (wave theory), and ultimately explains how the light produced by the lasers used in surgery interacts with different tissues.

Put simply, all matter has the potential to emit photons (quanta of electromagnetic radiation, including light). The number of photons emitted by, say, a glass of water on a desk is infinitesimally small; indeed, the number of photons emitted by a glass of water over time would be so small as to render them essentially invisible and to have minimal impact on matter that they subsequently encounter. In order to produce light with sufficient energy and of an appropriate wavelength to affect tissues, several things need to happen to the matter or medium used to produce the light.

A 'lasing medium' – that is, a medium that will emit a significant number of photons when stimulated – needs to be used. In the case of lasers used in surgery, a single element or compound, for example, yttrium aluminium garnet (YAG), carbon dioxide (CO_2) or a diode, is commonly used as the lasing medium. To augment the number of photons emitted by the lasing medium when it is stimulated, during the manufacture of the laser a small amount of an impurity is added, usually to the optical delivery system or to the lasing medium itself. This is known as 'doping'. These doping agents (also termed dopants), when combined with the appropriate lasing medium, will result in a more efficient laser that produces more photons per unit of energy inputted over time. Doping agents such as ruby, holmium (Ho), neodymium (Nd), erbium (Er) and thulium (Tm) are common. The introduction of each agent slightly changes the wavelength and momentum of the photons produced.

The lasing medium needs to be stimulated to encourage it to emit a greater number of photons. This is most commonly done by introducing electricity to the lasing medium. Any substance that would emit a meaningful number of photons without the introduction of additional stimulating energy would be dangerous and unsuitable for veterinary purposes. Such substances would be likely to be radioactive.

Lasers, whether for surgical or other purposes, produce a coherent beam of monochromatic light; that is, a beam of photons, all of the same wavelength, travelling in the same direction. As alluded to above, any lasing medium will be emitting photons even when it is not being stimulated. However, to produce the required coherent monochromatic light, a 'photon cascade' needs to be created (Figure 16.1).

When atoms of a given element are in an 'unexcited' stable state (called the ground state) they can and will spontaneously change from the ground state to an 'excited' or high-energy state. If energy – in the form of heat, light or electricity – is supplied to an atom, some of its electrons move from a low-energy orbit near the nucleus to a higher energy orbit further away from the nucleus. In the excited state, there is a chance that the atom will encounter another such atom and collide with it. This collision will produce a single photon. In the lasing medium, the introduction of electricity excites the atoms in the medium, causing more atoms to leave the ground state and enter an excited energy state. As the excited state is unstable, the natural tendency of these atoms is to return to their more stable ground state. As atoms in the lasing

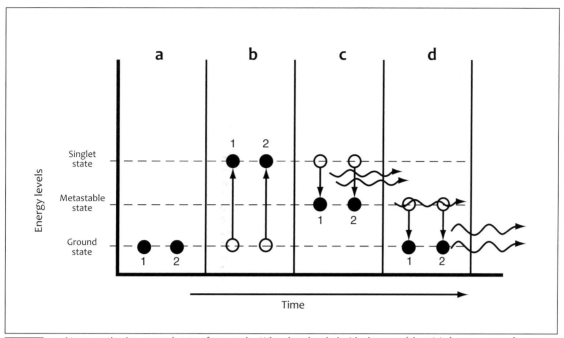

16.1 a = Atoms resting in a ground state of energy. b = When bombarded with electrons (electricity), atoms move from a ground state of energy. c = When excited, atoms drop from the singlet state to the metastable state of energy. This change in state results in the loss of energy in the form of a photon. d = If a photon collides with a metastable atom as it is dropping to the ground state (which invariably happens), energy is lost in the form of a photon. ⌇⌇⌇ = Photon.

medium move from a stable to an unstable state (and back again, repeatedly) under stimulation by electricity, more and more atoms in the medium collide and more and more photons are emitted. If the lasing medium is pure (apart from the dopant), the photons emitted will all be of the same wavelength, thus producing the desired mono-chromatic light.

The laser device itself is most simply understood as a 'box' containing the lasing medium. The interior of this box is covered by a highly reflective medium, and it has a single opening (the aperture) at one end. A series of lenses focuses the monochromatic but incoherent light produced by the lasing medium into a stream of photons, of the same wavelength, travelling at the speed of light in a uni-form direction. The amount of energy (in the form of elec-tricity) introduced to the device will have a more or less linear, although finite, effect on the energy produced by the laser beam.

The different wavelengths of light produced by different lasers will have different effects on biological tissues. This can be shown graphically in a coefficient of absorption curve (Figure 16.2). This graph illustrates how different wavelengths of light are absorbed by different tissues and other materials. Knowledge of this curve and the nature of the tissues that are expected to be encountered during a given surgical procedure will guide the veterinary surgeon in the choice of laser device for that procedure.

While there is a myriad of surgical lasers currently available for use in a wide range of applications, this chapter will focus on lasers with delivery systems that are suitable for use in minimally invasive surgery. For such purposes, the laser must have an optical delivery system that is compatible with endoscopes and endoscopic equipment. The most commonly used delivery system for this purpose is fibreoptic. Diode, Ho:YAG, Nd:YAG and Tm:YAG lasers all use some variant of a solid quartz glass fibre, with a solid but flexible core insulated by silicone or a similar cladding material. While there is an industry

standard for connection of the fibre to the laser device, known as an SMA connection, it should be noted that many fibres are proprietary to the laser manufacturer. This can be due to the nature of the dopant contained in the fibre and/or other proprietary features of the particular laser.

A large variety of diameters and shapes of fibres are available, but most commonly a 'flat beam' fibre is employed. This shape allows the light emitted by the fibre to travel in parallel with the long axis of the fibre itself. The diameter of the fibre has an impact on the maximum amount of light (and therefore the energy) delivered. If there is a chip, fracture or other defect at the fibre tip, the light emitted will be less coherent and therefore its energy will be attenuated as it leaves the fibre.

Power density, measured in watts (W)/cm², is the term used to describe the intensity of the laser beam. It is directly proportional to the power (in W) that the laser can deliver, and inversely proportional to the surface area (in cm²) that the beam strikes. Thus, doubling the power will double the power density if the same fibre is used, but doubling the diameter of the fibre (which will increase its surface area by a factor of four) will decrease the power density by three-quarters. Similarly, halving the fibre dia-meter will increase the power density for a constant power setting by a factor of four. The power density will be greatest when the laser beam is directed perpendicular to the tissue. If it is directed at an angle, the geometry of the laser spot will alter and the power density will diminish. The resultant power density will also be non-uniform and will be greatest at the point in the spot closest to the laser fibre.

As a very broad rule of thumb, the largest fibre that can be safely introduced into the endoscope via the instrument channel or some other port of ingress should be used. This will allow the operator the greatest range and control of energy imparted by the laser.

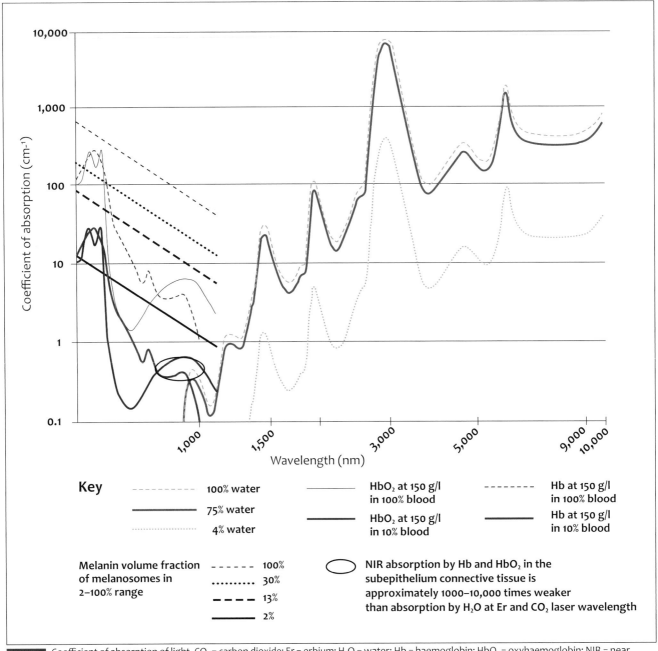

Key

– – – – – –	100% water
————	75% water
··············	4% water

————	HbO₂ at 150 g/l in 100% blood
————	HbO₂ at 150 g/l in 10% blood

- - - - - -	Hb at 150 g/l in 100% blood
————	Hb at 150 g/l in 10% blood

Melanin volume fraction of melanosomes in 2–100% range

- - - - -	100%
··········	30%
– – – –	13%
————	2%

NIR absorption by Hb and HbO₂ in the subepithelium connective tissue is approximately 1000–10,000 times weaker than absorption by H₂O at Er and CO₂ laser wavelength

16.2 Coefficient of absorption of light. CO_2 = carbon dioxide; Er = erbium; H_2O = water; Hb = haemoglobin; HbO_2 = oxyhaemoglobin; NIR = near infrared.

Types of laser

Carbon dioxide lasers

Historically, the CO_2 laser was the first surgical laser used routinely in small animal surgery. For many years, it was the most commonly used laser by small animal practitioners. These efficient, economical and highly effective lasers are excellent for general surgical use. However, the underlying physics of these lasers means that their use in endoscopic applications is limited. Most medical CO_2 lasers emit light in the 10,200–10,900 nm range. This has advantages in that the depth of penetration of the laser beam, assuming the same power output, is limited compared with diode lasers at surgically appropriate wavelengths. However, light in this range is highly attenuated by water and other fluid media and is poorly absorbed by biological

pigments. This makes the use of CO_2 lasers for endoscopic applications involving fluid irrigation and haemorrhage extremely limited. In addition, the delivery systems, often proprietary in nature, usually involve either some form of hollow semi-rigid internally reflective tube or a series of articulated arms with mirrors. These delivery systems make transmitting the light into endoscopes and related equipment very difficult and inefficient.

Neodymium:YAG lasers

The Nd:YAG laser was one of the earliest surgical lasers used in veterinary medicine. Nd:YAG is a crystalline material that uses neodymium as the dopant. It emits light in the infrared range at a wavelength of approximately 1064 nm. Many Nd:YAG lasers use a technology called Q-switching, which allows the laser to produce high-energy pulses. Historically, Nd:YAG lasers were adopted by equine practitioners for endoscopic procedures in the upper airway, with great success. In small animals, Nd:YAG lasers are used in upper airway surgery, uroendoscopy and, less commonly, in laser lithotripsy. These lasers have largely been replaced in small animal surgery by Ho:YAG and diode lasers.

Holmium:YAG lasers

The use of Ho:YAG lasers in veterinary practice has become more prevalent over the past 10 years as their cost has decreased. They have become the laser of choice for endourological procedures in humans, where laser lithotripsy and holmium laser enucleation of the prostate are now standard. Additionally, Ho:YAG lasers are approved in the USA for the resection of luminal strictures related to a variety of pathologies (in humans). They also are widely used 'off label' for a variety of surgical indications in both human and veterinary patients. Ho:YAG lasers produce light with a wavelength in the 2100 nm range, making them ideal for work in a fluid medium. (Light in the 2100 nm range is minimally attenuated by fluid. As such, they retain much of their original power at the surgical site.) These lasers produce a superpulse of light, creating an ultra-high-temperature plasma bubble at the tip of the fibre. This is a highly efficient source of laser energy with a reduced risk of collateral thermal injury. The plasma bubble causes significant vibration at the fibre tip, so much so that for a long time medical physicists theorized that Ho:YAG lasers exerted their physiological effect via a photoacoustic effect. However, it is now known that these lasers indeed produce a direct thermal effect on the tissues. The vibration has the unintended effect of pushing tissue (or calculi) away from the tip of the fibre. In the case of laser lithotripsy, this can be frustrating, as the stone will often be pushed away from the operator's field of view with each pulse. Newer Ho:YAG technologies for laser lithotripsy, such as MOSES™ (Lumenis), are designed to minimize this effect. Relative to the amount of energy generated, the risk of collateral thermal injury from Ho:YAG lasers is manageable. However, it should be remembered that the Ho:YAG laser is not a 'beginner' laser; the operator requires training and experience to use this device effectively and safely.

Thulium:YAG lasers

Tm:YAG lasers behave in a similar way to Ho:YAG lasers, producing light in the 2000 nm range. Clinically, they are used for many of the same applications as Ho:YAG lasers, and there is controversy regarding the advantages of thulium *versus* holmium lasers. Currently, Tm:YAG lasers are more expensive than neodymium or holmium lasers, but new manufacturers are introducing more cost-effective thulium lasers to the market.

Diode lasers

Diode lasers are the most commonly used lasers in small animal endoscopic surgery. Laser diodes are semiconductors that emit laser light at a given wavelength, which is determined by the construction of the particular diode. The production of laser diodes is very cost-effective, and the devices currently available have a high degree of reliability, require minimal maintenance and produce excellent power output relative to their cost and size. The most commonly used laser diodes are contained in small lightweight boxes with a simple user interface and are available at prices within the budget of many veterinary practices.

Diode lasers commonly used in veterinary surgery usually produce light at a wavelength of 980 nm or 810 nm, with maximum power ranging from 5 to 50 W. Each wavelength has unique benefits and limitations, and it is important that the veterinary surgeon understands the laser:tissue interactions specific to each (see below). The 810 nm diode laser is extremely useful for endoscopic surgery as it functions very well in in both air and fluid (e.g. saline irrigation during surgery), as well as in highly pigmented tissues (e.g. those containing haemoglobin or melanin). The minimal attenuation of the laser and its excellent absorption by pigmented tissue mean that it can provide haemostasis very effectively with minimal loss of power. Thus, masses in the nasal cavity or urinary tract, for example, can be excised or ablated very effectively with an 810 nm diode laser. The 980 nm diode laser behaves similarly but with somewhat less efficacy in pigmented tissue and greater attenuation in water. However, this wavelength penetrates tissue less deeply, allowing a relatively safer procedure with less concern over the depth of the surgical lesion.

Diode lasers can be used both in non-contact mode, with the fibre held a few millimetres from the surgical site, and in direct contact with the tissue. When used in non-contact mode, the laser behaves similarly to other types of laser (e.g. YAG, CO_2). In contact mode, a thin layer of char or carbon is burned into the tip of the fibre. This can be done in a proprietary fashion by the manufacturer, or by the operator activating the laser against a piece of pigmented paper, or even a tongue depressor with a dot of ink on it; when doing this, caution should be exercised not to ignite the material. Some manufacturers offer a liquid ceramic material that can be annealed to the surface of the tip before use.

Some practitioners suggest that diode lasers used in contact mode are not performing laser surgery at all; rather, the surgery is being done by the 'hot tip' of the fibre. However, it is the author's [DS] opinion that this argument is irrelevant, as both contact and non-contact methods offer different and equally important surgical techniques.

Laser:tissue interactions

It is essential for the veterinary surgeon to have a basic knowledge of laser:tissue interactions in order to be able to choose the equipment and techniques that will be most effective for a particular procedure. Each wavelength of light interacts with a variety of tissues and media differently during minimally invasive surgery, and knowledge of these interactions will guide the operator in selecting the right tool for the job.

Put simply, laser light acts as a form of thermal energy when it is in contact with a fluid or solid tissue. When the laser light meets tissue at the surgical site, the immediate effect is superheating of the tissue. The laser energy rapidly (in milliseconds) heats the intracellular water to well above boiling point. As the laser heats and vaporizes the intracellular water, the cell membrane proteins are denatured and the cell essentially explodes. This results in complete ablation of the tissue closest to the laser light. Radiating from the central point of light are zones of thermal ablation, irreversible cellular necrosis and reversible cellular injury (Figure 16.3). The thermal effect of the

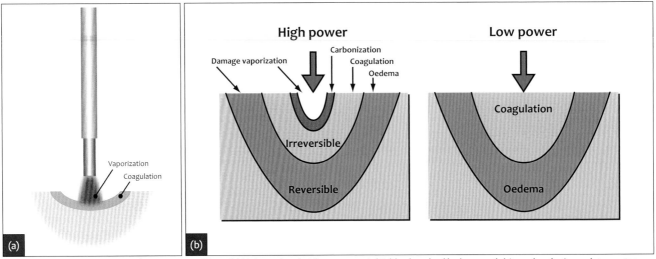

16.3 Tissue interaction with non-contact fibres. (a) Light emitted at 810–900 nm is highly absorbed by haemoglobin and melanin, and generates high temperatures at the tissue surface. This results in rapid vaporization with underlying coagulation of up to 3 mm. (b) The effects of high power (left) and low power (right) on the surrounding tissue.
(Courtesy of Diomed Ltd)

laser will radiate in three dimensions, so it is important for the surgeon to be aware of the impact on tissue that is not immediately visible at the surface of the surgical site. Depending on the anatomical area of interest, this may be of critical importance. For instance, the wall of the urethra is quite thin and excessive energy will potentially compromise its integrity deep to the point of contact in the lumen. In contrast, other areas, such as the rhinarium, are more resilient to thermal injury.

The variables controlling the thermal effect of a specific laser/fibre combination are: the wavelength of light it produces; its power (in W), representing the energy input; the mode of use (pulse *versus* continuous); and the length of time for which the laser is fired and the distance between the fibre tip and the tissue in non-contact mode. The coefficient of absorption curve (see Figure 16.2) will guide the surgeon in predicting the thermal effects of a given laser. For instance, 810 nm diode lasers produce light that is highly absorbed by haemoglobin and melanin. This effect, which is specific to the wavelength, will produce a magnified thermal impact. This can be beneficial, as it means that the surgeon can decrease the amount of power and the contact time to maximize the tissue-ablating efficacy of the laser while minimizing collateral thermal injury. However, if the surgeon should try to replicate the power and mode settings of a CO_2 laser, for example, the thermal injury would be potentially devastating.

Most lasers allow the operator to select a continuous firing mode or a pulse mode with different on/off intervals. In pulse mode, the heat is given a few milliseconds to dissipate into the surrounding tissues or the irrigation fluid between pulses; this allows the tissues to relax and minimizes collateral thermal injury. In continuous mode, the laser has a more rapid effect, which can reduce the operative time. Different tissues, pathologies and anatomical locations will respond to different wavelengths of light applied in different ways.

Laser safety

While the use of any form of thermal energy device in surgery warrants attention to safety issues, lasers have some particular characteristics that need to be considered.

When being used for surgical purposes, the laser should be active only when the fibre tip is visible and correctly placed in the surgical field; inadvertent firing of the laser poses a danger to personnel and the patient.

The operating theatre must be adequately equipped for laser surgery. Ideally, a room with few or coverable windows should be used. This will minimize the risk of inadvertent exposure of people outside the room to laser light. In addition, most surgical lasers are equipped with a remote interlock device, also known as a 'dead-man switch'. This device links the doors of the operating theatre to the laser. Essentially, when the operating theatre doors are opened, the circuit is broken and the laser will not fire. This ensures that anyone entering the room will not inadvertently be exposed to the laser beam. However, this device is rarely used in veterinary hospitals, and a small circuit connector can be used to override the interlock function. In any case, the door to the operating theatre should be labelled with appropriate signage indicating the use of the laser, the wavelength in use, and advising personnel entering to wear masks and appropriate eye protection.

The wavelengths of light used in endoscopic laser surgery fall in the infrared or near-infrared range, and as such are invisible to the human eye. Many lasers are equipped with an aiming diode that emits visible (usually red or green) light. Most lasers are also equipped with some form of audible signal that sounds when the laser is active and firing. While the aiming beam should not be pointed towards the eye, the greater concern is the active laser beam. Despite being invisible, the laser beam can still have a damaging impact on the eye, so appropriate eye protection must be worn. All personnel in the operating theatre should wear laser goggles. The goggles are wavelength-specific and are usually labelled with the wavelength against which they provide protection. It is imperative that the surgeon ensures that all personnel in the theatre are wearing eye protection specific to the wavelength of laser light being used. It is also important to protect the patient's eyes. Ophthalmic eye lubricants applied liberally, cotton wool or gauze moistened with saline, or purpose-made contact lenses all can be used to protect the patient's eyes. It is also worth noting that the laser beam can reflect off a variety of surfaces, including surgical instruments. While the risk is considerably lessened when the laser light is visualized on a monitor while being used within the patient, care should be taken to ensure that the laser is never fired without specific surgical intention.

If the endoscopic procedure is being performed 'dry' (i.e. without significant saline irrigation or within the lumen of dry viscera), the smoke or 'plume' created as the laser vaporizes tissue is a potential hazard. Studies have found fragments of viable DNA within the plume created (Hallmo and Naess, 1991; Pierce *et al.*, 2011) and, while there have been no documented cases of iatrogenic disease resulting from the inhalation of the plume, it is prudent to avoid exposure. Surgical masks with a pore size that is less permeable to the plume are available. In addition, smoke-evacuating devices are available that remove the plume from the surgical site.

Collateral thermal injury is a common safety concern and complicating factor in laser surgery. Fortunately, with proper training and education this risk can be minimized, but it cannot be eliminated. Selection of the appropriate type of laser, power level and mode, and conservative use of energy can help maintain healthy surgical margins. As any form of thermal energy can result in delayed tissue healing, this must be considered when planning the procedure. Accidental burns from the laser should be treated immediately by irrigation with cold fluids (where feasible), any haemorrhage should be controlled and the tissues should be kept moist. External laser wounds, whether surgical or iatrogenic, should be kept moist and protected by the frequent administration of topical lubricating antibiotic ointments.

Uses of laser endosurgery

Respiratory tract

The use of lasers together with endoscopy allows a range of conditions to be treated in a curative or palliative manner, especially in the upper respiratory tract. Three types of laser are mainly used: diode, Ho:YAG and CO_2 lasers. Each type has its advantages and disadvantages for each type of intervention.

Indications

Laser endoscopy is indicated for certain congenital conditions, inflammatory diseases and tumours, as well as removal (by vaporization) of polyps, stenosis and granulomas. Brachycephalic obstructive airway syndrome (BOAS) is the most complex pathology of the upper respiratory tract, and more than one type of laser can be used to treat the anatomical abnormalities and secondary problems that are characteristic of the syndrome. The interventions may be undertaken in an endoscopically assisted or purely endoscopic fashion, depending on the anatomical location.

Instrumentation

In addition to the various types of laser equipment, an endoscope is required in order to perform laser surgery in the respiratory tract. Both rigid and flexible endoscopes can be used for procedures in the respiratory tract. Flexible endoscopes range in diameter from 2.5 mm to 10 mm; the selection is dependent upon the size of the patient and the cavity to be explored (see below). If a rigid endoscope is to be used, normally a 9.5 Fr operating endoscope or a 2.7 mm, 30-degree endoscope with a sheath is sufficient to access the cavities where interventions may be required.

To some extent, the choice of endoscope is dictated by the location in the respiratory tract where the procedure is to be carried out:

- Nasal cavity – a rigid endoscope is recommended
- Nasopharynx – for an anterograde approach via the nasal cavity, a rigid endoscope is recommended; for a retrograde approach, either a flexible endoscope or a 120-degree rigid endoscope can be used
- Larynx and pharynx – a rigid endoscope or exoscope (video-telescopic operating microscope) is recommended
- Trachea and bronchi – for tracheobronchoscopy, a flexible endoscope is usually used as it allows access to the whole trachea and the bronchi. A rigid endoscope can be used for interventions in the trachea and sometimes, depending on the size of the patient, at the entrances of the mainstem bronchi.

However, the surgeon's experience and preference will ultimately determine the equipment selected for each procedure.

Anaesthetic considerations

The main precaution when using a laser in the interior of an airway is to avoid ignition, as oxygen and inhalational anaesthetic agents are flammable. The anaesthetist must ensure that the patient is at the correct level of anaesthesia and is adequately oxygenated, and that CO_2 is eliminated, while taking measures to reduce the risk of ignition and possible postoperative consequences. Various strategies can be used to reduce the risk of ignition. The use of an endotracheal tube resistant to laser action is recommended, as is the use of total intravenous anaesthesia (TIVA) with propofol/alfaxalone, fentanyl or a combination of both, rather than inhalational anaesthesia. However, it can be difficult to maintain a stable plane of anaesthesia with TIVA, and so careful monitoring, and adjustment of the infusion as needed, is essential. In addition, the inspired fraction of oxygen should be kept below 30% to reduce the risk of ignition. A wet gauze should be placed in the larynx to prevent any leaked oxygen or (if an inhalational protocol is used) anaesthetic agent from coming into contact with the laser. If the procedure is being carried out in the larynx, trachea or bronchi, a smaller diameter endotracheal tube can be used to maintain the airway during the entire procedure. However, in some situations this can hinder access to the surgical field and generate greater resistance in the airways. In these cases, TIVA should be used and supplemental oxygen supplied via a tracheal catheter.

Brachycephalic obstructive airway syndrome

BOAS is a respiratory disorder of dog breeds with shortened skulls and muzzles (e.g. French Bulldogs, Pugs, English Bulldogs). Dogs with BOAS have a range of anatomical abnormalities, such as an elongated soft palate, stenosis of the nares and nasal cavity, excessive protrusion of the turbinates into the nasopharynx, tracheal hypoplasia and tracheobronchomalacia, which make them prone to secondary abnormalities and disorders including everted laryngeal saccules, laryngeal, tracheal and bronchial collapse, pharyngeal obstruction and nasopharyngeal sialocoeles. Some of these abnormalities can be treated by laser surgery with endoscopy or exoscopy.

Elongated soft palate: The conventional approach to an elongated soft palate uses a scalpel or pair of scissors to excise the excess tissue. However, a CO_2 laser, diode laser or bipolar sealing device can also be used; with these devices, haemostasis is improved and there is no need to suture the tissue. If a CO_2 laser is used, a power of between 15 and 20 W is used in continuous mode. With a diode laser, 5 W of power in contact mode with a 400 μm fibre is sufficient. The power can be increased if necessary, but it is advisable not to increase it to more than 10 W to ensure that the heat from the laser does not spread beyond the incision line. The use of an endoscope or exoscope is not always necessary, but some veterinary surgeons prefer to use one or the other to improve the visibility of the soft palate and pharynx.

Laryngeal collapse: Laryngeal collapse is a form of obstruction of the upper airways resulting from loss of rigidity of the laryngeal cartilages leading to medial deviation. This condition has a high incidence among brachycephalic breeds of dog but can also occur in other breeds.

There are three stages of laryngeal collapse:

- Stage I – eversion of the laryngeal saccules
- Stage II – medial displacement of the cuneiform and corniculate processes, which appear to enter the lumen
- Stage III – collapse of the corniculate processes close to the dorsal arch of the glottis.

Laryngeal sacculectomy can be performed using scissors, since there is usually little bleeding from the laryngeal saccules, and a laser can be used only on the bleeding points to provide haemostasis. While it is possible to use a laser to perform the entire procedure, this is not recommended as the first option, as the dispersion of heat from the surgical site can cause laryngeal oedema.

Laryngeal collapse at stages II and III can be treated by laser surgery consisting of vaporization of the cuneiform processes to remodel the larynx. If a CO_2 laser is used, the cuneiform process should be incised at an angle of 60 degrees over the apex to avoid the corniculate process. A power of 12 W is used in superpulsed mode at a distance of between 5 and 10 cm (Llinás, 2017). A diode laser at a power of 5–10 W with the fibre in continuous or pulsed contact with the cartilage can also be used. The use of an endoscope or exoscope is optional, but may improve visibility of the surgical site in severe cases.

Nasopharyngeal sialocoeles: Sialocoeles have been found in the oral cavity and pharynx, and were recently also described in the nasopharynx of English Bulldogs, French Bulldogs and Pugs (De Lorenzi *et al.*, 2018). Nasopharyngeal sialocoeles may develop as a consequence of chronic non-physiological mechanical stress that results in changes in the minor nasopharyngeal salivary glands. They can be located ventrally or dorsally. Nasopharyngeal sialocoeles can be classified as occlusive or non-occlusive, and single or multiple sialocoeles may develop. Ablation can be performed with a diode laser (980 nm wavelength) (Figure 16.4). The laser fibre should be introduced through the working channel of a flexible endoscope that is retroflexed to access the nasopharynx. No complications during the procedure have been reported and no recurrences after surgery have been described.

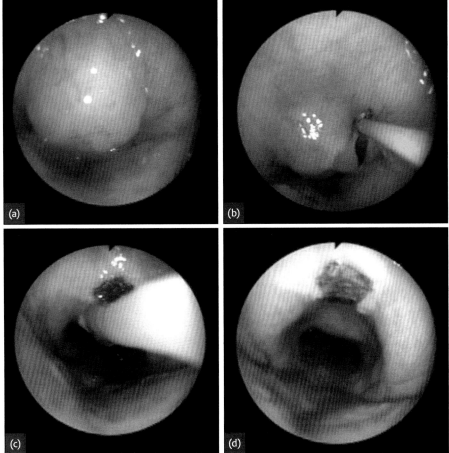

16.4 Laser ablation of a nasopharyngeal sialocoele. (a) Sialocoele. (b) Laser fibre in contact with the sialocoele. (c) Introduction of a probe to aspirate saliva from the opened sialocoele. (d) Final result of ablation.
(Courtesy of D. De Lorenzi)

Enlarged tonsils: In severe cases of BOAS, large tonsils can protrude into the nasopharynx. These can be removed using a laser, with or without the use of an endoscope or exoscope as required. This procedure also allows the space at the entrance to the nasopharynx to be increased.

Abnormal turbinates and intranasal airway obstruction: In a study of 132 brachycephalic dogs with severe respiratory distress due to BOAS, it was observed that all dogs had abnormal conchal growth that resulted in obstruction of the intranasal airways (Oechtering *et al.*, 2016a). Rostral aberrant turbinates (Figure 16.5) were very common in Pugs (90.9%) and less frequent in French Bulldogs (56.4%) and English Bulldogs (36.4%). Caudal aberrant turbinates (Figure 16.6) obstructing the nasopharyngeal meatus were commonly found in all breeds examined (66.7%). Deviation of the nasal septum was observed in almost all Pugs (98.5%) but was less common in Bulldogs. The abnormal turbinates had multiple points of mucosal contact that were responsible for the intranasal airway obstruction;

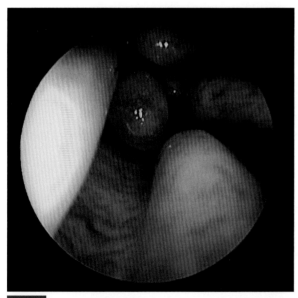

16.5 Rostral aberrant turbinate.

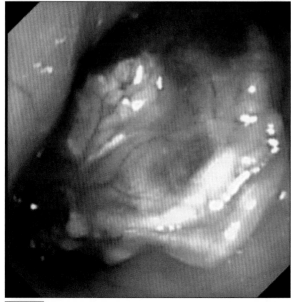

16.6 Caudal aberrant turbinate.

interconchal and intraconchal mucosal contacts were evident in 91.7% of dogs. These obstructions are an important factor in the exercise and heat intolerance that is characteristic of dogs with BOAS, as they compromise the pulmonary ventilator and thermoregulatory functions of the nose. Failure to relieve intranasal obstruction may be a reason for the lack of therapeutic success of conventional surgery for BOAS in some dogs.

Laser-assisted turbinectomy (LATE) is an effective method for creating a patent nasal airway. It consists of ablation of:

* The turbinates that narrow or obstruct the airway through the interior of the nasal cavity
* Rostral aberrantly growing turbinates
* The ventral nasal concha
* Caudal aberrantly growing turbinates.

LATE is a complex procedure that requires good knowledge of the anatomy of the nasal cavity. A 980 nm diode laser with a 400 μm fibre is used, together with a 2.7 mm diameter, 30-degree rigid endoscope with a sheath or a 9.5 Fr operating endoscope. Irrigation and suction systems are also required that connect to the endoscope or to suction tubes, to remove surgical smoke, blood and debris.

For transection of the turbinates, the laser is used in near-contact mode (3–4 W in a pulsed mode); the tip of the fibre should not touch the turbinate tissue but be kept at a distance of approximately 0.5 mm. In this way, a cut with coagulation is achieved. The turbinate can be mobilized with the aid of forceps or a suction tube to facilitate access of the laser fibre during the transection process. Finally, ridged forceps are inserted parallel to the endoscope to extract the excised turbinate and any remaining carbonized tissues. Alternatively, ablation can be performed by using the diode laser in contact mode to completely vaporize the aberrant turbinate (Figure 16.7).

LATE is considered to be a safe procedure; no major complications have been reported, although minor bleeding has been described. Bleeding from peripheral vessels during transection of the conchal tissue can complicate the surgical procedure, but the view of the surgical field is generally not compromised and the procedure can continue without the need for additional suction or flushing. Some patients will have ongoing and chronic serous nasal discharge as a sequela to LATE. The severity and duration of this is related to the magnitude of the resection performed.

Laryngeal and pharyngeal masses

The ablation of laryngeal (Figure 16.8) and pharyngeal masses can be performed endoscopically or assisted using an exoscope. The use of an endoscope or exoscope facilitates visualization of the mass, including its margins and vascularization, particularly for lesions that penetrate into the trachea. The mass can be completely ablated with a CO_2 or diode laser (either a 980 nm or 810 nm wavelength), using the lowest effective power for vaporization. However, excessive heat generated during the procedure can lead to laryngeal oedema and the serious consequences associated with this condition. Therefore, it is advisable to perform a mixed procedure, with the mass removed using scissors and the laser used only to coagulate areas of haemorrhage. This approach considerably reduces the possibility of heat dispersing from the laser into the surrounding tissues.

In many cases, the procedure must be performed without the use of endotracheal intubation because the

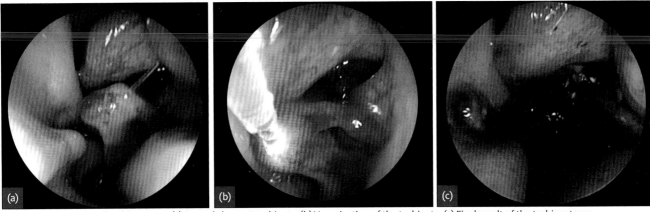

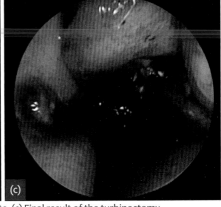

16.7 Laser-assisted turbinectomy. (a) Rostral aberrant turbinate. (b) Vaporization of the turbinate. (c) Final result of the turbinectomy.
(Courtesy of D. L. Casas)

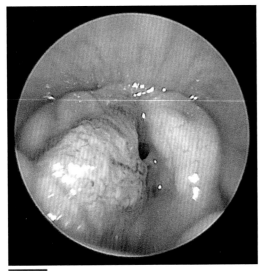

16.8 Laryngeal mass.

endotracheal tube would block the view of the mass, particularly if it is located in the larynx. In these circumstances, TIVA should be used. Oxygen should be supplied to the anaesthetized patient by introducing a catheter connected to the oxygenation equipment into the trachea. The laser must not be activated while oxygen is being supplied, as this could result in ignition and tissue burns, which could have serious consequences. The oxygen supply is cut off and the patient is allowed to take a few breaths, which will expel the residual oxygen; after this, the laser can be activated.

Trachea and bronchi

There are three conditions of the lower respiratory tract for which laser surgery may be appropriate: masses; tracheal stenosis; and granulation secondary to a tracheal stent. As with laryngeal masses, the use of oxygen should be approached with caution when undertaking procedures involving lasers.

Tracheobronchial masses: Tracheobronchial masses can be ablated using a laser (980 nm wavelength) (Figure 16.9). The laser fibre should be introduced via the working channel of the endoscope. Rigid grasping forceps and a flexible loop or basket can also be introduced via or parallel to the working channel, depending on the point in the procedure at which they are introduced and the surgeon's

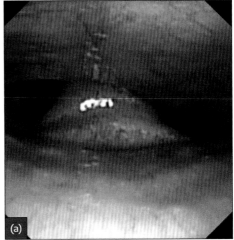

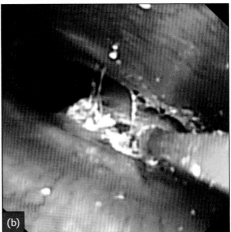

16.9 (a) Tracheal chondroma. (b) Ablation of the tracheal chondroma using a Ho:YAG laser.

preference. These instruments can be used to hold the mass during surgery and then to extract it at the end of the procedure. If the mass is located in a bronchus, rigid grasping forceps cannot be used (in this case, graspers and laser fibres must be used through the working channel of a flexible endoscope. The patient can be endotracheally intubated if the location of the mass and the working space required for the endoscope and instruments allow this. Where endotracheal intubation is not possible, oxygen should be delivered via a catheter placed in the trachea, and a second catheter should be used for aspiration of the smoke generated by the procedure.

Tracheal granulation: Tracheal stents can occasionally result in the proliferation of granulation tissue in the wall of the trachea. This can lead to infection, the accumulation of mucus and progressive airway obstruction. A diode laser can be used to vaporize the granulation tissue. It should be noted that this is a palliative rather than a curative treatment, but it can help to prevent occlusion of the tracheal lumen.

Nasal cavity and nasopharynx

It is very common to find abnormalities in the nasal cavity and nasopharynx that obstruct the airway or produce bleeding, mucus or chronic infections. In most cases, these clinical signs are due to tumours or polyps, hypertrophy of the turbinates, stenosis or aspergillosis.

A diode or Ho:YAG laser can be used to transect or vaporize the abnormal tissues. The diode laser produces very thin cuts that enable precise ablation, and has a good coagulation capacity. A power of between 5 and 15 W should be used, depending on the type of tissue to be ablated. In general, these lasers should be used when the area of tissue to be ablated is not very large and there is good visibility. The Ho:YAG laser vaporizes and cuts in a less precise manner when in contact with the tissue. A power of 2–12 W can be used for coagulation, while a power of 12–20 W is required for cutting. Ho:YAG lasers are useful for vaporizing large structures, but their coagulation efficiency is less than that of the 810 nm diode but equal to that of the 980 nm. Treatment can be curative in some patients but may be only palliative in others.

Intranasal masses and polyps: Primary intranasal tumours (Figure 16.10) represent approximately 1% of all neoplasms in dogs and cats; they are mainly carcinomas and sarcomas. They show progressive local invasion and have a low metastatic rate. For these reasons, and because they have a high recurrence rate, local treatment is very important. Radiotherapy is the treatment of choice, but chemotherapy or non-steroidal anti-inflammatory drugs (NSAIDs), or a combination of these treatments, can be used, with differing degrees of effectiveness.

It is unclear whether adjunctive removal of tumour tissue by laser rhinoscopy or open surgery decreases the rate of recurrence or increases the survival time. Empirically, local clinical signs appear to reduce with surgical treatment, especially in cases for which radiotherapy is not possible.

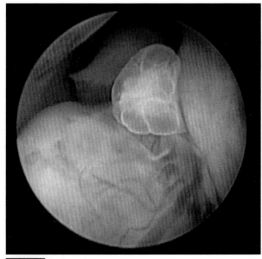
16.10 Rostral nasal carcinoma.

After laser turbinectomy, there is an evident reduction in the clinical signs associated with nasal masses (e.g. epistaxis, mucus and sneezing). Most importantly, it is possible to increase the size of the airway to improve the patient's breathing.

Laser surgery to remove intranasal masses (Figure 16.11) should be carried out with continuous irrigation with fluids and/or insufflation and aspiration of air. The fluids will prevent overheating of the tissues and help to clear the nasal cavity of blood, smoke and debris, to maintain good visibility. If continuous irrigation is not used, then insufflation and aspiration of air are required to prevent irritation of the tissues by the smoke and to ensure a clear surgical field.

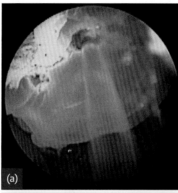
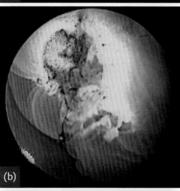
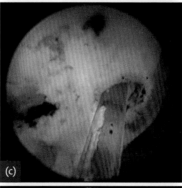
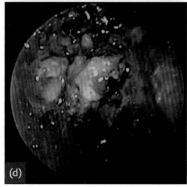

16.11 Turbinectomy to remove a nasal mass. (a) Laser fibre in contact with the mass. (b) Effect of firing the laser on the tissue. (c) Devascularization of the tissue following laser firing. (d) Appearance of the surgical site on completion of the turbinectomy.

When performing a turbinectomy, it is advisable to start the procedure at the most posterior part of the mass and move in an anterior direction; this ensures that the surgical field remains visible for the duration of the surgery. If the procedure is started at the anterior part of the mass, it may be difficult to visualize the posterior limits of the mass because of bleeding and debris obstructing the surgical field. Depending on the structure of the mass, it can be transected or vaporized using the laser. All vaporized tissues should be removed by flushing the surgical site with fluid or air and aspiration, and grasping, biopsy or basket forceps should be used to retrieve pieces of tissue.

The procedure for removing polyps or polypoid structures is the same as that for intranasal tumours, although it is usually a simpler process because the abnormal tissue is usually smaller (just a few millimetres) and therefore easier to transect or vaporize completely. If the mass or polyp is located within the nasopharynx (Figure 16.12), the procedure is more complex. Rigid or flexible endoscopy can be used to gain access to the mass from the nasal cavity and the nasopharynx (Figure 16.13). It is usually easiest to approach the mass from the nasal cavity; however, in some cases, due to the size, shape and location of the mass, it is necessary to perform the procedure via both cavities (Figure 16.14).

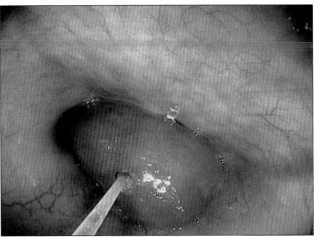

16.14 Retroflexed laser endoscopy for ablation of a nasopharyngeal mass.

Nasopharyngeal stenosis: The procedure of choice for nasopharyngeal stenosis in dogs is balloon dilation followed by the placement of a stent. In cats, laser incision followed by balloon dilation is usually sufficient. However, in cases where the stenosis is located caudally and the stenotic wall is very thin (Figure 16.15), the use of laser endoscopy may be sufficient; this is particularly the case in cats. The use of the laser to make two lateral cuts from the stenotic opening allows a more controlled balloon dilation and preserves the edges of the wound, facilitating re-epithelialization. The laser can also be used to control any haemorrhage following dilation.

Canine aspergillosis: Sinonasal aspergillosis is a relatively common disease in dogs. The main clinical signs are a profuse mucoid to haemorrhagic chronic nasal discharge, epistaxis and ulceration of the external nares with crusting. Diagnostic imaging (computed tomography (CT) and rhinoscopy) is mandatory to locate the fungal plaques and to assess the sinuses and the destruction of the nasal turbinates and, in severe cases, the cribriform plate.

Treatment involves using a diode or Ho:YAG laser to 'burn off' the fungal plaques and perform a partial turbinectomy around them (Figure 16.16). However, it should be noted that if the fungal plaques are located on the cribriform plate, a laser cannot be used. Following surgery, a topical antifungal agent should be instilled into the nasal cavity via a catheter that is inserted either through the

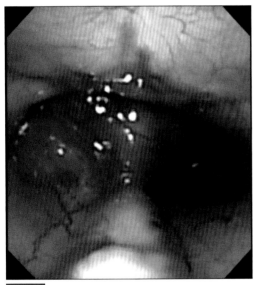

16.12 Nasopharyngeal mass.

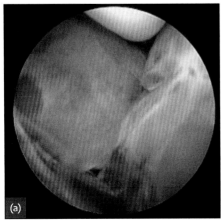
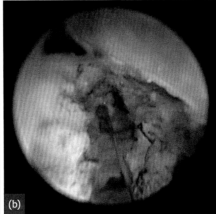
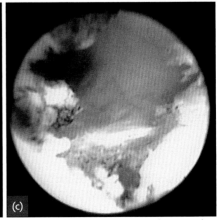

16.13 Ablation of a nasopharyngeal mass. (a) Rostral view of a nasopharyngeal tumour. (b) Effect of firing the laser on the tissue. Note that rostral access is required for this procedure. (c) Appearance of the surgical site on completion of the ablation.

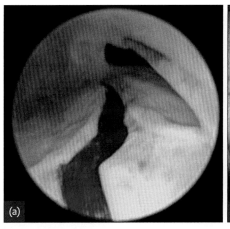
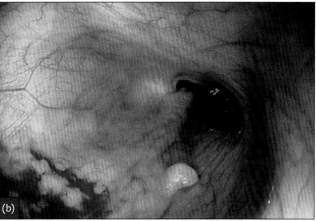

Nasopharyngeal stenosis. (a) View of nasopharyngeal stenosis from the nasal cavity. (b) View of nasopharyngeal stenosis during retroflexed endoscopy.

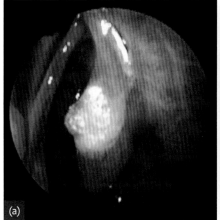
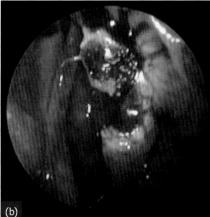
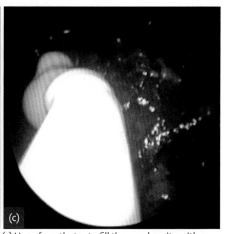

16.16 Nasal aspergillosis. (a) *Aspergillus* plaque. (b) Partial laser turbinectomy around the plaque. (c) Use of a catheter to fill the nasal cavity with clotrimazole cream.

working channel of the endoscope or parallel to it. The drug of choice is enilconazole, although clotrimazole (1% cream) or miconazole may also be used. The instillation should be visualized via the endoscope to ensure that the antifungal agent reaches all parts of the nasal cavity. In some cases, where there has been significant destruction of the nasal turbinates, direct access to the sinuses via rhinoscopy may be possible (see Chapter 9). In these instances, the antifungal agent can also be instilled into the sinuses. If the frontal sinuses are severely affected but cannot be accessed via rhinoscopy, then trephination should be performed to allow them to be cleansed with fluid irrigation and to instil the antifungal medication.

Rhinoscopy should be performed every 3 weeks to reassess the nasal cavity. If new fungal plaques or the remains of previous ones are present, then the procedure should be repeated. Normally, between one and three treatment cycles are required; however, if the condition is not very advanced and the plaques have been adequately debrided, a single treatment is often effective.

Postoperative considerations

In general, the patient does not need to be hospitalized after the procedures described above, unless complications occur (this is most likely in brachycephalic animals). Medical treatment involves the administration of NSAIDs or corticosteroids for a few days, depending on the extent of inflammation resulting from the procedure, and antibiotics as required. In some cases, bronchodilators and antitussives may be necessary.

Urinary tract

Uroliths

Uroliths can be fragmented with a Ho:YAG laser. The mechanism of stone fragmentation is mainly photothermal and involves a thermal drilling process rather than a shockwave effect. Energy from the Ho:YAG laser crystal is transmitted to the urolith via a flexible quartz fibre. To achieve the best results, the quartz fibre tip is guided with the aid of a cystoscope so that it is in direct contact with the surface of the urolith (see also Chapter 11).

Transurethral laser lithotripsy in bitches and queens: In female animals, laser lithotripsy is performed via urethro-cystoscopy with the patient anaesthetized (Figure 16.17). Although patient positioning is the choice of the surgeon, bitches and queens tend to be positioned in dorsal recumbency. A rigid cystoscope is passed into the vestibule and along the urethral lumen to allow visualization of the uroliths (Figure 16.17a). The urinary tract is lavaged and then refilled with sterile saline. During lithotripsy, continuous irrigation is provided to flush urolith fragments and debris away from the visual field and to absorb stray laser energy.

Laser energy is delivered via a quartz lithotripsy fibre that is passed through the working channel of the cystoscope (Figure 16.17b). The size of the fibre depends on the size of the working channel but is usually 365–400 μm. The cystoscope is used to guide the tip of the fibre into direct contact with the surface of the urolith. A foot-operated switch activates the laser lithotriptor. The laser energy selected varies depending upon the size and

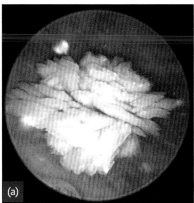 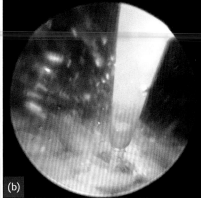 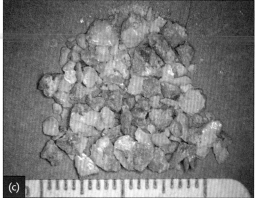

16.17 Intraoperative images of a calcium oxalate urolith (a) before and (b) during laser lithotripsy. (c) Following the procedure, the fragments were removed with a stone basket and by voiding urohydropulsion.

location of the urolith; however, for most uroliths the initial settings are typically between 0.8 and 1 J at 8–10 Hz. The laser energy can be adjusted for efficiency based on the operator's experience and the desired fragmentation process. After fragmentation, the larger urolith fragments are removed with a stone basket to verify that they are small enough to pass unimpeded through the urethra. The remaining smaller fragments are removed by voiding uro-hydropulsion (Figure 16.17c).

In some instances, bladder inflammation and trauma during lithotripsy result in the extravasation of blood and subsequent clot formation. If the clot adheres to the bladder wall and entraps small fragments of the uroliths, complete removal of all urolith material is unlikely to be possible. In the author's [JL] experience, the blood clots detach from the bladder wall within 24 hours. The residual stone burden can then be removed by voiding urohydro-pulsion or allowed to pass spontaneously during urination.

Transurethral laser lithotripsy in male dogs: The size of the os penis and flexure of the urethra in male dogs limit the size and deflectability of cystoscopes that can be introduced into the bladder. However, small-diameter (7.5–8.5 Fr) flexible endoscopes designed for the evaluation

of human ureters will pass easily through the urethra of most male dogs weighing more than 6–8 kg.

Some veterinary surgeons prefer to capture uroliths in the bladder with a basket and place them in the urethra before fragmentation. Urethroliths are readily fragmented because the small size of the urethral lumen prevents them from moving out of the laser field. To help prevent urethro-liths from travelling back into the bladder during lithotripsy, the energy (in J) of the laser lithotriptor can be reduced.

Transurethral laser lithotripsy cannot be performed in male cats because of the small diameter of the urethral lumen.

Potential complications: It is logical to consider whether lasers capable of shattering uroliths would be likely to damage the urinary tract. Because the laser energy is delivered in a pulsed fashion during the procedure and is readily absorbed by water, most complications are rare, rapidly reversible or clinically unimportant (Figure 16.18). Continuous irrigation of the bladder during lithotripsy ensures that stray energy is quickly absorbed and dispersed. Under these conditions, the thermal effect of the Ho:YAG laser is localized to within approximately 1–2 mm of the laser fibre tip. In a prospective study of 598 human

Complication	Occurrence	Avoidance
Bladder rupture	Rare	Bladder perforation is possible during excessive or forced overdistension with fluid, or by direct trauma via careless advancement of cystoscope. Proper patient positioning will minimize iatrogenic trauma, even in bladders with pre-existing weakness. Bladder perforation can also occur when incorporating voiding urohydropulsion to remove urolith fragments. Keeping the size and volume of urolith fragments to a minimum, and ensuring adequate anaesthesia to promote complete urethral relaxation will minimize intravesicular pressure during manual compression. If the integrity of the bladder wall is questionable, the urolith fragments should be removed with a stone retrieval basket
Cyanide production	Rare	Thermal decomposition of uric acid to cyanide can occur during lithotripsy. However, attempts to detect cyanide in the effluence during lithotripsy of uroliths composed of purines have been unsuccessful. Nonetheless, continuous irrigation of saline and frequent evacuation of the urinary bladder during lithotripsy is recommended
Mucosal haemorrhage	Common	Haemorrhage obscures working visibility. In addition to strategies recommended to minimize urethral swelling, lower laser power settings (0.6 J and 6 W) should be used to minimize urolith recoil during fragmentation
Mucosal perforation	Rare	Mucosal perforation is rare because Ho:YAG laser energy is delivered in 350 μs pulses and is quickly dispersed in the fluid surrounding the tip of the laser fibre. Care should be taken to ensure that the laser is activated only when the fibre is in contact with the surface of the stone. This will help to avoid urothelial perforation
Retention of small urolith fragments	Common	Urolith fragments approximately 0.5 mm or less in diameter can become trapped in blood oozing from and attached to denuded urothelium. If not passed, fragments may serve as a nidus for future uroliths. Voiding urohydropulsion 24 hours or longer following lithotripsy is often sufficient to completely evacuate the bladder. In some cases, these minute fragments will spontaneously pass during routine urine voiding

16.18 Potential complications of transurethral laser lithotripsy. (continues) ▶

Complication	Occurrence	Avoidance
Urethral obstruction	Rare	Complete obstruction is rare because irregular-shaped fragments are unlikely to form an occlusive seal within the urethral lumen. However, urethral obstruction may occur when a large number of fragments are voided through the urethra simultaneously. If this occurs, the laser should be used to break up the fragment conglomeration and reduce fragment size. If anticipated, a portion of the fragments can be removed with a stone basket before voiding urohydropulsion
Urethral swelling	Common	Urethral swelling impedes evacuation of uroliths and increases the likelihood of urethral obstruction. The degree of swelling is proportional to the frequency with which cystoscopes are passed and urolith fragments removed through the urethral lumen. To minimize this complication, well lubricated endoscopes should be passed gently, endoscopes with a smaller working diameter than the urethra should be chosen, the stones should be fragmented into smaller fragments before removal, and any infections should be corrected before lithotripsy. If urethral obstruction is imminent, a short period (24 hours) of continuous transurethral catheterization should be considered until the swelling subsides

16.18 (continued) Potential complications of transurethral laser lithotripsy.

patients with kidney or ureteral stones fragmented by laser lithotripsy, complications (consisting of ureteral trauma) were observed in only one patient (Sofer *et al.*, 2002). These results suggest that when properly performed, laser lithotripsy can be safely used in dogs and cats.

Ectopic ureters

The ureters originate at the hilum of the kidneys, travel caudally through the retroperitoneal space, enter the caudal bladder and travel intramurally between the tunica muscularis and the tunica mucosa before entering the bladder lumen at the cranial trigone. Ectopic ureters do not follow this normal path and open distally in the caudal trigone, bladder neck, urethra or, less commonly, the genital tract. Typically, dogs with ectopic ureters present with continuous leakage of urine. However, in cases where the terminal ureteral opening remains closed or the urinary sphincters override urine loss, the condition may appear asymptomatic and the patient may show hydroureter and hydronephrosis without urine leakage.

Ectopic ureters are classified as:

- Intramural – these tunnel through the caudal bladder, and comprise approximately 95% of ectopic ureters in dogs
- Extramural – these do not tunnel through the caudal bladder, and are typical in cats.

This distinction allows the veterinary surgeon to select the most appropriate treatment for the patient. Both types of ectopic ureter can be corrected surgically; however, only intramural ectopic ureters can be managed by laser ablation of the wall between the ureter and the urethra during cystoscopy (Figures 16.19, 16.20 and 16.21).

Cystoscopy is the most accurate method for diagnosing ectopic ureters. However, fluoroscopic-aided contrast urography, CT with contrast urography, or cystoscopic-assisted retrograde contrast ureteropyelography with fluoroscopy permit the identification of a transmural orientation of intramural ectopic ureters.

Preoperative considerations	
Patient positioning	Females – dorsal recumbency. The hindlimbs should be secured laterally and cranially. Alternatively, the patient should be placed in sternal recumbency with the hind legs hanging off the end of the table
	Males – lateral or dorsal recumbency. With a perineal approach, the patient should be positioned in dorsal recumbency and the hindlimbs secured laterally and cranially. Patient position varies with the surgeon's preference
Antibiotic treatment	Usually none required
Faeces removal	If present, digitally remove faeces from the rectum
Site preparation	Clip the hair around the vulva or penis. Aseptically prepare the perineal skin and vestibule/preputial cavity
Cystoscopy	Carefully evaluate the urethra (and vestibule in female animals) for the number and position of ectopic ureteral openings, including multiple fenestrations, and any additional anomalies (e.g. paramesonephric remnant, vaginal duplication, ureterocoele). If intramural tract orientation has not been confirmed, perform retrograde contrast ureteropyelography
Ureteral cannulation	Ureteral cannulation is usually achieved without guidewire assistance Females: • Pass a 4–6 Fr ureteral catheter or 8 Fr red rubber feeding tube into the vestibule • Pass the cystoscope into the vestibule • Digitally compress the labia around the sheath of the cystoscope to seal the vestibule • To improve visualization of the anatomy, dilate the vestibular cavity by gravity feeding sterile fluid through the cystoscope channel • Advance the ureteral catheter into the urethral opening and along the urethra • Follow with the cystoscope; this assists passage of the catheter into the ectopic ureteral opening. If the ectopic ureteral opening is obliquely deviated or inaccessible, use an angle-tipped ureteral catheter or place the ureteral catheter using a guidewire. If using a guidewire, pass the guidewire through the channel of the cystoscope into the ectopic ureter. Slide the cystoscope off the guidewire and pass the ureteral catheter over the guidewire into the ureter, then remove the guidewire Males: • Pass the ureteral catheter down the urethra • Follow with the cystoscope to assist insertion into the ureter by either a retrograde approach or a perineal approach

16.19 Procedure for ablation of ectopic ureters. (continues)

Procedure	
Ureteral ablation	• Load the laser fibre into the biopsy channel of the cystoscope • Position the cystoscope near the opening of the ectopic ureter • Extend the laser fibre sufficiently beyond the tip of the cystoscope and ablate the common wall between the ureter and urethra, 'unzipping' it until the ureter opens into the bladder • With a unilateral ectopic ureter, extend the opening to the level of the normal contralateral ureteral opening • With bilateral ectopic ureters, ablate the ureter with the more proximal opening first to minimize inflammation that may distort the anatomical orientation during repair of the ureter that opens more distally During activation of the laser, a sufficient flow of fluid is needed to prevent damage to the lateral walls of both structures. A catheter placed in the urethra can also be used to block laser energy from damaging the lateral wall of the urethra
Postoperative considerations	
Antibiotics	Co-amoxiclav (15–20 mg/kg q12h) for 1–3 days
Pain medication	Opioids or non-steroidal anti-inflammatory drugs for 3–5 days
Assessment of the procedure	Perform retrograde or anterograde contrast ureteropyelography to assess whether repositioning of the ureteral openings is sufficient, and whether urine leakage is present, immediately following the procedure, or 1–4 weeks later. When performed weeks after ectopic ureter ablation, abatement of hydroureter and hydronephrosis can also be evaluated

16.19 (continued) Procedure for ablation of ectopic ureters.

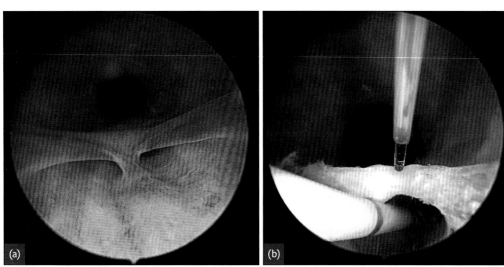

16.20 (a) Preoperative and (b) intraoperative images of laser ablation of bilateral intramural ectopic ureters in a bitch. A catheter is placed in the lumen of the left ectopic ureter to shield the outer wall while the wall shared between the urethra and ureter is ablated cranially until the ureter opens in the urinary bladder.

Complication	Management
Urethral/ureteral perforation	Experienced practitioners familiar with cystoscopy and laser use should not experience this problem unless an extramural ectopic ureter was incorrectly diagnosed as intramural. If perforation occurs, the ectopic ureter and the perforation can be repaired surgically, or a catheter can be placed in the urethra for several days to allow the perforation to close through normal tissue healing
Ureteral stenosis/stricture	Although rare, some ureters may show exuberant tissue proliferation during remodelling. Follow-up ultrasonography performed 1–2 months after ablation is recommended to assess the outcome and the need for a subsequent procedure
Continued urinary incontinence	Approximately, 50% of bitches and most male dogs are continent following ectopic ureter ablation. If incontinence persists or returns, urinary tract infection and polyuria should be excluded as contributing factors before trying phenylpropanolamine or reproductive hormone therapy. If the animal is still incontinent, consider urethral bulking agents to increase urethral closure pressure, or colposuspension to reposition a pelvic bladder. Placement of a urethral occluder may be needed for persistent and severe cases. With bilateral ectopic ureters, it is difficult to determine how far forward to move the ureteral openings into the urinary bladder; some dogs with bilateral ectopic ureters may require a second laser procedure to position the ureteral openings deeper (i.e. more cranial) in the urinary bladder
Urinary tract infection	Urinary tract infection is uncommon in dogs that did not have an infection before ectopic ureter ablation. Correction of other urogenital anomalies (e.g. ablation of paramesonephric remnants) and of structural (e.g. perivulvar dermatitis) and functional (e.g. endocrinopathies, obesity) risk factors may reduce the risk of urinary tract infection. Antibiotic therapy should be selected on the basis of urine culture and antimicrobial susceptibility testing

16.21 Potential complications of laser ablation of ectopic ureters.

Intraluminal bladder and urethral polyps

Most polyps in the urinary tract are benign (lympho-plasmacytic or eosinophilic) and form because of chronic irritation associated with urinary tract infection or urolith-iasis. Some, but not all, inflammatory polyps regress when the causative infection or urolithiasis is treated. However, polyps that are associated with haematuria, dysuria, urinary obstruction or recurrent infection, or those that have a malignant appearance or show continued growth, should be removed and submitted for histopathological analysis.

Polyps are removed cystoscopically by:

- Directing laser energy at their base, above and parallel to the bladder wall
- Forcibly plucking the polyp free from the mucosa after securely snaring it with a flat-wire stone-retrieval basket (flat-wire baskets cut tissue better than routine stone-retrieval baskets)
- Cauterizing the polyp free with a polypectomy snare attached to a cautery with the loop placed around the base of the polyp.

Malignant polyps (rhabdomyosarcoma, carcinoma *in situ*, transitional cell carcinoma, metastatic neoplasia) should be surgically removed when they are located in the body and dome of the bladder, with the goal of reducing the tumour burden and the likelihood of metastasis. While outcome-based prospective studies are lacking, there is significant anecdotal evidence to support endosurgical ablation or debulking of transitional cell carcinoma. While not likely to be curative in most cases, the resultant improvement in owner reported clinical signs and quality of life suggests the utility of these procedures. Endosurgical ablation as a stand-alone palliative operation, or as adjunctive therapy with other modalities, has significant merit (Cerf and Lindquist, 2012). Laser ablation did not improve the mean survival time, but severe complications were rare. Laser ablation of transitional cell carcinoma and other malignant tumours is a palliative treatment that primarily benefits dogs with tumours obstructing the urethra. Tumours in the urethral lumen should be carefully ablated parallel to the wall and towards the lumen. Diode lasers offer better operator control than pulsed holmium lasers when ablating such tissue.

Stenotic ureteral openings

Not all stenotic ureters (Figure 16.22) require surgical widening. Those associated with urinary incontinence, progressive dilatation, hydronephrosis and a decline in kidney function should be widened. However, those that are static and not associated with abnormalities can be monitored until it becomes apparent that intervention is warranted. The procedure is the same as that for the abla-tion of ectopic ureters. As stenotic ureters are primarily seen in male dogs, a perineal approach should be consid-ered to facilitate access and repair.

Ureterocoeles

Ureterocoele is a congenital abnormality where the distal ureter balloons at its opening into the lumen of the bladder. When the ureter is ectopic, the ureterocoele extends within the bladder neck or the urethra. Imaging (ultrasonography, retrograde urethrocystography and CT contrast urography) facilitates the diagnosis; a smooth, thin-walled cystic structure within the lumen of the bladder is seen.

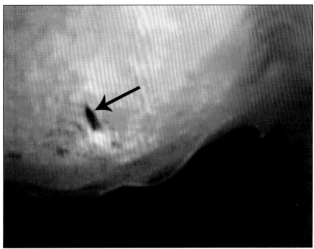

16.22 Stenotic distal ureteral orifice (arrowed) at the vesicourethral junction in a male dog.

Ureterocoeles can be ablated with a laser by incising over the dome as it bulges into the bladder lumen. Once the ureterocoele is open, the distal ureteral orifice can be visualized. If the orifice is stenotic or intramural and ectopic, the laser can be used to widen the opening and extend it to a normal position within the bladder. In some cases, the distal ureteral orifice may be identified distal to the ureterocoele. If there is an identifiable ureteral opening, the ureter can be catheterized and the uretero-coele ablated over the catheter.

Persistent paramesonephric remnants

Vestibulovaginal septal remnants can distort or block the vaginal and urethral openings (see also Chapter 11). Their clinical significance varies, but some are associated with urinary tract infection or interfere with mating. Most rem-nants are narrow and easily broken digitally. Remnants that are more difficult to detach can be freed from their dorsal and ventral attachments by laser ablation (Figure 16.23).

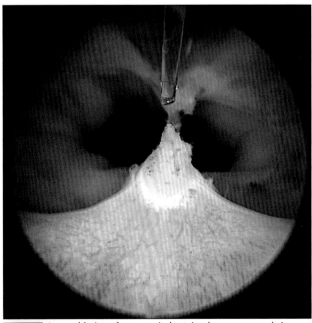

16.23 Laser ablation of a congenital retained paramesonephric remnant bridging the dorsal and ventral vestibulovaginal junction.

References and further reading

Berger NA and Eeg PH (2006) *Veterinary Laser Surgery: A Practical Guide.* Blackwell Publishing, Oxford

Bommarito DA, Kent MS, Selting KA *et al.* (2011) Reirradiation of recurrent canine nasal tumors. *Veterinary Radiology and Ultrasound* **52**, 207–212

Cancedda S, Sabattini S, Bettini G *et al.* (2015) Combination of radiation therapy and firocoxib for the treatment of canine nasal carcinoma. *Veterinary Radiology and Ultrasound* **56**, 335–343

Casas DL and Santana AJ (2018) *Técnicas de Mínima Invasión en Pequeños Animales.* Multimédica Ediciones Veterinarias, Barcelona

Cerf DJ and Lindquist EC (2012) Palliative ultrasound-guided endoscopic diode laser ablation of transitional cell carcinomas of the lower urinary tract in dogs. *Journal of the American Veterinary Medical Association* **240**, 51–60

De Lorenzi D, Bertoncello D and Mantovani C (2018) Nasopharyngeal sialoceles in 11 brachycephalic dogs. *Veterinary Surgery* **47**, 431–438

Hallmo P and Naess O (1991) Laryngeal papillomatosis with human papillomavirus DNA contracted by a laser surgeon. *Eur Arch Otorhinolaryngol* **248**, 425–427

Lhermette P and Sobel D (2008) *BSAVA Manual of Canine and Feline Endoscopy and Endosurgery, 1st edn.* BSAVA Publications, Gloucester

Liu NC, Oechtering GU, Adams VJ *et al.* (2017) Outcomes and prognostic factors of surgical treatment for brachycephalic obstructive airway syndrome in 3 breeds. *Veterinary Surgery* **46**, 271–280

Llinás J (2017) Diagnóstico y tratamiento con láser CO_2 del colapso laríngeo en braquicefálicos. *Clincirvet* **1**, 2–8

Morgan MJ, Lurie DM and Villamil AJ (2018) Evaluation of tumor volume reduction of nasal carcinomas *versus* sarcomas in dogs treated with definitive fractionated megavoltage radiation: 15 cases (2010–2016). *BMC Research Notes* **11**, 70

Oechtering GU, Pohl S, Schlueter C *et al.* (2016a) A novel approach to brachycephalic syndrome. 1. Evaluation of anatomical intranasal airway obstruction. *Veterinary Surgery* **45**, 165–172

Oechtering GU, Pohl S, Schlueter C and Schuenemann R (2016b) A novel approach to brachycephalic syndrome. 2. Laser-assisted turbinectomy (LATE). *Veterinary Surgery* **45**, 173–181

Pierce JS, Lacey SE, Lippert JF *et al.* (2011) Laser-generated air contaminants from medical laser applications: a state-of-the-science review of exposure characterization, health effects, and control. *Journal of Occupational and Environmental Hygiene* **8**, 447–466

Schuenemann R, Pohl S and Oechtering GU (2017) A novel approach to brachycephalic syndrome. 3. Isolated laser-assisted turbinectomy of caudal aberrant turbinates (CAT LATE). *Veterinary Surgery* **46**, 32–38

Sofer M, Watterson JD, Wollin TA *et al.* (2002) Holmium:YAG laser lithotripsy for upper urinary tract calculi in 598 patients. *Journal of Urology* **167**, 31–34

Weisse C and Berent A (2015) *Veterinary Image-Guided Interventions.* Wiley-Blackwell, Oxford

Winkler CJ (2019) *Laser Surgery in Veterinary Medicine* pp. 3–13. Wiley-Blackwell, Oxford.

Chapter 17

Evolving trends and future developments

Fausto Brandão and Alexander Chernov

Introduction

Endoscopy and minimally invasive surgery have developed rapidly over the past 5 years. This chapter highlights some of the evolving trends and potential future developments in the field. (Note: some of the techniques described are currently considered investigational and the reader should refer the editors' note below for further information).

Specialized instrumentation

Rigid endoscopes with integrated working channels

In an attempt to reduce the number of approaches to, and entry sites in, the body cavities, the use of rigid endoscopes with an integrated working channel (Figure 17.1) has become increasingly popular. These endoscopes allow the veterinary surgeon (veterinarian) to perform some minimally invasive procedures (e.g. laparoscopic parenchymatous organ biopsy) with only one entry site. However, it should be noted that by combining the working channel with the shaft of the endoscope, the size of the working area is effectively reduced. In addition, these rigid endoscopes have a reduced ability for movement and some visual field loss. They are also somewhat large and cumbersome for small patients <10–15 kg and do not train the surgeon in the triangulation and manipulation skills required for more complex procedures.

Current research interests include the use of integrated endoscopes for minimally invasive neuro-endoscopy and neurosurgery. A team of veterinary surgeons in Argentina has described a tentative approach to the third ventricle for the treatment of hydrocephaly and cauterization of the choroid plexus using a neuro-endoscope (Peyrelongue *et al.*, 2018); however, this technique has yet to be validated for clinical use. The small size of many dogs presenting

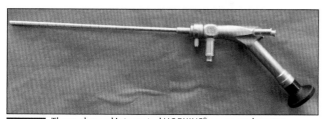

17.1 Three-channel integrated HOPKINS® neuro-endoscope. (Courtesy of Dr F Lillo)

with hydrocephalus present challenges in adapting human paediatric neuro-endoscopes for this purpose.

Video-assisted trans-sphenoidal hypophysectomy has also been described (Meij *et al.*, 1997a; Meij *et al.*, 1997b; Meij *et al.*, 1998; Meij *et al.*, 1999; Meij *et al.*, 2001; Meij *et al.*, 2002; Hanson *et al.*, 2005; Hanson *et al.*, 2007; Meij *et al.*, 2010); however, recent research has focused on developing a fully endoscopic procedure. A pilot study on the neuro-endoscopic approach to canine pineal tumours described the use of a three-channel integrated rigid endoscope (Figure 17.2) (Lillo *et al.*, 2016). Further research and clinical studies are required before this technique can be routinely implemented.

Miniature endoscopes

Special miniature endoscopes, such as the 1 mm x 20 cm x 0-degree semi-rigid endoscope, were originally designed for urethrocystoscopy in male cats to document lesion patterns in cases of idiopathic cystitis, but recently their use has been expanded to include other procedures such as the dual approach to feline imperforate nasopharyngeal stenosis (NPS) (Berent, 2016). This technique involves simultaneous fluoroscopically guided flexible nasopharyngoscopy and semi-rigid rhinoscopy via a rostral approach through the ventral meatus to the choanae (Figure 17.3). The use of a Veress optical needle as a sheath not only protects the endoscope, but also allows perforation of the NPS. Perforation of the NPS provides a rostral view of the tissue and permits the endoscope to be fluoroscopically guided through the ventral meatus to the caudal area of the nasal cavity. Posterior perforation of the NPS exiting in the common choanae is ensured by direct visualization using a 1 mm semi-rigid endoscope, as well as via video-assisted retroflexed nasopharyngoscopy. The integration of imaging modalities with dual endoscopic approaches is becoming more popular for specific conditions.

120-degree rigid endoscopes

Optimal image quality is required for endoscopic nasopharyngeal procedures and cavity evaluation. Flexible fibreoptic and video-endoscopes are used by many small animal surgeons performing minimally invasive procedures, but the use of retroverted 120-degree endoscopes is becoming more popular for high-detail nasopharyngoscopy (Figure 17.4). These endoscopes can also be used for grasping, cutting and obtaining biopsy

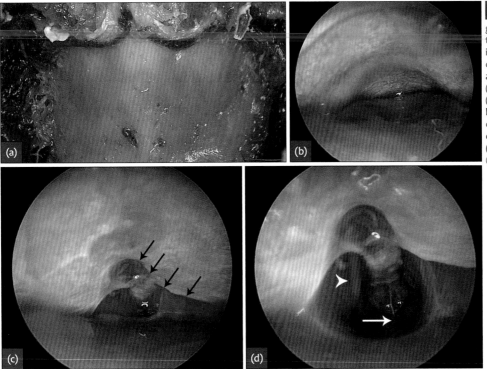

17.2 Neuro-endoscopic approach to the pineal gland in a dog. (a) Squamous part of the occipital bone. Neuro-endoscopic images showing: (b) the tentorium cerebelli membranaceum (dorsally) and the vermis of the cerebellum (ventrally); (c) the subtentorial space (the edge of the tentorium is denoted by the arrows); and (d) the left caudal cerebral artery (arrowhead) and dorsal aspect of the diencephalon (arrowed).
(Courtesy of Dr F Lillo)

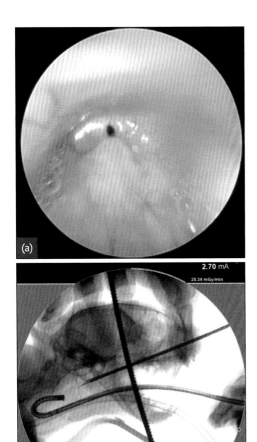

17.3 (a) Rostral view of the nasopharyngeal stenosis (NPS) in a cat using a 1 mm endoscope protected by an optical Veress needle. (b) Simultaneous fluoroscopic-guided flexible nasopharyngoscopy and rostral semi-rigid rhinoscopy for the treatment of imperforate NPS.
(Courtesy of Dr C Ifteme)

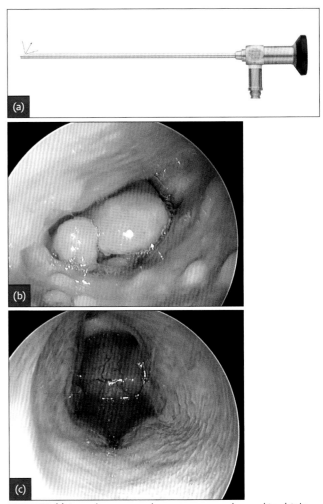

17.4 (a) A 120-degree nasopharyngoscope can be used to obtain high-quality images in cases of (b) feline lymphoma and (c) canine transmissible venereal tumour (TVT; round cell tumour).
(a, © Karl Storz SE & Co. KG; bc, courtesy of Dr C Ifteme)

samples using specialized retroflexed instruments. A dedicated sheath with a smooth round hook is available, which can be used to pull the soft palate cranially and manipulate the tissues with minimal trauma, extending the visual field.

These endoscopes are particularly useful in cases of brachycephalic obstructive airway syndrome (BOAS), where a high-detail non-insufflating modality is required for the evaluation of dynamic changes in the caudal part of the nasopharynx, for accurate anatomical evaluation of the caudal choanae and to carry out surgical procedures (Oechtering 2010; Schuenemann and Oechtering, 2014; Vilaplana *et al.*, 2015; Oechtering *et al.*, 2016a; Oechtering *et al.*, 2016b; Pohl *et al.*, 2016; Schuenemann *et al.*, 2017). The use of 120-degree rigid endoscopes for this purpose is likely to increase, as brachycephalic medicine and surgery is expanding with the popularity of these breeds.

Dynamic-range viewing endoscopes

A variety of dynamic-range endoscopes with variable viewing angles have been developed (EndoCAMeleon®, Karl Storz) and widely adopted for use in human ear, nose and throat endoscopy, thoracoscopy and laparoscopy. The major advantage of this type of endoscope is that it provides an expanded field of vision, especially in deep and narrow spaces, compared with the fixed distal tip angle of rigid endoscopes. In addition, these endoscopes have been shown to minimize iatrogenic injuries, due to the reduced need for manoeuvring within the body cavity.

There are three different types of endoscope currently available:

- A 4 mm diameter, 18 cm length endoscope with a variable direction of view from 15–90 degrees
- A 10 mm diameter, 32 cm length endoscope with a variable direction of view from 1–120 degrees
- A 10 mm diameter, 42 cm length endoscope with a variable direction of view from 1–120 degrees.

It has been suggested that the first two types of endoscope listed above would be of greatest benefit to veterinary practice, with the 4 mm diameter endoscope being used for thoracoscopy and laparoscopy in cats and small- to medium-sized dogs. Unfortunately, due to the limit of 90-degree angulation, this endoscope is not of use for nasopharyngoscopy.

A recent pilot study, conducted at North Carolina State University, looked at the use of variable angle endoscopes during thoracoscopy to avoid the visual impediments encountered when one lung ventilation is not clinically feasible (Diamond *et al.*, 2019). The study also revealed that the time taken to complete exploratory thoracoscopy procedures was significantly shorter with this type of endoscope compared with a standard fixed distal 30-degree angle endoscope. No statistically significant differences were found in cases where one lung ventilation was performed.

It is clear that variable angle endoscopes will be of use for thoracoscopic, cranial abdominal and pelvic laparoscopic procedures in veterinary patients.

In human medicine, these endoscopes are also being used for lachrymal and neuro-endoscopic procedures (Ebner *et al.*, 2015; Ali and Naik, 2016).

Techniques

Miniature laparoscopy and needle endoscopy

With the growing popularity of toy and miniature canine breeds, as well as cats and other small mammals, the demand for smaller instruments has increased, along with a trend towards miniature laparoscopy and needle endoscopy (Figure 17.5). Endoscopes with diameters between 1.9 mm and 3 mm are now available, allowing the entry points into the body cavities to be reduced in size to 3–3.9 mm with the use of miniature trocars. Needle entry instruments are also available.

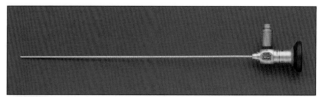

17.5 A 2 mm endoscope used in needlescopic laparoscopy.
(© Karl Storz SE & Co. KG)

Miniature laparoscopic and 'needlescopic' procedures have been described in human medicine since the early 2000s, but it is only in the last decade that they have become established as standard practice, particularly in paediatric and cosmetic minimally invasive surgery. From organ biopsy to more advanced procedures, such as myotomy and hernia repair, miniaturized techniques are becoming the gold standard for elective clinical procedures (Gagner and Garcia-Ruiz, 1998; Look *et al.*, 2001; Beck *et al.*, 2003; Cabral *et al.*, 2008; Carvalho *et al.*, 2009; Carvalho *et al.*, 2011; Turial *et al.*, 2011; Agresta and Bedin, 2012; Carvalho *et al.*, 2012; Fanfani *et al.*, 2012; Sajid *et al.*, 2012; Cai and Liu, 2013; Carvalho *et al.*, 2013; Krpata and Ponskin, 2013; Loureiro *et al.*, 2013; Bulian *et al.*, 2015; Inoue *et al.*, 2016; Lawall *et al.*, 2016; Ravikumar *et al.*, 2016; Lawall *et al.*, 2017; Ravikumar and Osborne, 2017).

In veterinary medicine, miniature laparoscopy and the use of needle instrumentation are becoming more popular. For example, the use of 'needlescopic' instruments (i.e. needle graspers) during two-port laparoscopic ovariectomy and cryptorchidectomy avoids the need for transabdominal suture fixation of the ovarian pedicle or testis. The needle graspers are introduced into the body cavity under capnoperitoneum using a single puncture technique (similar to the Tru-Cut technique), and the ovary or testis is dissected free whilst the tissue is held with the grasping tips. This technique has also been used for minor procedures, such as the dissection of ovarian remnants and for obtaining biopsy samples from multiple abdominal organs.

For manipulation of the gallbladder, these smaller instruments may be insufficient and could possibly induce rupture, thus 3 mm or 5 mm rubber-tipped graspers are preferred for this purpose. However, canine and feline 'needlescopic' cholecystectomy using 2 mm or 3 mm instruments has recently been demonstrated to be a relatively safe procedure in clinical practice (Ehara, 2017). In addition, the introduction of barbed suture material has meant that veterinary surgeons performing laparoscopic procedures can place intracorporeal sutures in routine cases, without the need to use smaller instruments such as 3 mm needle holders (Sánchez-Hurtado *et al.*, 2017).

The potential advantages associated with performing miniaturized procedures in clinical practice include reduced perioperative morbidity, better cosmetic effect and an increased range of instrument movement in small spaces. The current major limitation to miniature laparoscopy is the lack of access to advanced electrosurgical instruments for tissue and vessel sealing. However, the recent introduction of disposable miniature electrosurgical instruments with tissue sealing abilities in human medicine (e.g. JustRight™ Vessel Sealing System, Bolder Surgical) may overcome this limitation and broaden the range of procedures that can be performed using this technique (Quitzan *et al.*, 2019).

Dual camera system procedures and hybrid techniques

The use of dual camera systems is becoming more popular in small animal endoscopy and endosurgery, as they enable the veterinary surgeon to view the target tissues from two different anatomical points (Figure 17.6). A combination of an endoluminal and an endocavitary approach, or two endocavitary approaches, is typical for the procedures performed using this type of system. Two complete imaging equipment set-ups are required.

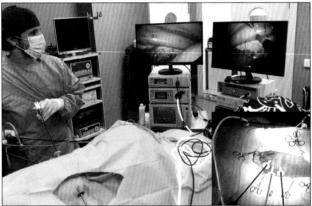

17.6 Dual camera imaging system set-up for a bilateral thoracic approach for the treatment of chylothorax with *en bloc* ligatures.
(Courtesy of Dr F Pérez-Duarte and J Gutierrez)

There has also been significant interest amongst veterinary practitioners in natural orifice transluminal endoscopic surgery (NOTES; see below). A number of different procedures using this technique have been cited in the veterinary literature, although few have become routine in clinical practice. This may be, in part, due to the longer procedural times and the requirement for specialized equipment, which can be expensive. To overcome these limitations, hybrid techniques using a combination of NOTES and a simplified laparoscopic approach have been developed. These hybrid techniques have proved popular, as they have the advantage of decreased operating times, possibly reducing both intraoperative complications and technical difficulties, and they require less specialized equipment, thereby reducing the costs associated with the procedure.

Although it is envisaged that the number of procedures performed using hybrid techniques will increase in the future, there are two techniques that are being widely adopted:

- Double endoscopic access to the nasal cavity (i.e. nasopharyngeal retroflexion combined with a rostral approach, as previously discussed)
- Bilateral thoracoscopy for the treatment of chylothorax (see Figure 17.6).

In cases of chylothorax, a standard approach is used for the right hemithorax followed by a left hemithorax approach to enhance visualization of the tissues and assist with *en bloc* suturing. This technique also allows complete ligation of the thoracic duct and its branches (Figure 17.7) (Radlinski *et al.*, 2002; MacDonald *et al.*, 2008; Allman *et al.*, 2010; Sakals *et al.*, 2011; Haimel *et al.*, 2012; Mayhew *et al.*, 2012).

The major disadvantages of both dual camera systems and hybrid techniques are the cost associated with the imaging systems and the variety of endoscopes and instruments required. However, as these minimally invasive surgical procedures gain widespread adoption, the cost of the equipment may become more affordable.

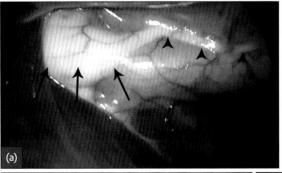
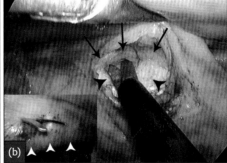
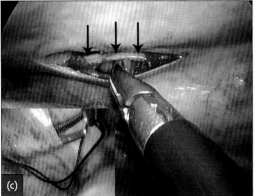
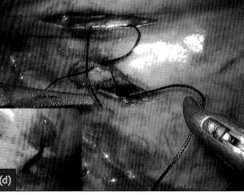

17.7 (a) Cisterna chyli prolongation into the thoracic cavity (arrowed). The thoracic duct is denoted by the arrowheads. (b) Complete mediastinal dissection ventral to the thoracic duct (arrowed) and dorsal to the aorta (arrowheads). (c) Complete mediastinal dissection ventral to the sympathetic trunk (arrowed). Note the double sutures through the dissection plane. (d) Double sutures incorporating all caudal mediastinum structures (*en bloc*) between the aorta and the sympathetic trunk.

Enhanced contact endoscopy

A routine endoscopic evaluation uses white light to illuminate the tissues. However, this type of light is not helpful when attempting to identify early lesions in the epithelial or subepithelial layers, or for determining accurate margins of macroscopic lesions. This information is critical for planning and carrying out procedures. Thus, over the last 10 years, research and development has focused on methods to enhance surface contrast to aid early detection of mucosal and submucosal lesions and margin demarcation. These methods include:

- Autofluorescence
- Conventional chromoendoscopy
- Image enhanced endoscopy.

Autofluorescence

Autofluorescence modalities are limited because they rely on tissue emission, and this can change under certain conditions, such as tissue granulation, telangiectasia, tissue scarring, necrosis, inflammation and epithelial keratosis (Arens *et al.*, 2004; Jacobson *et al.*, 2012).

Chromoendoscopy

Chromoendoscopy uses contrast dyes to enhance the visual characteristics of the mucosa and to highlight dysplastic and malignant changes that might not be detectable by white light endoscopy alone. The most commonly used dye in veterinary medicine is methylene blue. The dye is sprayed over the mucosa using a catheter and is selectively absorbed by the tissues, resulting in a colour change detectable by the endoscopist. At present, the use of chromoendoscopy is limited in small animal practice and lesion patterns are not well established (Rey Caro *et al.*, 2014).

Image enhanced endoscopy

A major advancement in the aim for greater image definition, both in conventional white light endoscopy and video-endoscopy, was seen with the introduction of high-definition television (HDTV) camera systems. These systems provide a resolution of at least 1080 pixels, which is far superior to standard systems. More recent technological advancements in the field include the development of a variety of three-dimensional (3D) endoscopic systems and the introduction of Ultra HD systems, which have a horizontal screen display resolution of approximately 4000 pixels.

The main focus of current research and development is on image-enhanced endoscopy (IEE) systems (e.g. i-scan, Narrow Band Imaging (NBI) and IMAGE1 S™). These systems allow detection and enhanced characterization of lesions in terms of microvascular and endocystoscopic abnormalities, such as dilatation, twisting and irregularities of the small vessels and capillaries in neoplastic tissues (Ni *et al.*, 2011). The IMAGE1 S™ (Karl Storz) is a versatile digital full HD video system, which provides specific colour rendering of the acquired broad visible spectrum within the HD camera system. Since spectral separation is obtained within the camera system and amplified by adapted colour processing algorithms, the IMAGE1 S™ does not require a dedicated narrow band light source but operates with a standard white light source. Thus, in addition to the standard white light mode, this system has five different predefined spectral ranges:

- CLARA
- CLARA + CHROMA
- CHROMA
- SPECTRA A
- SPECTRA B.

IEE can facilitate diagnosis of early neoplastic and preneoplastic lesions, which is key to minimally invasive endoscopic resection. For example, when IEE is performed using a standard HOPKINS® rod-lens endoscope, in conjunction with an HD video system, it is possible to identify the vascularity associated with preneoplastic areas or neoplastic lesions as 'endoscopic mucosal spots'. In addition, some epithelial changes such as hyperkeratosis can mask deeper epithelial and vascular abnormalities that may be identified using IEE.

Enhanced contact endoscopy is based on the dynamic fusion of IEE and contact endoscopy, but without the need for vital staining, thus combining the advantages of both modalities. This technique has been widely adopted for the investigation of gastrointestinal, respiratory and urinary tract disorders (Figure 17.8). It has the advantage of enhancing the margins of neoplastic lesions (e.g. of transitional cell carcinomas), allowing ultrasound-guided endoscopic laser ablation (UGELAB) to be performed in a safer manner and with a higher degree of accuracy compared with standard video imaging systems.

Three-dimensional endoscopy

Thoracoscopy and laparoscopy are the techniques of choice for an increasing number of surgical procedures, as they have the benefit of faster recovery rates and shorter hospitalization times, improved cosmesis, decreased blood loss and less postoperative pain. The standard endoscopic systems provide the veterinary surgeon with an indirect monocular view of the operating field, meaning that the surgeon is denied the binocular depth cues that provide a sense of stereopsis (i.e. the perception of depth and the 3D structure obtained on the basis of visual information, which is derived from two eyes by individuals with developed binocular vision). In addition, the loss of binocular vision on a two-dimensional (2D) display can cause visual misconceptions, particularly loss of depth perception.

Thus, the greatest challenge facing endoscopic surgeons is hand–eye coordination within a 3D environment observed on a 2D screen. Experienced surgeons learn to use monocular depth cues, such as light and shade, the relative size of objects, object interposition, texture gradient, aerial perspective and motion parallax instead of stereovision. By using these monocular cues, all endoscopic surgical procedures can be successfully accomplished; however, time and accuracy may be lost as these cues do not compensate completely for stereoscopic depth perception.

The use of a high-definition 3D view overcomes these limitations, providing greater depth perception and tactile feedback (Figure 17.9). It also improves surgical precision and hand–eye coordination with the use of conventional instruments. The depth perception afforded by this view allows for precise measurement of the dimensions of anatomical spaces, leading to more accurate placement of instruments for tissue manipulation, dissection and placement of intracorporeal sutures, as well as improvement in the design of surgical procedures. In addition, studies have reported that 3D systems place less eye strain and fatigue on the surgeon compared with 2D systems (Blavier *et al.*, 2006; Izquierdo *et al.*, 2012; Currò *et al.*, 2015).

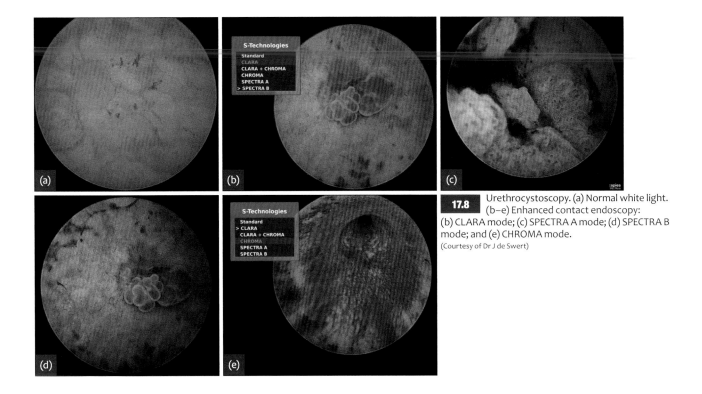

17.8 Urethrocystoscopy. (a) Normal white light. (b–e) Enhanced contact endoscopy: (b) CLARA mode; (c) SPECTRA A mode; (d) SPECTRA B mode; and (e) CHROMA mode.
(Courtesy of Dr J de Swert)

- Depth perception
- Tactile feedback
- Accuracy
- Safety
- Surgical precision
- Improved hand–eye coordination
- Low capital expenditure
- Low maintenance costs
- Conventional and new straight stick instruments can be used
- Shorter learning curve

17.9 Benefits of the use of 3D systems for laparoscopic surgery.

Recent technological advances have led to sophisticated high-resolution systems and light polarizing glasses that are lighter and more comfortable to wear. A dual channel optical endoscope is connected to two video cameras, which deliver two images that are shown to the endoscopist on a stereoscopic display. When the veterinary surgeon wears the circular light polarizing 3D glasses, the two images are merged by the brain into one, giving the perception of depth (Figure 17.10). Studies have shown that the use of stereoscopic displays improves accuracy during laparoscopic procedures performed by less experienced surgeons (manifested as a reduction in the number of repetitions and errors reported).

Very few 3D systems are currently used in veterinary endoscopy, but they are increasing in popularity as costs decrease. Individual practices will need to determine if these enhanced imaging platforms provide reasonable return on investment (Kunert *et al.*, 2013; Sinha *et al.*, 2013; Alaraimi *et al.*, 2014; Özsoy *et al.*, 2015; Sinha *et al.*, 2017; Kunert *et al.*, 2018; Nomura *et al.*, 2019a; Nomura *et al.*, 2019b).

Robotic platforms

Laparoscopic surgery has certain limitations, including 2D imaging, restricted range of motion of the instruments and poor ergonomic positioning of the veterinary surgeon. Robotic surgical systems were introduced to overcome these limitations and provide the surgeon with improved

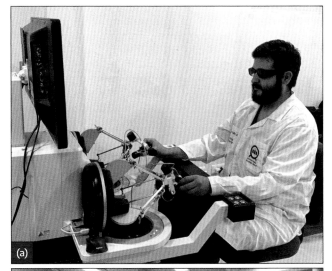

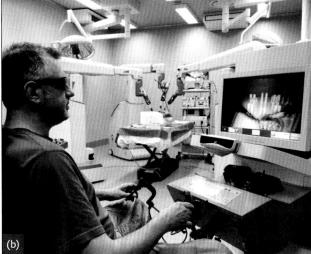

17.10 (a) 3D single port ColubrisMX robotic platform. (b) Senhance® robotic platform.
(a, Courtesy of Dr F Lillo; b, Courtesy of Dr L Formagini)

visualization and greater dexterity. This emerging modality has many technical advantages compared with conventional laparoscopy, including 3D imaging, tremor filters and articulated instruments. The disadvantages of robotic-assisted surgery include a lack of tactile feedback to the surgeon, the inability to move the surgical table once the arms of the robot are fixed, and the costs associated with the robot and semi-disposable instruments, as well as those related to installation and training.

The most commonly used systems include:

- da Vinci (Intuitive Surgical)
- Senhance® (TransEnterix)
- REVO-I (Meerecompany).

The oldest and most widely used robotic platform is the da Vinci system. The system uses 3D visualization and EndoWrist technology, which facilitates instrument rotation through tiny incisions. The robotic instruments replicate the surgeon's hand, wrist and finger movement. This allows for an extended range of motion and improved manipulation during procedures.

Robot-assisted techniques are well documented in human medicine and are becoming standard for many urological, gynaecological and gastrointestinal procedures. It has been demonstrated that for even demanding visceral surgical procedures, the perioperative complication rate for robotic surgery is not higher than that for open or laparoscopic surgical procedures. In cases of neoplasia, the accuracy of robotic resection for gastric, pancreatic and rectal lesions has been demonstrated to be adequate. The operating time is generally longer for robotic surgery compared with standard laparoscopic and open procedures; on the other hand, there is less blood loss, lower conversion rates to open surgery and shorter hospitalization times.

Current trends suggest that robotic procedures will become a permanent fixture in human surgery. In veterinary medicine, the use of robotic platforms for surgical procedures is anecdotal, but may become more widely adopted in the future (Giulianotti *et al.*, 2003; Aggarwal *et al.*, 2004; Herron *et al.*, 2008; Nezhat, 2008; Wilson, 2009; Aggarwal *et al.*, 2010; Sodergren and Darzi, 2012; Halabi *et al.*, 2013; Hyun *et al.*, 2013; Liao *et al.*, 2013; Salman *et al.*, 2013; Xiong *et al.*, 2013; Bailey *et al.*, 2014; Kim *et al.*, 2014; Diana and Marescaux 2015; Aaltonen and Wahlström 2018). There has been one report of a robotic-assisted adrenalectomy in a lioness (Figure 17.11) performed by a group of veterinary surgeons at the University of Lodi (Italy) using a Senhance® (ALF-X) platform.

Fluorescence techniques and targeted tissue dyeing

Fluorescence is the property of certain molecules (fluorochromes) to emit fluorescent radiation when excited by a laser beam or exposed to near-infrared light (NIR) at specific wavelengths (Alander *et al.*, 2012). As light energy is absorbed by the fluorochromes, electrons move from a ground state to an excited state or higher energy level. Upon return to the ground state, energy is emitted in the form of photons, reaching the eye of the observer as fluorescence of a specific wavelength. Indocyanine green (ICG) dye was developed for NIR photography by Kodak Research Laboratories in 1955 and was introduced into clinical practice in 1956 (e.g. for cirrhotic liver resection).

ICG has been shown to have relatively few side effects when injected into the bloodstream and thus can be safely

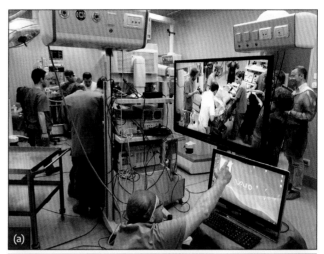

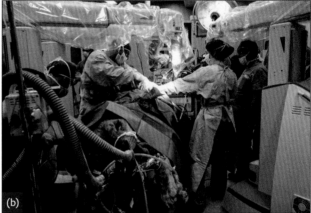

17.11 (a) Senhance® (ALF-X) robotic platform prepared for a robotic-assisted procedure. (b) Robotic-assisted left adrenalectomy in a lioness.
(Courtesy of Dr L Formagini)

used in veterinary medicine. Furthermore, ICG rapidly binds to plasma proteins following intravascular injection, resulting in minimal leakage into the interstitial compartment. Once excited by light at a specific wavelength, ICG becomes fluorescent and can be detected using specific filters and cameras and displayed on a screen. This allows tissues that accumulate ICG to be visualized, which may not be possible with normal white light endoscopy. Endoscopic systems can be switched from standard white light to NIR/ICG, and *vice versa*, via foot pedal control. When used in NIR/ICG fluorescent mode, images of the tissues can be shown in blue or green; the blue mode reveals highly perfused areas, whereas the green mode allows delineation of specific areas against the surrounding tissue (Johnson *et al.*, 2009; McAnulty, 2011; Ando *et al.*, 2012; Mayhew *et al.*, 2012; Nakajima *et al.*, 2018; Steffey and Mayhew, 2018; Kanai *et al.*, 2019).

Fluorescence techniques are becoming more widely adopted, both in open and minimally invasive surgery. NIR technology can be beneficial in oncological open surgery, as it can be used to map neoplastic tissues and the associated lymphatic drainage, allowing identification of lymph nodes for surgical removal and histopathological analysis. For example, hepatic neoplasia can be assessed intraoperatively (via an open approach) using an exoscope and NIR technology (Figures 17.12 and 17.13). Examination of the neoplastic tissue using this technique allows the surgeon to accurately delineate the margins for resection, whilst preserving vital anatomical structures where possible (Lida *et al.*, 2013).

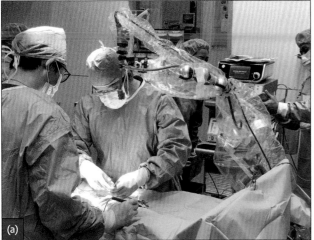

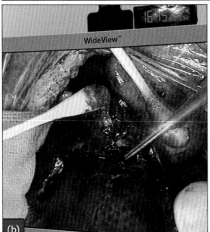

17.12 Video-exoscopic-assisted fluorescence procedure for hepatic neoplasia. (a) Prior to surgery. (b) Intraoperative assessment of neoplastic lesions for planning surgical removal.
(Courtesy of Dr C Hsien-Chieh)

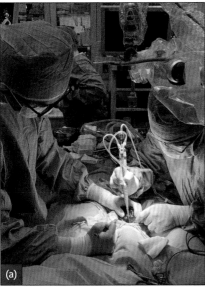

17.13 (a) Video-exoscopic-assisted hepatic mass resection using an ultrasonic aspirator. (b) Postoperative view of complete mass removal.
(Courtesy of Dr C Hsien-Chieh)

In recent years, NIR/ICG techniques have been used during thoracoscopy for mapping and resection of thoracic neoplastic lesions, as well as chylothorax resolution. By injecting ICG into the popliteal lymph node, or mesenteric vasculature, fluorescence lymphangiography can be performed, allowing real-time intraoperative differentiation of the thoracic duct and its branches (Figure 17.14). The accurate identification of these structures means that they can be completely ligated (Figure 17.15). This development has also led to the use of fluorescence for *en bloc* thoracic duct ligation, in conjunction with pericardiectomy and cisterna chyli ablation (Lida *et al.*, 2013; Kanai *et al.*, 2019).

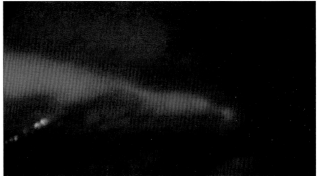

17.14 Fluorescent image of the thoracic duct obtained using a D-light (NIR/ICG) IMAGE1 S™ system.
(Courtesy of Dr K Ishigaki and Dr K Asano)

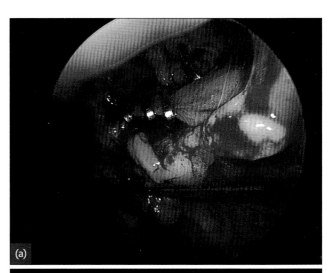

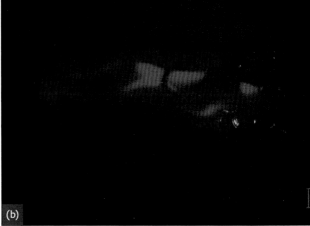

17.15 (a) White light thoracoscopy for thoracic duct ligation. (b) Post-thoracoscopic assessment of thoracic duct ligation using ICG fluorescence.
(Courtesy of Dr C Hsien-Chieh)

Future uses for fluorescence tissue enhancement imaging will depend on the research and development of antibody binding or specific tissue binding dye techniques. These techniques have the potential to be helpful in oncological surgery, where they could be used to identify specific areas of tissue for excision.

Integrated advanced imaging modalities

The increasing popularity of integrated operating and/or endoscopy suites with advanced imaging modalities, such as fluoroscopy, endoluminal ultrasonography, computed tomography (CT), magnetic resonance imaging (MRI) and, more recently, fusion imaging modalities, presents the opportunity to combine these imaging modalities with endoscopy and endosurgery. For example, CT lymphangiography before thoracoscopy (Figure 17.16) and laparoscopy has been described. Contrast media is injected into the patient and a CT study performed. Images are acquired for 3D reconstruction of the lymphatic system, which enables accurate surgical planning. This can be combined with fluorescence techniques to assist dissection of the relevant structures (see above). The advantage of using an integrated system is the accuracy it provides. The limitations of integrated systems include the high cost of investment in terms of equipment and the need for highly skilled personnel to perform the procedures and interpret the results.

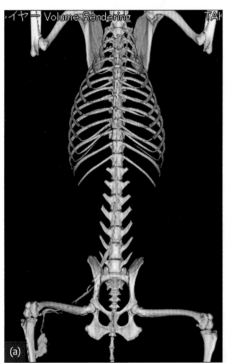

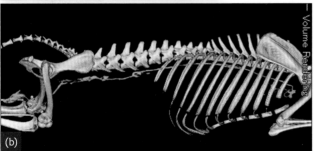

17.16 (a,b) 3D image rendering of presurgical CT lymphangiography in a dog for the treatment of idiopathic chylothorax.
(Courtesy of Dr K Ishigaki and Dr K Asano)

Natural orifice transluminal endoscopic surgery

Editors' note

Many of the procedures described in this chapter and in the accompanying video library are considered investigational. As such they should NOT be considered appropriate for routine clinical use. The practitioner is advised that these new and novel interventions should only be performed, at the time of publication, under the appropriate professional, ethical and legal guidelines relevant to the professional body that prevails in the jurisdiction within which they are practising. The practitioner is advised to consult with legal and professional regulatory bodies in their local jurisdiction to ensure that they are operating within professional, safe and ethical investigational guidelines. The health and welfare of the patient should remain the primary focus when deciding whether or not to undertake new and novel interventions and, where applicable, it should be ensured that owners are fully informed as part of the decision-making and consent process

Natural orifice transluminal endoscopic surgery (NOTES) is a relatively new concept of surgery, and it shows promise for both diagnostic and therapeutic surgical endoscopy (Kalloo and Datlner, 2006; Lima *et al.*, 2006; Kalloo, 2008; Sugimoto *et al.*, 2009; Mayhew, 2014; Freeman *et al.*, 2015).

In NOTES surgery, access is described as a 'first order portal', the animal's natural orifices (e.g. nose, mouth, anus, vagina, urethra), (Figure 17.17) (Isariyawongse *et al.*, 2008; Freeman *et al.*, 2010; Brun *et al.*, 2011; Chernov and Inykin, 2011; Mayhew, 2014; Chernov, 2018b), or a 'second order portal', an internal approach, traversing the wall of a hollow viscus or organ using a rigid or flexible endoscope (Nieponice *et al.*, 2006; Flora *et al.*, 2008; Metzelder *et al.*, 2009a).

Endoscopic surgery using natural orifices is effective and has many potential advantages, including less postoperative pain, reduced risk of inflammatory reactions, significantly lower risk of postoperative herniation and a relatively fast recovery period without skin scars (Giday *et al.*, 2007; Elmunzer, 2009; Giday *et al.*, 2010). These attributes allow successful laparoscopic endosurgery even if all the soft tissues of the abdominal wall are infected.

Adoption of NOTES procedures

The author [AC] has conducted interviews with approximately 50 veterinary surgeons (who have access to laparoscopy) regarding their preference for laparoscopic ovariectomy *versus* a NOTES procedure. Only 20% of those interviewed preferred the NOTES technique to traditional transabdominal laparoscopy. Reported reasons for this preference include the fact that the techniques are currently still under development, the equipment available is limited and the perception of risk of complications is higher. However, all participants noted the advantages of low postoperative pain and lack of scar tissue associated with the NOTES technique

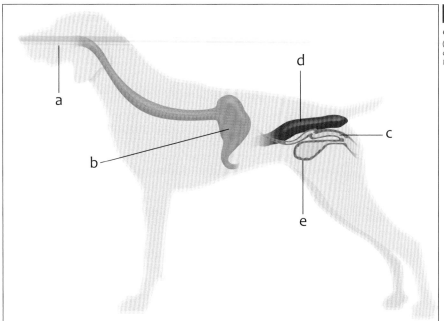

17.17 Approaches for NOTES procedures.
a = Peroral; b = Transgastric;
c = Transvaginal; d = Transrectal; e = Transvesical.
(Reproduced with permission from García and González, *Manual de técnicas de mínima invasión en pequeños animales*, Multimédica Ediciones Veterinarias (2018))

Owner expectations and consent

During 2015–2016, the author [AC] conducted a preoperative survey of 50 owners of dogs undergoing traditional laparoscopic surgery *versus* a transvaginal laparoscopic procedure. Owner expectations relating to NOTES procedures included less pain, reduced postoperative recovery times, reduced risk of complications and lower costs. It was reported that 70% of the owners surveyed preferred a NOTES procedure rather than laparoscopic surgery for their pet. In addition, it was found that owner consent for a NOTES procedure was easier to obtain than that for an open or laparoscopic procedure. There was also a perception amongst owners that surgeons performing NOTES procedures were more experienced

Transvaginal laparoscopy and endosurgery

A transvaginal approach to the abdomen was the first NOTES technique described in both human and veterinary medicine (Reuter *et al.*, 1999; Grady, 2007; Bakhtiari *et al.*, 2012; de Souza *et al.*, 2014). The advantage of this approach is that it allows visualization of the entire abdominal cavity. A transvaginal approach can be used for diagnostic and surgical procedures involving the ovaries, liver, biliary tract, kidneys, spleen and diaphragm (Figure 17.18; Video 17.1). The procedures most commonly performed via this approach in dogs and cats are ovariectomy and ovariohysterectomy (see below) (Chernov and Inykin, 2011; Chernov, 2013; Luz *et al.*, 2014). Other procedures that can be performed via a transvaginal approach include biopsy, gastropexy, cholecystectomy, ovarian cyst removal, hernioplasty and endoscopic haemostasis (Zorrón *et al.*, 2007).

- Both rigid and flexible endoscopes (with associated equipment) can be used (Jagannath *et al.*, 2005; Pader *et al.*, 2011a) for procedures via this approach.
- Use of a special rotary mechanism on the operating table will enable the position of the patient to be quickly changed, if required.
- Prophylactic antibiotics are advisable in the event of contamination of the surgical field.

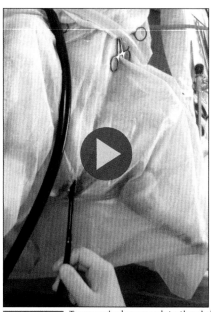

Video 17.1 Transvaginal approach to the abdomen using a flexible endoscope.

Transvaginal ovariectomy and ovariohysterectomy in dogs

- Patient preparation for a transvaginal procedure includes:
  - Ensuring that the bladder is empty
  - Cleaning the area with saline
  - Dilation of the vagina with blunt-pointed bougie dilators, if the diameter of the vagina is smaller than the diameter of the trocar. The author [AC] typically uses a 12mm optical trocar
  - Insufflating the peritoneal cavity with carbon dioxide using a Veress needle inserted through the abdominal wall in the midline in the umbilical area. The author [AC] recommends an abdominal pressure of 5–6 mmHg for all surgical procedures.
- The patient should be placed in either left or right lateral recumbency.

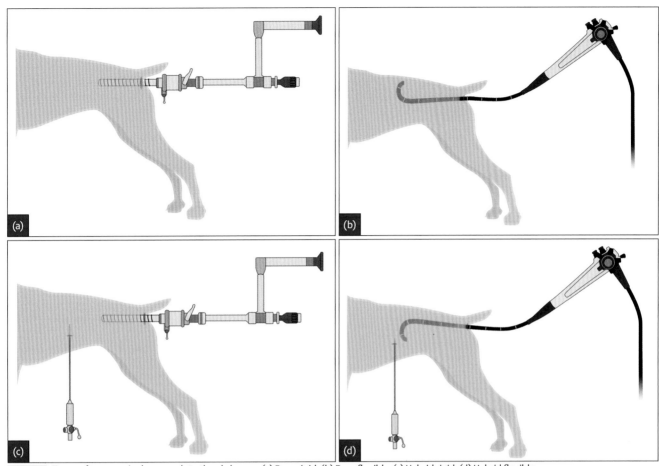

17.18 Types of transvaginal approach to the abdomen. (a) Pure rigid. (b) Pure flexible. (c) Hybrid rigid. (d) Hybrid flexible.
(Reproduced with permission from García and González, Manual de técnicas de mínima invasión en pequeños animales, Multimédica Ediciones Veterinarias (2018))

- The endoscope should be inserted into the vagina and the site for transvaginal laparocentesis identified. The typical site for laparocentesis is the middle of the vagina dorsally, deviating from the midline to the left or right depending on the recumbency of the animal (Chernov, 2018b).
- A trocar should then be introduced to facilitate insertion of the endoscope into the abdominal cavity. The use of an optical trocar allows this procedure to be visualized. The stylet should be advanced from the trocar to penetrate the vaginal wall. The stylet should then be withdrawn and the endoscope advanced into the abdominal cavity.
- Once inside the abdominal cavity, the nearby internal organs (e.g. bladder, loops of the small intestine, colon, body and horns of the uterus) can be used to aid orientation.
- The ovaries and uterus should be identified. The first ovary can then be ligated, dissected and mobilized ready for removal via the vagina. The remaining ovary should then be removed.
- If the uterus is to be removed, then this should be performed *en bloc* with the uterine horns and ovaries. Once exteriorized, the uterine body is clamped and ligated prior to transection. The wound is then closed before the uterine stump is returned to the abdomen.
- The endoscope can then be removed. The vaginal defect is typically left to heal without suturing.

Videos 17.2 and 17.3 show transvaginal ovariectomy in a dog, whilst Video 17.4 demonstrates the procedure for ovariohysterectomy.

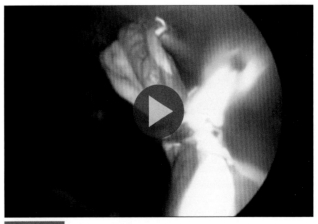

Video 17.2 Transvaginal ovariectomy in a dog.

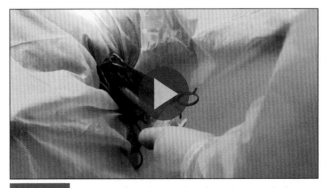

Video 17.3 Transvaginal ovariectomy in a dog using an optical trocar.

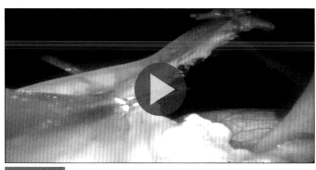

Video 17.4 Transvaginal ovariohysterectomy in a dog.

Transvaginal ovariectomy and ovariohysterectomy in cats

The procedure for transvaginal ovariectomy and ovario-hysterectomy in cats (Video 17.5) is similar to that in dogs, with the following exceptions:

* Rigid instruments are required to carry out these procedures in cats due to the anatomical features of the vagina and abdomen (Chernov, 2018b)
* The site for laparocentesis is in the proximal vagina, to the side of the urethral ostium
* The vaginal wall is dissected using a laser or monopolar electrosurgery
* The trocar is inserted into the abdominal cavity under visualization from the endoscope and insufflation with carbon dioxide via the cannula.

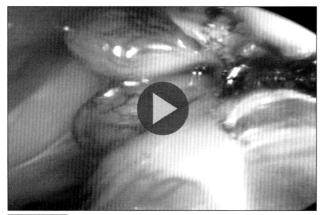

Video 17.5 Transvaginal ovariectomy in a cat using a diode laser.

Transgastric laparoscopy

Percutaneous endoscopic gastrostomy (PEG), performed by Ponsky in 1979, can be considered as the first proce-dure carried out using a transgastric approach to the abdomen. The advantage of this type of approach is that the endoscope can be manoeuvred into any area of the abdominal cavity. A transgastric approach can be used for diagnostic and surgical procedures involving the gastro-intestinal, urinary and reproductive tracts, as well as the abdominal organs. Procedures that can be carried out via this approach include ovariectomy, cholecystectomy, gastrostomy and gastroenterostomy.

* A flexible video-endoscope with a diameter of 7.9–13 mm, length of at least 1 m and a working channel of at least 2.8 mm in diameter is recommended for

transgastric procedures. The length of the endoscope used is dependent upon the size of the patient. A variety of endoscopic instruments are required for transgastric procedures, including needles, blades, loops and clips.
* Insufflation with carbon dioxide is required throughout the procedure. An abdominal pressure of 5–6 mmHg (and no greater than 14 mmHg) is recommended.

A transgastric approach to the abdominal cavity is pos-sible via any region of the stomach (Figure 17.19), with the exception of the area comprising the main blood supply.

* Patient preparation for a transgastric procedure includes ensuring that the stomach is empty. Any food remnants should be washed out using saline prior to the procedure.
* The patient should be placed in dorsal recumbency.
* The endoscope should be inserted into the mouth and advanced into the stomach.
* The site for transgastric laparocentesis should then be identified. The typical site for laparocentesis is the ventral wall in the distal part of the body of the stomach.
* Once the site has been selected, laparocentesis can be performed under visualization. The methods for transgastric laparocentesis include:

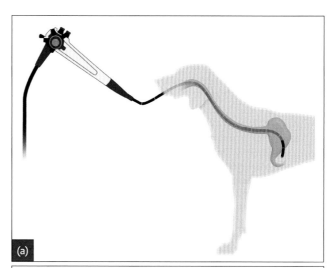

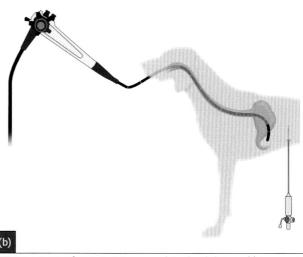

17.19 Types of transgastric approach to the abdomen. (a) Pure flexible. (b) Hybrid flexible.
(Reproduced with permission from García and González, Manual de técnicas de mínima invasión en pequeños animales, Multimédica Ediciones Veterinarias(2018))

- Direct dissection of the layers of the stomach using monopolar or bipolar electrosurgery. Further enlargement of the site is possible using a balloon dilator or sphincterotome
- Electrosurgical dissection (using a T-knife and graspers) of the mucosal and submucosal layers, creating a tunnel with a 'lid', continuing through the muscular and serosal layers until penetration into the abdominal cavity is achieved.

Direct visualization of the procedure helps to avoid any unexpected haemorrhagic complications. The main difficulty associated with port formation is orientation of the flexible endoscope in the stomach due to the constantly changing volume.

- The endoscope should then be advanced into the abdominal cavity and the required surgical procedure performed.
- Closure of the transgastric laparocentesis site is the most difficult part of the procedure and has limited application of the technique to date. Several methods for closure have been described (Isariyawongse *et al.*, 2008; Giday *et al.*, 2010; Guarner-Argente *et al.*, 2010) including:
  - Endoscopic clips (one of the most popular methods) (Video 17.6)
  - Full-thickness sutures:
    - Using a U-shaped pattern
    - Using an over-the-top pattern (Video 17.7) (von Delius *et al.*, 2007b). This is the most reliable technique for complete closure of the defect
  - Suturing the mucosal and submucosal layers using a fixing endoloop.

The future adoption of NOTES techniques using a transgastric approach is dependent upon the development of a safe and reliable method for closing the laparocentesis site in the stomach.

Porcine models

NOTES techniques via a transgastric approach were first described in porcine models (Simopoulos *et al.*, 2009). The procedures that have been reported include:

- Peritoneoscopy (Kalloo *et al.*, 2000; Kalloo *et al.*, 2004)
- Splenectomy (Kantsevoy *et al.*, 2006)
- Hernia repair (Hu *et al.*, 2007; Kantsevoy, 2009a; Earle *et al.*, 2010; Earle *et al.*, 2012)
- Gastrojejunostomy (Kantsevoy *et al.*, 2009b)
- Full-thickness gastric resection and closure (Ikeda *et al.*, 2005)

Transgastric ovariectomy in dogs

Transgastric ovariectomy (Video 17.8) allows the removal of the ovaries via the mouth, thus negating the need to dissect the abdominal wall. This procedure is achieved through electrosurgical ligation of the ovary and surrounding tissue using a polypectomy loop.

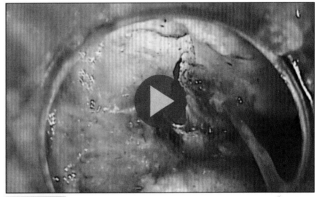

Video 17.8 Transgastric ovariectomy in a dog.

Transgastric cholecystectomy

As cholecystectomy is becoming somewhat more common in small animal surgery, a transgastric approach may be an advantageous alternative to traditional laparoscopic cholecystectomy (Video 17.9).

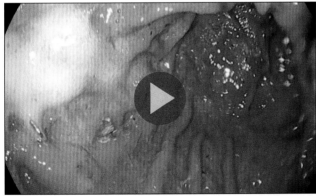

Video 17.6 Dog 1 year after transgastric laparoscopy with closure of the laparocentesis site using endoscopic clips.

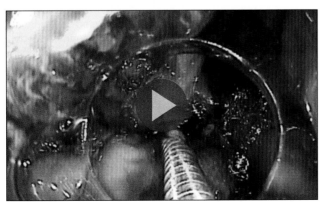

Video 17.7 Closure of the transgastric laparocentesis site using an over-the-top technique.

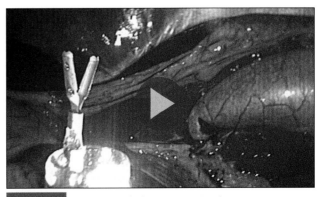

Video 17.9 Transgastric cholecystectomy in a dog.

Transgastric gastropexy

Acute and chronic gastric torsion, along with transient gastroparesis are common complications associated with open and percutaneous laparoscopic gastropexy. In order to prevent these complications, the author [AC] has proposed a method of transgastric gastropexy (Videos 17.10 and 17.11) that avoids large incisions in the abdominal wall.

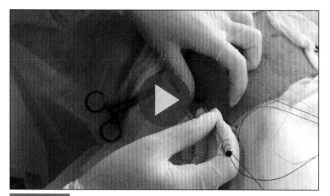

Video 17.10 Transgastric gastropexy in a dog (case 1).

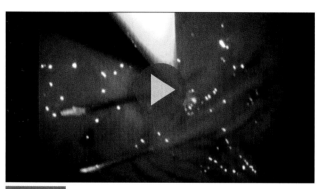

Video 17.11 Transgastric gastropexy in a dog (case 2).

Transgastric gastroenterostomy

Transgastric gastroenterostomy is indicated when the normal passage of food from the stomach to the small intestine is prevented. This technique involves anastomosis of the body of the stomach with the small intestine (Park, 2005).

- Transgastric exploration of the abdominal cavity should be undertaken to identify the site in the small intestine for anastomosis.
- The relevant section of the small intestine should be grasped and brought to the site of the laparocentesis in the stomach.
- The anastomosis should then be completed using stents and stay sutures as required.

In the future, transgastric gastroenterostomy and anastomosis may become the preferred technique for this type of procedure.

Transvesical laparoscopy

Laparoscopy via a transvesical approach to the abdominal cavity is currently under development. It involves the passage of the endoscope along the urethra and through the bladder wall (Sawyer *et al.*, 2008; Metzelder *et al.*,

2009a; Metzelder *et al.*, 2009b; Sawyer *et al.*, 2009). This approach allows examination of, and procedures to be carried out within, the abdominal cavity. Experimental procedures that have been carried out via a transvesical approach in pigs include cholecystectomy and nephrectomy (Lima *et al.*, 2006).

Transanal (transcolonic) laparoscopy

A transanal approach to the abdominal cavity for extracting resected masses following percutaneous laparoscopic colectomy was first described in human medicine in the early 1990s (Pai *et al.*, 2006). This type of approach can be used for diagnostic and surgical procedures within the abdominal cavity, including resection and removal of specific organs and tissues (Rajan *et al.*, 2002), sigmoidectomy (Whiteford *et al.*, 2007; Guarner-Argente *et al.*, 2010; Cho *et al.*, 2011) and nephrectomy (Bazzi *et al.*, 2013). A transanal approach to the abdominal cavity for NOTES procedures in veterinary medicine is not currently widely used.

- Both rigid and flexible endoscopes and instruments can be used (Fong *et al.*, 2007). However, it should be noted that there is only a limited range of instruments available for transanal procedures.
- Patient preparation for a transanal procedure includes evacuation of the colon and rectum to prevent contamination of the abdominal cavity with faecal material and subsequent infection (Raju *et al.*, 2006).
- The patient should be placed in left or right lateral recumbency.
- The endoscope should be inserted into the rectum and the site for transanal laparoscopy identified. The typical site for laparocentesis is the border of the rectum and descending colon, or anywhere along the length of the descending colon.
- Once the site has been selected, laparocentesis can be performed. The methods for transanal laparocentesis include:
  - Direct dissection of all the layers of the colon with further enlargement of the site using a balloon dilator
  - Layer by layer dissection of the intestinal wall until penetration into the abdominal cavity is achieved.
- The endoscope should then be advanced into the abdominal cavity and the required surgical procedure performed. No difficulties with spatial orientation within the abdominal cavity have been reported with this type of approach (Kono *et al.*, 2013).
- The methods for closure of the transanal laparocentesis site are similar to those used for the transgastric approach (Edwards *et al.*, 1999; Pham *et al.*, 2006).

The author [AC] has successfully used a transanal approach to laparoscopy in dogs for experimental purposes (Video 17.12). In these cases, clinically significant infection associated with the laparocentesis site was not observed and no antibiotics were administered (only in premedication).

Transoesophageal approach to the thorax

A transoesophageal approach has been recognized as the shortest route to gain access to the chest cavity (Fritscher-Ravens *et al.*, 2009; Fritscher-Ravens *et al.*, 2010a). This type of approach has been described in both porcine (von Delius *et al.*, 2007a; von Delius *et al.*, 2007b) and canine (Radu *et al.*, 2004; Badylak *et al.*, 2005;

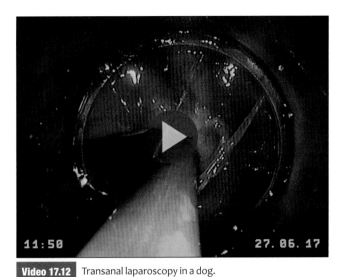

Video 17.12 Transanal laparoscopy in a dog.

Bessler, 2007; Bakhtiari *et al.*, 2012) models. The difficulty in this approach is associated with creating and maintaining pneumothorax within the thoracic cavity whilst performing the required procedure.

A transoesophageal approach can be used for diagnostic and surgical procedures. The procedures that have been described using this approach include thoracoscopy, mediastinoscopy, lymphadenectomy, pleural biopsy, thoracic injections, pericardial window formation, cardiomyotomy, oesophagomyotomy, vagotomy, sympathectomy, oesophagectomy and anastomosis, and lobectomy (Fritscher-Ravens *et al.*, 2007; Pasricha *et al.*, 2007; Sumiyama *et al.*, 2008). The author [AC] has performed several transoesophageal diagnostic thoracoscopy procedures without complications (Video 17.13).

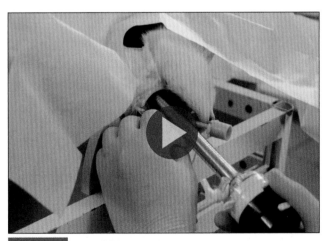

Video 17.13 Peroral thoracoscopy in a cat.

Hybrid NOTES procedures

In some cases, it may be beneficial to combine a standard percutaneous approach to endoscopy with a NOTES procedure. These are commonly referred to as hybrid NOTES techniques (Brun *et al.*, 2011; Bazzi *et al.*, 2013; de Souza *et al.*, 2014; Chernov, 2018b). Procedures that have been described using a hybrid NOTES technique include transvaginal ovariohysterectomy (Video 17.14) and a transgastric approach to the abdomen (Video 17.15). More recently, hybrid procedures have been described using two different NOTES approaches.

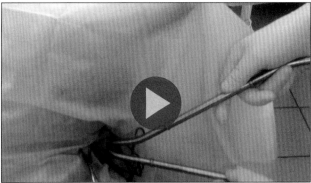

Video 17.14 Transvaginal ovariohysterectomy in a dog using a hybrid NOTES procedure.

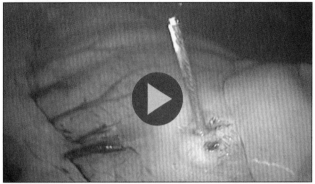

Video 17.15 Transgastric approach to the abdominal cavity in a dog using a hybrid NOTES procedure.

Endoscopic submucosal dissection and peroral endoscopic myotomy

As more techniques are adapted from human endoscopic surgery and implemented in small animal MIS, our options for surgical intervention continue to increase.

Endoscopic submucosal dissection

Endoscopic submucosal dissection (ESD) has proven to be a valuable technique to facilitate excision of mass or polypoid lesions in several clinical settings. *En bloc* excision of masses in the stomach, proximal small intestine and colon/rectum is greatly simplified. Even with appropriate energy sources (bipolar/monopolar, harmonic devices, lasers) aggressive excision can be largely incomplete without the ability to dissect lesions below the mucosal surface.

In ESD, an incision is made around the lesion using either sharp dissection or some form of energy. The incision should be made from 180 to 270 degrees around the lesion with a diameter sufficient to maximize the likelihood of clean surgical margins.

The goal of ESD is to provide separation between the mucosa/submucosa and the underlying muscularis. Blunt dissection, particularly in thin-walled hollow viscus structures, can be incomplete and dangerous. Several techniques are commonly employed to provide this separation. The simplest method uses saline, injected via a laparoscopic injection needle (in cases of rigid endoscopy) or a flexible injection needle, such as a sclerotherapy needle (in the case of flexible endoscopy) into the submucosal space. This provides separation between the lesion and the underlying tissues. With adequate separation the incision can be completed in a circumferential manner for safer more complete excision.

The same basic procedure can be performed similarly with balloon dilation catheters. ESD balloon dissectors are available in a variety of sizes to accommodate different endoscopes although standard endoscopic balloon dilation catheters can easily be employed. Following the initial incision as described above, the balloon is inserted into the submucosal space and slowly inflated per the manufacturer's instructions. With adequate separation the procedure can easily be completed with a greater likelihood of achieving clean surgical margins.

A further adaptation of this procedure is facilitated in endoscopic surgery of the colon and rectum by use of a transanal access platform (GelPOINT Path Transanal Access Platform, Applied Medical). These devices, similar in design and concept to a SILS™ device (as discussed elsewhere in this volume), allow for an airtight seal at the rectum, insufflation to allow for maintenance of bowel distention and improved visualization as well as the use of more robust rigid laparoscopic instrumentation.

ESD can be employed in the management of cricopharyngeal or oesophageal achalasia. While this disease is more common in humans, in canine patients it can be difficult to manage in the long term. Long term, this condition can lead to megaoesophagus, dysphagia, reflux oesophagitis and aspiration pneumonia. Canine patients often fail medical management as well as home management strategies, resulting in the need for alternative enteral access or, ultimately, euthanasia.

Peroral endoscopic myotomy

POEM is an endoscopic dissection technique that releases or resects the circular smooth muscle fibers of the lower oesophageal sphincter (LOS), allowing for increased ease of passage of ingesta to the stomach. This procedure can obviate the need for the more aggressive Heller Myotomy and its associated increased morbidity. The most common technique is creating a tunnel in the muscular layer and cutting the LOS under visual endoscopic control, by using a flexible endoscope.

Acknowledgements

The authors would like to thank David Sobel for his contribution on 'Endoscopic submucosal dissection and peroral endoscopic myotomy' to this chapter.

References and further reading

Aaltonen IE and Wahlström M (2018) Envisioning robotic surgery: surgeons' needs and views on interacting with future technologies and interfaces. *The International Journal of Medical Robotics and Computer Assisted Surgery* **14**, e1941

Aggarwal R, Darzi A and Yang GZ (2010) Robotics in surgery – past, present and future. In: *Medical Sciences, Volume II*, ed. BP Mansourian, A Wojtczak and BMcA Sayers, pp. 86–109. Eolss Publishers Co. Ltd., Oxford

Aggarwal R, Hance J and Darzi A (2004) Robotics and surgery: a long-term relationship? *International Journal of Surgery* **2**, 106–109

Agresta F and Bedin N (2012) Is there still any role for minilaparoscopic-cholecystectomy? A general surgeons' last five years experience over 932 cases. *Updates in Surgery* **64**, 31–36

Alander JT, Kaartinen I, Laakso A *et al.* (2012) A review of indocyanine green fluorescent imaging in surgery. *International Journal of Biomedical Imaging* **2012**, 940585

Alaraimi B, El Bakbak W, Sarker S *et al.* (2014) A randomized prospective study comparing acquisition of laparoscopic skills in three-dimensional (3D) vs. two-dimensional (2D) laparoscopy. *World Journal of Surgery* **38**, 2746–2752

Ali MJ, Singh S and Naik MN (2016) The usefulness of continuously variable view rigid endoscope in lacrimal surgeries: first intraoperative experience. *Ophthalmic Plastic and Reconstructive Surgery* **32**, 477–480

Allman DA, Radlinsky MG, Ralph AG and Rawlings CA (2010) Thoracoscopic thoracic duct ligation and thoracoscopic pericardectomy for treatment of chylothorax in dogs. *Veterinary Surgery* **39**, 21–27

Ando K, Kamijyou K, Hatinoda K *et al.* (2012) Computed tomography and radiographic lymphography of the thoracic duct by subcutaneous or submucosal injection. *Journal of Veterinary Medical Science* **74**, 135–140

Arens C, Dreyer T, Glanz H and Malzahn K (2004) Indirect autofluorescence laryngoscopy in the diagnosis of laryngeal cancer and its precursor lesions. *European Archives of Oto-Rhino-Laryngology and Head and Neck Surgery* **261**, 71–76

Badylak SF, Vorp DA, Spievack AR *et al.* (2005) Esophageal reconstruction with ECM and muscle tissue in a dog model. *Journal of Surgical Research* **128**, 87–97

Bailey JG, Hayden JA, Davis PJ *et al.* (2014) Robotic *versus* laparoscopic Roux-en-Y gastric bypass (RYGB) in obese adults ages 18 to 65 years: a systematic review and economic analysis. *Surgical Endoscopy* **28**, 414–426

Bakhtiari J, Khalaj AR, Aminlou E and Niasari-Naslaji A (2012) Comparative evaluation of conventional and transvaginal laparoscopic ovariohysterectomy in dogs. *Veterinary Surgery* **41**, 755–758

Bazzi WM, Stroup SP, Cohen SA *et al.* (2013) Comparison of transrectal and transvaginal hybrid natural orifice transluminal endoscopic surgery partial nephrectomy in the porcine model. *Urology* **82**, 84–89

Beck CAC, Pippi NL, Brun MV *et al.* (2003) Criptoquidectomia em coelhos: modelo experimental para tratamento laparoscópico. *Ciência Rural* **33**, 331–337

Berent A (2016) Diagnosis and Management of Nasopharyngeal Stenosis. *The Veterinary Clinics of North America. Small Animal Practice* **46**, 677–689

Bessler M, Stevens PD, Milone L *et al.* (2007) Transvaginal laparoscopically assisted endoscopic cholecystectomy: a hybrid approach to natural orifice surgery. *Gastrointestinal Endoscopy* **66**, 1243–1245

Blavier A, Gaudissart Q, Cadière GB and Nyssen AS (2006) Impact of 2D and 3D vision on performance of novice subjects using da Vinci robotic system. *Acta Chirurgica Belgica* **106**, 662–664

Brisson BA, Holmberg DL and House M (2006) Comparison of mesenteric lymphadenography performed via surgical and laparoscopic approaches in dogs. *American Journal of Veterinary Research* **67**, 168–173

Brun MV, Silva MAM, Mariano MB *et al.* (2011) Ovariohysterectomy in a dog by hybrid NOTES technique. *Canadian Veterinary Journal* **52**, 637–640

Buck L, Michalek J, Van Sickle K *et al.* (2008) Can gastric irrigation prevent infection during NOTES mesh placement? *Journal of Gastrointestinal Surgery* **12**, 2010–2014

Bulian DR, Knuth J, Cerasani N *et al.* (2015) Transvaginal/transumbilical hybrid–NOTES–*versus* 3-trocar needlescopic cholecystectomy: short-term results of a randomized clinical trial. *Annals of Surgery* **261**, 451–458

Cabral PH, Silva IT, Melo JV *et al.* (2008) Needlescopic *versus* laparoscopic cholecystectomy: a prospective study of 60 patients. *Acta Cirurgica Brasileira* **23**, 543–550

Cai Y and Liu X (2013) Feasibility and safety of minilaparoscopy-guided spleen biopsy. *Surgical Endoscopy* **27**, 3499

Carvalho GL, Cavazzola LT and Rao P (2013) Minilaparoscopic surgery – not just a pretty face! What can be found beyond the esthetics reasons? *Journal of Laparoendoscopic and Advanced Surgical Techniques* **23**, 710–713

Carvalho GL, Loureiro MP, Bonin EA *et al.* (2011) Renaissance of minilaparoscopy in the NOTES and single port era. *Journal of the Society of Laparoendoscopic Surgeons* **15**, 585–588

Carvalho GL, Loureiro MP, Bonin EA *et al.* (2012) Minilaparoscopic technique for inguinal hernia repair combining transabdominal pre-peritoneal and totally extraperitoneal approaches. *Journal of the Society of Laparoendoscopic Surgeons* **16**, 569–575

Carvalho GL, Silva FW, Silva JS *et al.* (2009) Needlescopic clipless cholecystectomy as an efficient, safe, and cost-effective alternative with diminutive scars: the first 1000 cases. *Surgical Laparoscopy Endoscopy & Percutaneous Techniques* **19**, 368–372

Chernov AV and Inykin VV (2011) One port laparoscopy technology. *Vestnik of Veterinary Medicine* **2**, 6–9

Chernov AV (2013) Transvaginal access to diagnostic and surgical laparoscopy in female dogs. *Russian Veterinary Journal* **2**, 23–26

Chernov AV (2018a) NOTES is a new concept in the veterinary surgery. *Russian Veterinary Journal* **1**, 27–31

Chernov AV (2018b) NOTES. In: *Tecnicas de Minima Invasion en Pequenos Animales*, ed. DL Casas Garsia and AJ Santana Gonzales, pp. 447–468. Grafica IN-Multimedica S.A.U., Barcelona, Spain

Cho YB, Park JH, Chun H-K *et al.* (2011) Natural orifice transluminal endoscopic surgery applied to sigmoidectomy in survival animal models: using paired magnetic intra-luminal device. *Surgical Endoscopy* **25**, 1319–1324

Currò G, La Malfa G, Lazzara S *et al.* (2015) Three-dimensional *versus* two-dimensional laparoscopic cholecystectomy: is surgeon experience relevant? *Journal of Laparoendoscopic and Advanced Surgical Techniques* **25**, 566–570

Dawson DL, Coil JA, Jadali M and Garrett G (1992) Use of skin staplers in experimental gastrointestinal injuries. *Journal of Trauma, Injury, Infection and Critical Care* **32**, 204–209

de Souza FW, Brun MV, de Oliveira MT *et al*. (2014) Ovariohysterectomy for videosurgery (hybrid vaginal NOTES), celiotomy or mini-celiotomy in bitches. *Ciência Rural* **44**, 510–516

Diamond DM, Mathews KG, Chiu KW and Scharf VF (2019) Fixed *versus* variable-angle endoscopy for exploratory thoracoscopy. *Scientific Presentation Abstracts, Veterinary Endoscopy Society 16th Annual Scientific Meeting, 29 April–1 May, Lake Tahoe, California, USA*

Diana M and Marescaux J (2015) Robotic surgery. *British Journal of Surgery* **102**, e15–e28

Earle DB, Desilets DJ and Romanelli JR (2010) NOTES transgastric abdominal wall hernia repair in a porcine model. *Hernia* **14**, 517–522

Earle DB, Romanelli JR, McLawhorn T *et al*. (2012) Prosthetic mesh contamination during NOTES(®) transgastric hernia repair: a randomized controlled trial with swine explants. *Hernia* **16**, 689–695

Ebner FH, Roser F, Roder C *et al*. (2015) Rigid, variable-view endoscope in neurosurgery: first intraoperative experience. *Surgical Innovation* **22**, 390–393

Edwards DP, Warren BF, Galbraith KA and Watkins PE (1999) Comparison of two closure techniques for the repair of experimental colonic perforations. *The British Journal of surgery* **86**, 514–517

Ehara EA (2017) Potentials for needlescopic veterinary surgery. Maneuverability of under 2mm outer diameter graspers and surgical indications. *Veterinary Endoscopy Society Scientific Annual Meeting 20–22 June, Los Cabos, México*

Elmunzer BJ, Schomisch SJ, Trunzo JA *et al*. (2009) EUS in localizing safe alternate access sites for natural orifice transluminal endoscopic surgery: initial experience in a porcine model. *Gastrointestinal Endoscopy* **69**, 108–114

Enwiller TM, Radlinsky MG, Mason DE and Roush JK (2003) Popliteal and mesenteric lymph node injection with methylene blue for coloration of the thoracic duct in dogs. *Veterinary Surgery* **32**, 359–364

Fanfani F, Fagotti A, Rossitto C *et al*. (2012) Laparoscopic, minilaparoscopic and single-port hysterectomy: perioperative outcomes. *Surgical Endoscopy* **26**, 3592–3596

Flora ED, Wilson TG, Martin IJ *et al*. (2008) A review of natural orifice translumenal endoscopic surgery (NOTES) for intra-abdominal surgery: experimental models, techniques, and applicability to the clinical setting. *Annals of Surgery* **247**, 583–602

Fong DG, Ryou M, Pai RD *et al*. (2007) Transcolonic ventral wall hernia mesh fixation in a porcine model. *Endoscopy* **39**, 865–869

Freeman LJ, Al-Haddad M, McKenna DM *et al*. (2015) *NOTES approach to endoscopic gastropexy: feasibility study in dogs*. Purdue University School of Veterinary Medicine, West Lafayette, IN, USA

Freeman LJ, Rahmani EY, Al-Haddad M *et al*. (2010) Comparison of pain and postoperative stress in dogs undergoing natural orifice transluminal endoscopic surgery, laparoscopic, and open oophorectomy. *Gastrointestinal Endoscopy* **72**, 373–380

Freeman LJ, Rahmani EY, Sherman S *et al*. (2009) Oophorectomy by natural orifice transluminal endoscopic surgery: feasibility study in dogs. *Gastrointestinal Endoscopy* **69**, 1321–1332

Fritscher-Ravens A, Cuming T, Eisenberger CF *et al*. (2010a) Randomized comparative long-term survival study of endoscopic and thoracoscopic esophageal wall repair after NOTES mediastinoscopy in healthy and compromised animals. *Endoscopy* **42**, 468–474

Fritscher-Ravens A, Hampe J, Grange P *et al*. (2010b) Clip closure *versus* endoscopic suturing *versus* thoracoscopic repair of an iatrogenic esophageal perforation: a randomized, comparative, long-term survival study in a porcine model. *Gastrointestinal Endoscopy* **72**, 1020–1026

Fritscher-Ravens A, Cuming T, Jacobsen B *et al*. (2009) Feasibility and safety of endoscopic full-thickness esophageal wall resection and defect closure: a prospective long-term survival animal study. *Gastrointestinal Endoscopy* **69**, 1314–1320

Fritscher-Ravens A, Patel K, Ghanbari A *et al*. (2007) Natural orifice transluminal endoscopic surgery (NOTES) in the mediastinum: long-term survival animal experiments in transesophageal access, including minor surgical procedures. *Endoscopy* **39**, 870–875

Gagner M and Garcia-Ruiz A (1998) Technical aspects of minimally invasive abdominal surgery performed with needlescopic instruments. *Surgical Laparoscopy and Endoscopy* **8**, 171–179

Giday SA, Dray X, Magno P *et al*. (2010) Infection during natural orifice transluminal endoscopic surgery: a randomized controlled study in a live porcine model. *Gastrointestinal Endoscopy* **71**, 812–816

Giday SA, Magno P, Gabrielson KL *et al*. (2007) The utility of contrast-enhanced endoscopic ultrasound in monitoring ethanol-induced pancreatic tissue ablation: a pilot study in a porcine model. *Endoscopy* **39**, 525–529

Giulianotti PC, Coratti A, Angelini M *et al*. (2003) Robotics in general surgery: personal experience in a large community hospital. *Archives of Surgery* **138**, 777–784

Grady D (2007) *Testing scarless surgery: doctors remove a gallbladder through the vagina*. New York Times April 20, A14

Guarner-Argente C, Cordova H, Martinez-Palli G *et al*. (2010) Yes we can: reliable colonic closure with the Padlock-G clip in a survival porcine model study. *Gastrointestinal Endoscopy* **72**, 841–844

Haimel G, Liehmann L and Dupré G (2012) Thoracoscopic *en bloc* thoracic duct sealing and partial pericardectomy for the treatment of chylothorax in two cats. *Journal of Feline Medicine and Surgery* **14**, 928–931

Halabi WJ, Kang CY, Jafari MD *et al*. (2013) Robotic-assisted colorectal surgery in the United States: a nationwide analysis of trends and outcomes. *World Journal of Surgery* **37**, 2782–2790

Hanson JM, Hoofd MM, Voorhout G *et al*. (2005) Efficacy of transsphenoidal hypophysectomy in treatment of dogs with pituitary-dependent hyperadrenocorticism. *Journal of Veterinary Internal Medicine* **19**, 687–694

Hanson JM, Teske E, Voorhout G *et al*. (2007) Prognostic factors for outcome after transsphenoidal hypophysectomy in dogs with pituitary-dependent hyperadrenocorticism. *Journal of Neurosurgery* **107**, 830–840

Hayashi K, Sicard G, Gellasch K *et al*. (2005) Cisterna chyli ablation with thoracic duct ligation for chylothorax: results in eight dogs. *Veterinary Surgery* **34**, 519–523

Herron DM, Marohn M and SAGES-MIRA Robotic Surgery Consensus Group (2008) A consensus document on robotic surgery. *Surgical Endoscopy* **22**, 313–325

Honda M, Nakamura T, Hari Y *et al*. (2010) Process of healing of mucosal defects in the esophagus after endoscopic mucosal resection: histological evaluation in a dog model. *Endoscopy* **42**, 1092–1095

Hu B, Kalloo AN, Chung SS *et al*. (2007) Peroral transgastric endoscopic primary repair of a ventral hernia in a porcine model. *Endoscopy* **39**, 390–393

Hyun MH, Lee CH, Kim HJ *et al*. (2013) Systematic review and meta-analysis of robotic surgery compared with conventional laparoscopic and open resections for gastric carcinoma. *British Journal of Surgery* **100**, 1566–1578

Ikeda K, Fritscher-Ravens A, Mosse CA *et al*. (2005) Endoscopic full-thickness resection with sutured closure in a porcine model. *Gastrointestinal Endoscopy* **62**, 122–129

Inoue S, Kajiwara M, Teishima J and Matsubara A (2016) Needlescopic-assisted laparoendoscopic single-site adrenalectomy. *Asian Journal of Surgery* **39**, 6–11

Isariyawongse JP, McGee M, Ponsky LE *et al*. (2008) Pure natural orifice transluminal endoscopic surgery (NOTES) nephrectomy using standard laparoscopic instruments in the porcine model. *Journal of Endourology* **22**, 1087–1091

Ishigaki K, Sakurai N, Nagumo T *et al*. (2019) Preoperative computed tomographic lymphangiography and intraoperative indocyanine green fluorescence imaging for triple combination endoscopic surgery in canine idiopathic chylothorax. *Scientific Presentation Abstracts 2019 Veterinary Endoscopy Society 16th Annual Scientific Meeting, 29 April–1 May, Lake Tahoe, California, USA*

Izquierdo L, Peri L, García-Cruz E *et al*. (2012) 3D advances in laparoscopic vision. *European Urological Review* **7**, 137–139

Jacobson MC, deVere White RW and Demos SG (2012) *In vivo* testing of a prototype system providing simultaneous white light and near infrared autofluorescence image acquisition for detection of bladder cancer. *Journal of Biomedical Optics* **17**, 036011

Jagannath SB, Kantsevoy SV, Vaughn CA *et al*. (2005) Peroral transgastric endoscopic ligation of fallopian tubes with long-term survival in a porcine model. *Gastrointestinal Endoscopy* **61**, 449–453

Johnson EG, Wisner ER, Kyles A *et al*. (2009) Computed tomographic lymphography of the thoracic duct by mesenteric lymph node injection. *Veterinary Surgery* **38**, 361–367

Kalloo AN (2008) *Natural Orifice Transluminal Endoscopic Surgery, an Issue of Gastrointestinal Endoscopy Clinics (The Clinics: Internal Medicine)*, Saunders

Kalloo AN and Datlner D (2006) ASGE/SAGES Working group on Natural Orifice Translumenal Endoscopic Surgery. White Paper October 2005. *Gastrointestinal Endoscopy* **63**, 199–203

Kalloo AN, Kantsevoy SV, Singh VK *et al*. (2000) Flexible transgastric peritoneoscopy: a novel approach to diagnostic and therapeutic interventions in the peritoneal cavity. *Gastrointestinal Endoscopy* **118**, A1039

Kalloo AN, Singh SB, Jagannath SB *et al* (2004) Flexible transgastric peritoneoscopy: novel approach to diagnostic and therapeutic interventions in the peritoneal cavity. *Gastrointestinal Endoscopy* **60**, 114–117

Kanai H, Hagiwara K, Furuya M *et al*. (2019) Effectiveness of *en bloc* thoracic duct ligation and conventional clipping by video-assisted thoracoscopic surgery in canine idiopathic chylothorax cases. *Scientific Presentation Abstracts 2019 Veterinary Endoscopy Society 16th Annual Scientific Meeting, 29 April–1 May, Lake Tahoe, California, USA*

Kantsevoy SV, Dray X, Shin EJ *et al*. (2009a) Transgastric ventral hernia repair: a controlled study in a live porcine model (with videos). *Gastrointestinal Endoscopy* **69**, 102–107

Kantsevoy SV, Hu B, Jagannath SB *et al*. (2006) Transgastric endoscopic splenectomy: is it possible? *Surgical Endoscopy* **20**, 522-525

Kantsevoy SV, Jagannath SB, Niiyama H *et al*. (2009b) Endoscopic gastrojejunostomy with survival in a porcine model. *Gastrointestinal Endoscopy* **62**, 287–292

Kawasaki R, Sugimoto K, Fujii M *et al*. (2013) Therapeutic effectiveness of diagnostic lymphangiography for refractory postoperative chylothorax and chylous ascites: correlation with radiologic findings and preceding medical treatment. *American Journal of Roentgenology* **201**, 659–666

Kim CW, Kim CH and Baik SH (2014) Outcomes of robotic-assisted colorectal surgery compared with laparoscopic and open surgery: a systematic review. *Journal of Gastrointestinal Surgery* **18**, 816–830

Kiyonaga M, Mori H, Matsumoto S *et al*. (2012) Thoracic duct and cisterna chyli: evaluation with multidetector row CT. *The British Journal of Radiology* **85**, 1052–1058

Kono Y, Yasuda K, Horoishi K *et al*. (2013) Transrectal peritoneal access with the submucosal tunnel technique in NOTES: a porcine survival study. *Surgical Endoscopy* **27**, 278–285

Krpata DM and Ponsky TA (2013) Needlescopic surgery: what's in the toolbox? *Surgical Endoscopy* **27**, 1040–1044

Kunert W, Auer T, Storz P *et al.* (2018) How much stereoscopic effect does laparoscopy need? Controlled, prospective randomized trial on surgical task efficiency in standardized phantom tasks. *Surgical Innovation* **25**, 515–524

Kunert W, Storz P and Kirschniak A (2013) For 3D laparoscopy: a step toward advanced surgical navigation: how to get maximum benefit from 3D vision. *Surgical Endoscopy* **27**, 696–699

Lai L, Poneros J, Cantil J *et al.* (2004) EUS-guided portal vein catheterization and pressure measurement in an animal model: a pilot study of feasibility. *Gastrointestinal Endoscopy* **59**, 280–283

Lawall T, Beck CAC, Gonçalves MC *et al.* (2016) Minilaparoscopia: outra abordagem para a laparoscopia em pequenos animais–revisão de literatura. *Revista Veterinária em Foco* **13**, 87–98

Lawall T, Beck CAC, Queiroga LB and Santos FR (2017) Minilaparoscopic ovariohysterectomy in healthy cats. *Ciência Rural* **47**, 1–7

Liao G, Chen J, Ren C *et al.* (2013) Robotic *versus* open gastrectomy for gastric cancer: a meta-analysis. *PLoS One* **8**, e81946

Lida G, Asano K, Seki M *et al.* (2013) Intraoperative identification of canine hepatocellular carcinoma with indocyanine green fluorescent imaging. *Journal of Small Animal Practice* **54**, 594–600

Lillo F, Borroni, C, Silva F *et al.* (2016) Design of an endoscopic subtentorial supracerebellar approach in dogs; a cadaveric pilot study. Veterinary Endoscopy Society 13th Annual Scientific Meeting, 12–14 June 2016, Jackson Hole, Wyoming

Lima E, Rolanda C, Pêgo JM *et al.* (2006) Transvesical endoscopic peritoneoscopy: a novel 5 mm port for intra-abdominal scarless surgery. *The Journal of Urology* **176**, 802–805

Lomano D, Dhir U, So JB *et al.* (2009) Total transvaginal endoscopic abdominal wall hernia repair: a NOTES survival study. *Hernia: the Journal of Hernias and Abdominal Wall Surgery* **13**, 415–419

Look M, Chew SP, Tan YC *et al.* (2001) Post-operative pain in needlescopic *versus* conventional laparoscopic cholecystectomy: A prospective randomized trial. *Journal of the Royal College of Surgeons of Edinburgh* **46**, 138–142

Loureiro MP, Trauczynski P, Claus C *et al.* (2013) Totally extraperitoneal endoscopic inguinal hernia repair using mini instruments: pushing the boundaries of minimally invasive hernia surgery. *Jounal of Minimally Invasive Surgical Sciences* **2**, 8–12

Luz MJ, Ferreira GS, Santos CL *et al.* (2014) Ovariohisterectomy in dogs by transvaginal hybrid NOTES: prospective comparison with laparoscopic and open. *Archivos de Medicina Veterinaria* **46**, 23–30

MacDonald NJ, Noble PJ and Burrow RD (2008) Efficacy of *en bloc* ligation of the thoracic duct: descriptive study in 14 dogs. *Veterinary Surgery* **37**, 696–701

Mayhew PD (2014) Recent advances in soft tissue minimally invasive surgery. *The Journal of Small Animal Practice* **55**, 75–83

Mayhew PD, Culp WT, Mayhew KN and Morgan OD (2012) Minimally invasive treatment of idiopathic chylothorax in dogs by thoracoscopic thoracic duct ligation and subphrenic pericardiectomy: 6 cases (2007–2010). *Journal of the American Veterinary Medical Association* **241**, 904–909

McAnulty JF (2011) Prospective comparison of cisterna chyli ablation to pericardectomy for treatment of spontaneously occurring idiopathic chylothorax in the dog. *Veterinary Surgery* **40**, 926–934

Meij BP (1999) Hypophysectomy in dogs: a review. *Veterinary Quarterly* **21**, 134–141

Meij BP, Auriemma E, Grinwis G *et al.* (2010) Successful treatment of acromegaly in a diabetic cat with transsphenoidal hypophysectomy. *Journal of Feline Medicine and Surgery* **12**, 406–410

Meij BP, Mol JA, van den Ingh TS *et al.* (1997a) Assessment of pituitary function after transsphenoidal hypophysectomy in beagle dogs. *Domestic Animal Endocrinology* **14**, 81–97

Meij BP, Voorhout G, van den Ingh TS *et al.* (1997b) Transsphenoidal hypophysectomy in beagle dogs: evaluation of a microsurgical technique. *Veterinary Surgery* **26**, 295–309

Meij BP, Voorhout G, van den Ingh TS *et al.* (1998) Results of transsphenoidal hypophysectomy in 52 dogs with pituitary-dependent hyperadrenocorticism. *Veterinary Surgery* **27**, 246–261

Meij BP, Voorhout G, van den Ingh TS and Rijnberk A (2001) Transsphenoidal hypophysectomy for treatment of pituitary-dependent hyperadrenocorticism in 7 cats. *Veterinary Surgery* **30**, 72–86

Meij BP, Voorhout G and Rijnberk A (2002) Progress in transsphenoidal hypophysectomy for treatment of pituitary-dependent hyperadrenocorticism in dogs and cats. *Molecular and Cellular Endocrinology* **197**, 89–96

Metzelder ML, Vieten G, Gosemann J *et al.* (2009a) Rigid NOTES: The transurethral approach in female piglets. *Journal of Laparoendoscopic and Advanced Surgical Techniques Part A* **19**, 581–587

Metzelder ML, Vieten G, Gosemann J *et al.* (2009b) Endoloop closure of the urinary bladder is safe and efficient in female piglets undergoing transurethral NOTES nephrectomy. *European Journal of Pediatric Surgery* **19**, 362–365

Millward IR, Kirberger RM and Thompson PN (2011) Comparative popliteal and mesenteric computed tomography lymphangiography of the canine thoracic duct. *Veterinary Radiology & Ultrasound* **52**, 295–301

Mora MC, Kowalski R, Desilets DJ *et al.* (2016) NOTES transgastric ventral hernia repair in a porcine survival model. 95th Annual Meeting September 12–14, 2014, Stowe Mountain Lodge VT, USA

Naganobu K, Ohigashi Y, Akiyoshi T *et al.* (2006) Lymphography of the thoracic duct by percutaneous injection of iohexol into the popliteal lymph node of dogs: experimental study and clinical application. *Veterinary Surgery* **35**, 377–381

Nakajima Y, Asano K, Mukai K *et al.* (2018) Near-Infrared fluorescence imaging directly visualizes lymphatic drainage pathways and connections between superficial and deep lymphatic systems in the mouse hindlimb. *Scientific Reports* **8**, 7078

Nezhat F (2008) Minimally invasive surgery in gynecologic oncology: Laparoscopy *versus* robotics. *Gynecologic Oncology* **111**, S29–S32

Ni XG, He S, Xu ZG *et al.* (2011) Endoscopic diagnosis of laryngeal cancer and precancerous lesions by narrow band imaging. *The Journal of Laryngology & Otology* **125**, 288–296

Nieponice A, Gilbert TW and Badylak SF (2006) Reinforcement of esophageal anastomoses with an extracellular matrix scaffold in a canine model. *The Annals of Thoracic Surgery* **82**, 2050–2058

Nomura K, Kikuchi D, Kaise M *et al.* (2019a) Operational effectiveness of three-dimensional flexible endoscopy: an *ex vivo* study using a new model. *Surgical Endoscopy* **33**, 3612–3615

Nomura K, Kikuchi D, Kaise M *et al.* (2019b) Comparison of 3D endoscopy and conventional 2D endoscopy in gastric endoscopic submucosal dissection: an *ex vivo* animal study. *Surgical Endoscopy* **33**, 4164–4170

Oechtering GU (2010) Brachycephalic syndrome–new information on an old congenital disease. *Veterinary Focus* **20**, 2–9

Oechtering GU, Pohl S, Schlueter C *et al.* (2016a) A novel approach to brachycephalic syndrome. 1. Evaluation of anatomical intranasal airway obstruction. *Veterinary Surgery* **45**, 165–172

Oechtering GU, Pohl S, Schlueter C *et al.* (2016b) A novel approach to brachycephalic syndrome. 2. Laser-assisted turbinectomy (LATE). *Veterinary Surgery* **45**, 173–181

Ohki T, Yamato M, Murakami D *et al.* (2006) Treatment of oesophageal ulcerations using endoscopic transplantation of tissue-engineered autologous oral mucosal epithelial cell sheets in a canine model. *Gut* **55**, 1704–1710

Özsoy M, Kallidonis P, Kyriazis I *et al.* (2015) Novice surgeons: do they benefit from 3D laparoscopy? *Lasers in Medical Science* **30**, 1325–1333

Pader K, Lescun TB and Freeman LJ (2011a) Standing ovariectomy in mares using a transvaginal natural orifice transluminal endoscopic surgery (NOTES) approach. *Veterinary Surgery* **40**, 987–997

Pader K, Freeman LJ, Constable PD *et al.* (2011b) Comparison of transvaginal natural orifice transluminal endoscopic surgery (NOTES) and laparoscopy for elective bilateral ovariectomy in standing mares. *Veterinary Surgery* **40**, 998–1008

Pai RD, Fong DG, Bundga ME *et al.* (2006) Transcolonic endoscopic cholecystectomy: a NOTES survival study in a porcine model [with video]. *Gastrointestinal Endoscopy* **64**, 428–434

Park PO (2005) Experimental studies of transgastric gallbladder surgery: cholecystectomy and cholecystogastric anastomosis (videos). *Gastrointestinal Endoscopy* **61**, 601–606

Pasricha PJ, Hawari R, Ahmed I *et al.* (2007) Submucosal endoscopic oesophageal myotomy: a novel experimental approach for the treatment of achalasia. *Endoscopy* **39**, 761–764

Pauli EM, Moyer MT, Haluck RS and Mathew A (2008) Self-approximating transluminal access technique for natural orifice transluminal endoscopic surgery: a porcine survival study. *Gastrointestinal Endoscopy* **67**, 690–697

Peyrelongue D, Rojas C, Echevarria M *et al.* (2018) Anatomia endoscopica de la pared caudal del III ventrículo del canino: *Implicacions quirúrgicas para el abordaje del acueducto mesencefálico*. XX Congreso de Anatomía del Cono Sur. XVI Simposio Iberoamericano de Terminología Anatómica, Histológica y Embriológica, XVI SILAT. XII Jornadas Chilenas de Anatomia IV Encuentro Regional de Morfología, 4–6 October 2018, Pucón, Chile

Pham BV, Raju GS, Ahmed I *et al.* (2006) Immediate endoscopic closure of colon perforation by using a prototype endoscopic suturing device: feasibility and outcome in a porcine model (with video). *Gastrointestinal Endoscopy* **64**, 113–119

Pohl S, Roedler FS and Oechtering GU (2016) How does multilevel upper airway surgery influence the lives of dogs with severe brachycephaly? Results of a structured pre- and postoperative owner questionnaire. *Veterinary Journal* **210**, 39–45

Quitzan JG, Singh A, Beaufrere H *et al.* (2019) Evaluation of the Performance of a 3 mm bipolar vessel sealing device intended for single use following multiple reuse and resterilization cycles. Scientific Presentation Abstracts 2019 Veterinary Endoscopy Society 16th Annual Scientific Meeting, 29 April–1 May, Lake Tahoe, California, USA

Radlinsky MG, Mason DE, Biller DS and Olsen D (2002) Thoracoscopic visualization and ligation of the thoracic duct in dogs. *Veterinary Surgery* **31**, 138–146

Radu A, Grosjean P, Fontolliet C and Monnier P (2004) Endoscopic mucosal resection in the esophagus with a new rigid device: an animal study. *Endoscopy* **36**, 298–305

Rajan E, Gostout CJ, Burgart LJ *et al.* (2002) First endoluminal system for transluminal resection of colorectal tissue with a prototype full-thickness resection device in a porcine model. *Gastrointestinal Endoscopy* **55**, 915–920

Raju GS, Ahmed I, Xiao SY *et al.* (2006) Controlled trial of immediate endoluminal closure of colon perforations in a porcine model by use of a novel clip device (with video). *Gastrointestinal Endoscopy* **64**, 989–997

Ravikumar S and Osborne G (2017) *Needlescopic scissor end effector and methods of use.* U.S. Patent Application 15/329, 370

Ravikumar S, Ravikumar V and Osborne G (2016) *Needlescopic instrument with reusable handle and detachable needle assembly.* U.S. Patent Application 14/784, 886

Reuter MA, Engel RME, Reuter HJ and Edward Potts Cheyney Memorial Fund (1999) *History of endoscopy: an illustrated documentation*. Stuttgart

Rey Caro DG, Rey Caro EP and Rey Caro EA (2014) Chromoendoscopy associated with endoscopic laryngeal surgery: a new technique for treating recurrent respiratory papillomatosis. *Journal of Voice* **28**, 822–829

Ryou M, Fong D, Pai R *et al.* (2008) Transluminal closure for NOTES: an *ex vivo* study comparing leak pressures of various gastrotomy and colotomy closure modalities. *Endoscopy* **40**, 432–436

Ryou M, Pai R, Fong D *et al.* (2007) Dual-lumen distal pancreatectomy using a prototype endoscope and endoscopic stapler: a NOTES survival study in the porcine model. *Endoscopy* **39**, 881–887

Sajid MS, Ladwa N, Kalra L *et al.* (2012) Single-incision laparoscopic cholecystectomy *versus* conventional laparoscopic cholecystectomy: meta-analysis and systematic review of randomized controlled trials. *World Journal of Surgery* **36**, 2644–2653

Sakals S, Schmiedt CW and Radlinsky MG (2011) Comparison and description of transdiaphragmatic and abdominal minimally invasive cisterna chyli ablation in dogs. *Veterinary Surgery* **40**, 795–801

Salman M, Bell T, Martin J *et al.* (2013) Use, cost, complications, and mortality of robotic *versus* nonrobotic general surgery procedures based on a nationwide database. *The American Surgeon* **79**, 553–560

Sánchez-Hurtado MÁ, Sánchez-Margallo FM, Usón-Casaús J *et al.* (2017) Closure of gastric incision with a barbed suture after needlescope-assisted hybrid NOTES. *Endoscopy* **49**, E138–E140

Sanduleanu S, Jonkers D, De Bruine A *et al.* (2001) Non-*Helicobacter pylori* bacterial flora during acid-suppressive therapy: differential findings in gastric juice and gastric mucosa. *Alimentary Pharmacology and Therapeutics* **15**, 379–388

Sawyer MD, Cherullo EE, Elmunzer BJ *et al.* (2009) Pure natural orifice translumenal endoscopic surgery partial cystectomy: intravesical transurethral and extravesical transgastric techniques in a porcine model. *Urology* **74**, 1049–1053

Sawyer MD, Cherullo EE, Marks JM *et al.* (2008) Endoscopic closure of vesicotomy/bladder wall defects with intravesical or extravesical endoscopic clips in a porcine model. *Journal of Endourology* **22**, A86

Schuenemann R and Oechtering GU (2014) Inside the brachycephalic nose: intranasal mucosal contact points. *Journal of the American Animal Hospital Association* **50**, 149–158

Schuenemann R, Pohl S and Oechtering GU (2017) A novel approach to brachycephalic syndrome. 3. Isolated laser-assisted turbinectomy of caudal aberrant turbinates (CAT LATE). *Veterinary Surgery* **46**, 32–38

Seaman DL, de la Mora Levy J, Gostout CJ *et al.* (2007) An animal training model for endoscopic treatment of Zenker's diverticulum. *Gastrointestinal Endoscopy* **65**, 1050–1053

Sherwinter DA, Gupta A, Eckstein JG (2011) Natural orifice translumenal endoscopic surgery inguinal hernia repair: a survival canine model. *Journal of Laparoendoscopic and Advanced Surgical Techniques Part A* **21**, 209–213

Sicard GK, Waller KR and McAnulty JF (2005) The effect of cisterna chyli ablation combined with thoracic duct ligation on abdominal lymphatic drainage. *Veterinary Surgery* **34**, 64–70

Simopoulos C, Kouklakis G, Zezos P *et al.* (2009) Peroraltransgastric endoscopic procedures in pigs: feasibility, survival, questionings, and pitfalls. *Surgical Endoscopy* **23**, 394–402

Singh A, Brisson BA, Nykamp S and O'Sullivan ML (2011) Comparison of computed tomographic and radiographic popliteal lymphangiography in normal dogs. *Veterinary Surgery* **40**, 762–767

Singh A, Brisson B and Nykamp S (2012) Idiopathic chylothorax: pathophysiology, diagnosis and thoracic duct imaging. *Compendium* (Yardley, PA) **34**, E2

Sinha RY, Raje SR and Rao GA (2017) Three-dimensional laparoscopy: Principles and practice. *Journal of Minimal Access Surgery* **13**, 165–169

Sinha RY, Sundaram M, Raje SR *et al.* (2013) 3D laparoscopy: technique and initial experience in 451 cases. *Gynecological Surgery* **10**, 123–128

Sisson S, Grossman JD and Getty R (1975) *Sisson and Grossman's The anatomy of domestic animals Vol. 2. 5th.* WB Saunders, Philadelphia

Sodergren MH and Darzi A (2012) Robotic cancer surgery. *British Journal of Surgery* **100**, 3–4

Sporn E, Astudillo JA, Bachman SL *et al.* (2009) Transgastric biologic mesh delivery and abdominal wall hernia repair in a porcine model. *Endoscopy* **41**, 1062–1068

Steffey MA and Mayhew PD (2018) Use of direct near-infrared fluorescent lymphography for thoracoscopic thoracic duct identification in 15 dogs with chylothorax. *Veterinary Surgery* **47**, 267–276

Sugimoto M, Yasuda H, Koda K *et al.* (2009) Evaluation for transvaginal and transgastric NOTES cholecystectomy in human and animal natural orifice translumenal endoscopic surgery. *Journal of Hepatobiliary Pancreatic Surgery* **16**, 255–260

Sumiyama K, Gostout CJ, Rajan E *et al.* (2008) Pilot study of transesophageal endoscopic epicardial coagulation by submucosal endoscopy with the mucosal flap safety valve technique (with videos). *Gastrointestinal Endoscopy* **67**, 497–501

Turial S, Enders J and Schier F (2011) Microlaparoscopic pyloromyotomy in children: initial experiences with a new technique. *Surgical Endoscopy* **25**, 266–270

Vilaplana Grosso F, Haar GT and Boroffka SA (2015) Gender, weight, and age effects on prevalence of caudal aberrant nasal turbinates in clinically healthy English bulldogs: A computed tomographic study and classification. *Veterinary Radiology & Ultrasound* **56**, 486–493

von Delius S, Feussner H, Wilhelm D *et al.* (2007a) Transgastric in vivo histology in the peritoneal cavity using miniprobe-based confocal fluorescence microscopy in an acute porcine model. *Endoscopy* **39**, 407–411

von Delius S, Karagianni A, Henke J *et al.* (2007b) Changes in intra-abdominal pressure, hemodynamics, and peak inspiratory pressure during gastroscopy in a porcine model. *Endoscopy* **39**, 962–968

Whiteford MH, Denk PM and Swanström LL (2007) Feasibility of radical sigmoid colectomy performed as natural orifice translumenal endoscopic surgery (NOTES) using transanal endoscopic microsurgery. *Surgical Endoscopy* **21**, 1870–1874

Wilson EB (2009) The evolution of robotic general surgery. *Scandinavian Journal of Surgery* **98**, 125–129

Xiong J, Nunes QM, Tan C *et al.* (2013) Comparison of short-term clinical outcomes between robotic and laparoscopic gastrectomy for gastric cancer: a meta-analysis of 2495 patients. *Journal of Laparoendoscopic and Advanced Surgical Techniques* **23**, 965–976

Yoshizumi F, Yasuda K, Kawaguchi K *et al.* (2009) Submucosal tunneling using endoscopic submucosal dissection for peritoneal access and closure in natural orifice transluminal endoscopic surgery porcine survival study. *Endoscopy* **4**, 707–711

Zorrón R, Filgueiras M, Maggioni LC *et al.* (2007) NOTES. Transvaginal cholecystectomy: report of the first case. *Surgical Innovation* **14**, 279–283

▶ Video extras

- **Video 17.1**   Transvaginal approach to the abdomen using a flexible endoscope
- **Video 17.2**   Transvaginal ovariectomy in a dog
- **Video 17.3**   Transvaginal ovariectomy in a dog using an optical trocar
- **Video 17.4**   Transvaginal ovariohysterectomy in a dog
- **Video 17.5**   Transvaginal ovariectomy in a cat using a diode laser
- **Video 17.6**   Dog 1 year after transgastric laparoscopy with closure of the laparocentesis site using endoscopic clips
- **Video 17.7**   Closure of the transgastric laparocentesis site using an over-the-top technique
- **Video 17.8**   Transgastric ovariectomy in a dog
- **Video 17.9**   Transgastric cholecystectomy in a dog.
- **Video 17.10**   Transgastric gastropexy in a dog (case 1)
- **Video 17.11**   Transgastric gastropexy in a dog (case 2)
- **Video 17.12**   Transanal laparoscopy in a dog
- **Video 17.13**   Peroral thoracoscopy in a cat
- **Video 17.14**   Transvaginal ovariohysterectomy in a dog using a hybrid NOTES procedure
- **Video 17.15**   Transgastric approach to the abdominal cavity in a dog using a hybrid NOTES procedure

Access via QR code or: bsavalibrary.com/endoscopy2e_17

Index

Note: Page numbers in *italics* refer to figures
(●) indicates video clip in the BSAVA Library

BSAVA Manual of Canine and Feline Endoscopy and Endosurgery, second edition. Edited by Philip Lhermette, David Sobel and Elise Robertson. ©BSAVA 2020